Review Questions

for the

Speech-Language Pathology

PRAXIS™ Examination

Edited by

Dennis M. Ruscello, PhD
Professor
Department of Speech Pathology and Audiology
College of Human Resources and Education
West Virginia University
Morgantown, West Virginia

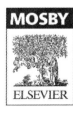

3251 Riverport Lane
Maryland Heights, Missouri 63043

MOSBY'S REVIEW QUESTIONS FOR THE SPEECH-LANGUAGE
PATHOLOGY PRAXIS™ EXAMINATION

ISBN: 978-0-323-05904-6

Copyright © 2010 by Mosby, Inc., an affiliate of Elsevier Inc.

Notices

Knowledge and best practice in this field are constantly changing. As new research and experience broaden our understanding, changes in research methods, professional practices, or medical treatment may become necessary.

Practitioners and researchers must always rely on their own experience and knowledge in evaluating and using any information, methods, compounds, or experiments described herein. In using such information or methods they should be mindful of their own safety and the safety of others, including parties for whom they have a professional responsibility.

With respect to any drug or pharmaceutical products identified, readers are advised to check the most current information provided (i) on procedures featured or (ii) by the manufacturer of each product to be administered, to verify the recommended dose or formula, the method and duration of administration, and contraindications. It is the responsibility of practitioners, relying on their own experience and knowledge of their patients, to make diagnoses, to determine dosages and the best treatment for each individual patient, and to take all appropriate safety precautions.

To the fullest extent of the law, neither the Publisher nor the authors, contributors, or editors, assume any liability for any injury and/or damage to persons or property as a matter of products liability, negligence or otherwise, or from any use or operation of any methods, products, instructions, or ideas contained in the material herein.

Library of Congress Cataloging-in-Publication Data
Mosby's review questions for the speech-language pathology Praxis™ examination / edited by Dennis M. Ruscello. – 1st ed.
    p. ; cm.
Includes bibliographical references and index.
    ISBN 978-0-323-05904-6 (pbk. : alk. paper) 1. Speech therapy–Examinations, questions, etc. I. Ruscello, Dennis M. II. Title: Review questions for the speech-language pathology Praxis examination.
    [DNLM: 1. Speech-Language Pathology–Examination Questions. WL 18.2 M8935 2010]
    RC423.M598 2010
    616.85′50710076–dc22   2009035660

Vice President and Publisher: Linda Duncan
Executive Editor: Kathy Falk
Managing Editor: Jolynn Gower
Publishing Services Manager: Anitha Rajarathnam
Project Manager: Mahalakshmi Nithyanand
Designer: Maggie Reid

Printed in United States of America

Last digit is the print number: 9 8 7 6 5 4 3 2

This book is dedicated to Claire and Ava, my two precious grandchildren. I also want to acknowledge and remember Adele, Tom, Tony, and Bob for their friendship and contributions to the profession.

Contributors

Richard D. Andreatta, PhD
Associate Professor
Division of Communication Sciences and Disorders
Department of Rehabilitation Sciences
College of Health Sciences
University of Kentucky
Lexington, Kentucky

Shelly S. Chabon, PhD, CCC-SLP, FASHA
Professor
Speech and Hearing Sciences Department
Portland State University
Portland, Oregon

Michelle Ciucci, PhD
Department of Surgery
Division of Otolaryngology–Head and Neck Surgery
School of Medicine and Public Health
University of Wisconsin
Madison, Wisconsin

Carl Coelho, PhD
Professor
Department of Communication Sciences
University of Connecticut
Storrs, Connecticut

Anysia Ensslen, MS, CCC-SLP
Doctoral Student
Department of Rehabilitation Sciences
University of Kentucky
Lexington, Kentucky

John A. Ferraro, PhD
Professor and Chairman
Hearing and Speech Department
University of Kansas Medical Center
Kansas City, Kansas

Kathleen Franklin, PhD, CCC-SLP
Associate Professor of Clinical Speech-Language
    Pathology and Director of Clinical Education
Associate Professor of Public Health Practice,
    Disability and Human Development
New York Medical College
Valhalla, New York

Leslie C. Graebe, MS, CCC-SLP
Externship Program Coordinator
Department of Speech Pathology and Audiology
West Virginia University
Morgantown, West Virginia

Karen B. Haines, MS, CCC-SLP
Clinical Assistant Professor
Department of Speech Pathology and Audiology
West Virginia University
Morgantown, West Virginia

Jacqueline Hind, MS, CCC-SLP, BRS-S
Department of Medicine
School of Medicine and Public Health
University of Wisconsin
Madison, Wisconsin

Audrey L. Holland, PhD
Regents Professor Emerita
University of Arizona
Tucson, Arizona

Yvette D. Hyter, PhD, CCC-SLP
Associate Professor
Western Michigan University
Department of Speech Pathology and Audiology
Kalamazoo, Michigan

David L. Irwin, PhD, CCC-SLP
Professor and Head
Department of Clinical Services
Director, Children's Center
School of Allied Health Professions
Louisiana State University Health Sciences Center
Shreveport, Louisiana

David L. Jones, PhD
Professor
Division of Communication Disorders
University of Wyoming
Laramie, Wyoming

Ashwini Joshi, MS
Doctoral Student
Department of Rehabilitation Sciences
University of Kentucky
Lexington, Kentucky

Mary R. T Kennedy, PhD
Associate Professor
Department of Speech-Language-Hearing Sciences
University of Minnesota
Minneapolis, Minnesota

Dorian Lee-Wilkerson, PhD
Coordinator of Graduate Studies
Department of Communicative Sciences and Disorders
Hampton University
Hampton, Virginia

Nidhi Mahendra, PhD, CCC-SLP
Assistant Professor
Department of Communicative Sciences and Disorders
California State University, East Bay
Hayward, California

Georgia Malandraki, PhD
Department of Medicine
School of Medicine and Public Health
University of Wisconsin
Madison, Wisconsin

Monica McHenry, PhD, CCC-SLP
Associate Professor
Department of Communication Sciences and Disorders
University of Houston
Houston, Texas

Paula Menyuk, EdD
Professor Emeritus
Department of Counseling and Development
School of Education
Applied Linguistics Program
Graduate School
Boston University
Brookline, Massachusetts

Benjamin Munson, PhD
Associate Professor
Department of Speech-Language-Hearing Sciences
University of Minnesota
Minneapolis, Minnesota

Diana B. Newman, PhD, CCC-SLP
Assistant Professor
Department of Communication Disorders
Southern Connecticut State University
New Haven, Connecticut

Mary Pannbacker, PhD
Professor, Speech-Language Pathology
Speech-Language Pathology Program
Department of Rehabilitation Sciences
Louisiana State University Health Sciences Center
Shreveport, Louisiana

Ashleigh A Payne, PhD
Assistant Professor
Department of Speech Pathology and Audiology
West Virginia University
Morgantown, West Virginia

Kay T. Payne, PhD, CCC-SLP
Associate Professor
Department of Communication Sciences and Disorders
Howard University
Washington, D.C.

Patricia A. Prelock, PhD, CCC-SLP
Professor and Chair
Department of Communication Sciences
University of Vermont
Burlington, Vermont

Lisa Hammett Price, PhD, CCC-SLP
Associate Professor
Department of Special Education and Clinical Services
Indiana University of Pennsylvania
Indiana, Pennsylvania

JoAnne Robbins, PhD, CCC-SLP, BRS-S
Professor
Departments of Medicine and Radiology
School of Medicine and Public Health
University of Wisconsin
Associate Director for Research
Geriatric Research Education and Clinical Center
William S. Middleton Memorial Veterans Hospital
Madison, Wisconsin

Tommie L. Robinson, PhD, CCC-SLP
Director
Scottish Rite Center for Childhood Language Disorders
Associate Professor of Pediatrics
George Washington School of Medicine
Washington, D.C.

Susan Rvachew, PhD
Associate Professor
School of Communication Sciences and Disorders
McGill University
Montreal, Quebec Canada

J. Anthony Seikel, PhD
Chair and Professor
Department of Communication Sciences and Disorders
Idaho State University
Pocatello, Idaho

Linda I. Shuster, PhD
Professor
Department of Speech Pathology and Audiology
College of Human Resources and Education
West Virginia University
Morgantown, West Virginia

Steven L. Skelton, PhD
Associate Professor of Speech-Language Pathology
Department of Communicative Disorders and Deaf Studies
California State University
Fresno, California

Joseph Stemple, PhD, CCC-SLP
Professor
Division of Communication Sciences and Disorders
College of Health Sciences
University of Kentucky
Lexington, Kentucky

Edythe A. Strand, PhD
Department of Neurology
Mayo Clinic
Rochester, Minnesota

Nancy Tye-Murray, PhD, CCC-A
Research Professor
Department of Otolaryngology
Washington University School of Medicine
St. Louis, Missouri

Linda D. Vallino, MS, PhD, CCC-SLP/A, FASHA
Head of the Craniofacial Outcomes Research Laboratory
Research Laboratory
Center for Pediatric Auditory and Speech Sciences
Alfred I. duPont Hospital for Children
Wilmington, Delaware

Betsy Partin Vinson, MMSc, CCC-SLP
Program Director and UG/G Coordinator
Clinical Associate Professor
Department of Communication Sciences and Disorders
University of Florida
Gainesville, Florida

Preface

Licensing examinations are typically part of a process to ensure that an individual is a competent practitioner in a professional field. Individuals seeking the Certificate of Clinical Competence (CCC) in Speech-Language Pathology (SLP)—the "gold standard" in licensing for the profession—must pass the national PRAXIS™ II subject assessment examination administered by the Educational Testing Service (ETS). In general, candidates taking the examination either are completing their master's-level coursework or have recently graduated and are new practitioners. Most candidates prepare for the examination through some type of review, such as rereading course notes and relevant content literature. This book and CD-ROM, *Mosby's Review Questions for the Speech-Language Pathology PRAXIS™ Examination,* are excellent sources for additional in-depth review. There are approximately 1500 test questions and answer rationales, developed by practitioners who are content experts in the field. An individual can answer the questions and then read the rationales for the correct answers. This format simulates the actual test and also allows an individual to understand the reasoning behind the question and correct answer.

Candidates who prepare for the test, in comparison with those who do not, have a higher probability of success on the test. This is to be expected, because the test assesses content knowledge within a specific time period. ETS continually evaluates the performance of candidates and has identified seven areas of difficulty for individuals who do not receive a passing score:

- Deficiencies in content knowledge that is being assessed
- Misinterpretation of basic concepts that are being examined
- Deficient reading skills
- Insufficient information-processing skills
- Inadequate experience discussing concepts and general erroneous beliefs
- Insufficient review for the test
- Test-taking anxiety

It is clear that a number of factors come into play, and by using this text and accompanying CD-ROM, readers can review the knowledge base under simulated test conditions;

that is, readers can take an actual practice examination with 120 questions. The simulation is timed for 2 hours, like the actual examination. This feature enables individuals to examine their time management skills. In addition, quizzes may be formulated with randomly selected questions from all of the content areas or specific areas so that test takers may concentrate on the areas found to be most problematic for them. Preparation is the key to successful test performance, and the book and CD-ROM are designed to give test takers the practice and confidence they need to master this examination.

SUGGESTIONS FOR TEST TAKERS

Your job is to apply the content knowledge that you have acquired during your education. You must be able to evaluate, synthesize, and apply your knowledge of the profession to specific examples and scenarios. The key concept is application and not just the recall of facts. With this in mind, it may be helpful to consider the following questions when preparing for the examination:

- Which is the optimum treatment, according to the highest level of evidence?
- Which assessment tools are necessary for the correct diagnosis?
- What are the ethical implications of a particular scenario?
- What national or state policies apply to this situation?

Test-taking strategies are also important during the actual administration of the examination, and careful consideration of strategies can enhance performance. Suggested strategies include the following:

- Plan to review at least 6 to 8 weeks before the examination. This will allow you to review at a reasonable pace. Be sure to target areas that you feel may be your "weaker areas" of content knowledge.
- Be well rested for the examination, and be prepared with the appropriate supplies, such as pencils, pens, and erasers.
- Read each question very carefully, and watch for modifier words and phrases such as "best" and "least likely."
- Carefully mark your answer sheet. If you skip items and plan to return to those items, be careful to check them later. Leave an item blank until you are ready to answer the question.
- Always identify the best choice among the answer selections listed. In some cases, selection is very difficult, but choose the answer that you feel is correct.
- Time is very important. Keep track of time, and pace yourself, so that you will be able to complete the test. You are allotted 2 hours for the test.
- If you find yourself running out of time, don't leave any question blank. There is no penalty for guessing.
- Project a positive attitude for success as you prepare and take the test. You have chosen a profession that is very rewarding, and the examination is one of the final requirements in achieving your goal!

Contents

PART IV NEUROGENIC DISORDERS   147

PART V AUDIOLOGY AND HEARING   213

PART VI CLINICAL MANAGEMENT   235

PART VII PROFESSIONAL ISSUES, PSYCHOMETRICS, AND RESEARCH   313

PART I

Basic Human Communication Processes

CHAPTER 1

Language Acquisition and Cognition

Paula Menyuk

LANGUAGE DEVELOPMENT: PARALINGUISTICS

All the questions about paralinguistics are concerned with behaviors that speech-language pathologists should know about when working with clients from diverse cultures and, in particular, when working with children who are autistic or have Asperger syndrome. These groups of children have particular difficulty with the pragmatic aspects of language.

1. Intonation patterns of caregivers' speech help infants:
   a. Segment the stream of speech
   b. Identify their dialect
   c. Identify the speaker
   d. Decide what and who to listen to
   e. Perceive different phonetic features

2. Facial expressions of speakers are used by listeners to:
   a. React to messages
   b. Perceive truthfulness
   c. Comprehend irony
   d. Process the verbal message
   e. Perceive additional information from the speaker

3. Gesture in communication:
   a. Is universally recognized
   b. Is used differently in different cultures
   c. Involves use of the hands only
   d. Is used for emphasis
   e. Is used only by young children

4. The word or phrase receiving the most stress or emphasis in a declarative sentence can always be used by a listener to identify:
   a. The speaker
   b. The addressee
   c. The act in the message
   d. The important features of the message
   e. None of the above

5. The meaning of a spoken message is conveyed by:
   a. Stress
   b. Intonation
   c. Rhythm
   d. Facial expression
   e. All the above

6. Infants attend first to which of the following aspects of spoken communication?
   a. Loudness and pitch of speech
   b. Prosody of speech and facial expression of the speaker
   c. Individual phonemes in speech
   d. Phrase and clause structure
   e. All the above

7. In the literature, "style of speech" refers to:
   a. Formal and informal
   b. Teenagers' way of speaking
   c. Differences in way of speaking among different cultural groups
   d. Suprasegmental differences among speakers
   e. Dialect variation among different speakers

8. Learning the ways in which a culture communicates:
   a. Is developed over time
   b. Depends on practice
   c. Requires sensitivity to prosodic features
   d. Is shaped by environmental experience
   e. Is acquired unconsciously

9. Some children without any neurophysiological problems have difficulty in learning others' communication rules because of:
   a. Lack of experience
   b. Stubbornness
   c. Other interests
   d. Interference of own rules
   e. Socioeconomic differences

10. What aspects of the communication situation do young children use to help them acquire word knowledge?
    a. Speakers' pointing
    b. Eye gaze
    c. Word stress
    d. Phonological cues
    e. All the above

PHONOLOGICAL AND MORPHOLOGICAL ACQUISITION

The questions concerning phonology and morphology are designed to assess the speech-language pathologist's awareness of what is considered normal when assessing children's phonological abilities, when the pathologist is interpreting test findings in the area, and in determining the appropriate intervention techniques at appropriate times of life. Children with problems in speech production and perception are those frequently found in language-disordered populations.

11. Children begin to recognize words:
    a. At 15 months of age
    b. At 12 months of age
    c. At 24 months of age
    d. Before 12 months of age
    e. Between 24 and 30 months of age

12. Phonological rules:
    a. Refer to allowable segmental sequences in a language
    b. Play an important role in word production
    c. Are dependent on motor abilities
    d. Are dependent on perceptual abilities
    e. Refer to allophonic variations of a phoneme

13. Discrimination of distinctive features is necessary for word acquisition:
    a. Because minimal pair distinctions are needed
    b. Because it is used to mark differences between words
    c. Because of the need to produce accurate speech sounds
    d. Because of the need to develop auditory percepts of developing sounds
    e. For none of the reasons above

14. Recognition of the syllabic structures in a language has been found:
    a. To be the same in different languages
    b. To be the most important factor in speech sound acquisition
    c. To change as the child develops knowledge of the language
    d. Not to appear sometimes during the first year of life
    e. Not to occur in language acquisition

15. Some speech sound combinations are difficult for children to acquire and therefore appear later in development. Which of the speech sound combinations listed below generally appear later?
    a. Prevocalic consonant clusters
    b. Postvocalic consonant clusters
    c. Medial consonant clusters
    d. Clusters with /s/ as a component
    e. Clusters with /r/ as a component

16. Speech and language production can be delayed for a number of different reasons. What is one of the first things that should be determined in children who appear to be developing normally except for delayed speech and language?
    a. Hearing acuity
    b. Stage of fine motor development
    c. Stage of cognitive development
    d. Stage of gross motor development
    e. Stage of social development

17. Which of the plural markers listed is generally used first by a child acquiring speech and language normally?
    a. Plural /z/
    b. Plural /iz/
    c. Plural /s/
    d. Number words such as "two" or "more"
    e. None of the above

18. Children who are acquiring English as a second language may continue to have sound production problems, depending on which of the following?
    a. The age at which the second language is acquired
    b. Distinctions between the phonological elements of their first language and those of English
    c. The frequency with which their first language is spoken at home
    d. Confusion in speech perception
    e. All the above

19. A period of very rapid development of word production, a so-called vocabulary spurt, occurs for many children; however, some children do not experience it, although they are developing normally. Which of the following reasons have been found to best account for the difference between these two groups of children?
    a. Differences in phonological perception
    b. Sophistication of phonological production
    c. Types of words known
    d. Cognitive differences
    e. None of the above

20. Infants' perception of speech sound differences during the first year of life have been studied. Which of the following statements best describes this course of development in monolingual infants?
    a. A gradual expansion of speech sound differentiation across different languages during the first year of life
    b. An equal ability in detecting perceptual speech differences across similar languages during the first year of life
    c. A marked change in the latter part of the first year of life toward better discrimination of sounds in the native language

    d. An inability to perceive differences in nonnative languages beginning shortly after birth
    e. A preference for the native language at birth that does not change during the first year of life

SYNTAX DEVELOPMENT

Difficulty with syntax has been the problem most frequently found in the language development of children with language disorders. The problem represents what is commonly termed a *plateau* in language development. The difficulties in this area apparently arise as a result of the increasing length of sentences and the amount of ambiguity produced by interruptions in word order.

21. Researchers have found that children understand the basic relations of subject, verb, and object as given by the word order rules of their language by the time they are what age?
    a. Three years
    b. Five years
    c. Two years
    d. Ten years
    e. Seven years

22. Which choice best describes the word order rules of the basic relations among subject, verb, and object in different languages?
    a. The verb is always after the subject
    b. The verb is always before the object
    c. The verb is always in the middle of the sentence
    d. The order of these basic relations varies among languages
    e. None of the above

23. Why do children rapidly acquire knowledge of the word order of their language?
    a. The order of subject-object-verb of the language is the form least frequently used by caregivers
    b. Caregivers correct word order errors before other errors
    c. Caregivers do not stress the order of the words in a sentence
    d. Early sentences used in communication with the child are simple, are used frequently, and expose the child to exemplars that make clear the order in their language
    e. All the above

24. Imitation is an important strategy for language learning. Physical imitation requires which of the following?
    a. Turn-taking
    b. Attending to the action
    c. Replicating the features of the action
    d. a and b
    e. a, b, and c

25. Bilingual children learn the syntax or word order of both languages. Which of the following factors account for the order in which the syntax of the first or second language is acquired?
    a. The syntax of the language used by their caregivers
    b. The syntax of the language that is easiest
    c. The syntax of the language that they hear most frequently
    d. The syntax of the language used by the members of their family
    e. The syntax of the language used in the child's educational environment

26. What causes the differences in the syntactic structures of various dialects in the United States?
    a. Environmental differences
    b. Different histories of language change across language communities
    c. Impoverished grammars in certain language communities
    d. Speech sound differences among different language communities
    e. Differences in morphological use

27. What is the definition of a speech act?
    a. The production of an utterance
    b. The paralinguistics of an utterance
    c. The context in which an utterance is produced
    d. The communicative intent of an utterance
    e. The listener's comprehension of the message

28. When and how do children indicate differences in speech acts?
    a. At age 3 years, they use a basic grammar
    b. At age 2 years, they can express basic semantic relations
    c. During infancy, they use different intonation patterns to covey different meanings for single words
    d. When they can express different sentence particles for questioning or negative responding
    e. All the above

29. What is the minimal distance principle as it relates to the comprehension of utterances?
    a. How far away the speaker is from the listener
    b. The amount of distance between the subject and the main verb of the sentence
    c. How the main verb is related to the dependent clausal verb
    d. The distance between subject and object
    e. The distance between the subject and complement of the sentence

30. How do children create comprehensible question sentences early in development?
    a. By adding question markers to simple sentences
    b. By changing the stress pattern in words

c. By gesture and facial expression
d. By change in intonation
e. All the above

LEXICAL DEVELOPMENT

This aspect of development has been found to be most closely related to cognitive development and input. Intervention techniques should be guided by sequences of development in this area and by the cognitive developments that appear to be precursors to these developments, particularly categorization and association. In addition, the crucial role of input in this aspect of development is a challenge in designing intervention and including parents in that intervention.

31. What is the first category of words that English-speaking infants typically acquire in their lexicons?
    a. Possessives
    b. Nominals
    c. Verbs
    d. Locative words
    e. Function words

32. Which factor is thought to affect the rate of lexical acquisition after acquisition of the first 100 words?
    a. Frequency of use by caregiver
    b. Reference to the here and now
    c. Pointing to referent
    d. Growth in cognitive development
    e. Growth in social development

33. Word association tasks are frequently used to assess the development of the meanings of words. Which of the following sequences of word knowledge development is the one observed by researchers?
    a. Paradigmatic and then syntagmatic
    b. Syntagmatic and then paradigmatic
    c. Antonyms and then synonyms
    d. Referential meaning and then relational meaning
    e. None of the above

34. Word definitions change over time, which indicates interactions between language and cognitive development. Which of the following researchers studied word definitions over time?
    a. Lev Vygotsky
    b. Noam Chomsky
    c. Roman Jakobson
    d. Jean Piaget
    e. Lois Bloom

35. Tests of word recognition assess children's vocabulary skills. What specific vocabulary skill in fact do these tests assess?
    a. Vocabulary knowledge
    b. Word association knowledge

c. Lexical retrieval
d. Visual recognition
e. All the above

36. In instances of different types of vocabulary acquisition, different cognitive abilities are called upon. For example, knowledge of different kinds of verbs and their use has been found. Which type of verbs do children learn first?
a. Transitive verbs
b. Intransitive verbs
c. Modal auxiliaries
d. Stative verbs
e. All the above

37. Short-term memory has been found to be critically related to the number of units in a sequence that can be recalled. What is the number of units that can be recalled by anyone?
a. Thirteen
b. Five plus or minus two
c. Seven plus or minus two
d. Nine plus or minus five
e. Ten

38. What is the age at which children can use short-term memory effectively and recall the number of items said to be the limit?
a. During preadolescence
b. During infancy
c. After infancy
d. Before adolescence
e. During adulthood

39. The ability to categorize words on the basis of their semantic relatedness is necessary to the understanding of what?
a. Referential word meaning
b. The syntax of utterances
c. Relational word meaning
d. Morphological word differences
e. None of the above

40. Of the following long-term memory factors, which one or more are crucial in comprehension and production of connected discourse?
a. Remembering the meaning of words over time
b. Remembering how sentences are put together
c. Remembering the relation between what is seen and what is heard
d. Remembering the structure of different types of discourse
e. All the above

ANSWERS

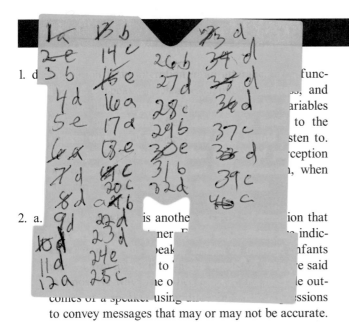

1. d. [...] func-
[...], and
[...] ariables
[...] to the
[...] sten to.
[...] ception
[...], when

2. a. [...] is anothe[...] ion that
[...]ner [...] indic-
[...] peak[...] nfants
[...] to [...] e said
[...] he o[...] e out-
comes of a speaker using [...] ssions
to convey messages that may or may not be accurate.

3. b. Gesture is a component of kinesics, which is the study of meaningful gestures and bodily movements during communication interactions. Gestures are different particularly from culture to culture. The other answers are different features of gesture but answer b is the most comprehensive answer.

4. d. Stress is used variably to indicate what the speaker wants the listener to attend to. The other answers are components of message processing that listeners utilize in the perception and comprehension of a message.

5. e. Stress, intonation, rhythm, and facial expression, in addition to other linguistic variables, are used by speakers to convey meaning in messages to others.

6. b. Initially, infants attend to the prosody and facial expression of the speaker. Prosody is the suprasegmental component of speech that includes such speech variables as intonation, rhythm, and stress patterns.

7. a. The term "style" usually refers to degree of formality in speech. Communication interactions are influenced by situational and contextual variables. Speakers unconsciously shift styles in different situations. For instance, contracted forms (e.g, "isn't") are used more frequently in informal use of English, such as verbal conversation, than in formal use in another context, such as reading.

8. b. Learning the communication of a particular culture is shaped by practice in listening to and using speech in that culture. The other choices are factors used in acquiring cultural communication differences; hence they are related to the answer (Q2). Culture is a very important component in communication interactions. In American culture, race, level of education, and socioeconomic class all help shape the communication experiences of a language learner.

9. d. Children from different cultures may have problems when communicating with speakers from another culture. Culture is an important component in the acquisition and use of a language, and because of dialect variation or bilingualism, the language learner may experience problems with the language rules of various cultural groups, which may differ.

10. e. Infants use multiple cues such as eye gaze, pointing, phonological cues, and word stress to learn what the speaker is referring to. This information, along with other input, is processed by the child to filter the speech stream and decode what is being said.

11. d. Children show some individual variation but, normally developing children should begin recognizing words during the first year of life. They are exposed to language from the moment of birth. Caregivers play an important role in language development, and both the child and caregiver develop a distinct pattern of communication interaction. They engage in shared communication through activities such as play and daily routines.

12. a. Although there are universals across languages that are allowable, phonological rules of different languages specify particular phonological sequences. Phonological rules are a component of language, which regulate the structure, distribution, and sequences of different speech sound patterns. They play a role in word production, but they more precisely refer to allowable segmental sequences in a language. Phonological rules are internalized and not dependent on various sensorimotor skills. Allophonic variations are phonetic variations of phonemes that are present in speech production.

13. e. Distinctive features consist of articulatory and acoustic features that differentiate one phoneme from another. Although distinctive feature differences mark distinctions between phonemes of a language and options a. through d. are related to feature development during acquisition, additional knowledge is necessary to differentiate words.

14. c. As found in recognition experiments, expectations about the structure of syllables change as the child develops language. In English, a syllable is a defined

unit that consists of a vowel and may have consonants that combine with the vowel in phonologically permissible patterns. A word can be a single syllable ("go") or multisyllabic ("baseball"). Syllables may be different in different languages and do appear during the first year of life. It is not established that the syllable is most important factor in speech sound acquisition.

15. c. Each type of cluster plays a different role in word generation. The use of medial clusters indicates use of words with more than one syllable, which is a later development than use of monosyllabic words. Prevocalic and postvocalic clusters may appear earlier than medial clusters. The /s/ and /r/ phonemes are later developing and may be problematic for clusters in any word position that contain these segments, but medial clusters are associated with multisyllabic words, a more advanced developmental marker.

16. a. One of the primary causes of speech and language delay is a history of hearing problems. Motor, cognitive, social, and communication domains develop in parallel. Delays in motor, cognitive, and social development can affect speech and language development. In the absence of such delays, however, a child with speech and language delays should be evaluated for a hearing loss. In the case of hearing loss, the language learner is deprived of auditory (sensory) input.

17. d. Children initially add to their lexicon words that are called *free morphemes*. Free morphemes such as "dog" and "cat" code individual meaning. The bound morphemes—plural /z/, plural /ɔz/, and plural /s/—are all used to denote pluralization but are used in combination with a free morpheme ("dog" + /z/ = dogs). Free morphemes such as number words are generally acquired before bound morphemes.

18. e. All the factors listed play a role and must be considered when the clinician evaluates a child who is learning English as a second language, because the first language is a foundation for acquisition of the second language.

19. b. Many children between the ages of 18 and 24 months experience a vocabulary spurt, or rapid growth in lexical development. The only difference between these children and those who do not experience this spurt has been found to be the sophistication of their phonological repertoires. Auditory perceptual skills, types of words acquired, and cognitive abilities are variables that do not differ significantly between the two groups.

20. c. Infants are able to discriminate between speech sounds from any language during their first months of life, which indicates that they are ready to acquire

any language early on. In general, by ages 10 to 12 months, they show a preference for the sounds of the native language and lose the ability to discriminate most sounds that are not part of their language.

21. c. One of the earliest rules of syntax that children learn is the order of subject, verb, and object in their language. Comprehension studies indicate that 2-year-old children use multiple cues in comprehending multiple-word utterances, and word order is one of those important cues used by children to comprehend the basic subject-verb-object sentence.

22. d. The word order of subject-verb-object relations varies among languages. In English, the basic order is subject-verb-object, but in some languages, such as German, the verb is at the end of the sentence.

23. d. Word order is a universal language learning principle and one of the earliest learned by children. It is thought that frequency of use is the factor that plays the most important role in learning this principle.

24. e. Imitation is an important skill for language development. It is an ability that enables the child to build internal representations of other's behavior and reproduce it. Successful physical imitation requires that the child engage in turn-taking, attend to the action, and replicate the features of the action.

25. c. Children are exposed to different syntactical structures through interactions with their caregivers and others in their environment. Although all the factors contribute to learning syntax, the major factor is how frequently the child hears a particular language.

26. b. A dialect is a rule-based system used by a specific group or language community that varies in any number of systematic ways from an ideal standard language. Dialect can vary as a function of variables such as geography, race and ethnicity, socioeconomic status, and peer influences. Syntactic differences can vary as a function of language change for a particular language community. Dialects signify differences among groups, not disorders.

27. d. Although the production, paralinguistics, and context of an utterance and the listener's comprehension of the utterance are involved in a speech act, the communicative intent of an utterance is the definition of a speech act. The speech act according to Searle is a basic unit of communication. It is an intentional message coded by a speaker and presented to a listener.

28. c. In terms of primitive speech act analysis, a preverbal or single word production is used by the child

to convey her or his intentions before the development of complex language patterns. The speaker's illocutionary element is often coded to a listener through suprasegmental intonation patterns. Infants learn very early the communicative intent of different intonation patterns on utterances and use them effectively with caregivers.

29. b. According to the minimal distance principle, speakers use comprehension strategies to relate subject to verb to understand the relation of actor and action. The further the subject is from the main verb of the sentence, the more difficult it is for the young listener to understand the sentence.

30. d. The earliest form of a question is signaled by a shift in intonation. A holophrase is produced in question form by an upward shift in intonation. The listener uses this cue to understand that the single-word utterance is a question.

31. b. The early lexicons of children consist of mainly of nominals. They are categorized into general nominals ("juice," "water," "dog") and specific nominals ("mama," "dada"). The other word categories, such as verbs or action words, are also acquired by the child but after nominals.

32. d. Frequency of use by the caregiver, reference to the here and now, and pointing to the referent are important factors in lexical acquisition, but a change in cognitive growth is thought to be responsible for the rapid spurt in lexical development that most children undergo after acquiring their first 100 vocabulary words.

33. b. Children initially acquire word meanings and associate those words with others in the same category. For instance, children are exposed to many types of dogs in their environmental interactions, and they would form lexical category of dogs. In a word association task, a word such as "boy" might elicit a response such as "play." This is a syntagmatic association wherein the target word elicits an action associated with the target word. As children become older, a different association strategy is used. In this case, a word such as "man" may elicit a response such as "boy." The paradigmatic response is based on the development of semantic categories, which consist of different semantic attributes. The syntagmatic-paradigmatic shift happens at approximately 7 years of age. The shift may be a function of either an alteration in and organization of semantic features or a transformation of general cognitive processing strategies.

34. a. All the individuals named have made important contributions to child language research. Vygotsky

formulated the associative hypothesis to explain concept formation and word learning. Accordingly, a child organizes word concepts in a specific way, using strategies that allow the child to recognize particular features of a referent. Each consecutive use of a particular word includes some attribute of the core concept.

35. e. All the skills listed are required in order for children to identify words that are part of their lexicon. Moreover, all these skills are required on most tests of children's word recognition.

36. a. Action (transitive) verbs can be related to utterances heard and observations made about an event or the environment and are therefore learned before other types of verbs. A sentence with a transitive verb also includes a direct object, although young children often use transitive verbs without the direct object. Another feature of transitive verbs is that they can be modified from active to passive voice. Intransitive verbs cannot take a direct object or be converted to the passive voice. Stative verbs like the copula ("to be") take a complement, rather than a direct object. A modal auxiliary (helping) verb is used to mark mood or attitude such as possibility ("might").

37. c. Studies of short-term memory have identified seven plus or minus two as the number of units that can be held in short-term memory. The key concept is "units," not an absolute number of items.

38. c. Children achieve the use of short-term memory capacity and recall the number of items said to be the limit by the end of infancy.

39. c. For a listener to comprehend the meaning of utterances, both the syntax of the utterance and the relational meaning of the words in it are necessary. In fact, some researchers suggest that children learn phrases in which subjects and verbs go together.

40. e. The long-term memory of the competent conversationalist is adequate for processing linguistic input and output. Memory is the ability that allows a speaker to recall different information that has been acquired and is in neural storage. Memory of the meaning of words, how sentences are put together, the relation between what is seen and what is heard, and the structure of different types of discourse play a crucial role in engaging in connected discourse. The more the child engages in conversation, the more long-term memory is used, inasmuch as linguistic information of all types is subject to rehearsal, constant repetition, and organization.

CHAPTER 2

Language Science

Lisa Hammett Price

Yvette D. Hyter

1. Of Piaget's (1983) stages, which of the following corresponds with the emergence of a normally developing child's first words?
   a. Preoperational
   b. Formal operations
   c. Sensorimotor
   d. Concrete operations
   e. Operational

2. Piaget (Owens, 2007) would support the following statement about language acquisition:
   a. The mind is a black box; we cannot see into it, and therefore we cannot speculate about what goes on within it
   b. Language is learned through environmental stimulation, imitation, selective reinforcement, and shaping of behavior
   c. The language acquisition device is a part of the brain specialized for language, and environmental stimulation triggers its development
   d. Language is part of a larger set of cognitive skills, and language acquisition therefore depends on the development of these cognitive processes
   e. Language is acquired through social interaction with adults and peers; therefore, both the child and the adult have active roles in driving language development

3. You are observing a clinician in private practice. He specializes in childhood language disorders and serves elementary school–aged children. You observe that this clinician has a well-structured reward system for each child. Some children receive a Froot Loop for each correct response they make; others work to earn stickers and even small toys. This clinician has written down each specific behavior that he wishes to elicit from each child with a percentage of accuracy

attached. For example, an objective for one child reads, "when presented with a picture of two or more objects, Jimmy will label the picture using plural 's' 80% of the time." This clinician probably subscribes to which of the following theories of child language development?
a. Nativist
b. Social interactionist
c. Universal grammar
d. Behaviorist
e. Cognitivist

4. Chomsky's (Owens, 2007) views on language acquisition:
a. Provided the foundation for Skinner's operant learning theory
b. Led to an emphasis on syntax in language intervention programs
c. Focused on the influence of memory and attention on language learning
d. Suggested a strong role for the environment in language acquisition
e. Led to the use of tangible reinforcers to shape specific behaviors

5. Of the following words, which contains three phonemes?
a. Choose
b. Fix
c. Toy
d. Know
e. Straight

6. Language form is made up of:
a. Phonology, morphology, and syntax
b. Semantics, phonology, and syntax
c. Pragmatics, semantics, and grammar
d. Content, use, and metalinguistics
e. Pragmatics, phonology, and semantics

7. Jeffrey is a 5-year-old who has Down syndrome. He lives with both parents and has a sister, aged 8, and a brother, aged 14 months. He participates in a regular kindergarten classroom for the majority of his day; during some activities, he receives paraprofessional support within the classroom. In addition to receiving speech language therapy, Jeffrey receives physical therapy and occupational therapy services once each week. Jeffrey communicates in single words and short phrases, in addition to using a few simple signs and "invented" gestures he learned in therapy (e.g., "please," "more"). He is very affectionate with the other students but is sometimes intrusive during group activities or disruptive during circle time, which often frustrates the other children. He does not always spontaneously share his toys and sometimes has tantrums during transitions between activities. He has had recurrent ear infections and bilateral tube placement, and he

also has a number of allergies. During a reevaluation of Jeffrey's language skills, his speech-language pathologist (SLP) collected a language sample, calculated his mean length of utterance (MLU), and analyzed how he was able to put words together to make sentences. Of the following domains of language, which was the SLP trying to assess?
a. Semantics
b. Pragmatics
c. Phonology
d. Receptive language
e. Syntax

8. Jeffrey is a 5-year-old who has Down syndrome. He lives with both parents and has a sister, aged 8, and a brother, aged 14 months. He participates in a regular kindergarten classroom for the majority of his day; during some activities, he receives paraprofessional support within the classroom. In addition to receiving speech language therapy, Jeffrey receives physical therapy and occupational therapy services once each week. Jeffrey communicates in single words and short phrases, in addition to using a few simple signs and "invented" gestures he learned in therapy (e.g., "please," "more"). He is very affectionate with the other students but is sometimes intrusive during group activities or disruptive during circle time, which often frustrates the other children. He does not always spontaneously share his toys and sometimes has tantrums during transitions between activities. He has had recurrent ear infections and bilateral tube placement, and he also has a number of allergies. An evaluation of Jeffrey's phonology reveals:
a. How he uses language in social interaction.
b. How he uses the sound system of language.
c. How he applies meaning to words.
d. How aware he is of what is appropriate in different communication situations.
e. How he orders words in sentence structure.

9. Jeffrey is a 5-year-old who has Down syndrome. He lives with both parents and has a sister, aged 8, and a brother, aged 14 months. He participates in a regular kindergarten classroom for the majority of his day; during some activities, he receives paraprofessional support within the classroom. In addition to receiving speech language therapy, Jeffrey receives physical therapy and occupational therapy services once each week. Jeffrey communicates in single words and short phrases, in addition to using a few simple signs and "invented" gestures he learned in therapy (e.g., "please," "more"). He is very affectionate with the other students but is sometimes intrusive during group activities or disruptive during circle time, which often frustrates the other children. He does not always spontaneously share his toys and sometimes has tantrums during transitions between

activities. He has had recurrent ear infections and bilateral tube placement, and he also has a number of allergies. Jeffrey has difficulty producing lingua-palatal sounds. Of the following sounds, which does he probably misarticulate?
a. /f/, /v/
b. /b/, /p/, /m/, /w/
c. /t/, /d/, /s/, /z/, /l/
d. /t∫/, /∫/, /ʒ/dʒ/ (as in *jump*)
e. /h/

10. Jeffrey is a 5-year-old who has Down syndrome. He lives with both parents and has a sister, aged 8, and a brother, aged 14 months. He participates in a regular kindergarten classroom for the majority of his day; during some activities he receives paraprofessional support within the classroom. In addition to receiving speech language therapy, Jeffrey receives physical therapy and occupational therapy services once each week. Jeffrey communicates in single words and short phrases, in addition to using a few simple signs and "invented" gestures he learned in therapy (e.g., "please," "more"). He is very affectionate with the other students but is sometimes intrusive during group activities or disruptive during circle time, which often frustrates the other children. He does not always spontaneously share his toys and sometimes has tantrums during transitions between activities. He has had recurrent ear infections and bilateral tube placement, and he also has a number of allergies. Jeffrey also makes the following errors on words: *stop* becomes "top"; *green* becomes "geen"; *blue* becomes "boo." This type of phonological error is called:
a. Cluster reduction
b. Initial consonant deletion
c. Postvocalic consonant deletion
d. Stopping
e. Fronting

11. Of the following utterances, which does *not* entail the use of grammatical inflectional morphemes?
a. "Daddy's cup"
b. "Mommy coming"
c. "Want up"
d. "I walked"
e. "He jumps"

12. A child produces the utterance "doggie eats." Of the following grammatical inflectional morphemes, which is used in this utterance?
a. Third-person singular present tense
b. Plural
c. Auxiliary
d. Present progressive
e. Possessive

13. How many morphemes does the utterance "Mommy likes the scarves and hats I knitted" contain?
a. 8 morphemes
b. 10 morphemes
c. 11 morphemes
d. 12 morphemes
e. 13 morphemes

14. Kiesha is an 18-month-old who is developing typically. In the past 6 month, Kiesha has slowly added more words to her lexicon. About how many words is she expected to use?
a. 10
b. 25
c. 50
d. 100
e. 200

15. A variation of a phoneme is called:
a. An allophone
b. A phone
c. A pause
d. A phoneme
e. A fricative

16. A toddler developing normally is hearing many new words in her environment every day and is rapidly learning to understand what they mean. She hears the word *spoon* and quickly attaches this symbol to its appropriate referent. She does so despite the fact that there are two other objects on the table, a cup and bowl, because she already knows the words *cup* and *bowl*. In this case, of the following learning strategies, which helped her learn the new word?
a. Extendability principle
b. Novel-name-nameless assumption
c. Semantic bootstrapping
d. Syntactic bootstrapping
e. Conventionality assumption

17. A preschool-aged child who is developing normally is playing with his toy trucks and tractors in the sand box. His mother is playing with him, modeling language, expanding and extending his utterances. He uses semantic bootstrapping to acquire new knowledge of language. Of the following examples, which best illustrates this strategy?
a. His mother said, "Look at the treads" and accompanied the utterance with a point to the treads; this signaled to him that the new word *treads* referred to a part rather than to the whole entity or object
b. His mother said, "The tractor dug a tunnel," and the child used his knowledge of subject-verb-object sentence structure to figure out the meaning of the word *tunnel* in his mother's utterance

c. His mother said, "My truck crashed!" and this child's knowledge of possessor-possession helped him to understand the noun phrase structure in the utterance

d. His mother said, "I'm tunneling through the sand"; this child's knowledge of the present progressive morphological marker "-ing" helped him recognize that *tunneling* was a verb in the sentence

e. After he said, "My dirt falled off," his mother said, "Uh oh, your dirt fell off"; the mother's recast of his utterance helped him learn the irregular past tense for the word *fall*

18. A toddler who is developing normally is playing with her dolls and dollhouse. Her father is playing with her, modeling language and being a good play partner. The child is using primarily two-word utterances. Of the following utterances, which is an example of the "demonstrative + entity" semantic relation?
    a. That baby
    b. My baby
    c. Little baby
    d. Baby cry
    e. Baby milk

19. Of the following treatment goals, which addresses a child's form of language?
    a. The child will maintain a topic for three verbal turns during play interactions 80% of the time
    b. The child will increase the number of different words used during narrative retelling to within one standard deviation of peers in samples of comparable length
    c. The child will use the correct regular past tense verb forms during conversational interactions 80% of the time
    d. The child will improve the ability to repair communication by increasing accuracy of answers to simple "who," "what," "where," and "when" questions to 80% during structured activities
    e. After instruction on a set of curricular vocabulary words, the child will use word-finding strategies to complete cloze sentences with 80% accuracy

20. Of the following interrogative utterances produced by a child, which is the most syntactically complex?
    a. "What did Daddy eat?"
    b. "I do it, okay?"
    c. "Where is Daddy?"
    d. "What is Daddy eating?"
    e. "Daddy going?"

21. Consider the following interaction:
    Child 1: What are you building?
    Child 2: A tower.

This is an example of which of the following linguistic features?
    a. Deixis
    b. Ellipsis
    c. Fast-mapping
    d. Anaphora
    e. Derivation

22. Consider the following text: "John and Maria were walking in the woods when they saw a large black bear on the path before them. It was eating berries. They quickly turned around and went back the way they had come." The use of the plural pronoun *they* to refer to John and Maria represents which of the following cohesive devices?
    a. Ellipsis
    b. Deixis
    c. Anaphora
    d. Conjunction
    e. Locative

23. Of the following utterances, which contains the use of a deictic term?
    a. "Once upon a time"
    b. "Where is the dog?"
    c. "After we eat"
    d. "Put that here"
    e. "It's on the table"

24. Read the following set of utterances from a child's language sample (E = examiner, C = child).
    E: Okay, now, tell me about what happened to Sadie (the child's cat).
    C: Sometimes she don't throw up.
    C: (Um) she went to the vet every time (um) we got her dry cat food.
    C: She don't like it, though.
    C: We got her something else at the vet.
    C: When I got outta school, she (um) got her some food for her.
    E: So you went after school to the vet.
    E: And he said she should have dry food?
    C: Because [4 second pause] she (um) throws up every time.
    E: She's been throwing up?
    C: Mm hm.
    C: Not every time, though.
    C: (She really) she's doing fine, though.
    E: But you said something about her fur coming back.
    E: Did she lose her fur?
    C: No.
    C: It's coming back, though.

The utterance "Did she lose her fur?" is which of the following sentence types?
    a. Declarative
    b. Interrogative

c. Imperative
d. Negative
e. Compound

25. Read the following set of utterances from a child's language sample (E = examiner, C = child).

    E: Okay, now, tell me about what happened to Sadie (the child's cat).
    C: Sometimes she don't throw up.
    C: (Um) she went to the vet every time (um) we got her dry cat food.
    C: She don't like it, though.
    C: We got her something else at the vet.
    C: When I got outta school, she (um) got her some food for her.
    E: So you went after school to the vet.
    E: And he said she should have dry food?
    C: Because [4 second pause] she (um) throws up every time.
    E: She's been throwing up?
    C: Mm hm.
    C: Not every time, though.
    C: (She really) she's doing fine, though.
    E: But you said something about her fur coming back.
    E: Did she lose her fur?
    C: No.
    C: It's coming back, though.

    Both the utterances "(She really) she's doing fine, though" and "Because [4 second pause] she (um) throws up every time" contain which of the following?
    a. Present progressive verb forms
    b. Third-person singular verb forms
    c. Mazes
    d. Contractible verb forms
    e. Root word errors

26. Calculate an MLU on the following utterances:
    C: My birthday was on Friday.
    C: We went to Daddy's work and picked him up.
    C: We hafta go get him every day because his car is broke.
    C: He (he) came with us to my party at Chuck E. Cheese.

    Of the following, which is the correct MLU for these utterances?
    a. 8.75
    b. 10
    c. 9.25
    d. 9.5
    e. 9.0

27. Samantha is a 5-year-old with language impairment. Her expressive and receptive language skills have improved substantially over the past year with intervention; however, her parents and preschool teacher are concerned that she is not developing literacy skills. According to ASHA's guidelines regarding the roles and responsibilities for SLPs with regard to reading and writing in children, which of the following is the best approach?
    a. Wait until she enters kindergarten to assess her early literacy abilities, and address them if necessary at that time; it is too early to address such skills in preschool
    b. Assess her early literacy skills now and give the results to her current classroom teacher so that these skills can be addressed in school
    c. Refer her for other special education services, because reading and writing are not in the SLP's scope of practice
    d. Assess early literacy and add appropriate goals to your treatment plan to address weaknesses, because children with language impairment are known to be at greater risk for difficulties learning to read and write
    e. Explain to the teacher and parents that Samantha has good articulation skills and, therefore, she should learn to read and write without any difficulty

28. Of the following, which best defines phonological awareness?
    a. A metalinguistic ability that includes awareness of different levels of the speech sound system, such as word boundaries, syllables, rhyming, phoneme segmenting, and blending
    b. The conscious awareness that words are made of smaller segments of speech, which can be represented with letters
    c. The rule system in a language that governs how phonemes are sequenced to make words
    d. The use of letters and letter combinations to represent phonemes in an orthography
    e. The prosodic features of speech, such as tone, stress, rhythm, intonation

29. Of the following, which is *not* true about the sentence "The boy threw the red ball"?
    a. "Threw" is a verb
    b. Both "the boy" and "the red ball" are noun phrases
    c. "The" is an article
    d. "The red ball" is the indirect object in this sentence
    e. "The red ball" contains an adjective modifier

30. In the sentence "My mother and I ate at a restaurant," the phrase "at a restaurant" is best described as a:
    a. Prepositional phrase
    b. Noun phrase
    c. Verb phrase
    d. Direct object
    e. Predicate

31. In the utterance "They were sad," the verb can be described as:
    a. A contractible copula
    b. A copula
    c. A contractible auxiliary
    d. An uncontractible auxiliary
    e. A passive verb

32. An SLP collected a language sample as part of an assessment of a school-aged child's syntax. Of the following syntactic forms, which is missing from this selection of the child's sentences?
    "Swimming is my favorite thing to do"
    "My green and blue swimsuit is pretty"
    "I am the team captain"

    a. Adjective phrase
    b. Adverbial phrase
    c. Gerund phrase
    d. Subject complement
    e. Infinitive

33. An SLP is evaluating a child's narrative by looking for the components of story grammar. She finds that in addition to other story grammar components, the child's narrative includes several attempts. This means that the narrative includes which of the following?
    a. Characters' success or failure at reaching their goals
    b. The characters' emotional responses to, thoughts about, or actions as a result of the outcome of the chain of events
    c. The characters' actions to attain their goals
    d. Characters' strategies for attaining their goals
    e. The event that induces the characters to act

34. Of the following, which is an example of a task of phonemic awareness skills?
    a. What is "cupcake" without "cup"?
    b. Do "cup" and "pup" rhyme?
    c. How many syllables are in the word "alligator"?
    d. How many words are in the sentence "I love pizza"?
    e. What is "cup" without /k/?

35. Of the following, which best describes the clause structure in the sentence "I can't play outside because I have too much homework"?
    a. Two independent clauses
    b. An independent clause followed by a dependent clause
    c. An independent clause and an adjective (or relative) clause
    d. A dependent clause and an adverb clause
    e. A dependent clause followed by an independent clause

36. It is important for a professional to have a sense of the historical development of his or her field. Of the following periods, in which did the field of speech-language pathology begin to become a recognized profession?
    a. 1975–2005
    b. 1965–1975
    c. 1900–1945
    d. 2000–2009
    e. 1800–1845

37. You believe that language is used primarily for communicating ideas and making connections with other people. Of the following, which best denotes the theoretical framework that will guide your clinical practice?
    a. Behaviorism
    b. Informational processing
    c. Linguistic theory
    d. Social interactionism
    e. Constructivism

38. Of the scholars listed as follows, who proposed that neural connections are made through language input and that language learning is possible when attention, perception, memory, and motivation are present?
    a. McWhinney
    b. Piaget
    c. Skinner
    d. Vygotsky
    e. Chomsky

39. Usage-based theory is a framework for understanding language learning. What are the primary underlying assumptions of this theory?
    a. Children's brains are hardwired to learn language, and children are born equipped with internal grammatical rules, regardless of the language; however, language input helps children learn the specific parameters of their own language
    b. Children are born with the cognitive abilities of reading others' intentions and finding patterns, both of which are fundamental to the origins of language
    c. Language is a network of connections that is transformed by language input
    d. Children's cognitive development occurs before language development
    e. Language is a behavior that is learned

40. Bloom and Lahey (1978) developed a theory in which language is viewed as an integration of form, content, and use. Bloom and Tinker (2001) expanded that model by embedding these three elements into what two domains?
    a. Pattern learning and intention reading
    b. Modular learning and egocentric perspectives
    c. Intersubjectivity and cognitive processes

d. Stimulus and responses

e. Axons and synapses

41. Several scholars have written about the relationship between thought and language. Of the following statements, which is consistent with the ideas of Vygotsky (Owens, 2007)?

a. Language is determined by cognition

b. Cognition is determined by language

c. Cognition initially influences language, and then language influences cognition

d. Language and cognition are related but independent skills

e. Language and cognition are not connected to each other

42. Nine-month-old Haleem vocalizes and persistently points at an object across the room while looking back and forth at the object and his mom. He is exhibiting intentionality because:

a. He is 9 months old

b. He is showing intersubjective awareness

c. He is attending to an object

d. He is vocalizing

e. He is exhibiting locutionary behavior

43. Gestures play an important role in communication and develop relatively early in life. Of the following types of gestures, which develops earliest?

a. Gestures that consistently convey a specific meaning across contexts

b. Gestures that track the rhythm of speech emphasizing ideas

c. Gestures that point to or show a referent

d. Gestures that convey a particular meaning based on social-cultural context

e. Gestures that mark the beginning of a story

44. Gestures and language share one cognitive skill, which is the:

a. Ability to decontextualize something represented in the mind

b. Ability to attend to important contextual information

c. Ability to remember past events

d. Ability to self-regulate behavior

e. Ability to perceive reality

45. What is primary relationship between language and symbolic play?

a. Play is a prerequisite skill for language development, in that a child must be able to play functionally before he or she is producing single word utterances

b. Language and symbolic play represent reality, and both tend to have similar developmental trajectories

c. Although both play and language are abstract, language is less abstract than symbolic play

d. Language is a prerequisite skill for play development, in that a child must be able to use age-appropriate language before he or she can play appropriately

e. There is no real relationship between language and play except that play helps children relax before an assessment

46. Children with specific language impairment may have general nonlinguistic representation disabilities such as those in:

a. Story retelling skills

b. Symbolic play skills

c. Closure skills

d. Inflectional morphology

e. Phonological skills

47. In many school systems, the relationship between play and literacy is not understood. What are the results of this limited understanding?

a. Some schools have increased play areas in classrooms

b. Some schools have minimized teacher-directed activities such as knowledge of alphabets

c. Some schools have reduced recess time

d. Some schools focus less on phonological awareness

e. Some schools include print awareness

48. Which 24-month-old described as follows is exhibiting an age-appropriate level of play?

a. Anthony is setting the stage for his play by assigning roles to his friends; for example, "You be the mommy and I'll be the baby"

b. James uses objects in a functional manner but does not spend much time with any object; for example, he may pick up a brush and touch it to his head before moving on to another object

c. Alicia picks up a toy and brings it to her mouth, and then bangs the toy on the table before returning it to her mouth

d. Marcia picks up the phone, dials it, pretends to talk on the phone, hands it to another person, and then hangs up the phone

e. Roberto pretends that he is a Teenage Mutant Ninja Turtle battling a Transformer and plays this game from different perspectives

49. Aly was a victim of prenatal exposure to alcohol, a teratogen. Furthermore, during the first 3 months of her life, Aly experienced severe neglect from her parents, both of whom suffered from alcoholism and depression. As a result of her birth history, Aly may have difficulty achieving which of the following important milestones that serves as a foundation for the development of cognition and linguistic skills?

a. Self-regulation

b. Sit without support

c. Engage in social interaction
d. Fine motor movements
e. Use of gesture

50. On your first day in your new position as SLP, you find that your school only has one formal assessment measure, the Test of Language Development Primary, Fourth Edition (TOLD-P:4). This assessment has nine subtests for measuring language. Specifically, the TOLD-P:4 is used to assess word meaning and relationships, word structures, and comprehension of sentence structure. Which aspect of language is not assessed with the TOLD-P:4?
    a. Syntax
    b. Semantics
    c. Pragmatics
    d. Speech
    e. Phonology

51. According to Brown (1973), young children produce eight prevalent semantic relations. The two-word utterance "more cookie" is which type of prevalent semantic relation?
    a. Action + object
    b. Agent + object
    c. Quantifier
    d. Recurrence
    e. Demonstrative + entity

52. The earliest pragmatic skill of a typically developing toddler (aged 12 to 36 months) is:
    a. Use of sarcasm
    b. Gestures and word combinations
    c. Taking turns
    d. Utterance repair
    e. Understanding jokes

53. Mirror neurons are important for language development because:
    a. They play a vital role in the connecting the Broca and Wernicke areas in the left hemisphere of the brain
    b. They play a vital role in the acquisition of language through the language acquisition device
    c. They play a vital role in the mental reenactment of actions when linguistic descriptions of those actions are processed
    d. They play a vital role in the ability of the Wernicke area to support language comprehension
    e. They play a vital role in gaze behavior

54. Of the following, which is the best example of the novel name-nameless category of word learning exhibited by toddlers?
    a. Johnny sees a cat and says, "dog"
    b. The only dog that Jasmine recognizes as a dog is her own pet poodle

c. A toddler can identify the blender when shown a ball, bottle, and a blender
d. When a mother points to a car and says, "Look a car," the toddler assumes that the word *car* refers to the whole object rather than to the wheel
e. Kathy sees any cat and labels it "cat"

55. One of the latest developing pragmatic skills in typical developing children is:
    a. Comprehending jokes
    b. Requesting by using pointing
    c. Clarifying requests
    d. Comprehending indirect requests
    e. Initiating conversation

56. Which phrase best describes what is meant by the term *culture*?
    a. African American
    b. Assumptions and world view
    c. Religious practices
    d. Family structure
    e. Socioeconomic status

57. Cultural reciprocity is important for
    a. Building rapport with a client
    b. Building collaborative relationships between clients and their families and the communication professional
    c. Building a treatment plan for the client to use at home
    d. Building relationships between professionals
    e. Building knowledge about language development.

58. You are conducting an ethnographic interview with Mrs. James, the mother of your client, Michael. Of the questions below, identify the most appropriate question to ask after this statement made by Mrs. James: "Michael gets all spastic when he is nervous":
    a. "Mrs. James, you stated that Michael gets spastic when he is nervous. What do you mean by 'spastic'?"
    b. "Mrs. James, you stated that Michael gets spastic when he is nervous. Does he get nervous often?"
    c. "Mrs. James, you stated that Michael gets spastic when he is nervous. Give me an example of what Michael does when he gets spastic."
    d. "Mrs. James, you stated that Michael gets spastic when he is nervous. What do you mean by 'spastic,' why do you think he gets nervous, and does this nervousness happen often?"
    e. "Mrs. James, you stated that Michael gets spastic when he is nervous. I'd like to now find out about how Michael makes friends."

59. In assessments of children who are learning English as a second language or who are speaking a social dialect

of English, which of the following assessment processes elicits the most accurate results?
a. Behavioral assessment processes
b. Standardized, norm-referenced assessments
c. Observational assessments
d. Dynamic assessment processes
e. The assessment measure without modifications

60. Of the following skills for an interpreter to possess in a bilingual assessment, which of the following would be insufficient?
a. Literacy in one language
b. Knowledge of two cultures
c. Familiarity with dialect difference
d. Knowledge of relevant terminology
e. Familiarity with the purpose of the assessment

61. Identify the statement below that is true:
a. Individuals who start learning a second language at a younger age usually achieve less proficient syntactic skills than those who begin learning a second language in adulthood
b. Second-language learners seldom experience language loss
c. Second-language learners may code switch within the same communicative interaction
d. Second-language learners do not exhibit dialectical variance
e. Second-language learning interferes with metalinguistic knowledge

62. Emergent literacy depends primarily on the child's:
a. Oral language and metalinguistic skills
b. Oral language and alphabet knowledge
c. Metalinguistic skills and print awareness
d. Alphabet knowledge and print awareness
e. Book awareness and environmental print

63. You are collecting a language sample from Angelique, aged 4 years, 6 months, when the following interaction occurs:
Angelique: I the mama and you the baby. I driving the car.
Clinician: Okay. Mama, where are we going? I'm hungry.
Angelique: I gonna buy you a fish sandwich. You be eating good stuff.
Clinician: Thanks, Mama, 'cause I didn't have lunch yet.

After reading the brief language sample, what can you say about Angelique's language?
a. Angelique's language may include features of Spanish-influenced English
b. Angelique's language may include features of African American English

c. Angelique's language may not include features of standard American English
d. Angelique might have a language disorder
e. Angelique might have a hearing impairment

64. You are collecting a language sample from Angelique, aged 4 years, 6 months, when the following interaction occurs:
Angelique: I the mama and you the baby. I driving the car.
Clinician: Okay. Mama, where are we going? I'm hungry.
Angelique: I gonna buy you a fish sandwich. You be eating good stuff.
Clinician: Thanks, Mama, 'cause I didn't have lunch yet.

Identify the grammatical markers of dialect exhibited in the utterance "I gonna buy you a fish sandwich. You be eating good stuff":
a. No auxiliary verb and habitual use of *be*
b. No copula and habitual use of *be*
c. Past tense and the copula *be*
d. Modal perfect and the auxiliary verb *be*
e. Future tense and the copula *be*

65. After completing a language sample on Angelique, aged 4 years, 6 months, who speaks African American English, you decide to use a criterion-referenced measure, the Minimal Competency Core (MCC) (Stockman, 1996). Of the following, which best describes what the MCC represents?
a. The most knowledge (or skill) needed for a child to be judged as typically developing
b. The range of morphosyntactic skills that young children are able to produce
c. The least amount of knowledge (or skill) needed for a child to be judged as typically developing
d. The alternative to language sample analysis
e. The range of communicative functions necessary for a child to be considered an age-appropriate language user

66. Michael produced a narrative that consisted of labels of objects, descriptions of events, and descriptions of actions. If Michael is developing typically, he is probably in what age range?
a. 4 to 5 years
b. 2 to 3 years
c. 5 to 7 years
d. 10 to 15 years
e. 20 to 25 years

67. In the following narrative, identify the statement that illustrates the narrator's ability to represent the landscape of action (subjectivity) of the story's characters:

"There was this boy who had a frog. He kept this frog in a jar in his bedroom. The boy and his family were going to a fancy restaurant, but the boy was worried about leaving the frog alone because he would have been lonely. So, the boy put the frog in his coat pocket, but his parents didn't know he had the frog with him. When they got to the restaurant and sat down, the frog caused all kinds of chaos."

a. "There was this boy, who had a frog."
b. "He kept this frog in a jar in his bedroom."
c. "The boy was worried about leaving the frog alone."
d. "The boy put the frog in his coat pocket."
e. "The frog caused all kinds of chaos."

68. All of the following concepts are part of the language component pragmatics, with the exception of:
    a. Intentions
    b. Narratives
    c. Register
    d. Lexicon
    e. Presupposition skills

69. How many t-units are present in the following passage?
    "There was this boy who had a frog. He kept this frog in a jar in his bedroom. The boy and his family were going to a fancy restaurant, but the boy was worried about leaving the frog alone because he would have been lonely. So, the boy put the frog in his coat pocket, but his parents didn't know he had the frog with him. When they got to the restaurant and sat down, the frog caused all kinds of chaos."

    a. Three
    b. Five
    c. Seven
    d. Nine
    e. Six

1. c. Piaget described the following four stages of development: sensorimotor (ages 0 to 2 years), peroperational (ages 2 to 7 years), concrete operations (ages 7 to 11 years), and formal operations (ages 11 years and older). Children use their first words in the sensorimotor stage. "Operational" (option e) is not one of the stages that Piaget described.

2. d. Piaget believed that language was part of a larger set of cognitive skills and that the development of language depended on the development of cognition. The idea that "the mind is a black box" (option a) is consistent with the behaviorist theory of language development proposed by B. F. Skinner (Owens, 2007). The idea that children learn language by hearing it in their environment, imitating it, and having others selectively reinforce and shape their language behaviors (option b) is one of the principles of behaviorism. The language acquisition device (option c) is a mechanism for learning language that applies to the nativist theory of language acquisition. According to the social interactionist theory of language acquisition (Vygotsky, Nelson, Bruner) (Pence, 2008), the environment offers opportunities for social interaction and language emerges because of a motivation to interact with others (option e).

3. d. This clinician is using tangible reinforcers to increase desired behaviors and decrease undesirable behaviors. He is also using an established and explicit criterion for success (80%). These are characteristics of a behaviorist approach to treatment. According to nativist theory (option a), such reinforcers would not have any affect on production. A social interactionist (option b) would arrange the natural environment in such a way as to encourage interaction and require the target language structure in order for the child to obtain what he or she wants, rather than creating such a rigid task oriented routine. Universal grammar (option c) is the formal system of rules that is genetically determined in its initial state and later affected by exposure to language; it is a feature of Chomsky's (Owens, 2007) nativist theory.

4. b. Chomsky outlined a nativist theory of language acquisition; infants are born with a language acquisition device or specialized language process that is part of the brain. This process allows them access to the universal rules of language. Exposure to a particular language then allows the language acquisition device to learn the rules specific for that language. For clinicians who subscribe to a nativist view of language acquisition, intervention therefore would focus on syntax. Skinner (option a) is associated with the theory of behaviorism, whereas Chomsky is associated with nativism. Information processing theories of language acquisition would focus treatment on memory and attention to improve language learning (option c). Behaviorists suggest a strong role for the environment in language acquisition (option d), and they would consider tangible reinforcers to be an appropriate therapeutic strategy (option e).

5. a. The word *choose* contains three phonemes: /t∫/, /u/, and /z/. The word *fix* (option b) contains four phonemes; *toy* (option c) contains two phonemes; *know* (option d) contains two phonemes; and *straight* (option e) contains five phonemes.

6. a. Language has been conceptualized as comprising three areas: form, content, and use. Language form consists of phonology, morphology, and syntax. Semantics (options b and c) includes vocabulary, or the content of language; pragmatics (options c and e) is the use of language in social contexts. Children need to learn metalinguistic skills (option d) in each of the domains of language.

7. e. Both MLU and analysis of sentence construction reveal information about syntax. If the SLP were interested in semantics (option a), she or he would have compiled a list of word types or the number of different words that Jeffrey used and would have analyzed semantic relationships within utterances. To analyze pragmatics (option b), the SLP would need to consider Jeffrey's use of initiations, responses, turn-taking, topic maintenance, and social appropriateness of his utterances. Phonology (option c) is analyzed not with a language sample but rather with a speech sample. Receptive language (option d) is not considered one of the five domains of language. The SLP could assess receptive and expressive abilities within each domain (e.g., receptive syntax or expressive syntax).

8. b. An evaluation of phonology would reveal the use of the sound system of the language. An evaluation of pragmatics would reveal how Jeffrey uses language in social interactions (option a) and whether he understands what is appropriate in different communication situations (option d). An evaluation of semantics would reveal how he applies meaning to words (option c), and an evaluation of syntax would reveal how he uses words in sentences (option e).

9. d. The sounds /tʃ/, /ʃ/, and /dʒ/ are all produced through contact between the tongue and the palate and are therefore lingual-palatal. The sounds /f/ and /v/ (option a) are labiodental sounds. The sounds /b/, /p/, /m/, and /w/ (option b) are bilabial sounds. The sounds /t/, /d/, /s/, /z/, /l/ (option c) are lingual-alveolar sounds. The sound /h/ (option e) is a glottal.

10. a. These errors reveal that Jeffrey exhibits the phonological process of cluster reduction, with /st/ becoming /t/, /gr/ becoming /g/, and /bl/ becoming /b/. Initial consonant deletion (option b) refers to the deletion of the consonant at the beginning of a word (e.g., *ton* becomes "on"). Postvocalic consonant deletion (option c) would be used if Jeffrey had deleted the final consonant sound in the word (e.g., *stop* becomes "ta"). Stopping (option d) would be used if the child substituted a stop-plosive sound for a continuous sound (e.g., *soup* becomes "tupe"). Fronting (option e) would be used if sounds made in the back of the mouth were produced with a substitution of a sound produced further forward in the mouth (e.g., *go* becomes "doe").

11. c. The utterance "Want up" does not contain any inflectional morphemes. "Daddy's cup" (option a) contains a possessive marker. "Mommy coming" (option b) contains a present progressive marker. "I walked" (option d) contains a regular past tense marker. "He jumps" (option e) contains a third-person singular present-tense marker.

12. a. The utterance "doggie eats" includes a third-person singular present tense /s/ marker on the word *eats.* An example of a plural marker (option b) would be an /s/ on the word *dogs.* An example of an auxiliary (option c) would be the word *is* in the utterance "doggie is eating." An example of a present progressive marker (option d) would be the "-ing" in the word *eating.* An example of a possessive (option e) would be the "-s" in the utterance "the dog's bone."

13. d. The utterance contains 12 morphemes. Each morpheme is separated with a slash: Mommy/like/s/the/scarv/es/and/hat/s/I/knitt/ed.

14. c. By 18 months of age, if a child is developing typically, he or she has about 50 words in his or her expressive lexicon.

15. a. A phone (option b) is a speech segment that has specific physical properties regardless of its place in the phonology. A phoneme (option d) is a set of phones that are perceptually equivalent; it includes all the variations of that phoneme that are still perceived to be within that category. An allophone is a variation of a phoneme. For example, the /r/ produced in the word *tray* is produced further forward in the mouth, and the /r/ produced in the word *gray* is produced further back in the mouth; however, these sounds are allophones, fitting into the category of the /r/ phoneme. A pause (option c) is a silent space within an utterance or after an utterance. A fricative (option e) is a category of consonant sounds made by forcing air through a narrow channel.

16. b. This child is using the novel-name-nameless assumption. This occurs when the child assumes that novel symbols are linked to previously unnamed and unknown referents. This child realizes that each referent has a unique symbol (novel); she already knows the names for the cup and bowl (name); and she does not know the name of the other object, a spoon (nameless). Therefore, the new word *spoon* must refer to the new object. The extendability principle (option a) would allow her to recognize this as a spoon even though it differs in some ways from previous spoons with which she is familiar. This spoon has shared perceptual features with other spoons; thus, even though this spoon may be slightly different in size, shape, or color, it is still called a *spoon.* Semantic bootstrapping (option c) involves the use of previously acquired semantic structures to understand the syntax of an utterance; in this example, however the learning that is described is semantic in nature. Syntactic bootstrapping (option d) involves the use of the syntax of the utterance to figure out a word meaning. In this example, it is unlikely that the child is relying on syntax when she is still learning single word meanings. The conventionality assumption (option e) would lead the child to assume that people use the same symbol over and over to refer to the same object; they do not use different symbols for the same object.

17. c. "My truck crashed" is an example of semantic bootstrapping because the child is using his semantic relations knowledge and applying it to understand syntax. In "Look at the treads" (option a), the mother is referring to a part rather than a whole entity, and so she accompanies the utterance with a gesture. This helps the child realize that the word she is using refers to a part. This, however, is not an example of semantic bootstrapping. "The tractor dug a tunnel" (option b) is an example of syntactic bootstrapping, which is using knowledge of syntax to help determine the meaning of a word. In "I'm tunneling through the sand" (option d), the child is using his knowledge of morphology to determine that the word is a verb. This would not be an

example of using semantic knowledge to facilitate syntactic learning. In "your dirt fell off," the child's mother recasts a sentence in a way that provides the correct morphology for the utterance; it is not an example of semantic bootstrapping.

18. a. "That baby" is an example of "demonstrative + entity." "My baby" (option b) is an example of a "possessor + possession" combination. "Little baby" (option c) is an example of an "attributive + entity" combination. "Baby cry" (option d) is an example of an "agent + action" combination. "Baby milk" (option e) is an example of an "agent + object" combination.

19. c. Use of correct regular past-tense verb forms represents a goal that addresses the child's form of language. Form includes phonology, syntax, and morphology. Maintaining a topic (option a) and increasing accuracy of answers to simple questions (option d) are goals that address the child's pragmatic use of language. Increasing the number of different words used (option b) and using word-finding strategies (option e) are goals that address the child's semantic abilities, or the content of language.

20. a. "Daddy going?" (option e) is the simplest involving the use of rising intonation rather than sentence form to indicate a question. In "I do it, okay?" (option b), a simple tag is added to a declarative sentence to turn it into a question. In "Where is Daddy?" (option c), the child must take the sentence "Daddy is _____ [location]" and invert the copula to precede the subject in order to form the question. Similarly, the child must take the sentence "Daddy is eating _____ [object]" and invert the auxiliary verb to precede the subject in order to form the question "What is Daddy eating?" (option d). Both of the latter two examples are acquired during Brown's stage IV (Owens, 2007). In the sentence "Daddy ate _____ [object]," the child must insert the proper form of the verb *do* before the subject because the sentence has no copula or auxiliary. This is learned during Brown's stage V, and it is the most complex interrogative form in the set.

21. b. Ellipsis is the omission of redundant information that was previously stated because the speaker can assume that the listener already knows that information. In this case, child 2 did not respond "*I am building* a tower" because it was contained in child 1's question. Deixis (option a) is the use of words for which the listener relies on the situational context to interpret their referent, such as in the phrase "that pencil right there," accompanied by a point.

Fast-mapping (option c) is a learning strategy used by a child to infer a connection between a word and its referent after only one exposure. Anaphora (option d) is the replacing of a noun, noun phrase, or sentence with a pronoun, as in the example "The castle has three towers on *it*," in which "*it*" refers to "castle." Derivation (option e) is the process of creating new words around a root whose meaning is modified by adding prefixes and suffixes. For example, the word *teacher* is derived from the root "teach" by adding the suffix "-er."

22. c. Anaphora is the replacement of a noun, noun phrase, or sentence with a pronoun. Thus, the use of *they* to refer to the subjects of the sentence, John and Maria, is an example of anaphora. Ellipsis is the omission of redundant information that was previously stated, as in the exchange "Where did you put the money?" "In the drawer." Deixis is the use of words for which the listener relies on the situational context to interpret their referent, as in the phrase "that pencil right there." Conjunction (option d) is the use of conjunctions as a cohesive device, as in the sentence "John went outside *and* Maria stayed in the house." Locative terms (option e) denote location, such as *in, on,* and *under.*

23. d. The utterance "Put that here" contains two deictic terms, *that* and *here;* for both, the listener relies on situational context in order to know their referents. "Once upon a time" (option a) contains a narrative device; "Where is the dog?" (option b) contains the interrogative term *where;* "After we eat" (option c) contains the temporal term *after;* and "It's on the table" (option e) contains the locative term *on.*

24. b. "Did she lose her fur?" is an interrogative sentence, or a question. Declarative sentences (option a) are statements, such as "I have the ball." Imperative sentences (option c) are those that demand or command that the listener perform some act, such as "Give me the ball." Negative sentences (option d) are those that contain a negative form, such as "I don't have the ball." Compound sentences (option e) are those that contain two complete sentences conjoined by a conjunction, such as "I have the ball and he has the bat."

25. c. These two utterances contain mazes, or filler words, pauses, and reformulations of the sentence. Only one of the sentences contains the present progressive ("doing"; option a), and only the other contains the third-person singular ("throws up"; option b). Only one of the sentences contains a contractible form ("she's"; option d). Neither utterance contains a root word error (option e), such as an error on

the root word "come" by using "comed" in place of "came."

26. c. Here are the correct morpheme counts for each sentence:

"My/birthday/was/on/Friday": 5 (compound words are counted as one morpheme)

"We/went/to/Daddy/'s/work/and/pick/ed/him/up": 11

"We/hafta/go/get/him/every/day/because/his/car/is/ broke": 12 ("hafta" is counted as one morpheme.)

"He (he)/came/with/us/to/my/party/at/Chuck E. Cheese": 9 (repetitions of words are counted as only one morpheme; irregular past-tense verbs such as "came" are counted as one morpheme; proper nouns such as "Chuck E. Cheese" are counted as one morpheme.)

To calculate the MLU, divide 37 total morphemes by 4 utterances, which is 9.25.

C: *My birthday was on Friday.*

C: *We went to Daddy's work and picked him up.*

C: *We hafta go get him every day because his car is broke.*

C: *He (he) came with us to my party at Chuck E. Cheese.*

27. d. There is considerable evidence that children with language impairment are at greater risk for difficulties with reading and writing and also that they can benefit from instruction in early literacy skills, including phonological awareness, alphabet knowledge, and concepts about print. A number of assessment measures can be used with preschoolers, and it would be quite appropriate to address early literacy skills in speech-language intervention during preschool (option a). Although it is appropriate for the preschool teacher to address early literacy skills (option b), it would be important for the SLP to also incorporate intervention for these skills into treatment sessions. ASHA's position paper on the roles and responsibilities of the SLP with regard to reading and writing specifically state that SLPs indeed should be knowledgeable in this area (option c) and should address these issues in therapy with children who need it. Children can have excellent articulation skills but nonetheless show difficulties in the area of phonological processing (option e).

28. a. Phonological awareness is a metalinguistic ability, and it includes a range of abilities. The conscious awareness of words as made up of smaller segments of speech (option b) is phonemic awareness, which is included in the category of phonological awareness; however, phonological awareness also includes a number of other skills. The rule system that governs how phonemes are sequenced to make

words (option c) is phonology. Phonological awareness is considered one skill within the domain of phonology; however, phonology includes a much wider array of abilities. The use of letters and letter combinations to represent phonemes (option d) is the alphabetic principle. The prosodic features of speech (option e) constitute the category of suprasegmentals.

29. d. In this sentence, the subject is "the boy," which is a noun phrase (option b); the verb is "threw" (option a); and the direct object is "the red ball." An indirect object is the recipient of the direct object; for example, in the sentence "The boy threw the red ball to his brother," the indirect object is "his brother." In addition, "the" is an article (option c), and "red" is an object modifier (option e).

30. a. The phrase "at a restaurant" is a prepositional phrase containing the preposition "at." "A restaurant" is a noun phrase (option b) containing an article "a" and a noun "restaurant"; however, this noun phrase is part of the prepositional phrase. The verb phrase (option c) is "ate at a restaurant," whereby "ate" is the verb and "at a restaurant" is the prepositional phrase that provides information about place. A predicate (option e) is the same as a verb phrase. The sentence contains no direct object (option d).

31. b. The verb in the sentence is "were," and it is a copula because it is the main verb denoting state of being. An example of a contractible copula (option a) would be "they're," in which "they are" is contracted. An auxiliary verb, sometimes called a *helping verb*, is one that is combined with the main verb; for example, in "they are walking" the verb phrase is "are walking" and the auxiliary verb "are" is contractible (option c), as in "they're walking." An uncontractible auxiliary verb (option d) is one that is unable to be contracted, as in "they were walking." An action verb (option e) is one in a sentence that signals an action such as "running" or "playing."

32. b. The only structure missing from this set of sentences is an adverbial phrase, which is a phrase that describes the verb in the sentence in terms of time, place, or manner. For example, the sentence "I can swim really fast" contains the adverbial phrase "really fast," which describes the verb "can swim." The sentence "My green and blue swimsuit is pretty" contains an adjective phrase (option a) describing the swimsuit ("green and blue"). The sentence "Swimming is my favorite thing to do" contains a gerund ("swimming"; option c). A gerund is the present participle form of a verb that is used in the sentence as a noun. Two sentences contain

subject complements (option d): In "I am the team captain," the complement "team captain" describes the subject "I", and in "My green and blue swimsuit is pretty," the complement "pretty" describes the subject "swimsuit." The sentence "Swimming is my favorite thing to do" contains the infinitive (option e) "to do." An infinitive is a verb form that is the bare stem of a verb preceded by "to."

33. c. Attempts in story grammar are the characters' actions to attain their goals. Characters' success or failure (option a) is the direct consequence of the attempts; responses, thoughts, and actions (option b) are the reactions of characters; strategies (option d) are the internal plans characters' have for achieving their goals; and what causes the characters to act (option e) is the initiating event.

34. e. Although all the options are examples of tasks that would address phonological awareness skills, only "What is 'cup' without /k/?" (option e) is an example of a task to practice phonemic awareness, or awareness of the individual sounds in words. "'Cupcake' without 'cup'" (option a) is an example of syllable deletion; "'cup' and 'pup'" (option b) is an example of rhyming; the number of syllables in the word "alligator" (option c) is an example of syllable segmenting; and the number of words in the sentence "I love pizza" (option d) is an example of word boundary awareness.

35. b. This sentence contains an independent clause "I can't play outside," which is the main clause and it can stand alone. It also contains a dependent clause "because I have too much homework," which must be attached to an independent clause; it cannot stand alone because it begins with a subordinating conjunction. The independent clause in the sentence is followed by the dependent clause. The sentence does not contain two independent clauses (option a). The second clause is not an adjective (or relative) clause (option c), which follows a noun or pronoun to modify it; for example, in the sentence "The girl who took my homework is going to get in trouble," the adjective clause "who took my homework" describes "the girl." An adverb clause (option d) provides information about time, place, manner, or condition; for example, in the sentence "We can't play if it keeps snowing," the adverbial phrase "if it keeps snowing" describes the conditions for playing. The ordering of the clauses is incorrect for option e.

36. c. The field of speech-language pathology took shape between 1900 and 1945, particularly through the 1930s with a major emphasis on speech. The

period between 1975 and 2005 (option a) marked a shift from a focus only on linguistics to inclusion of language use in social life (pragmatics). The period from 1965 to 1975 (option b) marked a focus on differentiating language from speech emphasizing linguistic structure.

37. d. One of the key assumptions of social interactionism is that the primary motivation for learning language is the proclivity of humans to interact socially and to communicate with others. According to behaviorism (option a), language is a behavior (verbal behavior) and, like any other behavior, is learned through modeling, imitating, practicing, and reinforcement. According to the theory of informational processing (option b), language is learned through attention, perception, memory, and motivation, and neural connections are made through language input. Proponents of linguistic theory (option c) assume that language is innate, that there is a universal grammar, and that aspects of a particular language are learned through the language acquisition device. A major assumption in constructivism (option e), proposed by Piaget, is that language emerges from a child's cognitive development; language represents cognitive schemas.

38. a. Brian McWhinney and other proponents of information processing (e.g., Bates et al., 1975) believe that language is learned through attention, perception, memory, and motivation and that neural connections are made through language input. Jean Piaget (option b), the primary proponent of cognitive constructivism, believed that language is composed of symbols for representing concepts. B. F. Skinner (option c), the primary proponent of behaviorism, believed that language is a behavior and, like other behaviors, is learned through modeling, imitating, practicing, and reinforcement. Lev Vygotsky (option d), a supporter of social interactionism, held the assumption that the primary motivation for learning language is the inclination of humans to interact socially and to communicate with others. Noam Chomsky (option e), the primary advocate of linguistic theory, believes that humans are particularly "wired" to acquire language and that language is innate.

39. b. The idea that children are born with cognitive abilities to understand intentions and find patterns is a major tenet of Tomasello's (2003) usage-based theory of language development. The idea of being innately equipped to understand language (option a) represents major assumptions of Chomsky's theory of universal grammar. The idea of language as a network of connections (option c) is an example of

informational processing (Bates et al., 1975; McWhinney in Owens, 2007). The idea that cognitive development occurs before language development (option d) is a major tenet of Piaget's cognitive theory. The idea that language is a learned behavior is a tenet of Skinner's theory of behaviorism.

40. c. Bloom and Tinker (2001) expanded the original Bloom and Lahey (1978) theory to include two superordinate domains: engagement and effort. *Engagement* is the child's ability to "determine what is relevant for learning" on the basis of the intersubjective relationship (social and emotional) that develops between the child and his or her caretaker. *Effort* is to the level of cognitive work it takes to learn a language.

41. c. Vygotsky believed that language and thought influenced each other, not that they were unrelated (option e). Linguistic determinism (option a) was proposed by Benjamin Whorf (1956). Cognitive determinism (option b) was put forward by Piaget. Chomsky views language and thought as being independent but related skills (option d).

42. b. Intentional communication emerges around 8 to 9 months of age and is demonstrated by interacting with others. Intersubjective awareness is the ability to recognize that one person focuses on the same thing as another person, which results in intentional communication.

43. c. Referential gestures develop during the transition from prelinguistic to linguistic stages of development. Gestures that identify or point to a referent are called *deictic gestures.* These gestures emerge before a child begins to talk and are a way of getting attention, requesting objects, or making a "comment" about an object or event. Gestures that consistently convey a specific meaning across contexts (option a) are called *referential gestures;* examples are holding your hand to the ear to indicate a telephone and holding up two fingers to represent a bunny. Gestures that follow the rhythm of speech (option b), called *beats,* do not convey meaningful information necessarily but are used frequently to emphasize ideas. Gestures that convey particular meaning (option d) usually agreed upon by the interlocutors are called *emblems;* examples are "thumbs-up" or "high-five" to represent a good job. Understanding of emblems is based on social-cultural context; for example, the "thumbs-up" gesture in one social-cultural context may not translate or may be offensive in another social cultural context. Gestures that mark the beginning of a story (option e) are called *metaphoric gestures.* According to McNeill (1996),

metaphoric gestures are those that encapsulate abstract ideas; they are used to mark that the content of what is being said by the speaker belongs together in a unit (e.g., narrative).

44. a. Important cognitive skills include the (1) symbolic ability to decontextualize some idea, thought, or event represented in one's mind; (2) ability to attend to the context; (3) the ability to recall past events, and (4) the ability to regulate one's behavior. Both gestures and language access the same memories (mental representations), and they share a symbolic ability to decontextualize those representations. Self-regulation of behavior may be a use of gesture (option d). Gestures do not involve attention to the context (option b), memory of past events (option c), or perception of reality (option e). Gestures, however, can be used as a memory aid.

45. b. Play is not a prerequisite skill for language development (option a), and language is not a prerequisite for play (option d). Similaiarly, language is not less abstract than symbolic play (option c), and both are cognitive-based behaviors that are used by children (option e). Moreover, cognitive prerequisites for symbolic play are not usually found in typical development. Instead, language and symbolic play tend to have similar developmental patterns, which occur at different points over the course of a child's development. For example, when a child is using single-word utterances, he or she is typically able to illustrate the use of objects for functional purposes (e.g., pushing a car). When a child is in the two-word stage of development, he or she is typically able to produce two themes with the same toy (e.g., hold the telephone, hand it to someone else to talk, and so forth).

46. b. Play is a nonlinguistic representation ability. Story retelling skills (option a), closure skills (option c), inflectional morphology (option d), and phonological skills (option e) are all linguistic abilities with which children with specific language impairment may have difficulty.

47. c. Unfortunately, because of the limited understanding of the relationship between play and literacy, some school systems have reduced or eliminated recess time, in accordance with the argument that play is a "waste of time" and prevents children from reaching literacy goals. Some schools also have increased a focus on memorization of facts.

48. d. Marcia's play skills exemplify those of a 24-month old, who is able to engage in multiple play episodes—pretend activities that represent her daily experiences—and to extend the actions from focus

on herself (e.g., pretending to eat from a spoon rather than feeding a doll) to a focus on others. Anthony (option a) is a good example of a child aged 3 to 4 years who is able to make hypotheses about future events and therefore plan out his play. James (option b) is an example of a 12-month-old who uses objects functionally (appropriately). Alicia (option c) is in the exploratory play stage and illustrates the typical manner used by 9- to 10-month-old children in the earliest stages of play. Roberto (option e) is involved in fantasy play and is playing from the perspectives of each character. This level of play is exhibited typically by children who are 5 years of age or older.

49. a. Self-regulation results from sensory integration and the child's ability to control sensory responses (homeostasis), which help regulate emotional state and ability to attend to the environment. The achievement of homeostasis is facilitated by the stable and organized relationship that infants develop with their caretakers. Self-regulation is an important function in learning and is related to adaptation (according to Piaget), the process of incorporating new information into what is already known (assimilation), and the development of new cognitive schemes when new information does not fit into what is already known (accommodation).

50. c. The TOLD-P:4 does not assess pragmatic language or language use, which involves the rules that govern what people say and how they say it. Syntax (language form that includes sentence structure; option a) is assessed with subtests about syntactic understanding and sentence imitation. Morphology, also language form, which encompasses speech (option d), is assessed on a subtest called morphological completion. Semantics (word meanings and relationships; option b) is assessed with subtests of picture vocabulary, relational vocabulary, and oral vocabulary. The TOLD-P:4 also assesses auditory discrimination and phonology (option e).

51. d. Recurrence is defined as a comment about or request for an "additional instance or amount, the resumption of an event, or the reappearance of a person or object" (Retherford, 2000, p. 52). Action (e.g., "eat") is an activity carried out by an agent (an animate that initiates an action, such as "Mom" or "Dad"; option b), and an object is a person or thing that is the recipient of an action (option a). Quantifiers (option c) are amounts or numbers of objects or people (e.g., one cookie, many cookies). Demonstrative pronouns (option e) are those that point to specific things. The demonstrative pronouns in English are *this, that, these,* and *those.*

52. c. Turn taking emerges quite early in life. Verbal turn taking emerges around the ages of 14 to 16 months. Gestures and word combinations (option b) emerge around 18 to 24 months of age; utterance repair (option d) emerges around 3 years of age; and understanding jokes (option e) emerges in later childhood and during early adolescence. The use of sarcasm (option a) occurs in later adolescence (ages 16 to 18 years).

53. c. Mirror neurons are specialized brain cells that activate when actions are observed, actions are performed, and actions are heard through linguistic descriptions. These mirror neurons play a critical role in language development, intersubjectivity, and empathy. With intact mirror neuron systems, children are able to mentally re-create actions that they see others performing and when they hear a description of those actions.

54. c. The novel name-nameless principle of language learning is the ability of children to select an object for which they have no name as the object that goes along with a new (unfamiliar) label. Calling a cat a "dog" (option a) is an example of an overextension, in which a child learned the word *dog* and then labeled all four-legged furry animals "dogs." Assuming that only a pet poodle is a dog (option b) is an example of underextension, in which a child learns a new word but uses that word only in reference to the objects with which she has personal experience. Assuming that "car" refers to the entire vehicle (option d) is an example of mapping words onto a whole object; this is the object scope principle, as described by Golinkoff and colleagues (1994). Kathy, who labels any cat a "cat" (option e), is an example of a child who has gone through the process of fast and slow mapping and has integrated the concept of "cat" into her cognitive schema.

55. a. Understanding jokes emerges during early adolescence. Making requests by using pointing (option b) is a relatively early development, when children become intentional (ages 9 to 10 months), and clarifying requests (option c) develops around the age of 3 years. Comprehending indirect requests (option d) emerges in later childhood (at approximately 7 to 8 years of age). Initiating conversations (option e) emerges relatively early in child development (at approximately 2½ years of age).

56. b. Assumptions and world view are the primary components of culture. "African American" (option a) identifies a person's ethnic or racial heritage. Religious practices (option c) and family structure

(option d) are practices and ways of organizing a person's life that are guided by the person's cultural underlying assumptions, world view, and values. Socioeconomic status (e) is a family's economic and social position in relation to other families, whereby comparison is based on income level, education, and occupation.

57. b. Cultural reciprocity is a person's ability to understand his or her own cultural self-awareness so that he or she can understand the cultural assumptions of the profession. This understanding about oneself and one's profession supports interactions with family members; helps the service providers identify the underlying assumptions, values, and priorities of the families they serve; and results in stronger collaborative relationships between clients, families, and the professional.

58. c. Asking for a clarification of behavior elicits more specific information about what Mrs. James means by "spastic" and may be helpful in identifying solutions for Michael's difficulties. In a response such as "What do you mean by 'spastic'?" (option a), the interviewer asks for meaning of a word, which may not provide sufficient information to understand the problem. Another ethnographic interviewing principle is to ask open-ended questions; a close-ended question (option b) elicits minimal information about the problem. Asking multiple questions at once (option d) overwhelms the interviewee. Changing the subject (option e) does not follow up on the term that Mrs. James used to describe Michaels behavior; as a result, important information may be missed.

59. d. The best option is the utilization of dynamic assessment processes, which entails the assessment of the child's ability to learn after experience or exposure with certain concepts. This type of assessment can provide significant information about a potential disorder, which can aid in intervention planning. It is well documented in the literature that standardized norm-referenced assessment carries inherent biases (e.g., linguistic bias or cultural bias), and therefore the SLP would need to modify those measures to engage in effective assessments of children learning English as a second language or speakers of a social dialect.

60. a. Interpreters need to be literate in both languages, not just one.

61. c. Second-language learners may code switch within the same communicative interaction. Code switching is a rule-governed communicative skill in which the speaker alternates between two languages during the same communicative interaction. The current literature has shown that young children learning a second language typically acquire more proficient oral and syntactic language skills than do adults who learn a second language (option a). Language loss (option b) can be experienced whenever the frequency of exposure to or relevance of a particular language has changed. All languages have dialectical variations (option d); for example, Spanish speakers from Mexico do not use the same dialectical variants as Spanish speakers from Puerto Rico. Dialectical variation can occur as a result of geographical location or social contexts such as education and income. Research shows that metalinguistic knowledge (option e) is facilitated by bilingualism.

62. a. Emergent literacy significantly depends on the child's oral language skills, which provide a foundation for the development of literacy. For example, a strong lexicon helps the child understand the meaning of written words. Emergent literacy also highly depends on the child's metalinguistic skills, which allows the child to think about language and make comments about it rather than just use it. Alphabet knowledge (children's understanding of the letters of the alphabet; options b and d), print awareness (an understanding of the forms and uses of written language, including environmental print; options c and d), and book awareness (option e) are important outcomes of emergent literacy abilities.

63. b. Angelique's language sample exhibits some features of African American English, including no copula, no auxiliary verb, and habitual use of be. Features of Spanish-influenced English are not prevalent in this sample (option a). In addition, speakers of African American English would also exhibit features of standard American English (option c). Finally, the information is insufficient to determine whether Angelique's language would be disordered (option d) or whether her hearing is impaired (option e).

64. a. Angelique's utterance contains no auxiliary verb (which would be am) and habitual use of be ("you be eating"). A copula (a verb, such as "to be," that serves as a main verb; options b and e), past tense (option c), and modal perfect verbs (option d) are not present in the targeted utterances.

65. c. Stockman (1996), who developed the MCC, stated that the MCC represents the "least amount of knowledge needed to be judged as normal in a given age range" (p. 358).

66. b. Narrative skills are acquired on a developmental basis. The earliest narrative stage occurs at the ages of 2 to 3 years, when children provide primarily descriptions and labels of objects, events, and actions. Children in the 4- to 5-year range produce narratives characterized by central characters (or object or event), an initiating event, an attempt, and a consequence. Children 5 years of age and older include all of the aspects included by children aged 4 to 5 years but also include character motivations and resolutions to the problems faced by the protagonist.

67. c. The landscape of action represents the subjective thoughts or consciousness of the characters and is frequently represented by concepts that convey the mental, emotional, or perceptual state of a character. In this narrative, mental states are conveyed in the following utterances, "The boy was worried," "he would have been lonely," and "his parents didn't know." The statement about the "fancy restaurant" is an evaluative comment from the perspective of the narrator.

68. d. Pragmatics, semantics, and structure are the interdependent components of language. Meanings and relationships of words and the structure of sentences or discourse are based on the social context. Nevertheless, pragmatic language skills generally are conceptualized to include communicative intentions (option a) or functions; discourse skills, such as conversations, narratives (option b), and expository text; and contextual variations of communicative style, such as communicative register (option c) and presupposition skills (option e). The lexicon is a concept typically associated with semantics, which pertains to word meanings and relationships.

69. c. A t-unit is one main clause with all the subordinate clauses attached to it or embedded in it. Coordinated clauses are segmented into two different t-units unless the coordinated clauses share a subject (e.g., "He runs and drops it"). Furthermore, clauses that begin with coordinating conjunctions (*and, but,* and *so*) are considered to start a new t-unit. The utterances are segmented into t-units as follows:
t-unit 1: "There was this boy who had a frog"
t-unit 2: "He kept this frog in a jar in his bedroom"
t-unit 3: "The boy and his family were going to a fancy restaurant"
t-unit 4: "(but) the boy was worried about leaving the frog alone because he would have been lonely"
t-unit 5: "(so) the boy put the frog in his coat pocket"
t-unit 6: "(but) his parents didn't know he had the frog with him"
t-unit 7: "When they got to the restaurant and sat down, the frog caused all kinds of chaos"

Bibliography

Anderson, R. T. (2002). Practical assessment strategies with Hispanic students. In A. Brice (Ed.), *The Hispanic child* (pp. 143–184). Boston, MA: Allyn & Bacon.

Applebee, A. (1978). *The child's concept of story: Ages 2–17*. Chicago, IL: Chicago University Press.

Bates, E., Camaioni, L., & Volterra, V. (1975). The acquisition of performatives prior to speech. *Merrill-Palmer Quarterly, 21,* 205–226.

Bloom, L., & Lahey, M. (1978). *Language development and language disorders*. New York: Wiley.

Bloom, L., & Tinker, E. (2001). The intentionality model and language acquisition. *Monographs of the Society for Research in Child Development, 66*(4), 267.

Brown, R. (1973). *A first language: the early stages*. Cambridge, MA: Harvard Univeristy Press.

Capone, N. C. (2010). Gesture development. In B. B. Shulman & N. C. Capone (Eds.), *Language development: Foundations, processes, and clinical applications* (pp. 177–196). Sudbury, MA: Jones & Bartlett.

Casby, M. (1997). Symbolic play of children with language impairment: A critical review. *Journal of Speech-Language-Hearing Research, 40,* 468–479.

Ezell, H., & Justice, L. M. (2005). *Shared storybook reading*. Baltimore, MD: Paul H. Brookes.

Goldin-Meadow, S., & Butcher, C. (2003). Pointing toward two-word speech in young children. In S. Kita (Ed.), *Pointing: Where language, culture, and cognition meet* (pp. 85–107). Mahwah, NJ: Erlbaum.

Goldstein, B. (2004). *Bilingual language development and disorders in Spanish-English speakers*. Baltimore, MD: Paul H. Brookes.

Golinkoff, R. M., Hirsh-Pasek, K. A., & Singer, D. G. (2007). Why play = learning: A challenge for parents and educators. In D. G. Singer, R. M. Golinkoff & K. Hirsh-Pasek (Eds.), *Play = learning: How play motivates and enhances children's cognitive and social-emotional growth* (pp. 3–14). New York: Oxford.

Golinkoff, R. M., Mervis, C. V., & Hirsh-Pasek, K. (1994). Early object labels: The case for a developmental lexical principles framework. *Journal of Child Language, 21,* 125–155.

Green, L. J. (2002). *African American English: A linguistic introduction*. New York: Cambridge University Press.

Hyter, Y. D., & Westby, C. E. (1996). Using oral narratives to assess communicative competence. In A. Kamhi, K. Pollock & J. Harris (Eds.), *Communication development and disorders in African American children* (pp. 247–284). Baltimore, MD: Paul H. Brookes.

Langdon, H. W., & Cheng, L. R. L. (2002). *Collaborating with interpreters and translators: A guide for communication disorders professionals*. Eau Claire, WI: Thinking Publications.

McNeill, D. (1996). *Hand and mind: What gestures reveal about thought*. Chicago, IL: University of Chicago Press.

Nelson, N. W., Bahr, C. M., & Van Meter, A. M. (2004). *The writing lab approach to language instruction and intervention*. Baltimore, MD: Paul H. Brookes Publishing.

Nelson, N. W., & Van Meter, A. M. (2002). Assessing curriculum-based reading and writing samples. *Topics in Language Disorders, 22*(2), 35–59.

Nippold, M. A., Hesketh, L. J., Duthie, J. K., et al. (2005). Conversational versus expository discourse. A study of syntactic development in children, adolescents, and adults. *Journal of Speech, Language, and Hearing Research, 48,* 1048–1064.

Owens, R. E. (2007). *Language development: an introduction*. Boston, MA: Allyn and Bacon.

Paul, R. (2001). *Language disorders from infancy through adolescence: Assessment and intervention* (2nd ed.). St. Louis, MO: Mosby.

Peña, E., Quinn, R., & Iglesias, A. (1992). The application of dynamic methods to language assessment: A non-biased procedure. *Journal of Special Education, 26,* 269–280.

Pence, K. L., & Justice, L. M. (2008). *Language development from theory to practice*. Upper Saddle River, NJ: Pearson.

Pence, K. L., & Justice, L. M. (2008). *Language development from theory to practice*. Columbus, OH: Pearson.

Piaget, J. (1983). *The child's conception of the world*. Totowa, NJ: Rowman and Allenheld.

Retherford, K. S. (2000). *Guide to the analysis of language transcripts* (3rd ed.). Eau Claire, WI: Thinking Publications.

Rizzolatti, G., & Craighero, L. (2004). The mirror-neuron system. *Annual Review of Neuroscience, 27*, 169–192.

Stockman, I. (1996). The promises and pitfalls of language sample analysis as an assessment tool for linguistic minority children. *Language, Speech, and Hearing Services in Schools, 27*, 355–366.

Ting-Toomey, S. (1999). *Communicating across cultures*. New York: Guilford.

Tomasello, M. (2003). *Constructing a language: A usage based theory of language acquisition*. Cambridge, MA: Harvard University Press.

Westby, C. E. (1980). Assessment of cognitive language abilities through play. *Language, Speech, and Hearing Services in Schools, 11*(3), 154–168.

Westby, C. E. (2007). Play: The roots of language and literacy development. Paper presented at the 27th Congress of the International Association of Logopedics and Phoniatrics, Copenhagen. Accessed July 9, 2009, at http://proceedings.ialp.info/FC23/FC23.1/%20Final%20Paper.pdf

Westby, C. E., Burda, A. N., & Mehta, Z. (2003). Asking the right questions in the right ways: Strategies for ethnographic interviewing. *The ASHA Leader Online*, Accessed July 9, 2009, at http://www.asha.org/publications/leader/archives/2003/q2/f030429b.htm.

Whorf, B. (1956). *Language, thoughts, and reality: selected writings*. Cambridge, MA: MIT Press.

CHAPTER 3

Learning Theory

Steven L. Skelton

1. The behavioral process of positive reinforcement is:
   a. The contingent presentation of a consequence that decreases the future occurrence of a behavior
   b. The contingent presentation of a consequence that increases the future occurrence of a behavior
   c. The contingent withdrawal of a consequence that decreases the future occurrence of a behavior
   d. The contingent withdrawal of a consequence that increases the future occurrence of a behavior
   e. The contingent removal of a reinforcer to decrease the future occurrence of a behavior

2. The behavioral process of negative reinforcement refers to:
   a. The application of a penalty to a person as a consequence of an undesirable behavior
   b. The removal of a reinforcer from a person as a consequence of an undesirable behavior
   c. The contingent presentation of a consequence, which increases the future occurrence of a behavior
   d. The contingent withdrawal of an aversive stimulus, which decreases the future occurrence of a behavior
   e. The contingent withdrawal of an aversive stimulus, which increases the future occurrence of a behavior

3. Extinction is a process in which:
   a. Continuous access to a reinforcer is no longer provided after a previously reinforced behavior, which results in the decrease of that behavior
   b. A new reinforcer is now provided after a previously reinforced behavior
   c. An event or stimulus is removed when a behavior occurs
   d. A punishment is now provided, instead of reinforcement, after a behavior
   e. The current consequences for behavior are not effective in changing that behavior

4. If you apply extinction to an undesirable behavior being produced by a client, you would expect occurrences of the behavior to:
   a. Decrease rapidly after the application of extinction procedures
   b. Decrease rapidly and then increase after the application of extinction procedures
   c. Increase after the application of extinction procedures
   d. Increase and then decrease after the application of the extinction procedures
   e. Start to decrease and then return to baseline levels

5. In behavioral analysis, "punishment" is:
   a. A consequence that, when contingent on performance of a behavior, results in the decrease of the future occurrence of a behavior.
   b. A consequence that, when contingent on performance of a behavior, results in the increase of the future occurrence of a behavior.
   c. The contingent presentation of a consequence known to be undesirable to a person.
   d. The application of timeout procedures.
   e. Any procedure that is an undesirable in routine clinical application.

6. According to social learning theory, the main process that modifies behavior is:
   a. Reinforcement and punishment
   b. Changing attitudes
   c. Observational learning
   d. Active involvement in small group activities
   e. Repeated trials of modeling and imitation

7. An operant behavior is one that:
   a. Is the result of a reflex
   b. Is controlled by environmental consequences
   c. Is controlled by genetic predispositions
   d. Results from the pairing of an unconditioned stimulus with a conditioned stimulus
   e. Results from a belief that a person can perform the behavior successfully

8. When a neutral stimulus is paired with an unconditioned stimulus, which elicits a reflex response, the process is called:
   a. Operant conditioning
   b. Instrumental conditioning
   c. Systematic desensitization
   d. Classical conditioning
   e. Paired stimuli technique

9. You are working with a client to decrease stuttering by having the client briefly stop speaking after each stutter. To encourage the client to do so, you use operant conditioning, applying:
   a. Positive reinforcement
   b. Negative reinforcement
   c. Punishment
   d. Extinction procedures
   e. Counseling

10. According to B. F. Skinner's behavioral analysis of language, when children request something, that requesting behavior is called:
    a. A tact
    b. A textual
    c. A mand
    d. An intraverbal
    e. An echoic

11. It was the view of Noam Chomsky (1986) that humans learn their first language as the result of:
    a. An innate language acquisition device
    b. A biologically developed language instinct
    c. Imitation of their parents' models that are reinforced
    d. Observational learning
    e. General neurological mechanisms

12. You are going to teach /r/ to an adolescent boy. To do so, you are going to start with /i/ and then gradually reinforce speech behaviors that move toward the production of /r/. From a behavioral perspective, this is called:
    a. Extinction
    b. Chaining
    c. Shaping
    d. Generalizing
    e. Self-monitoring

13. If you used a cognitive-behavioral perspective for treatment, then to change behavior, you must:
    a. Treat the client's thoughts, beliefs, and feelings without directly treating the behaviors
    b. Disregard the client's thoughts, beliefs, and feelings and provide direct treatment only for behaviors
    c. Treat the client's behaviors after the client has finished counseling or psychotherapy
    d. Only refer the client for counseling or psychotherapy
    e. Treat the client's thoughts, beliefs, and feelings in addition to behaviors

14. According to Piaget (1983), a normally developing child goes through several stages of cognitive development. Those stages are:
    a. Sensorineural, Preoperant, Abstract, Operational
    b. Sensory, Premotor, Concrete, Formal Operations
    c. Sensorimotor, Preoperational, Concrete, Abstract
    d. Sensorimotor, Preoperational, Concrete, Formal Operations
    e. Sensorimotor, Presystematic, Systematic, Formal Operations

15. According to Piaget's (1983) theory of cognitive development, accommodation occurs when a child:
    a. Integrates new information into an existing cognitive scheme
    b. Establishes an equilibrium between previously contradictory cognitive schemes
    c. Modifies new information to reconcile it with an existing cognitive scheme
    d. Uses new information to transform an existing cognitive scheme
    e. Responds to tasks from a later stage of development in a way that is consistent with an earlier stage of development

16. According to Piaget (1983), children apply new information to an existing cognitive scheme; that process is called:
    a. Accommodation
    b. Assimilation
    c. Transformation
    d. Application
    e. Internalization

17. According to Vygotsky's (1986) theory of cognitive development, the "zone of proximal development" is:
    a. What a child can do with adult assistance
    b. What a child can do without adult assistance
    c. The difference between what a child can do without adult assistance and with adult assistance
    d. The next stage of development after the termination of adult assistance
    e. A cognitive scheme that results from moving into the next stage of cognitive development

18. According to Vygotsky (1986), children learn through interactions with more experienced adults or peers who interpret the environment for them. Through this process, children learn to understand and interpret their environment. This process is called:
    a. An active learning experience
    b. A mediated cognition experience
    c. A mediated learning experience
    d. A generalized conditioning experience
    e. An assimilated learning experience

19. Scaffolding is a procedure in which:
    a. A clinician shapes a behavior to be learned
    b. A clinician models the strategy or task to be learned, then gradually shifts or removes instructional support for the child
    c. A child monitors his or her own performance of a behavior
    d. A child demonstrates the strategy or task to be learned and is then evaluated by the clinician
    e. The clinician uses the teaching process of successive approximations

20. If you teach the fricatives /f/, /z/, and /ʃ/ to a child and the child's pronunciation of other untaught fricatives begins to improve, this process is called:
    a. Maintenance
    b. Stimulus generalization
    c. Response generalization
    d. Discrimination
    e. Stimulus control

21. During a treatment session, a client produces a target behavior only when the speech-language pathologist shows a picture and asks, "What is this?" This response is an example of:
    a. Generalization
    b. Maintenance
    c. Stimulus control
    d. Observational learning
    e. Postreinforcement pause

22. You provide a token to a client after (on average) every five correct productions of the target behavior. This schedule of reinforcement is known as:
    a. Continuous
    b. Fixed interval
    c. Variable interval
    d. Fixed ratio
    e. Variable ratio

23. While two children are being taught during the same session, one child starts practicing the target language behavior. After a few minutes of this, without any direct teaching, the other child begins to respond with the same language behavior. This is an example of:
    a. Stimulus generalization across people
    b. Response generalization
    c. Stimulus discrimination
    d. Stimulus control
    e. Observational learning

24. The difference between a primary and a secondary reinforcer is:
    a. A primary reinforcer does not require learning (conditioning), and a secondary reinforcer is conditioned by prior experience
    b. A primary reinforcer is conditioned by prior experience, and a secondary reinforcer does not require learning (conditioning)
    c. A primary reinforcer is associated with classical conditioning, and a secondary reinforcer is associated with operant conditioning
    d. A primary reinforcer is associated with operant conditioning, and a secondary reinforcer is associated with classical conditioning
    e. A primary reinforcer is used on a continuous reinforcement schedule, and a secondary reinforcer is used on an intermittent reinforcement schedule

25. A client who stutters does not believe that he or she will be successful in using fluency shaping while speaking on the telephone. According to social learning theory, the belief that you can (or cannot) perform a behavior is called:
    a. Self-reinforcement
    b. Self-esteem
    c. Affirmation
    d. Self-efficacy
    e. Self-monitoring

1. b. A reinforcer is anything that, when made contingent on the occurrence of a behavior, increases the future occurrence of that behavior; thus, options a, c, and e are incorrect. In positive reinforcement, the consequence is presented to the person when the person performs the behavior. The removal of something contingent on the performance of a behavior is not positive reinforcement; thus, option d is incorrect. If the removal of a stimulus increases the future occurrence of a behavior, the process is called *negative reinforcement.*

2. e. A stimulus is removed or avoided, and as a result, the subsequent occurrence of the behavior increases. Because this is a reinforcement process, it increases the future occurrence of the behavior; thus, option d is incorrect. Options a (a penalty) and b (removal of a reinforcer as a consequence of an undesirable behavior) refer to the application of procedures without reference to their effect on the future occurrence of the behavior; it is not possible to determine whether something is a reinforcer without reference to the future occurrence of behavior. Option c refers to reinforcement, but the presentation of a consequence is positive reinforcement, not negative reinforcement, in which a stimulus is removed or avoided; as a result, the future occurrence of the behavior increases.

3. a. A reinforcer for an undesirable behavior must be identified and then withdrawn when the behavior occurs; this will eventually decrease the future occurrence of the behavior. Option b is incorrect because it states that a reinforcer is provided. Extinction, although decreasing behavior, must be distinguished from punishment, in which the occurrence or removal of a stimulus results in decreasing a behavior, not by continuously stopping a person's access to a reinforcer; therefore, options c and b are incorrect. Option e describes a condition in which the current procedures are ineffective.

4. d. Extinction typically results in an "extinction burst" in which the occurrence of the behavior being extinguished first increases and then (if not reinforced) begins to decrease gradually. This pattern of responding eliminates options a, b, and e, which refer to a decrease in the behavior after extinction begins. Option c does refer to an increase in the behavior but not an eventual decrease; therefore, option c is also incorrect.

5. a. Punishment, in behavior analysis, is any event that, when made contingent on the performance of a behavior, reduces the future occurrence of that behavior. Thus, option b, which refers to an increase in the behavior, is incorrect. Option c is based on a view that punishment is anything undesirable, which is a common perception of the word; in behavior analysis, however, the undesirability of a consequence (as subjectively perceived by a person) is not relevant to identifying the consequence as a punisher. Option d is incorrect because, although timeout can function as a specific punishment, punishment is broader than just timeout. Option e is incorrect because punishment (such as corrective feedback) can be very desirable in routine clinical applications.

6. c. Observational learning occurs when a person changes behavior by observing that behavior being performed by another person. Often in social learning theory (now called *social cognitive theory*), the observed consequences of the behavior are among the variables that influence whether the observer performs (or ceases to perform) the modeled behavior. Although social learning theory incorporates operant learning principles in its framework, these are viewed as secondary methods of behavior change; therefore, options a and e are eliminated. Social learning theory does address the role of a person's attitudes or beliefs about his or her ability to perform a behavior; however, a more general process of "changing attitudes" is not part of the behavior change process, and so option b is incorrect. Option d is irrelevant to social learning theory's principles of behavior change.

7. b. Operant behavior is behavior that "operates" on the environment, whereby future performance of the behavior is controlled by the resulting environmental consequences. This definition eliminates options a (referring to reflexes elicited by an unconditioned stimulus), c (genetic predisposition is not included in behavior analysis), d (referring to behavior developed through classical conditioning, not operant conditioning), and e (the concept of self-efficacy, which not part of operant conditioning).

8. d. The unconditioned stimulus elicits a reflex. When the unconditioned stimulus is paired with a neutral stimulus (one that elicits no response), the reflexive response begins to be elicited by the previously neutral stimulus. Then, the unconditioned stimulus can be removed and the previously neutral (now conditioned) stimulus will elicit the reflexive

response. The other options are different processes or techniques. Option a refers to a process of behavior change through contingent application of consequences to behavior. Option b is another name for operant conditioning. Option c is a procedure to reduce anxiety reactions to stimuli. Option e is an articulation therapy approach.

9. c. In behavior analysis, punishment is any contingent event that decreases the future occurrence of behavior, which is what is intended in this case to reduce stuttering. Options a and b are reinforcement procedures, which increase the future occurrence of behavior. Negative reinforcement is often confused with punishment, but it increases behavior by the contingent withdrawal or avoidance of an aversive stimulus. Option d is a procedure that identifies a behavior's reinforcer and then eliminates access to it; this does result in the eventual decrease in the behavior, but it is not the technique described in the question. Option e is not part of operant conditioning, which focuses on treating behaviors directly, not indirectly through counseling.

10. c. A "mand" is any verbal behavior that specifies its reinforcer (as is done in requesting). Although the other options are also categories of verbal behaviors from Skinner's (1957) analysis, they do not involve making requests (i.e., specifying verbally the desired reinforcer); therefore, they are incorrect. Tacts are verbal behaviors that comment on the environment. Textuals are verbal behaviors for which written text is the stimulus and speech is the response, or vice versa. Intraverbals are verbal behaviors for which the speaker's previous verbal behaviors are the stimulus. An echoic is the repetition of another person's verbal behavior.

11. a. Central to Chomsky's view of language is the innate language acquisition device, which contains the innate grammar that is the basis of language acquisition. Option b reflects Pinker's (1994) view of a language instinct that is the basis for the development and acquisition of language. Option c is the behaviorist perspective of language, which is the counterpoint to Chomsky's perspective. Option d reflects the social learning theory account of language development. Option e is a theory that was proposed by cognitive psychologists who believed that the human brain has species-specific cognitive or neurological abilities that make language possible, but these abilities are not used for language development alone.

12. c. Shaping is a behavioral process in which a target behavior is gradually formed from an established

behavior through operant conditioning techniques. All of the other options reflect processes that are used in behavior modification but do not reflect this situation. Option a is the process of restricting access to a reinforcer, which results in the eventual reduction of the previously reinforced behavior. Option b is a process of teaching a series of behaviors for which the preceding behavior is the stimulus and the succeeding behavior is the reinforcer, which leads to a final behavior in the chain and the final reinforcer. Option d refers to processes in which behavior is transferred to untaught stimuli or settings or processes in which taught behavior results in the changes in other similar behaviors. Option e is a process in which a person counts his or her own performance of a behavior with the goal of increasing or decreasing it.

13. e. Cognitive behaviorism views behavior as being controlled or influenced by an interaction of environmental variables (e.g., reinforcement) and internal thoughts and beliefs. In this perspective of treatment, both environmental and cognitive variables must be treated for behavior change to occur. Option a lists the cognitive but not the behavioral component of the treatment, and option b reflects the perspective of behaviorism, in which cognitive variables are not considered causes of behavior. Options c and d refer to the use of counseling, either followed by behavior modification or alone; neither of these options describe the full range of the treatment approach within cognitive behaviorism.

14. d. Piaget hypothesized that children's cognitive understanding of their world passes through four major stages: Sensorimotor, Preoperational, Concrete, and Formal Operations. The other options do not include all of these four stages.

15. d. Accommodation occurs when an existing cognitive scheme (a structure of understanding) is transformed by new information resulting from the child's interaction with the environment. Options a and b reflect part of Piaget's theory of how the child learns about the world, but not accommodation. Options c and e do not occur within Piaget's framework of cognitive development.

16. b. *Assimilation* is Piaget's term for the process described. Accommodation (option a) occurs when new information results in the change of the child's cognitive scheme. The other options do not reflect constructs from Piaget's theories.

17. c. The zone of proximal development is the difference in a child's performance between when it is aided

and when it is unaided. For any skill, task, or domain, the zone of proximal development is thought to be the range of a child's readiness to learn. Options a and b reflect the lower and upper limits of the zone of proximal development. Options d and e do not reflect constructs of Vygotsky's theories.

18. c. Feuerstein and colleagues (1991) explained that a "mediated learning experience" is one in which an adult assists in or mediates a child's learning from the environment. The adult intervenes between the stimulus to the child and the response from the child and thus assists the child's learning from the environment. The other options do not reflect learning constructs used to explain processes proposed by Vygotsky.

19. b. In learning theories based on Vygotsky's ideas, the instructional assistance a child receives from an adult or more competent peer is labeled *scaffolding*. The adult provides instruction to the child, and the result is an improvement in the child's performance. Then the adult gradually changes the instructional support so that the child continues to perform without dependence on the adult. Shaping a behavior (option a) is a behavior modification process to develop a new behavior. Option c is self-monitoring. Demonstration of the task, followed by evaluation by the clinician (option d), is the opposite of scaffolding. Scaffolding is not another term for successive approximations (option e), which has some similarity to shaping.

20. c. Response generalization occurs when teaching or modifying a behavior results in changes in other, similar behaviors; in this case, the three fricatives /f/, /z/, and /ʃ/ are taught, and without any treatment, the child's pronunciation of other fricatives begins to improve. Maintenance (option a) is the retention of a behavior after the completion of treatment and is not a generalization process. The other options refer to behavioral processes related to stimuli: Stimulus generalization (option b) is the use of a taught behavior in response to untaught stimuli; discrimination (option d) occurs when a behavior is performed in the presence of one stimulus and not another (and thus is the opposite of stimulus generalization); and stimulus control (option e) occurs when a stimulus sets the occasion for performing a behavior.

21. c. Stimulus control occurs when a stimulus sets the occasion for performing a behavior; therefore, the behavior is produced in the presence of the controlling stimulus. Generalization (option a) is the process in which treatment gains are transferred,

and maintenance (option b) refers to the retention of a behavior after the completion of treatment. Observational learning (option d) is learning from another person who is modeling a behavior. Postreinforcement pause (option e) occurs after reinforcement has been given on a fixed-ratio or interval reinforcement schedule. The postreinforcement pause is the interval that occurs between the delivery of a reinforcement and the resumption of responding.

22. d. There are several types of reinforcement schedules. Ratio schedules furnish reinforcement for a behavior after a certain number have been performed. Interval schedules provide reinforcement for the initial occurrence of a behavior after a period of time. Fixed schedules are those in which the ratio (number of responses) or interval (time period) is set and does not vary. Variable schedules are those in which the ratio or interval varies and is set to an average amount of reinforcement (e.g., on average, after five responses or after 1 minute). Therefore, what is described in the question is not a fixed interval (option b), variable interval (option c), or variable ratio (option e) schedule. A continuous schedule (option a) is one in which every occurrence of the behavior is reinforced.

23. e. Observational learning occurs when a behavior is modified by observing the performance of another person and the consequences that person receives for that behavior. It is a central component of social learning theory (Bandura, 1986). The other options are behavioral processes related to the direct treatment of behavior via operant conditioning techniques. Stimulus generalization and response generalization (options a and b) are generalization effects; the former is the behavior being used in the presence of people not associated with the original teaching, and the latter is the change in the untaught behavior as a result of treatment. Stimulus discrimination and stimulus control (options c and d) are stimulus processes in which a person differentially responds to dissimilar stimuli or a stimulus evokes a response.

24. a. A primary reinforcer does not need to be conditioned to be a reinforcer (e.g., food, sex, touch), whereas a secondary reinforcer arises from prior learning, such as pairing a neutral event (e.g., verbal praise) with a reinforcing event (e.g., food).

25. d. "Perceived self efficacy refers to beliefs in one's capabilities to organize and execute the courses of action required to produce given attainments" (Bandura, 1997, p. 3). It is a central component of the social learning theory of behavior change.

Self-reinforcement (option a) and self-monitoring (option e) are behavioral processes that do not relate to the person's belief about his or her capability to perform. Self-esteem (option b) and affirmation (option c) are vague and popular ideas that are not a part of social learning theory.

Bibliography

Bandura, A. (1986). *Social foundations of thought and action: a social cognitive theory.* Englewood Cliffs, NJ: Prentice-Hall.

Bandura, A. (1997). *Self efficacy: The exercise of control.* New York: Freeman.

Chomsky, N. (1986). *Knowledge of language: its nature, origin, and use.* New York: Praeger.

Feuerstein, R., Klein, P. S., & Tannenbaum, A. J. (1991). *Mediated learning experience: Theoretical, psychosocial and learning implications.* Tel Aviv, Israel: Freund.

Piaget, J. (1983). *The Child's conception of the world.* Totowa, NJ: Rowman and Allanheld.

Pinker, S. (1994). *Language and instinct: How the mind creates language.* New York: William Morrow.

Skinner, B. F. (1957). *Verbal behavior.* New York: Appleton-Century-Crofts.

Vygotsky, L. (1986). *Thought and language.* Translation and editing by Alex Kozulin. Cambridge, MA: MIT Press.

CHAPTER 4

Multicultural Awareness

Kay T. Payne

1. Research indicates that stuttering varies according to the social status of the speaker, the nature of the communication context, the type of language used by the speaker, and the attitude of the listener. A clinician who provides treatment by using a sociocultural approach would focus on which of the following?
   a. Operant conditioning
   b. Preparatory set
   c. Biofeedback
   d. Systematized desensitization
   e. Delayed auditory feedback

2. A test of language ability contains the item "The girl crossed the street" to examine a client's use of the past-tense grammatical morpheme. No alternative responses are permitted. The item is potentially biased against a speaker of African American English because:
   a. The test was not normed on an African American population
   b. The past-tense marker "-ed" is always absent for African American speakers
   c. African American speakers' development of past tense lags behind that of speakers of standard English
   d. African American speakers may pronounce "crossed" as "cross" because of the phonological rule of final consonant cluster reduction
   e. There is no opportunity for code switching

3. It is generally agreed that tests of English language ability should not be translated for speakers of other languages. Of the following statements in support of this position, which is *not* true?
   a. The order in which sounds are acquired and the stages at which they are acquired can vary among languages
   b. The types of interference from one language upon the other cannot be predicted

c. Children may know the labels for items in one language but not the other

d. Children acquiring a second language may experience language loss for the first language

e. All of the above

4. Of the following phonological processes, if present in the early stages of normal language acquisition and persistent in a 10 year-old African American child, which is indicative of a phonological disorder rather than a dialectal difference?
   a. Denasalization: "maybe" → "baby"
   b. Final consonant deletions: "man" → "[mã:]"
   c. Cluster reduction: "desk" → "des"
   d. Weak syllable deletion: "about" → "'bout"
   e. Fronting: "Keep" → "teep"

5. A clinician conducts a nonbiased assessment with a 7-year-old bilingual Latina student. The clinician gathers a language sample of 50 utterances made in different linguistic contexts and physical environments. Of the following utterances, which indicates the presence of a language disorder rather than first-language influence?
   a. "Did he bit somebody?"
   b. "He can no play no more."
   c. "He drop he glasses."
   d. "The boy are reaching."
   e. a and c.

6. An adult patient has recently sustained a cerebrovascular accident. A speech-language pathologist (SLP) conducts an assessment of this patient by using an interpreter who is a member of the hospital staff. The greatest challenge in employing a bilingual interpreter is:
   a. Breach of confidentiality
   b. Obtaining an exact translation of the patient's responses
   c. Scoring the patient's responses according to the test norms
   d. Describing the characteristics of the patient's language
   e. Describing the features of the patient's speech skills

7. An elementary school–aged child of Hmong descent has been evaluated by the local school district for consideration for placement in special education classes. Numerous letters have been sent to the home address in order to schedule the Individualized Education Plan (IEP) meeting, but the parents have never responded. Of the following procedures, which is the most professionally responsible and legally appropriate for securing the necessary educational services for the child?
   a. Place the child in regular education inasmuch as there is no consent for special education services
   b. Suspend the child from school until parents attend the IEP meeting

c. Place the child in special education without the consent of parents

d. Secure the services of a Hmong-speaking social worker to contact the parents

e. Refer the child to an outside agency for assessment/ treatment

8. Cheng is a 9-year-old who has been recommended for special education placement because of his difficulties with reading, writing, and math. Cheng and his family emigrated from Hong Kong when he was 5 years old. His family speaks Cantonese at home. He participates in a bilingual education program in his elementary school and attends a Chinese language school on weekends. For the SLP's evaluation, which of the following will be the strongest indicator of the presence of a language disorder?
   a. Difficulty in reading and writing in both English and Cantonese
   b. Substitutions of Cantonese words for English words
   c. Poor auditory memory skills
   d. Limited vocabulary in both Cantonese and English
   e. All of the above

9. A clinician provides a speech evaluation for a transgender male-to-female client and prepares a treatment plan for speech feminization. Of the following goals, which should receive the *lowest* priority as a treatment goal?
   a. Decreasing vocal intensity
   b. Increasing the vocal fundamental frequency (F_0) to the range of male/female overlap
   c. Increasing F0 to the female range
   d. Habituating voice parameters to public perceptions of passability
   e. None of the above

10. A person is learning English as a second language. This person has limited development of both the first language and English and no communication impairment. On the spectrum of bilingual language proficiency, how would this person be appropriately classified?
    a. Semilingual
    b. Ambilingual
    c. Bilingual
    d. Equilingual
    e. Sequential bilingual

11. Of the following issues, which can be given the *lowest* priority in assessment of infants and toddlers from low-income families who are at risk for the development of communication disabilities?
    a. Family-centered assessment
    b. Culturally oriented assessment
    c. Team assessment
    d. Standardized assessment
    e. Parent/child communicative interactions

12. An itinerant SLP services three separate schools in a suburban school district. In school 2, the demographic makeup is 85% African American, and the socioeconomic status for most families is below the poverty level. After screening first graders in all three schools for speech and language disorders, he notices that significantly more children in school 2 appear to have disorders. In this situation, the most appropriate action for the SLP is to:
    a. Arrange his schedule to accommodate the high caseload within school 2
    b. Service the children in school 2 who have the most severe needs
    c. Ask the classroom teachers in school 2 to confirm the presence of disorders
    d. Rescreen the children in school 2 with a different screening instrument
    e. Provide consultative services to the school

13. A preschool teacher expresses concern that Malik, a 4-year-old African American boy, has trouble articulating the sounds /s/, /tʃ/, /ʃ/, and /z/. Other African American children in the classroom have mastered these sounds. Therefore, the teacher refers Malik to the SLP. The SLP's best initial action should be to:
    a. Delay any intervention for 6 months and wait to see whether the child develops the sounds
    b. Conduct a speech sound and hearing screening
    c. Perform a diagnostic assessment to determine why the sounds are in error
    d. Tell the teacher that /s/, /tʃ/, /ʃ/, and /z/ are features of the child's dialect and no intervention is required
    e. Conduct a speech sound screening

14. An SLP working in an inner city public school system encounters a 10-year-old who is withdrawn and antisocial and refuses to communicate verbally. The child has been absent frequently for extended periods of time. Upon the child's return, the clinician notices bruises and scars on the child. Suspecting physical abuse, the clinician should:
    a. Begin to keep a journal documenting all evidence for reporting to the Child Protective Agency
    b. File a report of suspected child abuse with the principal
    c. Ask the child whether he is being abused and keep this information confidential
    d. Refer the child for psychological and physical examination in order to confirm suspicion
    e. None of the above

15. Of the following scenarios, which reflects interrater reliability for test administration with multicultural populations?
    a. A clinician notes that a child achieves the same results when tested by two different test administrators

b. A clinician administers a test strictly according to the test instructions
    c. A clinician allows more time to administer a test to a child who is bilingual
    d. A clinician finds that children receive the same scores on two different language tests
    e. A clinician administers the same test to a child within a 6-week period and records the same results

16. An SLP is employed in an urban school where the population is mainly Haitian Americans who speak in a dialect influenced by Haitian Creole. For placement in special education, the school system requires evaluation with standardized test results. The SLP knows that the required test instruments unfairly penalize the students because of their dialect and first language. In this situation, it is most appropriate for the SLP to:
    a. Continue to administer the test instruments because it is a school system requirement
    b. Refuse to administer the test instruments because they are not appropriate
    c. Devise self-made instruments that are sensitive to the dialect of the children
    d. Administer the instruments and report the results as tentative, supplementing the results with nonstandardized measurements
    e. Employ nonstandard measures exclusively

17. An 82-year-old bilingual Hispanic woman has presbycusis. Using phonetically balanced words for a speech discrimination task, an audiologist conducts a speech audiometry battery with the client. The client is asked to repeat a list of words presented at a comfortable level at the client's speech reception threshold. Of the following words, which would most probably result in an error of repetition?
    a. Sled
    b. Hive
    c. List
    d. Chip
    e. All of the above

18. Of the following utterances, which would be considered a true error of syntax and not a dialectal feature of African American English?
    a. "The baby shoe"
    b. "He like milk"
    c. "I might could go"
    d. "He wented home"
    e. None of the above

19. An African American child who uses the construction "I [ækst] her yesterday" is displaying which of the following rules?
    a. Omission of the past-tense construction
    b. Cluster simplification

c. Omission

d. Metathesis

e. Final consonant deletion

20. Of the following situations, which is an example of linguistic bias in a test battery administered to an African American child?

   a. The test items are pictures of objects unfamiliar to the child

   b. There were no African American children in the norming population for the test

   c. Mean length of utterance is scored according to Brown's (1973) developmental stages

   d. The test format is unfamiliar to the child

   e. All of the above

21. Of the following actions, which is the *least* appropriate in the attempt to eliminate test bias in English language instruments used with bilingual populations?

   a. Translate existing tests into the language spoken by the client

   b. Modify existing tests for the language spoken by the clients

   c. Restandardize existing tests for the bilingual population

   d. Use alternatives to testing such as naturalistic observations

   e. Include parental input in the assessment process

22. For alternative assessment of multicultural populations in which the focus is on processes of language conception rather than output of linguistic constructions, which of the following is useful?

   a. Inventories

   b. Work sample analysis

   c. Dynamic assessment

   d. Ethnographic interviews

   e. All of the above

23. For the purpose of speech and language assessment, which of the following is considered by law as the native language of a 2½-year-old deaf child whose parents are recent immigrants to the U.S. from Korea?

   a. American Sign Language

   b. Korean Sign Language

   c. Spoken Korean

   d. Spoken English

   e. Signed exact English

24. Chue is a 6-year-old English as a Second Language (ESL) student whose parents are recent arrivals from Cambodia. Hmong is the native language and the language spoken in the home. Chue's kindergarten teacher reports that he appears to be "nonverbal" in the classroom, and he failed a routine pure tone hearing screening. Of the following actions, which is the best initially for the SLP to determine a diagnosis?

   a. Refer Chue to the audiologist for a complete diagnostic battery with directions provided in Hmong

   b. Observe Chue's classroom performance and interaction with his peers

   c. Assess Chue's language performance with standardized tests in English and Hmong to determine language dominance

   d. Administer language tests to assess Chue's comprehension of English

   e. Rescreen hearing acuity

25. Of the following actions, which might be considered a violation of cultural rules by a female clinician providing treatment to a male client from a Middle Eastern Islamic country?

   a. Side-by-side seating close to a male client during the treatment session

   b. Direct eye contact by the clinician during conversation

   c. Addressing a male client by his first name

   d. Handing over materials with the left hand

   e. All of the above

26. Of the following scenarios, which cultural aspects are important enough to be considered by a clinician working on a Native American reservation?

   I. Therapy in small, same-gender groups

   II. Individual rewards for performance

   III. Extended time to answer questions

   IV. Cooperative learning exercises

   V. Individual drill and practice

   a. I, II, and IV

   b. III, IV, and V

   c. I, III, and IV

   d. II, IV, and V

   e. I, II, and III

27. An investigator wishes to construct a culturally fair and unbiased instrument to assess language disorders across a wide population of children that includes the major cultural groups represented in the national population. Of the following actions, which would be the most appropriate sampling mechanism to achieve inclusivity?

   a. Selecting individuals at random within the total population, including representatives of each cultural group

   b. Using a stratified random sample with an equal number of participants from all the cultural groups

   c. Using a stratified random sample that includes each cultural group in accordance with its census proportion within the national population

d. Using a stratified random sample that includes each cultural group in accordance with its proportion among the overall population of people with language disorders
e. None of the above

28. A 14-year-old bilingual Spanish speaker who says, "*I finish to watch television at 10 o'clock yesterday*" is most probably displaying which of the following types of language transference?
a. Interlanguage
b. Interference
c. Fossilization
d. Code switching
e. Positive transfer

29. Of the following statements, which is true with regard to English Language learners (ELL)?
a. In order for such people to learn English, their parents should speak only English at home
b. Reading skills from the first language are the skills most easily transferred to English
c. Learning a second language comes naturally with sufficient exposure and social interaction
d. After adolescence, the ability to learn a second language is severely reduced
e. Avoid language alternation

30. Researchers have formalized the distinction between the cognitively undemanding, automatic, surface aspects of language, known as basic interpersonal communication skills (BICSs), and more complex, higher level, cognitively demanding language necessary for classroom learning, known as cognitive academic language proficiency (CALP). A school-aged English Language learner (ELL) is able to function adequately with his English-speaking peers but exhibits difficulty in classroom tasks required for reading and writing. Of the following outcomes, which most probably reflect the child's abilities?
a. Adequate BICSs, adequate CALP
b. Marginal BICSs, adequate CALP
c. Inadequate BICSs, inadequate CALP
d. Adequate BICSs, inadequate CALP
e. Marginal BICSs, inadequate CALP

31. Mr. Tomatsu is a 40-year-old Japanese business executive who has engaged the services of an SLP for elective accent modification. The clinician wishes to establish a goal of focusing on initial sounds occurring with high frequency in English that are problematic for speakers of Japanese. Of the following words, which would be most appropriate for presenting the target sound?
a. "Door"
b. "Rice"
c. "Moon"
d. "Win"
e. "Pin"

32. It is recognized that standardized tests are not the most optimal for assessing multicultural populations. However, an advantage of using norm-referenced tests to measure language ability is that:
a. The potential for examiner error is minimized
b. Validity is confirmed
c. An individual's score can be compared with scores of other people of the same age
d. Scores for determining acceptable performance are preset
e. The test is standardized

33. A clinician conducts a treatment session with a 6-year-old Chinese boy with a speech sound disorder. Picture stimuli containing the target phoneme /l/ are presented in training strings wherein the child is required to say a key word and one target word and to repeat the key word. Correct productions are reinforced until a criterion is reached in two consecutive sessions. This approach to articulation training is known as the:
a. Paired stimuli approach
b. Minimal pair contrast approach
c. Phonological knowledge approach
d. Multiple phoneme approach
e. Multiple opposition approach

34. Of the following statements regarding children of multicultural backgrounds who have language disorders, which is *not* true?
a. Children from backgrounds of poverty display deficits in language learning ability
b. The effect of language disorders becomes more severe when carried over from childhood to adolescence
c. Children with language disorders usually have difficulties in phonology, morphology, syntax, semantics, and pragmatics
d. Children with language disorders have concomitant disorders of reading and writing
e. All of the above

35. A kindergarten teacher consults an SLP because he suspects that an African American boy in his classroom displays behaviors associated with attention deficit disorder (ADD). The teacher describes the characteristics displayed by the child, including difficulty remaining seated, lack of focus, and high distractibility. Of the following characteristics, which is *not* associated with ADD and therefore not essential for an appropriate differential diagnosis?
a. Difficulty following sequential instructions
b. Poor pragmatic skills
c. Poor listening skills
d. Lack of interest in interacting with others
e. Impulsivity

36. Of the following statements about the linguistic standard of a language community, which are true?
    I. *No one speaks the linguistic standard*
    II. *It is the written version of the language*
    III. *It is the only correct way to speak*
    IV. *It is the socially preferred dialect*
    a. I and II
    b. II and IV
    c. I, II, and IV
    d. II, III, and IV
    e. I, II, and IV

37. An SLP conducted a full diagnostic battery with a 6-year-old Native American boy for speech and language performance. A complete case history interview was conducted with the boy's mother; from this interview, the SLP determined that further testing and observation were required. Of the following characteristics, which might be a diagnostic "red flag" from the case history?
    a. History of sore throat
    b. Reluctance to speak in the classroom
    c. Frequent ear infections
    d. First word spoken at age 14 months
    e. Began to walk at 10 months

38. On the basis of predicted linguistic characteristics for speakers of African American English, there is a higher probability that a speaker will *not* delete /s/ for which of the following sentences?
    a. "He has two pencil*s*."
    b. "I have John's book."
    c. "The bu*s* is yellow."
    d. "The boy walk*s* to school."
    e. None of the above

39. A clinician is most likely to obtain naturalistic communication patterns of an African American school-aged child in which of the following communicative settings?
    a. Observation in the classroom
    b. Observation during play with peers
    c. Observation of responses to standardized language tests
    d. Observation of parent-child dyadic speech situations
    e. All of the above

40. An SLP is determining the primary language for intervention for a bilingual student who has a language disorder. Of the following possibilities, which is *least* important?
    a. Dominant language used by the student
    b. Availability of a bilingual clinician to provide the services
    c. The student's chronological age
    d. Amount of academic learning in the dominant language
    e. Language used in the home

41. Of the following audiological tests, which would *not* be affected by the clinician's and the client's accent or dialectal differences?
    I. *Temporal patterning tests*
    II. *Dichotic speech tests*
    III. *Speech recognition threshold*
    IV. *Uncomfortable loudness level*
    a. I and II
    b. II and III
    c. I and III
    d. II and IV
    e. I and IV

42. Cultural differences are most prominent in which of the following linguistic elements?
    a. Phonology
    b. Morphology
    c. Pragmatics
    d. Syntax
    e. Referential meaning

43. A bilingual SLP evaluates a 4-year-old child in both English and Tagalog. He notes that the child has been in the United States for 18 months and that Tagalog is the language spoken in the home. The child displays difficulties in both languages. Of the following scenarios, which are major indicators that the child's problems indicate a language learning disability?
    I. *The child fails to follow instructions*
    II. *The child uses Tagalog words in English sentences*
    III. *The child's errors are inconsistent*
    IV. *The child's performance in English is better than Tagalog*
    V. *The child has difficulty paying attention*
    a. I and IV
    b. III and V
    c. I and V
    d. III and IV
    e. II and IV

44. Of the following intervention objectives, which is *not* appropriate for helping a bilingual student develop expressive vocabulary in the silent period of second language acquisition?
    a. By January, Tito will identify objects in pictures in both English and Spanish with 80% accuracy
    b. By February, Tito will select the correct words from a list for sentence completion items with 90% accuracy
    c. By May, Tito will use the picture dictionary in completing his spelling assignments with 90% accuracy
    d. By December, Tito will use sound blending skills to identify words in English with 80% accuracy
    e. By April, Tito will use sound segmenting skills to identify words in English with 80% accuracy

45. A clinician consults with a fourth-grade teacher regarding a Native American student for possible special education placement. While observing in the classroom, the SLP notes that the student does not volunteer to speak and appears hesitant when called upon to answer questions. The student readily interacts with other children, especially when independent seatwork is required, which the teacher considers cheating. Of the following recommendations from the clinician to the teacher, which would be appropriate?

    I. *Allow additional time for reflection in answering questions*

    II. *Seat the child in the front of the class where the student's talking can be monitored*

    III. *Place the student in group learning situations in which free talk is allowed*

    IV. *Recognize the child's cultural differences that appear to be learning difficulties*

    a. I only
    b. I and II
    c. I, II, and IV
    d. I, III and IV
    e. I, II, and III

46. Juan was referred to the IEP team for evaluation and possible placement in the learning disabilities program. In the classroom, Juan displays grade-level delays in math and reading. A bilingual SLP completed standardized tests in Spanish that revealed the following results:
Overall language skills significantly delayed in comparison with intellectual functioning
Delayed receptive vocabulary skills
Difficulty following oral directions and responding to questions

    Of the following actions, which is the most appropriate next step for Juan?
    a. Placement in the learning disabilities program
    b. Complete further testing in English
    c. Complete classroom observations to verify test results
    d. Compare test results with the findings of other IEP team professionals
    e. All of the above

47. The American Speech-Language-Hearing Assocation's (ASHA's) position on social dialects provides for each of the following *except:*
    a. In order to provide services to individuals who speak social dialects, SLPs must have a thorough knowledge of the dialect
    b. SLPs providing services to individuals who speak a social dialect must preserve the original dialect
    c. SLPs are prohibited from providing clinical services to individuals who speak a social dialect
    d. For individuals who speak a social dialect and exhibit a communication disorder, the SLP must treat only those features that are disorders
    e. None of the above

48. A bilingual SLP works within a school district in which a large number of immigrant children who are English language learners are enrolled. The SLP is called upon to work in a role traditionally assigned to ESL instructors. To operate in accordance with ASHA's regulations, the SLP could appropriately perform all of the following functions *except:*
    a. Provide bilingual assessments of speech and language ability
    b. Provide ESL instruction
    c. Collaborate with the ESL instructor on issues such as language development
    d. Collaborate with the ESL instructor in developing an intervention plan
    e. b and d

49. Of the following statistics, which is an example of a criterion-referenced measurement outcome for a test of language ability administered to a Native American child?
    a. Percentile score
    b. Age level score
    c. Standard score
    d. Standard deviation
    e. Quartile

50. Ms. Martinez is a 58-year-old Hispanic school teacher who suffered a mild stroke. Although she spoke both Spanish and English fluently before the stroke, her Spanish skills are now stronger than her English skills. In determining which language to use for Ms. Martinez's rehabilitation, which of the following situations is *not* a factor?
    a. Ms. Martinez's need to return to her job setting
    b. Ms. Martinez's prognosis for recovery of English
    c. Ms. Martinez's prognosis for recovery of Spanish
    d. Whether Spanish and English were developed simultaneously or sequentially
    e. None of the above

1. d. A sociocultural approach addresses the secondary behaviors, attitudes, and environment of the speaker and listener. Systematized desensitization focuses on these aspects of interaction. Operant conditioning (option a), preparatory set (option b), biofeedback (option c), and delayed auditory feedback (option e) address issues not related to sociocultural contexts.

2. d. The question makes no reference to the norming population (option a). The statements about the past-tense marker "-ed" (option b) and about African American speakers' development of past tense (option c) are clearly false. Code switching (otion e) is the ability of a speaker to transfer between dialects or languages as a function of a listener, content, or topic.

3. b. Through linguistic comparisons, it is possible to predict the interference of one language on another. Research has revealed that patterns of acquisition do vary among languages (option a). Knowledge of labels in only one language (option c) and language loss (option d) are indeed frequently observed among learners of English as a second language.

4. a. Phonological processes are normal in the early stages of language acquisition but disappear as the child's linguistic system matures. African American English is a dialect wherein characteristics of normal development often reflect the rules of early development in standard English. Final consonant deletions (option b), cluster reduction (option c), weak syllable deletion (option d), and fronting (option e) are characteristic of African American English. Denasalization of /m/ is not a rule of African American English.

5. c. Confusion of possessive pronouns is not a feature of linguistic interference. Common forms of grammatical interference of Spanish on spoken English include auxiliary past-tense construction confusion (option a), use of double negatives (option b), and differing subject-verb agreement (option d).

6. b. When use of an interpreter becomes necessary for an aphasic client, the greatest challenge is obtaining an exact translation, because the patient's responses may or may not be impaired. Typically, interpreters attempt to convey the meaning of the communicator and, in doing so, unconsciously edit important information.

7. d. Although parental attendance at the IEP meeting is mandated under Individuals with Disabilities Education Act (IDEA), responsibility for providing notice to parents is the responsibility of the school system. When parents do not respond, it is often assumed that they are noncompliant, but issues of language or literacy may preclude response. Therefore, school systems must secure the services of translators.

8. c. Poor memory skills are suggestive of underlying cognitive dysfunction. Difficulty in reading and writing (option a) and limited vocabulary in both languages (option d) are typical in children learning a second language. Code switching (option b) is also a common behavior in people learning second languages.

9. a. Although it is generally believed that the feminine voice carries less intensity than the male voice, vocal intensity is a weak indicator of gender; therefore, it would receive less priority as a treatment goal.

10. a. An individual who is ambilingual (option b) has full development of both languages. An incipient bilingual person (option c) has full development of the first language and a developing proficiency in the second language. An individual who is equilingual (option d) has balanced proficiency but demonstrates influences of the first language on the second. In the case of sequential bilingualism (option e), the second language was acquired after the first language.

11. d. Few standardized instruments are available for assessment of infants and toddlers, and most commercial instruments are designed for structured observation of specific behaviors. Therefore, a comprehensive assessment of infants and toddlers involves a variety of general procedures underscored by a holistic approach.

12. d. The law stipulates that children must be evaluated with unbiased test instruments. Because the school is overwhelmingly African American, some children may speak a dialect to which the initial screening instrument was not sensitive. The children should be rescreened with another instrument to confirm the reliability of the results. This would need to be done before initiating any type of intervention.

13. b. Although /s/, /tʃ/, /ʃ/, and /z/ are developed later in phonological acquisition, the child is not on par with his peers. Because the sounds belong to the phoneme class of sibilants, misarticulation resulting from hearing loss should be confirmed or ruled out.

14. b. The law requires immediate reporting for suspected child abuse. The most appropriate authority is the school principal.

15. a. *Reliability* refers to the stability of a client's performance on the same test across different observations or observers. Interrater reflects test reliability across different observers.

16. d. The requirements of the school system should not be violated. However, according to law, children must not be placed in special education on the basis of biased instruments. Therefore, the legal and professional option is to supplement testing with the standardized tests by using nonstandardized tests that are sensitive the the students' dialect.

17. d. Because of Spanish influence on English, the client may confuse /tʃ/ and /ʃ/. "Chip" may be pronounced as "ship."

18. d. Syntactic features of African American English include unmarked possessive (option a), unmarked third-person singular verbs (option b), double modals (option c). Double irregular past tense such as "he wented" is not a feature of African American English.

19. d. The past-tense verb "asked," which in standard English is pronounced [æskt], would be pronounced in African American English as [ækst] as a result of metathesis of the /k/ and /s/. The present-tense pronunciation would follow the same metathesis rule and pronounced as [æks].

20. c. Although exclusion from the norming population (option b), unfamiliar test items (option a), and unfamiliar format (option d) might be types of biases, they are not linguistic biases. Shorter mean length of utterance is normal for some speakers of African American English; thus, this measure would represent a linguistic bias.

21. a. Although modifications of tests are considered temporary solutions, the optimal solution is the development of new tests. Parental input can be an important source of diagnostic information. The least desirable solution is to translate tests because these versions have not been validated with the bilingual population.

22. c. Dynamic assessment is a procedure recommended for multicultural populations using a test-teach-test approach, which allows the examiner to observe whether a client can grasp what is required for successful test performance, rather than a single-trial question/answer approach.

23. d. For a 2½-year-old, the native language is the language spoken by the parents, which would be spoken korean.

24. a. Failure of the pure tone hearing screening is a red flag that Chue's problems may arise from hearing difficulties. This is the initial concern and should be investigated before the concerns with Chue's language are addressed. A complete Audiological assessment with support is needed.

25. d. Although many actions of a female clinician do not need to vary from the usual Western practices, use of the left hand is considered rude in Middle Eastern Islamic countries.

26. c. Mainstream schools emphasize individual learning and learning by trial and error, but group and holistic learning is favored in many Native American cultures. Native American tend to groups and display longer wait times between conversation turns.

27. d. A culturally fair and unbiased instrument would include all the relevant cultural groups in proportion among the overall population of people with language disorders.

28. b. Language interference is marked by Spanish syntax superimposed on an English expression. The utterance reflects Spanish syntax interference.

29. b. Research has shown that reading transfers most readily from the first language to the second language and that reading enhances second language development. All the other statements are myths about second language learning.

30. d. Children in the process of second language acquisition may develop adequate BICSs in 2 years, whereas more than 5 years may be required for CALP to develop. A child with adequate BICSs can function well with peers, but classroom difficulty is an indicator of inadequate CALP.

31. b. Japanese speakers may have difficulty with /r/ and /l/.

32. c. Norm-referenced measurements enable comparison of an individual's score with those of a reference group.

33. a. In the paired stimuli approach, the clinician presents pictures of objects in whose names a target sound appears in initial or final position and key words are paired with target words. The others are phoneme-based approaches to speech sound treatment.

34. a. Although extreme poverty is often associated with a higher incidence of language disorders, the trend is not absolute. Therefore, it is not true that children from impoverished backgrounds display such disorders.

35. d. The social and pragmatic interactions of children with ADD are often inappropriate; however, they do interact with other people.

36. b. The linguistic standard (e.g., standard English) is the socially preferred (IV) and written (II) dialect of a language.

37. c. Frequent ear infections could be the result of chronic otitis media, which is common in Native Americans. Without treatment, chronic otitis media can cause delays in language development. Although a history of sore throat (option a) and reluctance to speak in the classroom (option b) are concerns, they have not been related to language development. Reluctance to speak in the classroom and speech beginning at age 14 months (option d) are cultural characteristics of Native Americans. Walking milestone (option e) is within developmental expectations.

38. c. According to the rules of African-American English, /s/ as a morphological marker, such as plural "-s" (option a), possessive "-s" (option b), and the third-person singular /s/ (option d), and the copula "be" are more likely to be deleted than the phoneme /s/ within words.

39. b. The most naturalistic environment for observation of a child's speech is during play with peers. Classroom (option a) and testing (option c) environments are not appropriate for naturalistic observation because the opportunities for language are restricted. Often dyadic speech between African-American parents and their children (option d) is unidirectional from parent to child.

40. b. A monolingual SLP should use a consultative model if a bilingual clinician is not available. The student's dominant language (option a), chronological age (option c), amount of academic learning in the dominant language (option d), and langauage used in the home (option e) are important considerations.

41. e. Objective tests in which pure tones (test I) or physiological responses (test IV) are used would not be affected by accent or dialectal differences. Tests that involve the recognition of speech (tests II and III) are subject to influences of accent or dialect.

42. c. Pragmatics is related to the use of language with regard to meaning and purpose. Therefore, it is most affected by cultural differences.

43. c. Using Tagalog words in English sentences (scenario II), inconsistent errors (scenario III), and better performance in English than in Tagalog (scenario IV) are indicative of normal second language acquisition. However, failure to follow instructions (scenario I) and difficulty paying attention (scenario V) are problems indicative of language learning disability.

44. d. Sound blending and sound segmentation are techniques to improve phonological awareness, not for building expressive vocabulary, exclusively.

45. d. The student's behaviors are typical of Native American culture. Corrective measures such as monitoring the child's talking (recommendation II) are ineffective and may further alienate the student.

46. c. First, test scores in Spanish should be compared with performance in English. Because scores based on standardized tests should be interpreted with caution, classroom observations should then be conducted to verify the test scores.

47. c. ASHA's position on social dialects does not restrict professionals from providing services to individuals who speak social dialects. Professionals may provide services if they have a thorough knowledge of the dialect (option a); they must preserve the dialect (option b); and an SLP may treat only the disorder, not the dialect (option d).

48. b. ASHA stipulates that SLPs can provide ESL instruction only if they have the required knowledge and skills. In the absence of this knowledge and skill, an SLP may instead act as a consultant.

49. b. A criterion-referenced score is a measurement outcome based on a preestablished criterion, such as age level. Percentile scores (option a), standard scores (option c), standard deviations (option d), and quartiles (option e) are based on comparisons of the individual's score with group scores.

50. d. Simultaneous or sequential bilingualism are important factors to be considered for children in the process of acquiring a second language. Because Ms. Martinez's Spanish is stronger than English, each of the other factors—her need to return to work (option a), her prognosis for recovery of English (option b), and her prognosis for recovery of Spanish (option d)—are important factors in the decision of whether to provide treatment in Spanish or English.

CHAPTER 5

Speech Science

Richard D. Andreatta

1. Which subset of the 12 cranial nerves is critically important during speech production?
   a. III, VI, X, and XI
   b. V, VII, X, and XII
   c. IV, V, VII, and XII
   d. I, V, X and XI
   e. IV, V, VI, and XI

2. Nuclei are groups of cell bodies (somas) that reside:
   a. Inside the central nervous system (CNS)
   b. Outside the CNS
   c. Inside the peripheral nervous system (PNS)
   d. Outside the PNS
   e. Within the layers of the cerebral cortex

3. The corticobulbar tract projects to most of the brainstem's motor nuclei in which manner?
   a. Ipsilaterally
   b. Contralaterally
   c. Rostrally
   d. Caudally
   e. Bilaterally

4. The _____ is the basic unit of the nervous system.
   a. Axon
   b. Dendrite
   c. Soma (cell body)
   d. Motor unit
   e. Neuron

5. Executive functions such as reasoning, planning, and problem solving are associated with the operation of the _____ lobe.
   a. Frontal
   b. Parietal
   c. Temporal
   d. Insula
   e. Occipital

6. A lesion to the lower motor neuron will result in which of the following symptoms?
   a. Spasticity
   b. Hyperactive reflexes
   c. Tremor
   d. Observed muscle effects on the contralateral side from the injury
   e. Flaccid paralysis or paresis

7. Ataxic dysarthria is related to a lesion of which of the following?
   a. Basal ganglia
   b. Broca area
   c. Cerebellum
   d. Facial motor nucleus
   e. Brainstem

8. The trigeminal lemniscal system transmits which of the following sensations from the face to the primary sensory cortex in the brain?
   a. Proprioception and touch
   b. Touch and vision
   c. Auditory input
   d. Olfactory sensation and taste
   e. Only painful sensations

9. Motor neurons innervating the muscles of mastication reside within which brainstem nucleus?
   a. The motor nucleus of the trigeminal system
   b. The facial motor nucleus
   c. The nucleus ambiguus
   d. The mandibular nucleus
   e. The nucleus retrotrigeminalis

10. Complete damage to the right and left hypoglossal nerves (cranial nerve XII) would result in:
    a. Inability to voluntarily move the lips
    b. Inability to voluntarily move the tongue
    c. Inability to taste
    d. Inability to trigger a swallowing reflex
    e. Inability to propel a bolus down the esophagus

11. The _____ nerve innervates the muscles of expression and mediates taste in the anterior segment of the tongue.
    a. Facial
    b. Vagus
    c. Glossopharyngeal
    d. Accessory
    e. Oculomotor

12. The Broca area and the Wernicke area are interconnected through the:
    a. Uncinate fasciculus
    b. Cingulum
    c. Arcuate fasciculus

    d. Internal capsule
    e. Internal arcuate fibers

13. Which efferent tract innervates all the motor nuclei of the cranial nerve systems in the brainstem?
    a. Corticobulbar tract
    b. Tectospinal tract
    c. Corticospinal tract
    d. Rubrospinal tract
    e. Vestibulobulbar tract

14. In the absence of the trigeminal nerve, what abnormalities would be observed?
    a. Loss of sensation to the larynx
    b. Loss of taste to the anterior portion of the tongue
    c. Loss of sensation to the skin of the face
    d. Loss of motor control to the muscles of the face
    e. Loss of salivary gland function

15. Which muscle, originating from the lateral and superior cricoid rim, is involved primarily in "medial compression" during vocalization and, when active, rotates the muscular process of the arytenoid laterally?
    a. Lateral cricoarytenoid
    b. Oblique inter arytenoids and lateral cricoarytenoid
    c. Cricothyroid
    d. Transverse interarytenoid and lateral cricoarytenoid
    e. Superior cricoarytenoid

16. Glottal abductors include the:
    a. Cricothyroid muscle with assistance from the thyroarytenoid muscle
    b. Posterior cricoarytenoid muscle
    c. Transverse interarytenoid and lateral cricoarytenoid muscles
    d. Interarytenoid and lateral cricoarytenoid muscles
    e. Hyothyroid and sternothyroid muscles

17. The _____ is the largest of the laryngeal cartilages.
    a. Thyroid
    b. Cricoid
    c. Arytenoid
    d. Hyoid
    e. Corniculates

18. The _____ is a free-floating and U-shaped bone that forms the upper extent of the laryngeal system.
    a. Thyroid
    b. Cricoid
    c. Arytenoid
    d. Hyoid
    e. Tragus

19. The thyrovocalis muscle:
    a. Abducts the vocal folds
    b. Slides the arytenoid cartilages toward the midline
    c. Decreases the distance between the cricoid and the arytenoid cartilages
    d. Contributes minimally to pitch adjustment during speech
    e. Forms the medial segment of the musculature of the vocal folds

20. The mentalis muscle originates from the anterior surface of the mandible and:
    a. Inserts into the upper lip to assist in upper lip elevation
    b. Inserts into the lower lip to assist in lower lip elevation
    c. Inserts into the oral angle to help draw the corners of the mouth posteriorly
    d. Inserts into the deep skin of the nostrils to assist in a flaring action
    e. Can function to depress inferiorly the skin of the chin and bottom lip

21. The buccinator muscle is a deep facial muscle that originates partially from the maxilla and:
    a. Makes its insertion by interdigitating with the nasalis muscle
    b. Makes its insertion by interdigitating with the muscles that constitute the oral angle
    c. Makes its insertion by interdigitating with the corrugator muscle
    d. Makes its insertion by interdigitating with the palatoglossus muscle
    e. Makes its insertion into the ramus of the mandible

22. The zygomaticus major and minor muscles operate together to:
    a. Retract the oral angle directly posterior
    b. Draw the lower lip directly upward and compress it against the upper teeth during speech
    c. Elevate the upper lip and draw the oral angle superiorly and posteriorly
    d. Compress the cheek tissue against the teeth
    e. Draw the oral angles downward, as in a frown

23. Originating from the temporal fossa, the temporalis muscle is capable of:
    a. Rapidly depressing the mandible
    b. Shearing and tearing actions
    c. Preventing lateral motion of the jaw to one side if contracted unilaterally
    d. Acting as an antagonist to the masseter muscle
    e. Opening the oral cavity by lowering the mandible

24. The medial pterygoid muscle plays an active role in closing the jaws during speech. Which muscle is

considered the direct antagonist of the medial pterygoid muscle during speech?
    a. Lateral pterygoid muscle
    b. Anterior belly of digastricus muscle
    c. Masseter muscle
    d. Mylohyoid muscle
    e. Stylohyoid muscle

25. The _____ muscle is responsible for the opening of the eustachian tube.
    a. Levator veli palatini
    b. Palatopharyngeus
    c. Palatoglossus
    d. Musculus uvulus
    e. Tensor veli palatini

26. High vowels have a higher oral impedance, which is correlated with a:
    a. Smaller velopharyngeal opening
    b. Larger velopharyngeal opening
    c. Velopharyngeal opening size that decreases with production of low vowels
    d. Velopharyngeal opening size that varies between small and large
    e. Larger nostril opening

27. The muscles of the velopharyngeal system include the:
    a. Levator veli palatini, tensor veli palatini, and superior pharyngeal constrictor
    b. Levator veli palatini, tensor veli palatini, and cricopharyngeus
    c. Tensor veli palatini, cricopharyngeus, and lateral cricoarytenoid
    d. Cricopharyngeus, lateral cricoarytenoid, and posterior cricoarytenoid
    e. Tensor veli palatini, cricopharyngeus, and superior pharyngeal constrictor

28. The levator veli palatini muscle is commonly referred to as the *velar sling*. The primary role of this muscle during velopharyngeal port closure is:
    a. To tense and stiffen the anterior velum at the border of the palatine bone
    b. To shorten and thicken the nasal surface of the velum along the midline
    c. To lower the velum
    d. To stiffen the nasal surface of the velar tissue
    e. To elevate and retract the velum posteriorly

29. The primary function of the musculus uvulae during velopharyngeal port closure is:
    a. To tense and stiffen the anterior velum at the border of the palatine bone
    b. To shorten and thicken the nasal surface of the velum along the midline

c. To lower the velum

d. Minimal and redundant with the action of the levator veli palatine

e. To elevate and retract the velum posteriorly

30. The tongue body is able to adjust its shape and perform complex three-dimensional changes because of the lack of an internal bony skeleton. Such a system is referred to as:
    a. An isovolume system
    b. A muscular hydrostat
    c. A hydroelastic system
    d. A hygrometer
    e. A skeletal muscle

31. The cranial plates of the skull are connected with the following type of joint:
    a. Synarthrodial
    b. Diarthrodial
    c. Gliding
    d. Pivot
    e. Saddle

32. Lateral deviation of the tongue body requires fine motor regulation of the:
    a. Transversus and verticalis muscles
    b. Genioglossus and thyrohyoid muscles
    c. Superior and inferior longitudinal muscles
    d. Verticalis and styloglossus muscles
    e. Transversus and styloglossus muscles

33. Changes to the surface shape of the facial skin is a consequence of the following condition:
    a. Elasticity of the basement membrane of the skin
    b. Tendinous attachment of muscle to the facial skin
    c. Direct insertion of muscle fascicles into the facial skin
    d. Compression of static tissues volumes during oral movement
    e. Edema

34. The maxilla and the palatine bone contribute to constitute what structure?
    a. The soft palate
    b. The hard palate
    c. The pre-maxilla
    d. The tertiary palate
    e. The temporomandibular joint

35. What is the fundamental importance of pleural linkage in the respiratory system?
    a. It allows for the translation of rib movement, through activation of the respiratory muscles, into lung volumes changes
    b. It prevents the collapse of the lung

c. It facilitates rib rotation through the bucket-handle and pump-handle maneuvers

d. It prevents the rib cage from expanding to an extremely large volume

e. It reduces heat produced by friction between the pleural membranes

36. Regulation of the respiratory system through rapid and controlled internal intercostal muscle activity allows a person to modulate different parameters of voicing, including:
    a. Phrasing
    b. Formant values
    c. Prosody
    d. Nasality
    e. Fluency

37. The vertebral column has the following number of vertebrae in each of its divisions:
    a. 5 lumbar and 7 sacral
    b. 6 lumbar and 8 cervical
    c. 12 thoracic, 5 lumbar, and 7 cervical
    d. 7 cervical, 1 lumbar, and 4 sacral
    e. 5 lumbar, 12 sacral, and 7 thoracic

38. Lung tissue and the deep surfaces of the rib cage are lined with two pleural membranes known as the:
    a. Vital and partial pleural
    b. Visceral and parietal pleura
    c. Vacuous and particulate pleura
    d. Reticular and mesothelial pleura
    e. Parenchyma and endothelia pleura

39. Lung volumes are affected by a variety of factors, including:
    a. Personality type
    b. Educational level
    c. Age
    d. Height
    e. Chest circumference

40. The volume of air inspired or expired during any given breath cycle is known as:
    a. Expiratory reserve volume
    b. Inspiratory reserve volume
    c. Tidal volume
    d. Residual volume
    e. Dynamic volume

41. Together, which abdominal muscles form the lateral abdominal wall?
    a. Rectus abdominis, transverse abdominal, and subcostal muscles
    b. External abdominal oblique, quadratus lumborum, and scalene muscles

c. Internal abdominal oblique, external abdominal oblique, and transverse abdominal muscles

d. Trapezius, latissimus dorsi, and serratus posterior muscles

e. Deltoid, serratus anterior, and sacrospinal muscles

42. The volume of air remaining in the pulmonary system at the end of maximum expiration is known as:
    a. Expiratory reserve volume
    b. Inspiratory reserve volume
    c. Tidal volume
    d. End-point volume
    e. Residual volume

43. The maximum volume of air that can be forcefully expired after a maximum inspiration is known as the:
    a. Inspiratory capacity
    b. Vital capacity
    c. Functional residual capacity
    d. Total lung capacity
    e. Total residual capacity

44. Which segment of the internal intercostal muscle group operates to lower the ribs?
    a. Interchondral segment
    b. Intrapulmonary branch
    c. Interpleural segment
    d. Bronchiole segment
    e. Interosseous segment

45. A lesion to the recurrent laryngeal nerve would result in what behavioral outcome?
    a. Loss of sensation in the larynx
    b. Loss of motor (muscle) activity to the extrinsic laryngeal muscles
    c. Paralysis of all the intrinsic muscles of the larynx, except the cricothyroid
    d. Paralysis of the cricothyroid
    e. Paralysis of the external laryngeal muscles

46. A spirometer is used to measure _____.
    a. Lung volumes
    b. Airflow
    c. Subglottal pressure
    d. Loudness
    e. Pleural pressures

47. The relaxation pressure curve is a graph that:
    a. Depicts the amount of active pressure generated during inhalation and exhalation
    b. Illustrates the concept that lung pressures can be created with the passive elastic recoil and rebounding forces of the lung-chest wall system

c. Demonstrates that the magnitude of lung pressure generated is not related or influenced by lung volumes

d. Demonstrates that negative lung pressures are generated when lung volumes are greater than volumes at rest

e. Illustrates the concept that all lung pressures necessary to support speech production must be actively generated

48. Bucket-handle rib rotation:
    a. Results in a large change in the mediolateral volume of the thorax
    b. Is generated by dorsoposterior rotation of the rib
    c. Results in a small mediolateral volume change during inhalation
    d. Occurs in the absence of any other form of rib motion
    e. Describes the expansion of the rib cage during quiet breathing

49. The vocal tract is modeled as a pliable tube with:
    a. One end open
    b. Both ends open
    c. Both ends closed
    d. A hard boundary on one end and a soft boundary on the other
    e. One end open and the other end either open or closed

50. A mathematical and structural theory relating the motion of the vocal folds to that of a spring-mass system was developed by:
    a. Bernoulli
    b. Titze
    c. Fant
    d. Fourier
    e. Stemple

51. The spectrographic patterns of nasalized vowels, in comparison with those of nonnasalized vowels, exhibit the following characteristic:
    a. A narrowing of the effective bandwidths around specific formant peaks
    b. An increase in overall sound energy
    c. An increase in specific formant peaks
    d. A perceived decrease in pitch
    e. An absence of sound energy at certain frequencies within the source spectrum

52. Peaks in a vowel output spectrum with maximal energy transfer are called:
    a. Crests
    b. Troughs
    c. Formants
    d. Harmonics
    e. Vowels peaks

53. _____ consonants start out like stop plosives, but the articulatory occlusion is released less abruptly, with a less vigorous burst of airflow.
    a. Nasal
    b. Fricative
    c. Affricate
    d. Glottal
    e. Glide

54. With regard to vowel formants, the vowel quadrilateral demonstrates which generality?
    a. First formant frequency (F_1) is affected mostly by the anterior-posterior position of the tongue
    b. Second formant frequency (F_2) is influenced mostly by the height of the tongue body
    c. Low vowels have higher F_1 values than do high vowels
    d. Third formant frequency (F_3) is influenced by the interaction of tongue position and height
    e. F_1 is affected most by the size of the oral opening

55. A low-pass filter is characterized by what property?
    a. It attenuates low-frequency components in a complex waveform
    b. It boosts the amplitude of low-frequency components in a complex waveform
    c. It boosts the intensity of high-frequency components in a complex waveform
    d. It has a flat frequency response
    e. It attenuates high-frequency components in a complex waveform

56. A fricative consonant's sound source consists of:
    a. Turbulent noise generated by forcing air through a narrow articulator constriction
    b. Vocal fold vibration
    c. The period of the stop-gap
    d. Antiresonance effects
    e. Complex voicing resonances during frication

57. If the difference in amplitude between the frequencies of 100 Hz and 1600 Hz is 100 dB, what is the roll-off rate of a filter?
    a. 25 dB/octave
    b. 0 dB/octave
    c. 20 dB/octave
    d. 10 dB/octave
    e. 15 dB/octave

58. What is the bandwidth of a formant if the upper and lower cutoff frequencies are equal to 1100 Hz and 700 Hz, respectively?
    a. 400 Hz
    b. 1100 Hz
    c. 900 Hz

d. 1800 Hz
e. 770 kHz

59. _____ occurs when the articulatory characteristics of an upcoming sound influence the characteristics of a currently produced sound.
    a. Phonation
    b. Resonance
    c. Coarticulation
    d. Articulation
    e. Unintelligible speech

60. Oscillation of a particle around its rest position as a result of recoil and inertial forces is called _____.
    a. Complex harmonic motion
    b. Simple harmonic motion
    c. Uniform circular motion
    d. Aperiodic motion
    e. None of the above

61. Resonance is the phenomenon in which an object tends to vibrate with _____ energy at _____.
    a. Minimum, a particular frequency
    b. Maximum, a particular frequency
    c. Minimum, minimal amplitude
    d. Maximum, minimal amplitude
    e. Maximum, all frequencies

62. Period and frequency are _____ related to each other.
    a. Directly
    b. Inversely
    c. Not
    d. Sometimes
    e. Nonlinearly

63. Formants are resonances of the vocal tract that:
    a. Change in value according to alterations in the shape of the vocal tract
    b. Remain constant with changes in the shape of the vocal tract
    c. Change in value without alteration in the shape of the vocal tract
    d. Remain constant with different vowels
    e. Characterize voiceless vowel sounds

64. The position of the second formant for a given vowel (relative to the first formant) is most related to changes in the:
    a. Volume of the oral cavity
    b. Volume of the nasopharynx
    c. Volume of nasal cavity
    d. Volume of the pharyngeal cavity
    e. Size of the oral opening

65. The three quantitative measures depicted by a spectro-gram are:
    a. Amplitude, frequency, and pitch
    b. Frequency, amplitude, and time
    c. Time, pitch, and amplitude
    d. Frequency, intensity, and phase
    e. Phase, attenuation rate, and harmonic effects

66. Skeletal muscle fiber is composed primarily of fila-ments known as:
    a. Fascia
    b. Myofibrils
    c. Collagen
    d. Epimysium
    e. Myoactin

67. The sarcomere:
    a. Represents the smallest structural unit of a muscle capable of decreasing its overall length
    b. Is bounded by the A-bands
    c. Represents a theory of muscle contraction and force development
    d. Is another name for a muscle fiber
    e. Is synonymous with the term *motor unit*

68. The smallest functional element controlled by the motor control system is the:
    a. Motor neuron
    b. Motor unit
    c. Motor cortex
    d. Muscle unit
    e. Sarcomere

69. The physiological classification of muscle fibers as "fatigue resistant" suggests that these fibers:
    a. Generate large amounts of force
    b. Operate for short time periods
    c. Are active during strenuous activities
    d. Are well suited to support rapid burst of force production
    e. Generate small levels of force during most routine behaviors

70. The myofibril is composed of two critical proteins whose interaction underlies the process of muscle contraction. These two proteins are:
    a. Myosin and tropomyosin
    b. Actin and cytoskeleton
    c. Myosin and actin
    d. Troponin and actin
    e. Myoactin and tropomyosin

1. b. Cranial nerves V, VII, X, and XII all participate during speech production. Cranial nerve V is sensory to the facial skin, cranial nerve VII provides motor innervation to the muscle of the facial mask, cranial nerve X provides both sensory and motor innervation to the laryngeal area, and cranial nerve XII innervates the intrinsic muscles of the tongue.

2. a. The cell body is the metabolic center of a neuron. Cell bodies cluster in groups within the CNS and are referred to as *nuclei*. Its counterpart in the PNS is called a *ganglion*.

3. e. The corticobulbar tract is a principle descending motor path originating from the primary motor cortex and innervating the majority of cranial motor nuclei within the brainstem in a bilateral manner. In other words, one side of the brain innervates both the left and right brainstem nuclei in parallel.

4. e. The neuron is the basic cell type of the nervous system. All the other structures listed are components of a neuron.

5. a. The frontal lobe regulates cognitive skills and the planning of motor performance. This lobe receives substantial input from other lobes of the brain and is thought to organize these various inputs to accomplish behaviors such as planning future activity and solving complex problems.

6. e. Because the lower motor neuron is the final common pathway to the musculature, an injury to this neuron deprives the ipsilateral muscle of neural input, which results in flaccid paralysis or paresis. Spasticity (option a) and hyperactive reflexes (option b) are caused instead by a lesion to the contralateral upper motor neuron. Tremor is involuntary movement generally due to a lesion of the basal ganglia (option c). Option d is indicative of damage in the CNS.

7. c. The cerebellum serves a comparator function during motor control and helps coordinate all movements underlying an action. Focal lesions to the cerebellar cortex result in articulatory overshoot or undershoot, dyscoordination, and degraded intelligibility of speech. This group of symptoms is referred to as *ataxic dysarthria*.

8. a. The trigeminal lemniscal system mediates somatosensory inputs from the face, including pain, temperature, touch, and proprioception. The trigeminal lemniscal system is considered the rostral extent of the dorsal column–medial lemniscal system. Visual (option b), auditory (option c), and olfactory and taste events (option d) are mediated by other brainstem cranial nerve systems.

9. a. The trigeminal system comprises multiple cranial nerves. The sensory component of this system will transmit pain, temperature, touch, and proprioceptive inputs to the central nervous system. In addition, the trigeminal system possesses a discrete motor nucleus that is involved in the voluntary control of mandibular skeletal muscles.

10. b. The hypoglossal nerve provides the motor innervation to the intrinsic muscles of the tongue body. Injury to these nerves therefore disrupts the integrity of signal transmission to these muscles, resulting in lingual paralysis or paresis.

11. a. The muscles comprising the facial mask (muscles of expression) are innervated by the motor branch of the facial cranial nerve system. The facial nerve system also possesses a sensory component that is responsible for the mediation of gustatory function from the anterior two thirds of the tongue dorsum.

12. c. The association fibers of the arcuate fasciculus are a white matter tract that interconnects the posterior part of the temporoparietal junction of the cerebrum with the frontal cortex of the brain. The arcuate fasciculus is sometimes considered a component of the larger superior longitudinal fasciculus.

13. a. The corticobulbar tract consists of projection fibers originating from pyramidal neurons residing with the primary motor cortex. These fibers have synapses with lower motor neurons within cranial nerve systems of the brainstem. The inputs carried by the corticobulbar tract are responsible for providing the central motor commands for behavior of neuromuscular systems of the head.

14. c. The trigeminal cranial nerve system is sensory to the skin of the face. A disruption of the trigeminal nerve produces facial skin anesthesia.

15. a. Of the intrinsic muscles of the larynx, only the lateral cricoarytenoid muscle originates from the superolateral cricoid rim and inserts into the arytenoid muscular process. The orientation of the lateral

cricoarytenoid muscle generates a lateralization of the arytenoid muscular process, thereby swinging the vocal processes toward midline and assisting to approximate the vocal fold margins.

16. b. The posterior cricoarytenoid muscle is positioned posterior between the cricoid and the arytenoid cartilages. The posterior cricoarytenoid muscle operates to pull the muscular processes of the arytenoid muscles in a medial trajectory, which in turn abducts the vocal folds away from the midline. The thyroarytenoid, interarytenoid, and lateral cricoarytenoid muscles are all adductor in function, whereas the cricothyroid muscle's role during laryngeal behavior is to adjust the tension level of the vocal fold in a more gross manner.

17. a. The thyroid cartilage forms the anterior extent of the laryngeal cartilaginous framework. The thyroid is typically described as looking like a "shield," with the dorsal aspect open-ended.

18. d. The hyoid bone is a U-shaped structure that lacks a ligamentous attachment to other bones of the skull and neck. The hyoid bone forms the uppermost extent of the laryngeal framework and is suspended above the larynx through its attachments with extralaryngeal musculature.

19. e. The thyrovocalis muscle is positioned between the deep surface of the thyroid cartilage at its angle and the vocal process of the arytenoid cartilage. It is the medial segment of the thyroarytenoid muscle and is believed to constitute one of the primary regulators of vocal fold stiffness.

20. b. The mentalis muscle is a powerful muscle situated between the incisor fossa of the mandible and the skin of the chin. Contraction of the mentalis muscle leads to an elevation and eversion of the lower lip.

21. b. The buccinator muscle (often referred to as the "bugler's" muscle) functions to compress the cheeks against the teeth to stabilize the lateral wall of the oral cavity during oral pressure development for tasks such as speech, chewing, and production of wind instrument sound. The buccinator muscle inserts into the muscles that constitute the oral angle. This insertion also enables the buccinator muscle to contribute to the direct lateral retraction of the oral angles.

22. c. Both the zygomaticus major and minor muscles originate from the zygomatic arch and follow a downward oblique path toward their insertion points into the muscle and skin of the upper lip. Synergistic activity of these muscle leads to smiling.

23. b. The temporalis muscle is a broad fan-shaped muscle positioned between the lateral surface of the cranium and the ramus of the mandible. Upon contraction, this muscle rapidly elevates the mandible, thus providing the required power to shear, tear, and snap items placed between the teeth.

24. b. The anterior belly of the digastricus muscle spans the space between the deep mandibular symphysis and the anterolateral hyoid. The functional potential of this muscle is to open the mandible, a maneuver that is antagonistic to the jaw-closing function of the medial pterygoid muscle.

25. e. The medial segment of the tensor veli palatini muscle originates from the nasopharyngeal opening of the eustachian tube. If the velar insertion of this muscle is held stable, the action of the muscle is to pull open the eustachian tube and normalize middle ear air pressure.

26. a. High vowels have a smaller velopharyngeal opening because of the close proximity of the tongue dorsum and the oral surface of the velum. The smaller opening is a compensatory strategy to prevent failure of the velopharyngeal port during high vowel production, a time when impedance forces around the velopharyngeal port are great.

27. a. The levator veli palatini, tensor veli palatini, and superior pharyngeal constrictor together constitute the major components of the velopharyngeal port. These muscles operate in concert to reduce the cross-sectional diameter of the velopharyngeal port.

28. e. The levator veli palatini muscle, upon contraction, draws the velum in a superoposterior manner. The anteroinferior oblique angle of this muscle contributes to this action.

29. b. The musculus uvulae accounts for the longitudinal convexity of the upper surface of the velum. It functions to shorten and lift the velum while thickening the nasal surface of the velum along the midline.

30. b. Hydrostats represent systems of muscular organs whose intrinsic organization functions as its internal framework. They are isovolumetric systems that reorganize their volume by shifting and altering the shape of the organ in three-dimensional space. Typical examples of muscular hydrostats include the truck of an elephant, tongues, and squid tentacles.

31. a. Synarthrodial joints are classified as fibrous joints and immovable. Diarthrodial (option b), gliding (option c), pivot (option d), and saddle joints (option e) provide for some degree of movement between each articulator of the joint complex.

32. c. The superior and inferior longitudinal muscles are positioned on either side of the midline and run the length of the tongue from root to apex. Unilateral contraction of these muscle groups causes the anterior segments of the tongue to turn toward the direction of contraction.

33. c. The muscles of the lower face insert directly into the overlying skin. Therefore, facial muscle contraction applies strain on the skin, which results in complex conformational changes that are important for speech sound production and facial gesturing.

34. b. The hard palate is a composite structure created by the fusion of the palatal processes of the maxilla and the palatine bone. The palatal processes of the maxilla make up the anterior two thirds of the hard palate, and the palatine bone constitutes the posterior third.

35. a. Pleural linkage arises as a function of the negative pressure within the intrapleural space caused by the opposing forces generated by the lung tissue and chest wall. The adherence of the lung tissue onto the chest wall through pleural linkage allows for rib motion to directly affect lung volumes.

36. c. Respiratory driving pressure adjustments directly influence the intensity of the voice. Generating rapid and pulselike lung pressure changes is the physiological correlate for prosody and intonation during running speech.

37. c. The vertebral column is divided into five distinct segments: cervical, thoracic, lumbar, sacral, and coccygeal. The vertebral column has 7 cervical, 12 thoracic, and 5 lumbar vertebrae. The sacral plate represents a fusion of 4 to 5 sacral vertebrae, and the coccyx is a vestigial segment.

38. b. The visceral and parietal pleura are mesothelial tissues that line or encapsulate the rib cage and lung tissues, respectively. These pleura form the outer and inner surfaces of the intrapleural space and are necessary components for the development of pleural linkage.

39. c. Lung volumes dramatically increase from childhood to adulthood and then slowly decrease throughout life. A variety of factors contribute to this decline, including stiffening of the chest wall, changes in lung tissue compliancy, reduced respiratory muscle drive, and pulmonary disease states.

40. c. Tidal volumes represent the amount of air moved in and out of the respiratory system during any given breath cycle. Tidal volumes vary according to the demands of a given task. For example, tidal volume increases with greater physical exertion, and decreases on cessation of physical activity.

41. c. The internal and external abdominal oblique muscles and the transverse abdominal muscles form a crisscrossing pattern of muscle fibers that generate compressive forces on the sides of the abdominal contents. These muscles are engaged during forced expiratory events.

42. e. Residual volume consists of the air that is essentially "trapped" with the open spaces of the pulmonary apparatus and that cannot be accessed by the individual by any means. Residual volume is typically estimated to equal 1 L of air.

43. b. The vital capacity is the summation of the inspiratory and expiratory reserve volumes and tidal volume. As such, vital capacity constitutes the usable lung volumes available to an individual.

44. e. The interosseous segment of the internal intercostal muscles is positioned between the osseous segments of the ribs. With their origin closer to the sternum and their insertion nearer the vertebral end, this muscle, on contraction, depresses the ribs.

45. c. The recurrent laryngeal nerve innervates all of the intrinsic muscles of the larynx except for the cricothyroid muscle. The cricothyroid muscle is innervated separately by the external branch of the superior laryngeal nerve. Recurrent laryngeal nerve lesions typically arise after neck surgery and are the cause of underlying vocal fold paralysis.

46. a. The spirometer is a measurement device for assessing lung volumes. Classical spirometers consist of an inverted bell floating in a container of water. A breathing tube is coupled to the underside of the inverted bell so that lung volumes generated by a subject are transduced into a vertical motion of the inverted bell. The inverted bell is linked to a scribe to record bell displacements onto a paper strip chart for subsequent examination.

47. b. The relaxation pressure curve depicts changes in alveolar pressure produced entirely by the passive

recoil and rebounding forces of the tissues that constitute the breathing apparatus. Relaxation pressure is an inherent background force that is influenced by voluntary (muscularly driven) pressure changes.

48. a. During the bucket-handle maneuver, the ribs rotate about a dorsoventral axis to elevate the rib shafts upward and outward. This allows for a large volume change at the thorax. This type of rib motion is so named because it resembles the movement of a handle on a pail or bucket when someone is lifting it off the ground.

49. a. The vocal tract is modeled as a flexible and stretchy tube that is sealed on one end. The sealed end represents the closed glottis, and the open radiating end represents the oral or nasal opening. This particular model has been useful for developing an understanding of the resonance phenomena generated during voice and speech.

50. b. Ingo R. Titze is a leading investigator examining the physics and engineering principles underlying voice production. He has played an instrumental role is the current view of vocal fold motion, emphasizing the importance of tissue elasticity and compliancy. His work has led to the conceptualization that vocal fold vibration is a self-sustaining dynamic process.

51. e. Nasalized vowels demonstrate an absence of acoustic energy at certain frequencies within the source spectrum. They also possess broad bandwidths around specific formant peaks (option a), a reduction in overall sound energy (option b), a decrease in specific formant frequency peaks (option c).

52. c. The formants of speech and vocalization reflect the primary resonance of the human vocal tract. Formants are simply peak intensity areas of the filtered source spectrum.

53. c. Affricate consonants include /t∫/ and /d3/. Both can be characterized as "stops" followed by "fricatives."

54. c. The vowel quadrilateral loosely represents the oral cavity and the position of the tongue within this cavity. During low vowel production, the descended positioning of the tongue effectively decreases the size of the pharyngeal resonator and thus raises the value of F_1. The size of the pharyngeal space is inversely correlated to the value of F_1.

55. e. In general, filters function to highlight certain frequencies and attenuate others in a complex waveform. The low-pass filter is tuned to allow for the transmission of low-frequency components unattenuated, and attenuating all frequency values above cutoff.

56. a. The fricative's sound source is generated by creating turbulent noise at the place of articulation. Depending on whether the place of articulation is anterior or posterior, the turbulence frequency range varies from high to low, respectively.

57. a. An octave is a doubling of frequency. There are four octaves between 100 Hz and 1600 Hz (100 to 200 Hz, 200 to 400 Hz, 400 to 800 Hz, and 800 to 1600 Hz). If the difference in amplitude over four octaves is 100 dB, the roll-off rate would be 25 dB/octave (100 dB/4 octaves).

58. a. Bandwidth is the difference between the upper and lower limits of the formant (i.e., $1100 - 700$ Hz $=$ 400 Hz bandwidth).

59. c. Coarticulatory effects reflect the physiological consequence of articulator motion on the acoustic features of sound transitions during speech.

60. b. Simple harmonic motion, or sinusoidal motion, is derived from the linear projection of uniform circular speed in time.

61. b. During resonance, an object vibrates at a given frequency with maximal energy and amplitude. Resonance arises when waves reflect back on to themselves and are allowed to constructively interfere with each other.

62. b. *Frequency* reflects the number of cycles in 1 second of time. Dividing 1 second by the frequency results in the total time for one cycle of the signal in seconds. This is known as the *period*. As frequency increases in value, the period time must decrease.

63. a. A formant is a peak of resonance in the vocal tract. Resonance changes are generated through alterations in the geometry of the vocal tract spaces. As the shape of the vocal tract changes, formants values are modified accordingly.

64. a. The position of the second formant is most responsive to changes in the size of the oral cavity. Changes in tongue position or lip configuration will affect this formant dramatically.

65. b. The spectrogram depicts how all formant peaks, generated during speech or vocalization, change in time. In a given spectrogram, time is reflected on the horizontal axis, frequency is reflected on the

vertical axis, and gray-scale levels depict the relative amplitude of a formant's bandwidth.

66. b. Myofibrils are intrinsic components of skeletal muscle fibers that extend along the entire length of the muscle cell.

67. a. Sarcomeres represent the smallest functional unit of the motor control system that can undergo contraction. It is the elemental structure that possesses all the necessary components (proteins) that allow for contraction to occur.

68. b. The motor unit is the smallest functional element controlled by the motor control system. It is composed of the lower motor neuron and all of the muscle fibers it innervates. The motor unit is considered the final common pathway for integrated signals from the central nervous system.

69. e. Fatigue-resistant muscle fibers are made of type IIA fibers and rely on oxidative methods of metabolism. Their contractions are of small force during most routine muscle movement. In contrast, fatigable muscle fibers are composed of type IIB fibers, rely on glycolytic methods of metabolism, and are capable of generating large forces for brief time periods.

70. c. Myofibrils are composed of thick and thin protein filaments known as myosin and actin, respectively. The excitation-coupling of these constituent proteins underlies sarcomere length changes.

PART II

Phonological and Language Disorders: Assessment and Treatment

CHAPTER 6

Phonological Disorders

Benjamin Munson

1. Of the following babbling sequences, which is an example of an infant using *pure frames* as discussed by MacNeilage (2008)?
   a. /dædi/
   b. /mami/
   c. /bʌbʌ/
   d. /gægæ/
   e. None of the above

2. Of the following babbling sequences, which provides evidence that the child is moving the tongue and the jaw independently from one another?
   a. /dædæ/
   b. /mʌmʌ/
   c. /bʌbʌ/
   d. /gægæ/
   e. All of the above

3. Young children are *least* likely to delete an unstressed syllable from which of the following words?
   a. *Police*
   b. *Giraffe*
   c. *About*
   d. *Catsup*
   e. *Above*

4. Young children are most likely to delete an unstressed syllable from which of the following words?
   a. *Tuba*
   b. *Color*
   c. *Kitty*
   d. *Giraffe*
   e. *Mommy*

5. A child demonstrates consistent velar fronting and initial voicing, inconsistent final consonant deletion, and inconsistent nasal harmony. How might this child produce the word *cat?*

a. /dæt/
b. /tæt/
c. /kæt/
d. /gæt/
e. All of the above

6. A child demonstrates consistent velar fronting and initial voicing, inconsistent final consonant deletion, and inconsistent nasal harmony. Of the following utterances, which is *least* likely to be this child's pronunciation of the word *cone?*
   a. /goʊ/
   b. /noʊn/
   c. /doʊn/
   d. /doʊ/
   e. None of the above

7. Of the following sounds, which is an example of a distortion error in English?
   a. Substituting /t/ for /k/
   b. A lateral lisp
   c. Final consonant deletion
   d. Addition of the vowel /ə/ to consonant clusters
   e. Stopping of fricatives

8. A child is acquiring African American English as her native language. Of the following pronunciations, which most reflects African American English, as opposed to developmental processes that occur across different dialects of American English?
   a. /ʃʌbəl/ for shovel
   b. /bæf/ for bath
   c. /doʊ/ for go
   d. /wæp/ for giraffe
   e. All of the above

9. A child is acquiring African-American English as her native language. Of the following pronunciations, which most reflects African American English, as opposed to developmental processes that occur across different dialects of American English?
   a. /sʌvəl/ for shovel
   b. /bæs/ for bath
   c. /goʊs/ for ghost
   d. /baʊt/ for about
   e. None of the above

10. Of the following, which is not a phonological characteristic of child-directed speech?
    a. Hyperarticulation of consonants (e.g., producing the word *kitty* as /kʰɪti/ rather than /kʰɪri/
    b. Higher fundamental frequency than that of conversational speech
    c. Greater pitch range than that of conversational speech
    d. Fast rate than that of conversational speech
    e. All of the above

11. Of the following sounds, which is likely to be produced last by children acquiring North American English?
    a. /s/
    b. /n/
    c. /d/
    d. /t/
    e. /m/

12. The phonological process of *stopping* would affect a child's pronunciation of which of the following words?
    a. *Cat*
    b. *Dome*
    c. *Phone*
    d. *Bee*
    e. *Tan*

13. The phonological process of *fronting* would affect a child's pronunciation of which of the following words?
    a. *Cat*
    b. *Dome*
    c. *Fly*
    d. *Bee*
    e. *Way*

14. Of the following, which is *not* a characteristic of the speech of preschool- and young school-aged children?
    a. Longer speech-sound durations than adults
    b. Faster rate of speech than adults
    c. Greater variability in formant frequencies for vowels than adults
    d. More variability in fundamental frequency than adults
    e. All of the above

15. Macken and Barton (1980) described four stages in the acquisition of the voicing contrast in stops. Of the following stages, which comes second in the development of the voicing contrast for initial stops in American English?
    a. Children produce an exaggerated contrast between voiced and voiceless stops
    b. Children produce a measurable difference in voice onset time between voiced and voiceless stops that is imperceptible to most adults
    c. Children produce adult-like differences between voiced and voiceless stops
    d. Children produce no measurable differences in voice onset time between voiced and voiceless stops
    e. Children produce a measurable difference in voice onset time between voiced and voiceless stops that is perceptible to most adults

16. Of the following, which is *not* a typical production for a speaker of African-American vernacular English?

a. /wɪf/ for *with*
b. /mɪn/ for *men*
c. /su/ for *zoo*
d. /hiə/ for *here*
e. /æks/ for *ask*

17. Which theory of phonological development makes the explicit claim that babbling and early speech are discontinuous?
   a. The frames-then-content model
   b. The structuralist model
   c. The behavioralist model
   d. The continuity model
   e. None of the above

18. Of the following words, which is *most* likely to undergo weak syllable deletion?
   a. *Alive*
   b. *Better*
   c. *Silly*
   d. *Mother*
   e. *Doctor*

19. Of the following choices, which is *not* a feature of child-directed speech?
   a. Slower rate than in conversational speech
   b. Smaller acoustic vowel space than in conversational speech
   c. Exaggerated voicing contrasts in comparison to conversational speech
   d. Higher average fundamental frequency (F$_0$) than in conversational speech
   e. All of the above

20. Of the following statements about infant speech perception, which is *not* true?
   a. Infants attend longer to infant-directed speech
   b. Infants prefer to listen to their native language
   c. Six-month old infants raised in English-speaking households can discriminate between /da/ and /ɖa/
   d. Six-week old English-speaking infants cannot discriminate between the /ba/ and /da/
   e. All are true

21. Werker and Stager (2000) studied the effect of object pairing on speech perception. Their results suggested which of the following?
   a. Infants' loss of sensitivity to fine phonetic detail is related to early word learning
   b. The development of speech perception is an innately guided process
   c. Infants' speech perception abilities at 8 months are adult-like
   d. Children with phonological disorders have poorer speech perception than typically developing children
   e. All of the above

22. Of the following, which is *not* an anatomical constraint on early speech production?
   a. The oropharynx is almost nonexistent in infants
   b. The receptive vocabulary in infants is small
   c. The larynx is positioned high in the infant vocal tract
   d. The tongue is large in relation to the rest of the oral cavity in infants
   e. All of the above

23. Of the following statements, which has been offered as an explanation for why some sounds are acquired later than others?
   a. Later acquired sounds are less frequent in the ambient language than early acquired sounds
   b. Later acquired sounds are more linguistically marked than early acquired sounds
   c. Later acquired sounds are motorically more difficult than early acquired sounds
   d. a and b
   e. a, b, and c

24. Of the following statements about dialects (and speakers of dialects), which is *not* true?
   a. Many individuals are bi-dialectal
   b. Dialects are mutually intelligible
   c. Speakers of a dialect are a homogeneous group
   d. There is a relationship between the prestige associated with a dialect and the prestige of the group speaking the dialect
   e. Some dialectal features are shared by many different dialects

25. Of the following sounds, which is *not* produced with a rapid ballistic movement of the tongue in /a/-consonant-/a/ sequences?
   a. /j/
   b. /ŋ/
   c. /k/
   d. /t/
   e. /m/

26. Rvachew (1994) provided speech perception training for three groups of children with /ʃ/ errors. Group 1 received identification training for correct and incorrect /ʃ/ (the "shoe-Xshoe" group). Group 2 received training for /ʃ/ and /m/ (the "shoe-moo" group). Group 3 received training on an unrelated contrast (the "cat-Pete" group). All children received traditional articulation treatment concurrent with perception training. After training, which of the following results did Rvachew obtain?
   a. Children in group 1 produced /ʃ/ more accurately than did children in group 2 or 3
   b. Children in groups 1 and 2 produced /ʃ/ more accurately than did children in group 3

c. Children in group 3 produced /ʃ/ more accurately than did children in groups 1 and 2, which suggests that speech perception training inhibits sound learning rather than facilitating it

d. Children in groups 1, 2, and 3 produced /ʃ/ with equally accuracy

e. No improvement was found with any of the groups

27. A child produces /bɪ/ for *bee*, /pɪp/ for *peep*, and /sɪt/ for *seat*; /sɛ/ for *say* and /fɛs/ for *face*; and /lɛs/ for *less*. Of the following, which describes the child's error patterns?
    a. Tensing
    b. Laxing
    c. Derhoticization
    d. Diphthongization
    e. Lip rounding

28. A child produces /bɪ/ for *bee*, /pɪp/ for *peep*, and /sɪt/ for *seat*; /sɛ/ for *say* and /fɛs/ for *face*; and /lɛs/ for *less*. The clinician wishes to train the vowel /i/ in the most facilitative context. Of the following words, which would be best for such training?
    a. *Bee*
    b. *Keep*
    c. *Peep*
    d. *Seat*
    e. *Sheet*

29. Of the following treatment programs, which includes auditory bombardment at the beginning of each therapy session?
    a. The Hodson-Paden Therapy for Unintelligible Children
    b. Programmed Conditioning for Articulation
    c. McDonald Sensory-Motor Program
    d. Motoric Automatization of Articulatory Performance
    e. Multiple Oppositions

30. In a 4-year-old child, a severe phonological disorder is diagnosed. She presents with the following phonetic inventory (assume that these sounds occur in both target and nontarget environments):

Bilabial	Alveolar	Palatal	Velar	Glottal
/b/	/d/			
				/h/
/m/				
		/j/		

According to Gierut's (2000) research, teaching which of the following new sounds will result in the most spontaneous generalization to untreated sounds?
    a. /p/
    b. /g/
    c. /s/
    d. /t/
    e. /w/

31. In a 4-year-old child, a severe phonological disorder is diagnosed. She presents with the following phonetic inventory (assume that these sounds occur in both target and nontarget environments):

Bilabial	Alveolar	Palatal	Velar	Glottal
/b/	/d/			
				/h/
/m/				
		/j/		

If the clinician were to teach two new sounds in contrast, per Gierut's (2001) research, which of the following pairs would likely result in the most spontaneous generalization to untreated sounds?
    a. /k/ and /g/
    b. /d/ and /t/
    c. /d/ and /f/
    d. /p/ and /z/
    e. None of the above

32. A child with a phonological disorder produces /ʃ/ incorrectly. The following productions are noted:

Word	Pronunciation
ship	dɪp
shell	dɛw
shark	daʊk
fishing	fɪtɪn
wishes	wɪtɪ
vicious	bɪtɪ
hush	hʌs
wish	wɪs
crash	kwæs

Of the following statements, which is true?
    a. If /ʃ/ is taught in initial position, spontaneous generalization to medial and final position will probably occur
    b. This child's errors are inconsistent within word positions
    c. If /ʃ/ is taught in final position, correct production in initial and medial position will probably not occur spontaneously
    d. This child will not benefit from a maximal contrast approach to therapy
    e. All of the above

33. Of the following sentences, which is an example of using a metaphor to teach the sound /s/?
    a. "Make the sound that the tea kettle makes when the water gets hot"
    b. "Put your tongue tip behind your upper teeth and breathe out"
    c. "Push your tongue against the cold place in your mouth" (following the application of lemon ice to the alveolar ridge)
    d. "Say the sound as I say it [sssss]"
    e. "Place your tongue behind your front teeth, smile and make the sound that I make"

34. Of the following techniques, which would most likely work when establishing /θ/ in a child with a /f/-for-/θ/ substitution and a strong aversion to tactile stimuli?
    a. Sitting next to the child in front of a mirror and demonstrating correct and incorrect /θ/ production with exaggerated acoustic cues
    b. Having the child hold a bite-block between his or her molars, which would making labiodental contact difficult
    c. Holding a tongue depressor in front of the child's mouth and instructing him or her to touch it with his or her tongue while breathing out
    d. Place your finger on the child's lips and instruct him not to bite his or her upper lip when he or she says the words *bath* and *think*
    e. All of the above

35. Of the following tests of phonological awareness, which is used to assess rapid automatized naming?
    a. Test of Phonological Awareness
    b. Phonological Awareness Test
    c. Comprehensive Test of Phonological Awareness
    d. Goldman-Fristoe Test of Articulation–2
    e. The Arizona Articulation Proficiency Scale–3

36. A certain child's phonetic inventory contains both voiced and voiceless stops in all word positions, but no fricatives. The clinician decides to help the child learn the earliest acquired fricative, /f/, to 90% accuracy in all word positions and at all levels of linguistic complexity. After this, she trains the child in the next earliest acquired sound, /s/ (according to the Iowa-Nebraska norming study; Smit et al, 1990), to 90% accuracy in all word positions and at all levels of linguistic complexity. The remaining fricatives are taught in a similar manner. This is an example of which of the following goal selection strategies?
    a. Cycles
    b. Maximum contrast
    c. Horizontal
    d. Vertical
    e. None of the above

37. A certain child's phonetic inventory contains both voiced and voiceless stops in all word positions, but no fricatives. The clinician decides to help the child learn the earliest acquired fricative, /f/, to 90% accuracy in all word positions and at all levels of linguistic complexity. After this, she trains the child in the next earliest acquired sound, /s/ (according to the Iowa-Nebraska norming study; Smit et al, 1990), to 90% accuracy in all word positions and at all levels of linguistic complexity. The remaining fricatives are taught in a similar manner. Of the following pairs of sounds, which differs in only one distinctive feature?

    a. /b/ and /p/
    b. /t/ and /ð/
    c. /m/ and /s/
    d. /p/ and /s/
    e. /k/ and /f/

38. Of the following characteristics of adults with a history of moderate-to-severe phonological disorders, which was *not* documented by Felsenfeld and associates (1992, 1994)?
    a. Adults with a history of phonological disorders had poorer receptive vocabulary skills (as measured by the Peabody Picture Vocabulary Test) than did adults without a history of phonological disorders
    b. Adults with a history of phonological disorders worked less skilled jobs than did adults without a history of phonological disorders
    c. Adults with a history of phonological disorders received lower grades in high school than did adults without a history of phonological disorders
    d. Adults with a history of phonological disorders were less satisfied with their education and employment than were adults without a history of phonological disorders
    e. All of the above

39. Phonological awareness tasks purportedly make use of which of the following cognitive skills?
    a. Speech perception
    b. Reasoning skills
    c. Memory
    d. All of the above
    e. None of the above

40. A child's does not produce /s/ in any phonetic contexts. In therapy, the child is taught /s/ in the words *seek, seat, seed*, and *seal*. After treatment, the child produces the sound correctly in those words, as well as in *soup, sad, song*, and *south*. This is an example of which of the following?
    a. Generalization across word positions
    b. Generalization across levels of linguistic complexity
    c. Generalization across phonetic contexts
    d. Generalization across sounds
    e. Generalization across a sound class

41. Of the following, which is an example of training clients to distinguish between fricatives and stops at the conceptual level, as would be done in phase I of the Metaphon program?
    a. Fricatives are "sounds you make by breathing warm air"; stops are "sounds you make by tapping your tongue or popping your lips"
    b. Fricatives are "hissy sounds, like a snake makes"; stops are "loud sound, like a balloon when it pops"

c. Fricatives are "long sounds"; stops are "short sounds"

d. All of the above

e. None of the above

42. Using a straw to provide feedback on the location of airflow is most useful in treating:
    a. A lateral lisp
    b. A frontal lisp
    c. An /r/ misarticulation
    d. Final consonant deletion
    e. Alveolar assimilation

43. According to Elbert and associates (1991), how many minimal word pairs were required for the majority (59%) of subjects with phonological disorders to generalize correct production to untreated word pairs?
    a. 3
    b. 5
    c. 7
    d. 10
    e. 12

44. A certain child's phonetic inventory does not contain any initial voiceless stops. The clinician chooses to target initial voicing in therapy. This is an example of which of the following approaches to goal selection?
    a. A segment approach
    b. A phonological process approach
    c. A contrast approach
    d. A motor approach
    e. None of the above

45. A clinician trains /ʃ/ in the sentences "I like the shoe," "I like the sheep," and "I like the shovel." After treatment, the child produces /ʃ/ correctly in those sentences, as well as in "I have a new shoe," "The sheep live on the farm," and "My daddy has a shovel." This is an example of which of the following?
    a. Generalization across word positions
    b. Generalization across levels of linguistic complexity
    c. Generalization across phonetic contexts
    d. Generalization across sounds
    e. Generalization across a sound class

46. Of the following techniques, which has proven most successful in promoting generalization of correct speech production to spontaneous speech outside of the therapy situation?
    a. Training a maximal contrast in 5 minimal pairs of words
    b. Adopting a cycles approach to goal attack
    c. Metaphon therapy
    d. Training self-monitoring and self-correction
    e. None of the above

47. The following is a clinician-client exchange during a therapy session. The client consistently simplifies initial consonant clusters and deletes final stop consonants. The clinician and client are playing with stuffed animals.
    Clinician [putting his teddy bear on a toy car]: My teddy bear is driving a car.
    Client [putting his teddy bear on a toy bike]: My teddy bear's riding a bike /maɪ dɛi bɛʊ waɪdɪ ə baɪ/.
    Clinician [putting his teddy bear on a bike]: So is mine! My teddy bear's riding a bike /maɪ tɛɾi berz raɪdɪŋ ə baɪk/. They both are!

    What technique is the clinician using?
    a. Recasting
    b. Adding events
    c. Response-contingent timeout
    d. Expansion
    e. Modeling

48. Which is the highest level of linguistic complexity of the following list?
    a. Conversational speech
    b. Sentences
    c. Phrases
    d. Words
    e. Syllables

49. According to the cycles approach (Hodson-Paden therapy for unintelligible children), when should auditory bombardment be provided?
    I. *In the beginning of the session, after picture cards from the previous week have been reviewed*
    II. *At the end of the session, after stimulability probes*
    III. *During home programming, to be administered by the parent*
    a. I
    b. I and II
    c. I, II, and III
    d. None of the above; this program explicitly rejects the notion that ear training is necessary
    e. Only used at discretion of the clinician

50. "Listen to what I say: boat, coat, bed, bridge. Which word doesn't start with the same sound as the other three?" This is an example of which of the following?
    a. A phoneme-blending task
    b. Awareness of alliteration
    c. A phoneme-segmentation task
    d. A sound comparison task
    e. A rhyming task

51. Of the following sound types, which is most difficult to train in isolation?

a. Voiceless
b. Voiceless fricatives
c. Nasal sounds
d. Vowels
e. Dipthongs

52. A child has a consistent vowel backing error: She produces /kɑt/ for *cat*, /tʌn/ for *ten*, and /buɪp/ for *beep* (in which /ɯ/ is the high back unround tense vowel). Front vowels should be taught in which of the following phonetic contexts?
    a. k _____ k
    b. p _____ p
    c. t _____ t
    d. g _____ g
    e. None of the above

53. Of the following tests, which does not provide separate normative scores for boys and girls?
    a. The Bankson-Bernthal Test of Phonology
    b. The Arizona Articulation Proficiency Scale–3
    c. The Goldman-Fristoe Test of Articulation–2
    d. All of the above provide norms for boys and girls
    e. None of the above because all three provide separate norms for boys and girls

54. A child produces the word *screaming* as /wimn/. According to the scoring guidelines for the Percent Consonants Correct test, how many consonant errors has the child made for this word? Note that *screaming* has stress on the first syllable.
    a. 2
    b. 3
    c. 4
    d. 5
    e. 6

55. Of the following standardized tests, which enables the measurement of vowel production accuracy?
    a. Percent Consonants Correct
    b. The Goldman-Fristoe Test of Articulation–2
    c. The Arizona Articulation Proficiency Scale–3
    d. The Bankson-Bernthal Test of Phonology
    e. The Fisher-Logemann Test of Articulation

56. A child with consistent cluster reduction is being taught initial /st/ clusters in therapy. The child and the clinician are playing with stuffed animals and a toy store. The child says, "Which one is going to the /stor/?" (i.e., he correctly produces the initial /st/ cluster.) Of the following clinician responses, which would conform to the principle of communicative reinforcement?
    a. "Hey! You said your /st/ sounds, just as we practiced! Great! You're working very hard."

b. "I like the way you said your /st/ sounds. Say them again. Tell me /stor/ five times."
c. "What did you just say? Say it again. I'm not sure I heard you."
d. "I think this guy is going to the /stor/, too. Yeah, this guy is going to the /stor/. Here's another guy. Let's see where he's going to go."
e. All of the above

57. Which is an example of a tensing error (per Pollock, 1990)?
    a. /hɪt/ for *heat*
    b. /ʃud/ for *should*
    c. /bɛk/ for *bake*
    d. /bʊt/ for *boot*
    e. All of the above

58. Of the following standardized, norm-referenced tests, which weights errors according to the frequency of the occurrence of sounds in the ambient language?
    a. The Scaffolding Scale of Stimulability
    b. The Goldman-Fristoe Test of Articulation–2
    c. The Arizona Articulation Proficiency Scale–3
    d. The Bankson-Bernthal Test of Phonology
    e. None of the above

59. Of the following children, for whom would the cycles approach (Hodsen-Paden therapy for unintelligible children) be most appropriate?
    a. A child with systematic errors who is not stimulable
    b. A child with systematic errors who is stimulable
    c. A child with nonsystematic errors who is not stimulable
    d. A child with nonsystematic errors who is stimulable
    e. None of the above

60. At the beginning of treatment, a child's phonetic inventory contained no fricatives. The child is being taught the sound /f/ in initial position in single-syllable words. In addition to monitoring the child's progress on initial /f/, the clinician has chosen to monitor word-initial /v/ as a generalization behavior and word-initial /l/ in monosyllables as an unrelated behavior. Data from 12 treatment sessions are given in Figure 6-1.
    What can you conclude about the efficacy of treatment?
    a. Treatment is facilitating only the target behavior, initial /f/
    b. Treatment is facilitating the target behavior, initial /f/, and the child is spontaneously learning the generalization behavior, /v/
    c. The child is learning the target sound, but no generalization learning has occurred

d. The child is not learning the target sound

e. No definitive conclusions can be drawn about treatment efficacy

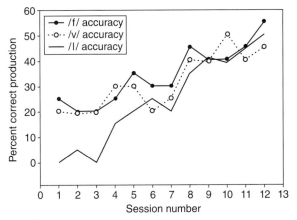

Figure 6-1

61. At the beginning of treatment, a child's phonetic inventory contained no fricatives. The child is being taught the sound /f/ in initial position in single-syllable words. In addition to monitoring the child's progress on initial /f/, the clinician has chosen to monitor word-initial /v/ as a generalization behavior and word-initial /l/ in monosyllables as an unrelated behavior. Data from 12 treatment sessions are given in Figure 6-1.

Of the following statements about this therapy scenario, which is true?

a. The clinician used a developmental approach to goal selection

b. The generalization behavior that the clinician chose to monitor, initial /v/, was not phonetically related to the target behavior, initial /f/

c. The unrelated behavior that the clinician chose to monitor, initial /l/, was phonetically very similar to the target behavior, initial /f/

d. The clinician selected a developmentally later acquired speech sound to treat

e. None of the above

62. Of the following, which is a *negative* prognostic indicator for a child with inaccurate production of velar stops?

a. The child produces a covert contrast between the /t/ that the child produces for target /t/ and the /t/ the child produces for target /k/

b. The client produces /k/ and /g/ correctly before /i/ but incorrectly elsewhere

c. For one third of the words with a target velar sound, the child produces an alveolar stop as a substitute; for one third, the child deletes the target velar; and for one third, the child produces a /j/ as a substitute for the velar

d. The child is able to produce /k/ and /g/ in words when given auditory and visual cues

e. None of the above

63. Of the following phonological processes, which changes a word's syllable structure?

a. Stopping

b. Velar fronting

c. Cluster reduction

d. Deaffrication

e. Backing

64. A child with a velar fronting error would produce which of the following words in error?

a. *Knight*

b. *Enough*

c. *Ghost*

d. *Rough*

e. *Through*

65. The instruction "Tell me what word these sounds make: /f/ /ɪ/ /ʃ/" is an example of which of the following types of phonological awareness tasks?

a. Phoneme segmentation

b. Phoneme comparison

c. Phoneme blending

d. Rhyming

e. Onset phoneme segmentation matching

66. Of the following sounds, which occurs least frequently in words in English?

a. /s/

b. /d/

c. /l/

d. /ʃ/

e. /z/

67. Of the following statements about children's word recognition, which is true?

a. To accurately recognize spoken words, children require less acoustic information than do adults

b. Two-year-old children are able to discriminate among all of the possible sound contrasts in the world's languages

c. Children's word recognition is not affected by the presence of background noise

d. In detecting misperceived words, children are less accurate than are adults

e. All of the above

68. Of the following words, which is not a phonological neighbor for the word *nip?*

a. *tip*

b. *gnat*

c. *map*

d. *snip*

e. a and d

69. Of the following phonemes, which is most difficult for children with high-frequency hearing loss to perceive?

a. /s/
b. /m/
c. /r/
d. /w/
e. /n/

70. Fletcher and Meldrum (1968) examined the relationships between the size of the lingual frenum and speech production accuracy and found which of the following?
    a. Children with short lingual frena have moderate to severe speech-sound disorders
    b. Children with short lingual frena produce no more speech-sound errors than do children with normal-length frena
    c. Short lingual frena cause /w/-for-/r/ substitutions
    d. Children with shorter frena make more speech-sound errors than do those with longer frena, although the number of errors is within normal limits
    e. Children with short frena showed a high frequency of velar point of articulation errors

71. Of the following error patterns, which is more likely to be associated with the speech of English-acquiring children with cleft palate than with the speech of children with phonological disorders?
    a. Velar fronting
    b. Glottal substitution
    c. Initial voicing
    d. Weak syllable deletion
    e. Stopping

72. Of the following phonological errors, which has the least effect on English-acquiring children's ability to produce phonologically normal regular plural nouns?
    a. Initial voicing
    b. Final consonant deletion
    c. Stopping
    d. Final consonant devoicing
    e. Cluster reduction

73. With regard to the relationship between speech-sound stimulability and speech-sound learning, Powell and coworkers (1991) found which of the following?
    a. Children learn stimulable and nonstimulable sounds at similar rates during treatment
    b. Stimulability affects the learning of some sounds (such as /s/) but not others (such as /r/)
    c. Stimulable sounds are more readily generalized than are nonstimulable ones
    d. Nonstimulable sounds are learned more readily than are stimulable ones
    e. Stimulability is not related to sound learning skills

74. Of the following conditions, which would preclude a relational analysis of a child's spontaneous speech?
    a. The child is highly unintelligible

b. The child has a vocabulary of only 200 words
c. The child has only a few sounds in error, and these are all later acquired sounds
d. The child makes errors only on fricatives and liquids
e. All of the above

75. If a child failed a 20-dB hearing screening at 4000 Hz and 8000 Hz, which of the following sound contrasts would probably be the hardest for the child to perceive?
    a. /b/ and /m/
    b. /m/ and /l/
    c. /w/ and /j/
    d. /s/ and /ʃ/
    e. /i/ and /e/

76. Of the following errors, which is an example of a progressive assimilation?
    a. /pop/ for *poke*
    b. /mi/ for *mean*
    c. /kok/ for *poke*
    d. /in/ for *mean*
    e. /ki/ for *ski*

77. Of the following utterances, which is an error metathesis?
    a. /ɑsk/ for *ox*
    b. /ɑks/ for *box*
    c. /sɑs/ for *socks*
    d. /tʃɛks/ for *chess*
    e. tʌn for *stun*

78. Of the following cluster reduction errors, which can be characterized as a coalescence error?
    a. /Φɑl/ for *small*
    b. /wɪm/ for *swim*
    c. /ti/ for *tree*
    d. /daɪ/ for *dry*
    e. None of the above

79. Of the following processes, which is most likely to disappear earliest in children's speech?
    a. Liquid gliding
    b. Depalatalization
    c. Final consonant deletion
    d. Final consonant devoicing
    e. Gliding of a liquid

80. Of the following words, which is a candidate for the phonological process of regressive nasal assimilation?
    a. *Moon*
    b. *Loon*
    c. *Mule*
    d. *Lull*
    e. *Note*

81. A child with childhood apraxia of speech is observed to have inconsistent production of the sound /p/, sometimes

producing it as /Φ/. In which of the following words might the child have the greatest difficulty producing /p/?
a. *Pie*
b. *Up*
c. *Peter*
d. *Pay*
e. *Ape*

82. Of the following sounds, which is a glide?
a. /j/
b. /r/
c. /s/
d. /l/
e. /f/

83. The first sound in which of the following sounds has a long-lag voice-onset time?
a. *Ten*
b. *Boy*
c. *Sing*
d. *Dog*
e. *Lion*

84. Of the following, which is the lowest level of linguistic complexity?
a. Conversational speech
b. Sentences
c. Phrases
d. Words
e. Syllables

85. Of the following sounds, the production of which is most likely to differ between blind and sighted children?
a. /t/
b. /k/
c. /p/
d. /s/
e. /g/

86. Acoustic analyses show that children who are perceived to substitute /t/ for /k/ sometimes produce a measurable acoustic difference between sounds that are transcribed as identical, whereas other children produce true substitutions of /t/ for /k/. How do these two groups differ?
a. Children in the former group have a more severe impairment than do children in the latter group
b. Children in the former group progress through therapy more quickly than do children in the latter group
c. Children in the former group show clear signs of childhood apraxia of speech
d. Children in the latter group have a severe language impairment
e. Children in the latter group progress through therapy more quickly than do children in the former group

87. A child who produces /dip/ for keep demonstrates which of the following two phonological processes?
a. Fronting and regressive place of articulation harmony
b. Initial voicing and coalescence
c. Fronting and initial voicing
d. Regressive place of articulation harmony and initial voicing
e. Stopping and metathesis

88. How does the sound /ð/ differ between Mexican Spanish and North American English?
a. It is an allophone in Mexican Spanish and a phoneme in North American English
b. It is a phoneme in Mexican Spanish and an allophone in North American English
c. This sound has the same phoneme status in North American English and Mexican Spanish
d. /ð/ does not occur in Mexican Spanish
e. None of the above

89. For a speaker with velopharyngeal incompetence, which of the following sounds would be most difficult to produce normally?
a. /m/
b. /s/
c. /l/
d. /j/
e. /i/

90. Morrisette and Gierut (2002) found that generalization of correct sound production to untrained words is greatest if sounds are taught in which of the following types of words?
a. Those that have high frequency of occurrence, have high phonological neighborhood density, and are stimulable
b. Those that have high frequency of occurrence and low phonological neighborhood density
c. Those that have low frequency of occurrence and high phonological neighborhood density
d. Those that have low frequency of occurrence and low phonological neighborhood density
e. Those that have low frequency of occurrence, have low phonological neighborhood density, and are stimulable

91. Children acquiring Japanese as a first language typically learn /k/ before /t/, and /k/-for-/t/ substitutions are more common than /t/-for-/k/ substitutions (Beckman et al, 2003). What does this finding imply?
a. Children acquiring Japanese are more likely to have cleft palates than are English-acquiring children
b. The rate of occurrence of phonological processes is language specific
c. The sound /t/ is linguistically unmarked

d. Children acquiring Japanese are more likely to have phonological disorders than are English-acquiring children

e. All of the above

92. Of the following vowels, which is most similar to the consonant /j/?
    a. /i/
    b. /u/
    c. /æ/
    d. /ɑ/
    e. None of the above

93. Of the following sounds, which can be characterized by the distinctive feature [+sonorant]?
    a. /f/
    b. /t/
    c. /z/
    d. /l/
    e. /b/

94. Of the following statements, which does *not* describe the perception abilities of infants in the first 6 months of life?
    a. An inability to discriminate phoneme contrasts not present in the language that the child has been exposed to
    b. The ability to discriminate place of articulation contrasts (e.g., /b/ versus /d/)
    c. The ability to discriminate the vowel /i/ from /u/
    d. A preference for listening to child-directed speech
    e. None of the above

95. Of the following words, which has a weak-strong stress pattern?
    a. *Kitty*
    b. *Mother*
    c. *Animal*
    d. *Alone*
    e. *Eating*

96. Of the following conditions, which is *not* a characteristic of children with childhood apraxia of speech?
    a. Weakness of the oral musculature
    b. Severely unintelligible speech
    c. Inconsistent error patterns
    d. Vowel distortions
    e. Prosodic variations

97. The phonological process of final consonant deletion would affect a child's pronunciation of which of the following words?
    a. *High*
    b. *Sigh*
    c. *Enough*
    d. *Guy*
    e. *Toy*

98. Of the following statements about African American English, which is true?
    a. It typically does not have /θ/ in word-final position
    b. It typically does not have /θ/ in word-initial position
    c. Most speakers of African American English cannot perceive differences between African American English and other mainstream dialects of American English
    d. It does not have /tʃ/ in word-final position
    e. All of the above

99. Of the following sound pairs, which differs in more than one distinctive feature?
    a. /p/ and /b/
    b. /t/ and /s/
    c. /m/ and /b/
    d. /v/ and /d/
    e. /n/ and /m/

100. Of the following English phonemes, which is not a phoneme in the majority of dialects of Spanish?
    a. [x]
    b. [m]
    c. [n]
    d. [dʒ]
    e. [i]

101. A certain child's phonetic inventory does not contain any initial voiceless stops. The clinician chooses to teach the sound /p/ in therapy. This is an example of which of the following approaches to goal selection?
    a. A segment approach
    b. A phonological process approach
    c. A contrast approach
    d. A distinctive features approach
    e. None of the above

Answers

1. c. The term *pure frames* refers to vocalizations made by holding the tongue in a fixed position and wagging the jaw up and down. In pure frame vocalizations, alveolar sounds always pair with front vowels, bilabial sounds with central vowels (as in /bʌb/ʌ/), and velar sounds with back vowels.

2. d. The vocalizations in /dædæ/ (option a), /mʌmʌ/ (option b), and /bʌbʌ/ (option c) could all be made by holding the tongue in a fixed position and moving the jaw up and down to achieve closure. The vocalization in /gægæ/ could be made by only moving the tongue from a relatively posterior closure for /g/ to a more anterior posture for /æ/ while simultaneously opening and closing the jaw.

3. d. Unstressed syllables are most likely to be deleted from words that have weak-strong stress patterns. *Police* (option a), *giraffe* (option b), *about* (option c), and *above* (option e) all have a weak-strong stress pattern. Only *catsup* has a strong-weak pattern.

4. d. Unstressed syllables are most likely to be deleted from words that have weak-strong stress patterns. *Tuba* (option a), *color* (option b), *kitty* (option c), and *mommy* (option e) all have a strong-weak stress pattern. Only *giraffe* has a weak-strong pattern.

5. a. In /dæt/, the child has applied velar fronting (changing the place of articulation from the velar to the alveolar position) and initial voicing (changing the voiceless stop to a voiced stop). Neither final consonant deletion nor nasal harmony have applied.

6. a. The utterance /goʊ/ is the least likely pronunciation because it fails to demonstrate velar fronting, which is described as an obligatory phonological process. The other choices—/noʊn/ (option b), /doʊn/ (option c), and /doʊ/ (option d)—are examples of velar fronting for this particular production error.

7. b. Distortions are defined as substitutions in which the substituted sound is not a phoneme of the language being acquired. The lateral fricatives and affricates characteristic of the "lateral lisp" are not phonemes of English, and hence lateral lisps are defined as distortions. The substitution of /t/ for /k/ (option a), final consonant deletion (option c), addition of a vowel (option d), and stopping of fricatives (option e) are substituted phonemes, not distortions of the intended phonemes.

8. b. Like many dialects of English, African-American English does not have a distinction between /f/ and /θ/ in syllable-coda position. The stopping in /ʃʌbəl/ (option a), fronting in /doʊ/ (option c), and syllable-deletion, w-for-r substitution in /wæp/ (option d) are not characteristic of African American English.

9. c. Apparent deletion of final consonants, particularly /t/ in final consonant-consonant sequences, is a characteristic of African-American English. The depalatalization in /sʌvəl/ (option a), /s/ for /θ/ substitution in /bæs/ (option b), and weak syllable deletion in /baʊt/ (option d) are not.

10. d. Child-directed speech is slower than conversational speech.

11. a. Across a variety of normative studies (Sanders, 1972; Smit et al., 1990; Templin, 1957), /s/ is found to be later acquired than /n/ (option b), /d/ (option c), /t/ (option d), or /m/ (option e).

12. c. *Stopping* the phonological process in which fricatives becomes stops, typically at the same place of articulation. The words *cat* (option a), *dome* (option b), *bee* (option d), and *tan* (option e) do not contain fricatives and therefore could not be targets for a fronting process.

13. a. *Fronting is* the phonological process in which velar stops becomes alveolar stops. The words *dome* (option b), *fly* (option c), *bee* (option d), and *way* (option e) do not contain velar stops and therefore could not be targets for a fronting process.

14. b. Children's speech is slower and more variable than that of adults.

15. b. The four stages in the development of the voicing contrast begin with no measurable differences in voice onset time between voiced and voiceless stops (option d), followed by measurable but mostly imperceptible differences in this time (option b), exaggerated contrast between voiced and voiceless stops (option a), and adult-like differences between voiced and voiceless stops (option c). One critical finding of Macken and Barton's (1980) study is that many children go through a stage in which they produce acoustic differences between voiced and voiceless stops that many adults cannot hear. Measurable difference in voice onset time that is mostly

perceptible (option e) is not part of the stages described by Macken and Barton.

16. c. The /f/-for-/θ/ substitution (option a), /ɪ/ raising before a coda nasal (option b), postvocalic /r/ deletion (option d), and metathesis (option e) are all characteristic of African American English. The devoicing of /z/ is not a characteristic of African American English.

17. b. According to Jakobson's (1971) classic structuralist model of acquisition, babbling and early speech were discontinuous, whereby babbling reflected only universal motoric and perceptual constraints, and early speech reflected the child's knowledge of language. According to more contemporary models, the two are continuous, in view of both evidence of language specificity in prelinguistic babbling and the phonological similarity of children's babbling and early words.

18. a. Weak syllable deletion is most likely to occur in words with weak-strong stress patterns. *Alive* is the only word that has a weak-strong pattern.

19. b. The acoustic vowel space in child-directed speech is larger than those of conversational speech. This is true across languages. Expanded vowel space makes individual vowels easier to tell apart. The other descriptions (options a, c, and d) are also features of child-directed speech.

20. d. Children across different cultures and different language backgrounds have the ability to discriminate among a wide variety of speech sounds from very early in life until about the end of the first year of life. Indeed, infants in English-language environments can discriminate pairs of sounds that are relevant to the language being acquired, as in the /ba/ and /da/ contrasts, as well as contrasts that are not in their ambient language, as in the alveolar-retroflex contrast (option c), which is phonemic in many languages, such as Hindi and Tiwi, but not in English. Moreover, infants prefer to listen to infant-directed speech (option a) and to their native language (option b).

21. a. Across a variety of experimental studies, Werker and Stager (2000) and other researchers have shown that developmental changes in speech perception are yoked to the infants' development of a rudimentary receptive lexicon.

22. b. Although all of the choices are constraints on early speech production, only receptive vocabulary is not related to anatomy.

23. e. There is substantial disagreement among theories in why some sounds are acquired later than others. All of the descriptions about later acquired sounds (options a, b, and c) have been offered as possible reasons for order-of-acquisition differences across languages.

24. c. Speakers of a dialect are not homogeneous; indeed, they are quite heterogeneous. Some demonstrate many features of the dialect, others demonstrate few. Some speakers of a dialect use some or all of its features consistently, whereas others use them only in specific social interactions in which they bear a particular social meaning. Many individuals fluently command different dialects (option a) and code-switch among them regularly. By definition, dialects are mutually intelligible. One criterion for considering two varieties of a language "dialects" is that they are mutually intelligible. A relationship does exist between dialect and social dominance (option d), and many dialects share some features (option e).

25. a. Stop consonants—including both oral and nasal consonants—are produced with rapid, ballistic movements of the tongue. Glides such as /j/ are produced with slower, ramped movements.

26. b. Rvachew (1994) found that any speech perception that involved tokens of /ʃ/ facilitated speech-production gains in correct production of /ʃ/. This result has been replicated in numerous studies since Rvachew's. It indicates that perceptual training directed to a production target results in improved production performance of that target.

27. b. The child produces the tense vowels /i/ and /e/ as their lax counterparts /ɪ/ and /ɛ/. Tenseness and laxness are features of vowels and pertain to degree of muscular tension in the vocal tract. Tense vowels are associated with muscular tension, particularly of the tongue, whereas lax vowels are not.

28. a. The word *bee* has a consonant-vowel structure, whereas the others have a consonant-vowel-consonant structure. Vowels in consonant-vowel-consonant syllables are shorter and more centralized than those in consonant-vowel syllables, and thus they are naturally more lax.

29. a. The Hodson-Paden program, also known as the "cycles program," includes auditory bombardment at the beginning of each therapy session. The other treatment programs emphasize either phonetic or phonemic teaching strategies.

30. c. Gierut (2001) found that introducing later developing sounds (i.e., ones that would typically be found in a child with more advanced phonological development) will facilitate spontaneous generalization learning of new sounds in children with less complex inventories. In this scenario, the sound /s/ would be a target because it is a later developing sound from a sound class not present in the child's inventory. It can be paired with a sound that is functional for the child or with another sound that is not part of the child's inventory.

31. d. The sounds /p/ and /z/ differ in place, manner, and voicing, and one sound, /z/, is characteristic of the sound inventories of children with more advanced phonological development. The other pairings are contrasts but not major class feature differences. Gierut (2001) developed the maximal opposition approach, and underlying this treatment is the fact that more complex linguistic input results in more extensive change to the client's sound system. Ideal word pairs are chosen to contrast major class features, as with /p/ and /z/.

32. c. Work by some researchers has shown that when children's errors are consistent within word position but not consistent across word position (as in this example), then correct production is not generalized to untreated word positions, and the children need to be taught the sound in each word position separately.

33. a. The sound of a boiling kettle (option a) is a metaphor. Tongue placement (options b and e) is a response to a phonetic placement cue, pushing the tongue (option c) is a response to a tactile cue, and repeating after someone (option d) is a response to an auditory stimulation cue.

34. a. Demonstrating in front of a mirror (option a) is a technique that does not involve a tactile cue. Holding a bite-block (option b), touching a tongue depressor (option c), and having a finger placed on the lips (option d) all involve sensory cues. Those three scenarios would not work well for children with a strong aversion to tactile cues.

35. c. Rapid automatized naming is a very strong predictor of literacy abilities, and deficits in this skill have been linked to reading disability. Of these tests, only the Comprehensive Test of Phonological Awareness enables measurement of rapid automatized naming. Both the Test of Phonological Awareness (option a) and the Phonological Awareness Test (option b) are only tests of phonological awareness, whereas the Goldman-Fristoe Test of Articulation–2 (option d)

and the Arizona Articulation Proficiency Scale–3 (option e) are tests of speech-sound production.

36. d. A vertical goal attack strategy is one in which a small number of targets—often just one—are trained intensively until a preset criterion is reached. The narrative describes a typical vertical response strategy.

37. a. The pair /b/ and /p/ differ in only one feature: voice. The pairs /t/ and /ð/ (option b) and /m/ and /s/ (option c) differ in three features (voicing, tongue placement, and manner of articulation), whereas the pairs /p/ and /s/ (option d) and /k/ and /f/ (option e) differ in two features (tongue placement and manner of articulation).

38. d. Felsenfeld and associates' (1992, 1994) long-term follow-up of adults who had phonological disorders as children revealed numerous differences between these subjects and adults who had not had childhood phonological disorders, including differences in receptive vocabulary (option a), in level of skill required in employment (option b), and in school grades (option c). However, a history of childhood phonological disorder was not associated with less satisfaction with educational or vocational outcomes.

39. d. As argued by McBride-Chang (1995), phonological awareness tasks are introspective activities that require speech perception (option a), reasoning (option b), and memory skills (option c).

40. c. In this hypothetical example, the child has been taught /s/ in the /i/ vowel context. Correct generalization to the /u/, /æ/, /ɔ/, and /aʊ/ contexts is evidence of generalization across phonetic contexts.

41. c. One unique facet of the Metaphon therapy program is that it teaches conceptual differences among sounds—such as calling fricatives "long" and stops "short"—before training clients in the production and perception of the sounds. The Metaphon approach targets phonological processes primarily through the use of metalinguistic awareness tasks; minimal attention is given to the production of phonological contrasts.

42. a. Lateral lisps are characterized by air flowing off the sides of the tongue, rather than through a central groove in the tongue. Straws are sometimes used to cue children to use a tongue posture that allows central airflow.

43. a. In their study of 19 misarticulating children, Elbert and associates (1991) found that a majority (59%) needed to be taught sound contrasts in only three

word pairs before they met criteria for generalization learning. An additional 21% of children generalized after learning contrasts in only five word pairs.

44. b. Targeting an entire class of errors—in this case, errors in which all voiceless stops are produced as voiced (often called the phonological process of *initial voicing*)—is an example of a phonological process approach to therapy. The other choices are additional treatment approaches that may be used but depend on the theoretical orientation of the clinician and the type of speech-sound error patterns that the child presents.

45. b. In this hypothetical example, the child has been taught /ʃ/ in the frame "I like the [X]." Correct generalization to the other simple phrases listed in this question is generalization to a new level of linguistic complexity. The other choices are types of generalization put the example is that of generalization across linguistic complexity.

46. d. Koegel and colleagues (1988) showed that generalization of correct production outside of the therapy room was best facilitated by training focused on self-monitoring and self-correction.

47. a. In this example, the clinician does not explicitly correct the child's erroneous production; instead, he repeats it with the errors corrected. This is an example of the clinical technique of recasting.

48. a. Of the five levels of complexity listed, conversational speech is the most complex. Speaking in syllables (option e) is the least complex.

49. c. The cycles approach is based partly on the assumption that one of the underlying factors in speech-production problems is the existence of incorrect "auditory images": perceptual targets for speech sounds. The program thus places a strong emphasis on auditory bombardment, a technique presumed to facilitate the building of these images. Auditory bombardment is meant to be administered multiple times during therapy sessions and during home programming.

50. d. All of the phonological awareness tasks listed enable the child to engage in language introspection. In sound comparison tasks, children must phonologically analyze the structure of spoken words and compare them, as in the task of segmenting off the initial sound of the one-syllable words spoken and determining that the second word begins with a sound that is different from that of the other three.

51. a. Because of their aerodynamic and articulatory characteristics, voiceless stops are both difficult to produce in isolation without a following or preceding vowel and impossible to sustain. They are thus the most difficult to train in isolation.

52. c. The /t/ sound is produced with a relatively anterior tongue position and thus serves as a good phonetic context for teaching front vowels. Because of their back tongue position, /k/ (option a) and /g/ (option d) are appropriate contexts for teaching back vowels to children with vowel-fronting errors, whereas the /p/ (option b) context is appropriate for teaching round vowels to children.

53. a. The Bankson-Bernthal Test of Phonology does not provide separate norms. The Arizona Articulation Proficiency Scale–3 (option b) and the Goldman-Fristoe Test of Articulation–2 (option c) provide separate normative scores for young boys and girls, as some studies have found the rate of speech-sound development to differ between sexes.

54. b. In the Percent Consonants Correct test (Shriberg and associates, 1997), this child would be said to have produced three errors: deleting of the /s/ and /k/ in the initial syllable and substitution of /w/ for the /r/. Production of the final /ŋ/ as /n/ is not considered an error in this system, as this pronunciation is common in normal children and adults' speech.

55. c. The Arizona Articulation Proficiency Scale–3 contains items that enable the clinician to evaluate the child's accuracy in producing different vowels. The other tests do not incorporate formal vowel assessment.

56. d. According to the principle of communicative reinforcement, children's correct productions should be reinforced by pragmatically appropriate, communicatively meaningful responses. The praise (option a) and request to repeat the word five times (option b) draw attention to the child's phonology, whereas asking the child what he said (option c) does not reinforce the correct production.

57. b. The production of the tense /u/ for the lax /ʊ/ is an example of a tensing error. In all of the other utterances, a target tense vowel is produced as lax. Tenseness and laxness are features of vowels and pertain to degree of muscular tension in the vocal tract. In this example, the tense vowel /u/ (note the muscular tension of your tongue) is substituted for the lax counterpart /ʊ/ (note lack of muscular tension).

58. c. In the scoring scheme for the The Arizona Articulation Proficiency Scale–3, errors for sounds that occur frequently in the ambient language are penalized more than errors for sounds that are less frequent.

59. b. The cycles approach is designed for children whose errors are very consistent—that is, whose errors reflect simplifying phonological processes—and who are stimulable for correct speech-sound production for at least some of the sounds that are targeted in therapy.

60. e. Because the child's production of all of the measured behaviors, including the control sounds (related sound /v/ and unrelated sound /l/), is improving, it is not clear whether the child's increases are resulting from therapy or whether the child is experiencing a "spurt" in speech development.

61. a. The clinician in this scenario chose to train the earliest acquired fricative, /f/. This is an example of a developmental approach to goal selection.

62. c. Children who produce inconsistent error patterns typically take longer to learn the target sounds than do children who produce consistent errors, children who are stimulable for correct production, or children who show phonetic knowledge of a contrast.

63. c. Cluster reduction changes the number of consonants in a word, which changes the word's syllable structure. Stopping (option a), fronting (option b), deaffrication (option d), and backing (option e) are all process substitution errors that change one sound to another sound.

64. c. Velar fronting is a phonological process that changes the velar sounds /k/, /g/, and /ŋ/ to their alveolar counterparts. Of the words listed, only *ghost* (/goʊst/) has a velar sound.

65. c. All of the choices are phonological awareness tasks and enable the child to engage in language introspection. Tasks in which children are given the component segments of a word and are told to produce them as a fully coarticulated word are called *phoneme blending* tasks.

66. d. Computational analyses of the content of spoken English words have revealed that /ʃ/ occurs less frequently than do the sounds /s/ (option a), /d/ (option b), /l/ (option c), and /z/ (option e).

67. d. To recognize words, children require more acoustic information than do adults; children's ability to discriminate sound pairs that do not occur in the language or languages they are acquiring disappears at approximately 12 months of age, and children's word recognition in noise is much poorer than their word recognition in quiet—even more so than adults'.

68. c. A *phonological neighbor* is typically defined as a word that can be created by adding, deleting, or substituting a single phoneme in a target word. The words *tip* (option a), *gnat* (option b), and *snip* (option d) can all be created by substituting or adding a phoneme to nip, whereas *map* cannot.

69. a. The sound /s/ is characterized acoustically by high-frequency noise. This noise is usually in the frequency range that is impaired in children (and adults) with high-frequency hearing loss. Not surprisingly, it is often a sound that children with hearing loss produce in error, too.

70. d. Fletcher and Meldrum's (1968) often-cited finding was based on data from 20 children with normal lingual frena and 20 with short frena. The frenum is a flap of mucous membrane that extends from the floor of the mouth to the midline of the underside of the tongue. A short frenum has frequently been associated with ankyloglossia (tongue-tie) and believed to be the cause of speech problems as a result of restricted lingual range of motion. However, ankyloglossia as a causal agent in speech-sound disorders occurs very infrequently. The fact that the number of errors is within normal limits indicates that the frenum was not a causal agent.

71. b. Although children with phonological disorders often have a variety of speech-sound errors, the substitutions of glottal sounds for sounds with a supralaryngeal constriction is considerably more prevalent among children with cleft palates than among children with phonological disorders who have normal orofacial structure and function.

72. a. English plurals are formed with a suffix whose phonetic form is /s/, /z/, or /əz/, depending on the phonetic shape of the noun to which it affixes. These forms would potentially be affected by some or all of the processes in final consonant deletion (option b), stopping (option c), final consonant devoicing (option d), and cluster reduction (option e) but not by initial voicing (option a).

73. c. Stimulability is the ability of the child to produce a target sound, in isolation or in context, in response to visual and auditory stimulation provided by the clinician. Powell and coworkers (1991) found that stimulability was the single best predictor of how readily a child generalized a sound during therapy and that this was true for a variety of sounds for many children.

74. a. Relational analyses compare the child's productions to the normal adult targets. If a child is highly unintelligible, it may be impossible to tell what the targets themselves are, and thus making a relational analysis would be impossible.

75. d. The /s/ and /ʃ/ sounds are characterized by (relatively) high-frequency energy and are voiceless. A child with a high-frequency hearing loss would probably have difficulty discriminating between them.

76. a. Assimilation is a phonological process error, represented by /pop/ for *poke*. Progressive assimilations are errors in which a feature for a sound that occurs early in a word shows up again in place of a sound later in the word. In /pop/, the regressive error is the retention of the labial place of articulation in the final sound of the word *poke*.

77. a. Metathesis is a phonological process error, represented by /ɑsk/. In metathesis errors, the order of two sounds in a word is switched, as in switching the order of /k/ and /s/ in *ox*.

78. a. Coalescence errors are ones in which characteristics of two sounds—typically adjacent in a word—are combined into a third sound. The /Φ/ (voiceless bilabial fricative) in this production of small retains the voicing and frication of the target /s/ and the labial place of the /m/.

79. c. In their review of studies of phonological processes in typical children's acquisition of English, Stoel-Gammon and Dunn (1985) identified processes that disappear relatively early and ones that disappear relatively later. Final consonant deletion was identified as one of the processes that disappear relatively earlier.

80. b. Assimilation is a phonological process wherein one sound influences another, so that the second sound assumes the features of the influencing sound. It is a normal developmental process that is generally suppressed early in phonological development. Regressive nasal assimilation can occur if a word has a final nasal consonant and a nonnasal consonant earlier in the word. If nasal assimilation were to apply to the word *loon*, it might be produced as /nun/.

81. c. Children with childhood apraxia of speech are often observed to make more errors on speech sounds in longer words than in shorter words. Of the four words in this question, *Peter* is the longest both in terms of number of phonemes (four) and number of syllables (two).

82. a. Of the sounds listed, /j/ is the palatal glide, as in the words *you* (/ju/) and *yes* (/jɛs/). The sounds /r/ (option b) and /l/ (option d) are liquids, and /s/ (option c) and /f/ (option e) are fricatives.

83. a. Voice-onset time is an acoustic variable that is important in understanding the production characteristics of stop sounds. When stops are produced, durational differences exist in the stop burst and start of the vowel articulation, which differ according to whether the stop is voiced or voiceless. Long-lag voice-onset times are characteristic of word-initial voiceless stops in English, such as the /t/ in the beginning of the word *ten*.

84. e. Of the five levels of complexity listed, syllables (option e) is the least complex. Conversational speech (option a) is the most complex.

85. c. Mulford (1988) showed that blind children produce a significantly lower proportion of bilabial sounds, such as /p/, than do sighted children. This is evidence that the occurrence of bilabial sounds in children with typical vision is related in part to their visual salience.

86. b. Children who show phonetic knowledge of a contrast (by making measurable acoustic differences between target sounds and their substitutions) progress through therapy more quickly than those who do not. This was shown by Tyler and associates (1993). Children who only apparently substitute /t/ for /k/ are marking differences acoustically that listeners do not perceive. This suggests that they have phonetic knowledge of the contrast and increased potential for change with treatment, in comparison with children who are not marking the differences acoustically.

87. c. The fronting error of the /d/ for /k/ changes the target velar stop to an alveolar stop, and the initial voicing changes the target voiceless stop /k/ to a voiced stop /d/. According to processes analysis, those two process rules explain the speech-sound pattern error described.

88. a. The sound /ð/ occurs as an allophone of /d/ in Mexican Spanish, whereas it is a phoneme (albeit a very infrequently occurring one) in North American English.

89. b. The production of obstruent consonants—stops, fricatives, and affricates—requires the build-up of oral air pressure. Building up oral air pressure is difficult for individuals with velopharyngeal incompetence. The sounds /m/ (option a), /l/ (option c),

/j/ (option d), and /i/ (option e) are speech sounds that do not require the generation of high pressure but are produced with a relatively open vocal tract.

90. b. Morrisette's and Gierut (2002) finding has clear implications for the selection of treatment targets in phonological therapy for preschool children with severe speech-sound disorders. Lexical complexity is a composite of word frequency and neighborhood word density. Word frequency is the regularity with which a particular word occurs in a language, and research findings suggest that individuals tend to identify high-frequency words more readily than low-frequency words. Neighborhood density is a word measure of the phonetic structure of similar words. For example, *tea, stow*, and *doe* are neighbors of the word *toe*, inasmuch as the items vary in terms of a single phoneme difference. Research indicates that words from low-neighborhood densities, which have limited phonetic linkages with other words, are typically easier to identify that are high-density words. Stimulability is a measure of phonetic skill and not lexical complexity.

91. b. This and similar findings illustrate that the phonological processes used by children reflect, in part, the structure of the language that they are acquiring.

92. a. The palatal glide /j/ is produced with a tongue posture that is similar to that of the vowel /i/, which is a high front tense vowel. The vowel /u/ (option b) is similar to the glide /w/, whereas neither of the low vowels, /æ/ (option c) and /ɑ/ (option d), is associated with a glide.

93. d. Sonorant sounds are voiced sounds produced with a relatively open vocal tract. Of the sounds listed, only the liquid /l/ is sonorant.

94. a. For most of the first year of life, children are able to discriminate among sound contrasts that are not present in the language to which the child has been exposed. This ability declines toward the end of the first year of life, whereas the ability to perceive contrasts that are present in the ambient language improves.

95. d. The first syllable in *alone* is unstressed and the second is stressed. The other four words have a strong-weak pattern.

96. a. By definition, children who have childhood apraxia of speech do not have muscle weakness. A finding that a child had muscle weakness would suggest that the child might have a dysarthria. Severely unintelligible speech (option b), inconsistent error patterns (option c), vowel distortions (option d), and prosodic variations (option e) have all been reported as features of childhood apraxia of speech.

97. c. Of the five words in this question, only *enough* has a final consonant (/f/). The words *high* (option a), *sigh* (option b), *guy* (option d), and *toy* (option e) have simple consonant-vowel syllable shapes with no final consonants.

98. a. As in many dialects of English, the contrast between /θ/ and /f/ in word-final position is neutralized in African-American English.

99. d. The subphonetic elements of speech sounds have distinctive features, and sounds are categorized according to feature bundles. One feature system is classification according to the traditional features of voice, place, and manner of production. The sounds /p/ and /b/ (option a) differ only in voicing; the sounds /t/ and /s/ (option b) and /m/ and /b/ (option c) differ only in manner of articulation; and the sounds /n/ and /m/ (option e) differ in terms of place of articulation. The sounds /v/ and /d/ differ in both place of articulation and manner of articulation.

100. d. The voiced palatoalveolar affricate [dʒ] is not a phoneme in most dialects of Spanish. The voiceless fricative phoneme [x] does occur in Spanish but not in most dialects of English. The phonemes [m], [n], and [i] occur in both Spanish and English.

101. a. Targeting a single sound (in this case, /p/) is an example of a segment approach to goal selection. A phonological process approach (option b), a contrast approach (option c), and a distinctive features approach (option d) are all examples of linguistics-based approaches. These approaches focus on teaching sound contrasts and patterns to children who have multiple speech-sound errors.

Bibliography

Beckman, M. E., Yoneyama, K., & Edwards, J. (2003). Language specific and language universal: aspects of lingual obstruent productions in Japanese-acquiring children. *Journal of the Phonetic Society of Japan*, 7, 18–28.

Elbert, M., Powell, T., & Swartzlander, P. (1991). Stimulability as a factor in the phonological generalization of misarticulating preschool children. *Journal of Speech and Hearing Research*, 34, 1318–1328.

Felsenfeld, S., Broen, P. A., & McGae, M. (1994). A 28-year follow-up of adults with a history of moderate phonological disorder: linguistic and personality results. *Journal of Speech and Hearing Research*, 35, 1114–1125.

Felsenfeld, S., Broen, P. A., & McGae, M. (1994). A 28-year follow-up of adults with a history of moderate phonological disorder: educational and occupational results. *Journal of Speech and Hearing Research*, 37, 1341–1353.

Fletcher, S. C., & Meldram, J. R. (1968). Lingual function and relative length of the lingual frenulum. *Journal of Speech and Hearing Research*, *11*, 382–390.

Gierut, J. (2001). Complexity in phonological treatment: clinical factors. *Language, Speech, and Hearing in Schools*, *32*, 229–241.

Jakobson, R. (1971). *Studies on child language and aphasia*. The Hague: Mouton.

Koegel, R. L., Koegel, L. K., Costello Ingham, J., & Van Voy, K. (1988). Within-clinic versus outside-clinic self-monitoring of articulation to promote generalization. *Journal of Speech and Hearing Disorders*, *53*, 392–398.

MacNeilage, P. F. (2008). *The origin of speech*. New York: Oxford University Press.

Maken, M. A., & Barton, D. (1980). The acquisition of the voicing contrast in English: the study of voice onset time in word-initial stop consonants. *Journal of Child Language*, *7*, 41–74.

McBride-Chang, C. (1995). What is phonological awareness? *Journal of Educational Psychology*, *87*, 179.

Morrisette, M. L., & Gierut, J. (2002). Lexical organization and phonological change in treatment. *Journal of Speech, Language, and Hearing Research*, *45*, 143–159.

Mulford, R. (1988). First words of the blind. In M. Smith & J. L. Locke (Eds.), *The emergent lexicon: the child development of a linguistic vocabulary* (pp. 293–338). New York: Academic Press.

Pollock, K. E., & Hall, P. K. (1991). An analysis of the vowel misarticulations of five children with developmental apraxia of speech. *Clinical Linguistics and Phonetics*, *5*, 207–224.

Powell, T. W., Elbert, M., & Dinnsen, D. A. (1991). Stimulability as a factor in the phonologic generalization of misarticulating preschool children. *Journal of Speech and Hearing Research*, *34*, 1318–1328.

Rvachew, S. (1994). Speech perception training can facilitate sound production learning. *Journal of Speech and Hearing Research*, *37*, 347–357.

Sanders, E. (1972). When are speech sounds learned? *Journal of Speech and Hearing Disorders*, *37*, 55–63.

Shriberg, L. D., Austin, D., Lewis, B. A., McSweeney, J. L., & Wilson, D. L. (1997). The percentage of consonants correct (PCC) metric: extensions and reliability data. *Journal of Speech, Language, and Hearing Research*, *40*, 708–722.

Smit, A. B., Hand, L., Freilinger, J. J., Bernthal, J. E., & Bird, A. (1990). The Iowa Articulation Norms Project and its Nebraska replication. *Journal of Speech and Hearing Disorders*, *55*, 779–798.

Stoel-Gammon, C., & Dunn, C. (1985). *Normal and disordered phonology in children*. Baltimore, MD: University Park Press.

Templin, M. (1957). *Certain language skills in children, monograph series no. 26*. Minneapolis, MN: Institute of Child Welfare, University of Minnesota.

Tyler, A. A., Figurski, G. R., & Langsdale, T. (1993). Relationships between acoustically determined knowledge of stop place and voicing contrasts and phonological treatment progress. *Journal of Speech and Hearing Research*, *36*, 746–759.

Werker, J. F., & Stager, C. L. (2000). Developmental changes in infant speech perception and early word learning: Is there a link? In M. B. Broe (Ed.), *J. B. Pierrehumbert papers in laboratory phonology acquisition and the lexicon* (pp. 181–193). New York: Cambridge University Press.

CHAPTER 7

Child Language Disorders

Patricia A. Prelock

Diana B. Newman

1. Carlos is a 3-year-old boy with a delay in expressive language of 18 months and a delay in receptive language of 12 months. During play with his mother, he was observed responding to his mother's initiations by using simple gestures or showing his understanding by responding to her simple requests. He waited for his mother to initiate play but imitated her actions. What should be the speech-language pathologist's (SLP's) primary treatment goal?
   a. Increase the social contexts in which the child responds to requests
   b. Decrease the verbal output of the adult until the child begins to use verbal language
   c. Create opportunities for initiation through the use of nonverbal and verbal means
   d. Encourage the use of socially appropriate responses
   e. Provide opportunities for play with age-matched peers

2. Of the following observations, which would be indicative of a possible language impairment?
   a. The child is producing words with only sounds that are consistent with the words he or she already knows
   b. The child is communicating intent nonverbally before speaking his or her first words
   c. The child is demonstrating some disfluency in early speech
   d. The child is beginning to put two words together at age 36 months
   e. The child is pointing to request what he wants and to comment on what he sees

3. You are working with the family of a young child with a language impairment. Of the following statements, which would be the most appropriate for you to say to the family?

a. Reassure the parents that their child is just a late talker and will catch up

b. Urge the parents to have genetic testing

c. Discourage the child's parents and siblings from talking for the child, because this may be a primary cause of a language impairment

d. Advise the parent to have their child's hearing tested

e. Explain that the child will probably require language intervention throughout his time in school

4. Of the following assumptions about language impairment in children, which would be the least appropriate?

a. Language impairments place children at risk for later academic difficulties

b. Children with language impairments have intellectual deficits

c. Children with learning disabilities are likely to have language impairments

d. Language impairments may manifest themselves at different stages of life

e. Early language intervention should be a consideration for children with or at risk for language impairments

5. You are examining a child who produces fluent and well-formed sentences with adequate articulation. His language content, however, is often odd, and he is usually verbose. Comprehension also seems to be overly literal and conversational maintenance is poor. What language subtype would you predict this child is demonstrating?

a. Phonological-syntactic deficit

b. Lexical-syntactic deficit

c. Semantic-pragmatic deficit

d. Phonological programming deficit

e. Verbal dyspraxia

6. According to research evidence, what is an SLP appropriate way to formulate a prognosis for a young child with a language delay?

a. The SLP should avoid providing prognostic information as questions; for instance, "Will my daughter outgrow her language impairment?" cannot be answered

b. Families and clinicians have little difficulty making decisions about whether a young child with early expressive language delay will benefit from therapy

c. Single evaluation measures can be used to determine the severity of a young child's language impairment and the prognosis for successful outcomes

d. Clinical judgment is most appropriate for determining the severity of a child's language impairment

e. Trial therapy during an assessment period is an appropriate strategy for forming a prognosis

7. George is 8 years old and in the second grade. His teachers have noted difficulties in his ability to learn to read. They reported that he has difficulties in word recognition and reading comprehension. An assessment of his nonverbal IQ indicates performance in the typical range. George's mother identified concerns at home as well. George seems to have trouble understanding what is being said (e.g., directions, questions). His mother also noted difficulties in his ability to tell a story and to find the right words to explain what he wants to share. She suspects that George's vocabulary is not as well developed as those of his peers. In your initial assessment of George, you observe that George makes frequent errors in how he formulates sentences, such as selecting the wrong forms for irregular past tense. George's difficulties described are most consistent with a possible diagnosis of:

a. Autism spectrum disorder

b. Intellectual disability

c. Specific language impairment

d. Language delay

e. Articulation disorder

8. Damian is a 5-year-old African American boy whom you evaluated in a kindergarten screening. His speech was extremely difficult to understand. Damian is a speaker of African American English; however, your experience with other young speakers of this dialect suggests to you that Damian's language is impaired. You learn that he and his parents have just moved from an impoverished community in Louisiana, where he attended an age-appropriate class in a school in which approximately 90% of his classmates were black; the school district that you are currently serving is composed almost entirely of white administrators, staff, and students. Damian's kindergarten teacher has expressed concerns about his language. She says he is hard to understand, has a limited vocabulary, cannot master letter-sound correspondences, and has trouble listening to and understanding others. Of the following occurrences, which would increase your suspicion of a possible diagnosis of language impairment?

a. Damian's mother reports that he has always talked differently than his siblings and peers

b. Damian's score on a test of articulation of standard English is in the 10th percentile

c. Damian becomes frustrated when you ask him to repeat himself

d. Damian frequently drops off the ends of the words he produces (e.g., he says "nes" instead of "nest")

e. Damian is hesitant to respond to the questions posed to him during the kindergarten screening

9. Damian is a 5-year-old African American boy whom you evaluated in a kindergarten screening. His speech

was extremely difficult to understand. Damian is a speaker of African American English; however, your experience with other young speakers of this dialect suggests to you that Damian's language is impaired. You learn that he and his parents have just moved from an impoverished community in Louisiana, where he attended an age-appropriate class in a school in which approximately 90% of his classmates were black; the school district that you are currently serving is composed almost entirely of white administrators, staff, and students. Damian's kindergarten teacher has expressed concerns about his language. She says he is hard to understand, has a limited vocabulary, cannot master letter-sound correspondences, and has trouble listening to and understanding others. In view of Damian's background, which of the following would suggest to you that Damian is exhibiting a language difference as opposed to a language impairment?

a. Damian is cooperative and responsive during the kindergarten screening

b. Damian's mother is equally difficult to understand, and she considers Damian to be competent in his language in comparison with his siblings

c. Damian's scores on a test of vocabulary standardized on a cross-section of North American native English speakers are in the 35th percentile

d. Damian's mother has no trouble understanding him

e. Damian knows when he is not being understood and tries to repeat what he has said

10. You are evaluating 18-month-old Ethan, whose mother expresses concerns about his speech and language development. She reports he is "not talking like other kids his age" and uses repeated vocalizations (e.g., "eh eh eh eh" while pointing) to communicate. Recently, Ethan has started to use some words, which are paired with a gesture. For example, he says "more" while pointing to something he wants, or he says "up" while raising his arms to be lifted up. In your interaction with Ethan, he looks at you, smiles, and follows your eye gaze to distal objects. He understands simple phrases that his mother directs to him and carries out two-step commands (e.g., "Pick up the ball and give it to me"). There are no reports of immediate or extended family members who have had language impairments. Ethan has no history of ear infections and passed a recent hearing screening. What would increase your suspicion of a diagnosis of language impairment?

a. Ethan demonstrated a limited ability to engage in symbolic play

b. Ethan used many more gestures than sounds or words

c. Ethan was only able to attend to tasks for a short period

d. Ethan exhibited a limited number of facial expressions

e. Ethan preferred to play with sensory (e.g., musical toys) and cause-effect toys

11. You are evaluating 18-month-old Ethan, whose mother expresses concerns about his speech and language development. She reports he is "not talking like other kids his age" and uses repeated vocalizations (e.g., "eh eh eh eh" while pointing) to communicate. Recently, Ethan has started to use some words, which are paired with a gesture. For example, he says "more" while pointing to something he wants, or he says "up" while raising his arms to be lifted up. In your interaction with Ethan, he looks at you, smiles, and follows your eye gaze to distal objects. He understands simple phrases that his mother directs to him and carries out two-step commands (e.g., "Pick up the ball and give it to me"). There are no reports of immediate or extended family members who have had language impairments. Ethan has no history of ear infections and passed a recent hearing screening. What should Ethan's mother expect with time if her child does not have a language impairment but is rather a "late talker"?

a. Ethan will begin to engage in unusual repetitive behaviors

b. Ethan will slowly add new words and begin to combine them into two-word utterances

c. Any new words that Ethan utters are likely to be distorted and difficult to understand

d. Ethan may develop aggressive behaviors to cope with his inability to communicate effectively

e. Ethan will probably lose words that he has heard previously in his speech

12. Amelia is a 19-month-old who has been monitored by a Birth to Three program in her area because she was born 8 weeks prematurely and her primary care physician referred her for developmental follow-up. As the SLP participating in her Birth to Three follow-up, you visited Amelia's home and noticed that Amelia demonstrated little eye contact, no jargoning, and a few screeching sounds when she was unhappy or wanted something. She tended to perform the same actions over and over again with her toys and preferred to play without an adult joining in. Noting that her daughter does not seem to like her, Amelia's mother has been frustrated in her efforts to get her daughter to respond. Amelia's mother also recently lost her job and has been raising not only Amelia but also a 4-year-old son with little support from her family. What would be your next step in supporting this family?

a. Tell the mother that her daughter has autism

b. Explain to the mother that the stress in her life is likely to affect her daughter's ability to connect

c. Remind her that Amelia was premature and is doing what might be expected of a younger toddler and that it will take some time to adjust

d. Acknowledge the mother's concerns and that you share those concerns, and suggest an assessment plan for addressing Amelia's needs and those of the family

e. Acknowledge the current stresses affecting the mother's situation and offer to find personal care or respite support to alleviate some of her immediate needs

13. Amelia is a 19-month-old who has been monitored by a Birth to Three program in her area because she was born 8 weeks prematurely and her primary care physician referred her for developmental follow-up. As the SLP participating in her Birth to Three follow-up, you visited Amelia's home and noticed that Amelia demonstrated little eye contact, no jargoning, and a few screeching sounds when she was unhappy or wanted something. She tended to perform the same actions over and over again with her toys and preferred to play without an adult joining in. Noting that her daughter does not seem to like her, Amelia's mother has been frustrated in her efforts to get her daughter to respond. Amelia's mother also recently lost her job and has been raising not only Amelia but also a 4-year-old son with little support from her family. A case manager, who is an early childhood special educator, is assigned to Amelia and her family. The case manager coordinates the services among the disciplines involved in Amelia's case, including the services of the SLP, a social worker, a developmental pediatrician, and a psychologist. It is determined that the SLP and the case manager will assess the child, and the social worker will assess the support needs of Amelia's mother. The psychologist and developmental pediatrician have agreed to be consulted about diagnostic, behavior, and medical or developmental questions and may or may not see Amelia individually. Of the following assessment team approaches, which is the case manager using to support Amelia and her family?
    a. Unidisciplinary team approach
    b. Multidisciplinary team approach
    c. Interdisciplinary team approach
    d. Transdisciplinary team approach
    e. Coordinated services approach

14. Of the following problems, which is the best predictor of autism in young children?
    a. Impairment in receptive language
    b. Impairment in expressive language
    c. Impairment in joint attention
    d. Impairment in pretend play
    e. Impairment in imitation

15. Theory of mind has been reported frequently as an area of deficit for children and adolescents with autism spectrum disorders. What assessment task could provide you with specific information about an individual's theory of mind?
    a. Assessment of figurative language use
    b. Assessment of word knowledge
    c. Assessment of the number of quality interactions
    d. Assessment of pitch, intensity, and intonation in conversation
    e. Assessment of narrative language and storytelling

16. You are working with a 7-year-old with a severe language disorder. Some members of the educational assessment team believe that the child does not have the cognitive abilities to perform as expected in the classroom or to fully benefit from the intervention plan being proposed. You recognize that the child's expressive language impairment is interfering with an adequate assessment of his potential. The child is able to point and respond to questions but has difficulty with oral and motor imitation. You believe his nonverbal intelligence is within normal limits. What measure of cognitive ability could you administer to provide support for your assumption about this child's potential?
    a. Leiter International Performance Scale−R
    b. Merrill-Palmer Scales of Mental Tests
    c. Cognitive Abilities Scale
    d. Test of Nonverbal Intelligence−3
    e. Swanson Cognitive Abilities Scale

17. An educational team is attempting to support the social communication of Jack, an 8-year-old with autism. They are making some decisions about the appropriateness of interventions that could be implemented in the general education classroom, in which Jack is included. They are asking you as the SLP to make a recommendation about an intervention that provides Jack with choices in the classroom, capitalizes on his interests in maps and dinosaurs, shares the control of teaching opportunities so that sometimes Jack takes the lead and sometimes the adult takes the lead, and is based on evidence of supporting social communication across communicative partners and learning contexts. What intervention would you recommend?
    a. Floor time training
    b. Pivotal response training
    c. Discrete trial training
    d. Social story training
    e. Sensory integration training

18. The use of imitation as an intervention strategy for children with language impairment is limited because it:
    a. Is clinician or adult controlled
    b. Is contextualized speech
    c. Relies on semantic knowledge

d. Lacks a focus on syntactic structure

e. Fails to account for communicative intent

19. Prelinguistic milieu teaching fosters a child's interest in communicating by:
    a. Placing desired objects out of reach, waiting expectantly, or sabotaging routines that violate an expectation
    b. Showing, pointing to, and commenting on objects of interest
    c. Modeling a desired production and reinforcing the child's attempts at communicating
    d. Following a child's lead in play and allowing the child to select toys of interest
    e. Differentially reinforcing responses, prompting responses, and fading responses

20. Michael is just beginning his freshman year in high school. He received speech and language therapy in kindergarten until the fifth grade but was dismissed from therapy before going to middle school. Michael's speech and language history was characterized by difficulty with syntactic structure, difficulty with identifying and communicating the most relevant information when interacting with adults and peers, poor attention to tasks, chronic ear infections, and poor social relationships. Although he had some early speech sound deficits, these have been resolved and sentence structure is appropriate. Michael has always been verbal, but his expressive language has often masked his difficulties in comprehension. He is a good reader, but his written language is unorganized and his spelling is poor. His written language is adequate when adaptations are made for keyboard use and extra time is given to complete the required tasks, although his expository writing is usually factual with few inferences or integration of ideas. Math performance has been inconsistent, and word problems continue to challenge him. Michael has had periodic tutoring in the summer for written language, reading comprehension, and math. His teachers are increasingly worried about his transition to high school. They have also noticed that his social problems have increased. He does not seem to recognize the nonverbal cues of his peers, fails to read their facial expressions and does not have a sense of idiomatic expressions. What do you suspect might explain Michael's current profile?
    a. Specific language impairment
    b. Asperger disorder
    c. Nonverbal learning disability
    d. Attention deficit/hyperactivity disorder (ADHD)
    e. Dyslexia

21. The most common phonological problem associated with a history of otitis media in young children during their first 2 years of life is:

a. Cluster reduction

b. Nasalization

c. Velar fronting

d. Stridency deletion

e. Gliding

22. In comparison with the narratives of children who do not have language impairment, those of children with language impairments include:
    a. A similar number of episodes but less story complexity
    b. More intrusions of irrelevant information but accurate use of cohesive devices
    c. Less use of conjunctions and of elaborated noun phrases
    d. Adequate use of personal pronouns and weak use of past-tense verbs
    e. Shorter and less complex communication units (C-units) but adequate word use and syntactic structure

23. Discrete trial teaching typically involves:
    a. Establishing meaningful communication
    b. Using differential reinforcement, modeling, and prompting
    c. Using more child-initiated than adult-initiated interactions
    d. Developing complex syntactic and semantic structures
    e. Using child choice and child-preferred materials

24. When developing intervention goal priorities for children with language impairment, what would be the highest priority consideration in language intervention?
    a. Forms and functions used in 50% to 90% of the required contexts
    b. Forms that a child does not use at all
    c. Forms that a child does not appear to understand in receptive task formats
    d. Forms and functions used in 1% to 10% of required contexts and understood in receptive task formats
    e. Forms and functions that a child uses in 10% to 50% of required contexts

25. Hybrid language intervention approaches include:
    a. Facilitated play
    b. Focused stimulation
    c. Drill
    d. Modeling
    e. Clinician-directed activities

26. You have established a goal for increasing a child's use of conventional gestures. To support your efforts to facilitate the meaningful use of gestures, you create a need for communication with which of the following activities?

a. A routine in which you present an object to the child, and then you wait expectantly for the child to look, vocalize, and gesture

b. A routine in which you present an object to the child, and then you give the child the object if the child looks at it

c. A routine in which the child looks at an object and then you give the child the object when the child points at it

d. A routine in which the child looks at an object and you verbally prompt the child for a gaze

e. A routine in which the child looks at an object and you model a related vocalization

27. Children with specific language impairment typically exhibit deficits in:
   a. Understanding word meanings
   b. Understanding short sentences
   c. Producing sentences with appropriate morphological endings and syntax
   d. Demonstrating adequate nonverbal cognitive abilities
   e. Managing the motor aspects of written language

28. If you are planning treatment for a 6-year-old child with a multiple speech-sound disorder, what would be an effective strategy for initiating your intervention with this child?
   a. Identify the child's phonological processes and begin to address them by using a minimal-pair approach
   b. Emphasize the child's auditory discrimination of error versus correct sounds
   c. Consider the developmental occurrence of each sound and address production sound by sound
   d. Begin with sounds that the child can say, and use those to facilitate production with error sounds
   e. Teach error sounds in isolation first, followed by nonsense syllables and then real words

29. Billy is a 4½-year-old with multiple speech sound errors. His error pattern includes final consonant deletion, gliding, cluster reduction, and stridency deletion. You are the SLP assigned to this child. Which is an appropriate recommendation for intervention?
   a. Refer Billy for a comprehensive evaluation to rule out a potential cognitive deficit
   b. Defer treatment because the phonological processes Billy is exhibiting are those typically seen in young children
   c. Consult with the family and provide informal support through storybook reading and emergent literacy activities that focus on Billy's error sounds
   d. Focus on the production of /m/ and /p/ because these are early acquired and frequently used sounds
   e. Initiate a language-based phonological approach beginning with the production of final consonants

30. What is an appropriate pragmatic language goal for facilitating a young child's use of language in meaningful contexts?
   a. During story retelling, the child will use irregular past tense in five targeted verbs 80% of the time
   b. During conversation, the child will produce final consonants in single-syllable words with 90% accuracy
   c. During play, the child will initiate a turn and respond to a request either verbally or nonverbally 80% of the time
   d. During play, the child will produce clusters with 75% accuracy
   e. During one-on-one intervention, the child will produce two- and three-word combinations 90% of the time

31. Early language intervention for infants at risk for language deficits should focus on:
   a. Creating readiness activities in the context of play
   b. Introducing storybook reading
   c. Teaching symbolic play
   d. Training primary caregivers to facilitate language
   e. Consulting with the infant's physician about indications of language impairment

32. Children with discourse problems are likely to require support for addressing challenges in:
   a. Morphology
   b. Vocabulary
   c. Cohesive devices
   d. Gesture use
   e. Phonology

33. ADHD can be differentiated from a language disorder because:
   a. ADHD and language disorders seldom co-occur
   b. The *DSM-IV-TR* (American Psychiatric Association, 2000) diagnostic criteria for ADHD clearly specifies the criteria for ADHD
   c. Children with ADHD seldom have learning disabilities, whereas children with language disorders often have learning disabilities
   d. ADHD is a more behaviorally based disorder, whereas language disorders are more cognitively based
   e. Tests designed to assess language are clearly focused on knowledge and use of language structures

34. The current literature in language and literacy suggests that phonological awareness is a skill that:
   a. Represents an ability to think about, reflect on, or come to a mental realization of the nature and functions of language
   b. Can help predict a child's ability to read words in second grade

c. Refers to letter-sound correspondence and linking written symbols with phonemes
d. Is best assessed through knowledge of the alphabet
e. Is unlikely to improve with intervention after second grade

35. SLPs are in a unique position to support children with or at risk for reading disabilities because:
a. SLPs work with developmental language problems
b. SLPs build word attack and word recognition skills
c. SLPs emphasize the development of phonics
d. SLPs support orthographic word identification
e. SLPs provide individual assessment and intervention

36. Children with learning disabilities are generally viewed as:
a. No more or less popular than their typically developing peers
b. Different by their teachers but not by their peers in their social skills
c. Having similar social skills as their peers according to their own self-report
d. Experiencing a more hostile communication environment with peers
e. Struggling with peer relationships in childhood but with little connection to later academic, vocational, or emotional behavior

37. You have just begun a job at a local high school as an SLP. You are reviewing historical records on students who were discharged from treatment in the past 2 years. You are surprised to note that Maria, a 17-year-old with developmental delays, had not been seen in therapy for at least 2 years. In your interactions with her in the hallway and the lunchroom, she continues to demonstrate a significant communication deficit. When you revisit her records, you find that Maria was no longer receiving treatment because test scores indicated that her cognitive ability and language ability were commensurate. You are disappointed in the decision to have her dropped from therapy and the former SLP's inappropriate use of:
a. Low achievement scores
b. Cognitive referencing
c. Response to intervention
d. A wait-to-fail formula
e. Verbal performance measures

38. Joshua is a second grader, and you are providing language intervention for him. He has some difficulty in spelling during written language tasks. Although he has knowledge of the alphabet and realizes that letters have names, he continues to omit vowels in many of his spellings and seems to encode only parts of the words he is writing. His spelling is at what developmental level?

a. Nonspelling
b. Invented spelling
c. Phonetic spelling
d. Mixed phonetic and visual spelling
e. Conventional spelling

39. How does the literature describe the written language of school-aged children with language impairments and learning disabilities (LLD)?
a. Written narratives are more challenging than expository summaries for children with LLD
b. Written language length for students with LLD is similar to that of typical peers, although complexity may differ
c. Morphological errors are common in the written language samples of children with LLD
d. Children with LLD are generally able to connect their ideas by using cohesive ties
e. The planning and revising skills of children with LLD are similar to those of children who are typically developing

40. You are working with a preschool-aged child who has a specific language impairment. You begin therapy by introducing a play scenario. You and the child are helping a farmer make sure all his animals are in the barn before he goes to bed. You take a cow, put it in the barn, and say, "The cow is in the barn." Then you find a horse and say, "The horse is in the barn." Then you ask the child, "What about the sheep?" The child says "Sheep." You say, "Yes, a sheep. Let's put the sheep in the barn." Now you say, "The cow is in the barn," "The horse is in the barn," and "The sheep is in the barn." Then you say, "How about the pig?" The child says, "Pig in barn." You say, "Yes he is. The pig is in the barn. Is the chicken in the barn? He is in the barn. Tell the farmer. Tell him, 'The chicken is in the barn.'" And the child says, "Chicken is in barn." You end by saying, "Yes, now everyone is in the barn. Now the farmer can go to bed." This approach to language facilitation is known as:
a. Vertical restructuring
b. Parallel talk
c. Focused stimulation
d. Expansion
e. Recasting

41. When distances between a child and a communication partner and between the child and a communication book or board are increased, and when responses (i.e., the child gets a picture, seeks a communication partner, and places the pictures in the partner's hand to get what he or she wants) are trained in new settings, in what phase of the Picture Exchange Communication System (PECS) is the child likely to be working?
a. Commenting phase
b. Physical exchange phase

c. Answering questions phase

d. Picture discrimination phase

e. Expanding spontaneity phase

42. Long-term memory is a complex cognitive process that involves both declarative knowledge, which is knowing the facts, and procedural knowledge, which is:
    a. Knowing that information fades over time
    b. Knowing how to perform an action
    c. Knowing how to retrieve information
    d. Knowing the extent and depth of available information
    e. Knowing the ease with which a word can be used spontaneously

43. Short-term memory has control processes that help an individual to remember information. One of these processes allows the person to place information into meaningful categories. This process is known as:
    a. Tagging information
    b. Relating information
    c. Using mnemonics
    d. Clustering
    e. Chunking

44. The American Speech-Language-Hearing Association (1988) defined three levels of prevention (primary, secondary, and tertiary) that can be applied to communication disorders. Of the following scenarios, which is an example of teritary prevention?
    a. Conducting neonatal hearing screening to detect hearing loss and to provide early amplification or cochlear implantation
    b. Setting up a language stimulation class for teenaged mothers to help them learn techniques for encouraging language development
    c. Offering low-cost speech and hearing screenings at community events
    d. Providing special education services to a child with autism spectrum disorder
    e. Offering language literacy workshops for parents of children at risk

45. If a child has mild to moderate mental retardation, dysmorphic facial features, a hoarse voice quality, hypersensitivities to sound, partial chromosome deletion, and relative strengths in verbal ability but delays in language development, what is likely to be diagnosed?
    a. Down syndrome
    b. Prader-Willi syndrome
    c. Angelman syndrome
    d. Williams syndrome
    e. Fragile X syndrome

46. Advanced audio coding (AAC) is an intervention that can be used to support children who are deaf-blind with higher cognitive abilities. An example of aided AAC is:
    a. Finger spelling
    b. Anticipatory cues
    c. Opticon
    d. Braille
    e. Communication board

47. Strategy instruction has a critical role in supporting students with language learning disabilities. Which strategy provides support, functions as a tool, extends the range of the student, allows the student to accomplish a task not otherwise possible, and is used selectively to aid the student when needed?
    a. Self-reinforcement
    b. Goal setting
    c. Self-instruction
    d. Self-monitoring
    e. Scaffolding

48. Jennifer has a qualitative impairment in social interaction with no clinically significant delay in her language or cognitive development, but she does have a specific interest in talking about storms, specifically hurricanes and tornadoes. It is likely she will be receive a diagnosis of:
    a. Asperger disorder
    b. Rett disorder
    c. Autistic disorder
    d. Childhood disintegrative disorder
    e. Pervasive development disorder, not otherwise specified (PDD-NOS)

49. A pragmatic difference typically reported for a child using African American Vernacular English (AAVE) in comparison with a child using standard American English might be described as follows:
    a. Interrupting a conversation is typically not done in standard American English, whereas it is often considered helpful to a conversation in AAVE
    b. Intense and dynamic verbal behavior in public conversations is consider acceptable in AAVE, whereas more restraint and less intensity is more typical of standard American English
    c. Narratives in AAVE are more topic-centered, whereas standard American English narratives are more associational
    d. Direct eye contact is considered proper speaking and listening behavior for children with AAVE, whereas indirect eye contact is considered proper listening behavior for children with standard American English
    e. Wit and sarcasm are important elements of interactions in standard American English but are less popular pragmatic characteristics in AAVE

50. When you identify a deficient or an emerging skill, intervene to teach principles of a particular task, and then reassess how modifiable a child's performance is, you are using what form of dynamic assessment?
   a. Testing the limits
   b. Interviewing on responses
   c. Graduated prompting
   d. Test-teach-retest
   e. Measure modifiability

51. Best practices for school-based SLPs include referring to state educational standards when identifying goals and objectives for students in their caseloads or workloads. The reason for such practice is:
   a. To make sure all students on the caseload or workload can master all standards
   b. To ensure that only linguistically based standards are addressed during therapy
   c. To identify the standards that cause students academic difficulty and work on only those standards
   d. To determine and work on underlying linguistic skills that hinder students from meeting the standards
   e. To facilitate the development of nonlinguistic standards in students with language disorders

52. In assessment of language skills, the high school planning and placement team urges the SLP to use cognitive referencing for eligibility for speech-language intervention. This is:
   a. Appropriate because language functioning cannot surpass cognitive levels even with intervention
   b. Appropriate because specific cognitive skills are prerequisites to language development
   c. Inappropriate because cognitive prerequisites are neither sufficient nor necessary for language development
   d. Inappropriate because cognitive referencing is suitable only for preschoolers
   e. Inappropriate because SLPs do not have knowledge of cognitive testing

53. Consider the three-tiered model of responsiveness to intervention (RTI). Which activity might a SLP consider for a tier 2 level of intervention in the general education classroom?
   a. Rereading the social studies chapter to a small group of students
   b. Previewing the social studies test with a small group of struggling students
   c. Identifying and practicing how to "look back" for key information in the social studies chapter with a small group of struggling students

d. Preteaching the social studies vocabulary to a small group of students
   e. Enlarging the print of the social studies study guide given by the classroom teacher

54. Of the following observations, which is an example of a well written present level of educational performance (PLEP)?
   a. Joe achieved a standard score of 100 on the receptive core of the Clinical Evaluation of Language Fundamentals—4
   b. Joe scored in the average range on the receptive core of the Clinical Evaluation of Language Fundamentals—4
   c. Joe becomes easily confused with multistep directions given orally in the classroom
   d. Joe appears unaware of directions
   e. Joe performed with a standard score of 75 on the receptive core of the Clinical Evaluation of Language Fundamentals—4

55. For a student with a word retrieval difficulty, providing a word bank for written assignments is an example of:
   a. A modification
   b. An accommodation
   c. An inclusion
   d. An objective
   e. All of the above

56. Which activity is the best example of strategy instruction?
   a. Preteaching the vocabulary
   b. Chunking key vocabulary words by significant features
   c. Repeating key vocabulary words 10 times each
   d. Reducing the number of vocabulary words necessary to learn
   e. None of the above

57. Questioning the oral direction given by a teacher (e.g., as being incomplete) is an example of:
   a. Pragmatics
   b. Phonological awareness
   c. Metalinguistic awareness
   d. Morphological awareness
   e. Syntax

58. An adolescent has significant difficulty with following oral directions of increasing length and complexity. The SLP introduces a method of visualization that has been identified as improving auditory memory. The young student is taught this strategy and has had guided practice each week for 6 weeks. The ability to follow oral directions is now retested. This format of assessment is known as:
   a. Narrative assessment
   b. Assessment of semantic development

c. Dynamic assessment

d. Assessment of language processing capacity

e. Norm-referenced assessment

59. The extent to which clinician-directed intervention should be used is debated; however, what is commonly agreed is that clinician-directed intervention is an appropriate model _____.

a. At the initial stages of therapy

b. At the middle stages of therapy

c. During transition and generalization in therapy

d. At the final stages of therapy, immediately before dismissal

e. At the initial and final stages of therapy

60. Although no single pattern of speech and language skills is specific to all children with Down syndrome, certain strengths and challenges are common for most of the children in this population. Of the following statements, therefore, which would be an example of a language profile common to an 8-year-old with Down syndrome?

a. Morphology is a relative strength

b. Phonology is commensurate with chronological age

c. Expressive language skills are more advanced than receptive language skills

d. Receptive language skills are more advanced than expressive language skills

e. Receptive and expressive skills are equivalent

61. You are working with a 10-year-old boy whose vocabulary is average, as measured on both standardized and criterion-referenced assessments. However, he often interrupts other speakers and irritates his listeners; as a result, he is avoided by many peers. Treatment should focus on:

a. Discourse

b. Syntax

c. Morphology

d. Semantics

e. Phonology

62. You are working with an adolescent who has receptive and expressive vocabulary problems. All other areas of language are appropriate. He is getting Ds in most of his content area classes in middle school and has few friends. In therapy, it would be best to focus primarily on:

a. Increasing auditory discrimination skills

b. Increasing his use of complex sentences containing subordination clauses

c. Increasing his social use of language

d. Increasing his ability to understand and use figurative language

e. Increasing his word definition and word retrieval skills

63. Of the following statements, which is *not* true about dynamic assessment?

a. The SLP actively intervenes during the assessment with the child with the goal of intentionally changing present level of language skills.

b. The assessment focuses on the child's processes of problem solving, including those that encourage as well as hinder successful communication.

c. The assessment provides a baseline for intervention but should not be used to monitor progress in a Response to Intervention model.

d. The most unique information from the assessment is information about how a child responds to intervention.

e. Dynamic assessment should be administered in a pretest-intervention-posttest format.

64. Of the following statements, which is *not* true?

a. Collaboration with classroom teachers is not important in assessment of children's language strengths and needs

b. A child's chronological age is not always the best predictor of what kind of treatment is appropriate; developmental level is a more reliable indicator

c. After taking a global standardized language assessment, some children referred for language difficulties require assessment of discourse skills

d. Criterion-referenced assessment may include teacher checklists

e. A combination of standardized measures and criterion-referenced assessment provides information for intervention baseline

65. For students with writing problems, argument text is typically more difficult than descriptive text because of:

a. Required length

b. Differences in grammar and punctuation

c. Knowledge about the topic

d. Planning and revising on the basis of expectations of the reader

e. Generating a story grammar

66. The assignment in science class requires students to compare oceans with lakes. On which level of Bloom's taxonomy of learning objectives is this assignment?

a. Knowledge

b. Comprehension

c. Analysis

d. Synthesis

e. Evaluation

67. In an assessment of the lexical diversity of a child's narratives, which of the following is the best measure?

a. Type-token ratio

b. Number of different words

c. Expressive Vocabulary Test

d. Mean length of utterance
e. Mean length of a C-unit

68. When standardized measures are used, which criterion is most appropriate in identifying the presence of a language disorder?
    a. 1.0 standard deviation on two tests
    b. 1.25 to 1.5 standard deviations on one test
    c. 1.25 to 1.5 standard deviations on two tests
    d. 2.0 or more standard deviations on one test
    e. 2.0 or more standard deviations on two tests

69. According to models of language production such as Bock and Levelt's (1994), which of the following is the order of levels in oral language production?
    a. Lexical-semantic level, conceptual level, phonological level, utterance
    b. Conceptual level, lexical-semantic level, phonological level, utterance
    c. Conceptual level, phonological form, lexical-semantic level, utterance
    d. Utterance, conceptual level, phonological form, lexical-semantic level
    e. Utterance, phonological form, conceptual level, lexical-semantic level

70. Of the following terms, which is *not* typically used to describe a 7-year-old who performs poorly in a language assessment?
    a. Language impairment
    b. Language disability
    c. Language disorder
    d. Language delay
    e. Childhood aphasia

71. Of the following models of child language disorders, which provides the most information for planning intervention for a child with a language-learning disability?
    a. Systems
    b. Categorical
    c. Specific disabilities
    d. Descriptive-developmental
    e. Medical

72. The assignment in science class requires students to define different bodies of water such as oceans, lakes etc. On which level of Bloom's taxonomy of learning objectives is this assignment?
    a. Knowledge
    b. Comprehension
    c. Analysis
    d. Synthesis
    e. Evaluation

73. Of the following activities, which is an example of a working memory task?

    a. Sharing a story about a childhood experience
    b. Blending phonemes into words
    c. Listing animals that live in the forest
    d. Repeating a phone number
    e. Repeating sentences verbatim

74. The difference between phonological awareness and phonics is that:
    a. Phonological awareness involves sounds in written words, and phonics involves the relationship between sounds and spoken symbols
    b. Phonological awareness involves sounds in spoken words, and phonics involves the relationship between sounds and written symbols
    c. Phonological awareness involves syllables in spoken words, and phonics involves the relationship between syllables and written symbols
    d. Phonological awareness involves syllables in written words, and phonics involves the relationship between syllables and spoken symbols
    e. Phonological awareness involves sounds in spoken words, and phonics involves the relationship between syllables and spoken symbols

75. Elicited imitation ("Say what I say") and elicited production is part of:
    a. Classroom observation
    b. Criterion-referenced procedures
    c. Developmental scales
    d. Child-centered activities
    e. Play-based assessment

76. _____ requires a listener to recognize a discrepancy between what is being said and what is really meant and to realize the purpose in making that comment.
    a. Persuasion
    b. Sarcasm
    c. Negotiation
    d. Conversation
    e. Narration

77. Of the following strategies, which has *not* been suggested for use by a speaker to improve retrieval of known words?
    a. Mnemonic cueing
    b. Rehearsal
    c. Pausing
    d. Attribute-cueing
    e. Word bank

78. As content of the lexicon improves with age, there is typically improvement in _____ of retrieving words.
    a. only speed
    b. only accuracy
    c. either speed or accuracy
    d. both speed and accuracy
    e. neither speed nor accuracy

79. An adolescent often substitutes a similar-sounding real or nonsense word for a word that he or she very well comprehends: for example, "tethoscope" for "stethoscope." This is an example of:
    a. A word-finding disorder when the semantic aspects of a target word are inaccessible
    b. A receptive vocabulary weakness
    c. A word-finding disorder when the phonological features of a target word are blocked
    d. An expressive vocabulary weakness
    e. Both a receptive and expressive vocabulary weakness

80. Divergent naming tasks require a broad lexical search. Of the following questions, which is an example of such a task?
    a. "Tell me all the animals you can think of"
    b. "Tell me the name of this animal"
    c. "Tell me a sentence with the word *animal* in it"
    d. "Name the pictures" (e.g., in the Boston Naming Test)
    e. "Name these pictures as quickly as you can" (e.g., in the Rapid Naming subtests of the Comprehensive Test of Phonological Processing)

81. Dyslexia is conceptualized as a specialized language-based reading disorder characterized by difficulty in decoding, usually reflecting insufficient phonological processing. This description is the basis for which of the following learning disability theories?
    a. Core phonological deficit hypothesis
    b. Matthew effect
    c. Simple view
    d. Whole-language theory
    e. Phonological processes

82. The National Reading Panel (2006) identified important components of learning to read. These include phonemic awareness, fluency, vocabulary, and text comprehension. Of the following SLP-led activities, which is an example of simultaneously targeting phonemic awareness and vocabulary?
    a. Orally presenting words from the classroom curriculum and asking the children to discuss what each word means
    b. Orally presenting words from the classroom curriculum and asking the children to identify the words that have three or more syllables
    c. Orally presenting words from the classroom curriculum and asking the children to use two of them in one sentence
    d. Orally presenting words from the classroom curriculum, asking the children to identify the words that begin with a target phoneme, and asking the children to use those words in sentences
    e. Reading words from the classroom curriculum several times while having the children read them along with the SLP

83. Of the following descriptions, which is *not* an example of a semantic-pragmatic deficit characteristically seen in autism spectrum disorders?
    a. Literal interpretation of figurative language
    b. Poor turn-taking and topic maintenance
    c. Poor ability when reading to sound out words that are not recognized
    d. Problems initiating or responding to questions
    e. Difficulty with verbal and nonverbal cues of conversational partners

84. Deficits in theory of mind are applicable to the population of individuals with which communication disorders?
    a. Language-learning disabilities
    b. Autism
    c. Hearing loss
    d. Intellectual deficits
    e. Dyslexia

85. A child produces this narrative: "My dog woke up. Then he runned outside. Then he eated his food." In assessing story structure, you would consider this narrative at which level?
    a. Heaps
    b. Descriptive sequence
    c. Action sequence
    d. Reactive sequence
    e. True narrative

86. In transcribing a language sample to be scored by hand, transcribing the examiner's comments verbatim is:
    a. Never necessary
    b. Necessary if the examiner's comments are part of a dialogue or leading
    c. Always necessary
    d. Necessary if the examiner's comments are not part of a dialogue or are nonleading
    e. In question; there is no consensus about transcribing the examiner's comments

87. Spelling involves which process or processes?
    a. Alphabetic, orthographic, and morphological knowledge
    b. Alphabetic and orthographic knowledge
    c. Alphabetic and morphological knowledge
    d. Only alphabetic knowledge
    e. Only orthographic knowledge

88. In child language therapy, intervention approaches are considered along a continuum of naturalness. Of the following types of therapy, which is an example of the least natural approach?
    a. Focused stimulation
    b. Script therapy
    c. Daily activities

d. Facilitated play

e. Drill play

89. Which technique may be most effective in facilitative play with a young child who is extremely limited in verbal expression?

a. Self-talk and parallel talk

b. Imitations

c. Expansions and extensions

d. Buildups and breakdowns

e. Recasts

90. Of the following actions, which is *not* an advantage of a criterion-referenced procedure?

a. Controlling the linguistic stimuli

b. Examining a particular form of communication behavior with reference to other children's achievement

c. Establishing baseline function

d. Identifying targets for intervention and measuring whether intervention goals have been met

e. Measuring progress

91. Functional outcomes in language therapy are _____ as a result of intervention.

a. Performances on "high-stakes" (state or national) examinations

b. Evidence of progress in academics or life skills

c. Scores on standardized tests

d. A list of objectives mastered

e. A list of academic goals not mastered

92. Of the following patterns listed, which represents a hierarchy in phonological awareness training?

a. First rhyming, then sound matching, followed by phoneme blending; phoneme substitution is the most difficult

b. First rhyming, then phoneme substitution, followed by phoneme blending; sound matching is the most difficult

c. First sound matching, then rhyming, followed by phoneme blending; phoneme substitution is the most difficult

d. First phoneme substitution, then rhyming, followed by sound matching; phoneme blending is the most difficult

e. First rhyming, then sound matching, followed by phoneme substitution; phoneme blending is the most difficult

93. A 12-year-old has a weakness in vocabulary as measured by the Expressive Vocabulary Test. Frequent "disruptions in speech" (mazes) are noted in conversation. Of the following actions, which would probably be the next step in assessment?

a. Assessing rapid automatized naming skills

b. Analyzing speech disruptions in discourse for word-finding difficulties

c. Using a criterion-referenced measure of lexical diversity

d. Identifying ability to formulate syntactically correct sentences when given target words

e. Measuring rate of speech

94. Joe is a 10-year-old with a history of speech and language delay. He continues to have difficulty with syntax, articulation, and phonological processes such as final consonant deletion. He also demonstrates "soft" neurological signs (e.g., clumsiness and poor visual-motor integration) and has received a diagnosis of attention deficit disorder. Pragmatic deficits are related more to comprehension difficulties than to deficits in theory of mind. Of the following conclusions, which can be inferred from the information given?

a. Joe's reading and writing skills are likely not delayed

b. Joe is able to quickly and efficiently process auditory information

c. Joe will require a behavior modification plan to address pragmatic weaknesses

d. As Joe continues to outgrow obvious linguistic deficits, remaining deficits will surface in academic situations that necessitate complex language skills (e.g., narrative tasks)

e. Joe's semantic-pragmatic language skills will suggest a change in diagnosis to have an autism spectrum disorder

95. Joe is a 10-year-old with a history of speech and language delay. He continues to have difficulty with syntax, articulation, and phonological processes such as final consonant deletion. He also demonstrates "soft" neurological signs (e.g., clumsiness and poor visual-motor integration) and has received a diagnosis of attention deficit disorder. Pragmatic deficits are related more to comprehension difficulties than to deficits in theory of mind. Of the following objectives, which would be appropriate for his treatment plan?

a. In a class discussion, Joe will demonstrate appropriate turn-taking skills

b. When given core curriculum vocabulary, Joe will demonstrate the ability to use these in grammatically correct sentences during classroom discussion

c. During silent reading activities, Joe will attend to the task, as measured by completion of a teacher-made worksheet

d. When given target verbs, Joe will identify these in his textbooks

e. When given multisyllabic words, Joe will repeat these after they are modeled by the clinician

1. c. Creating opportunities for initiating communication so that the child can increase the spontaneity of his communication would be the appropriate initial treatment goal. Because Carlos is already responding to requests, increasing the contexts in which he responds (option a) does not address his current challenge of initiating. Decreasing adult verbal output (option b) also does not address the child's current need to initiate communication. Although socially appropriate responses are always encouraged (option d), the child is already responding; therefore, this goal does not address the child's priority need. Facilitating the child's play with peers (option e) is a future goal but would not be a priority, because the child must first successfully initiate communication.

2. d. Young children typically begin to put two words together between ages 18 and 24 months; this child is demonstrating almost a year's delay in putting words together. Early on, children commonly select words to say that use sounds they know and can produce and avoiding words with sounds they do not know or cannot produce (option a). Children as young as 9 months use eye gaze, gestures, and pointing to regulate an adult's behavior, interact socially, and establish joint attention (option b) well before they say their first words. It is common for young typically developing children to exhibit some disfluencies in their speech (option c), such as repeating words or parts of words, as the complexity of their language increases. Young developing children typically point to communicate (option e) in the first year of life; this is an important skill for establishing joint attention before they can use words.

3. d. The first condition to rule out as a potential cause of a speech and language delay is hearing impairment. Reassuring a family that a child is a late talker (option a) is appropriate because although 10% to 15% of young children in middle-income families are identified as "late bloomers," a little less than half of these children with early expressive language delay continue to have problems and are at risk for academic failure. Advising the parents to have genetic testing (option b) is also inappropriate because in most cases, no specific genetic abnormality accounts for the range of speech-language impairments among young children. Despite the tendency of a parent or older sibling to sometimes talk for a younger child (option c), this is not a primary reason or cause for a child's language delay. Although

children with speech and language impairment are at risk for ongoing challenges (option e), it would be inappropriate to suggest this without some evaluation of the child's response to intervention and to consider the type of speech and language impairment presented.

4. b. Although many children who have intellectual disabilities have language impairments (option c), most children with specific language impairments have nonverbal intelligence that is within normal limits. Young children with language impairments are indeed more likely to have reading deficits when they reach school age (option a). When the language impairments of young children are not corrected, such children often demonstrate learning disabilities in school; basic skills areas (i.e., reading, writing, math, oral and written expression) all require sophistication in speech and language. Language impairments can be congenital or acquired and occur throughout childhood and into adulthood (option d). Early language intervention and even prevention strategies are encouraged to support the language of children at risk for or with demonstrated impairments (option e) because children with sustained language impairments are at even greater risk for ongoing academic failure if their language disorder is not addressed or improved by the second grade.

5. c. According to Rapin and Allen's (1987) description of clinical language subtypes, a child with adequate speech and sentence formation but with more bizarre content, use of echolalia or unanalyzed scripts, and literal language use with poor conversation skills has a semantic-pragmatic deficit. Phonological-syntactic deficit (option a) is characterized by a speech sound disorder, more disfluent speech with short and grammatically incorrect utterances, and some comprehension challenges when the speaker is faced with complex language. Lexical-syntactic deficit (option b) is characterized by adequate articulation with challenges in word finding, difficulty formulating connected conversation and narration, and poorer understanding of abstract rather than concrete language. Phonological programming deficit (option d) is characterized by age-appropriate conversation and fluent speech with long utterances that are difficult to understand. Childhood apraxia of speech (option e) is typically characterized as adequate comprehension but impaired articulation and short utterances.

6. e. Trial therapy during an assessment period is an appropriate strategy for forming a prognosis, inasmuch as clinicians often probe a child's response to intervention strategies to determine the child's responsiveness to treatment and to develop a potential treatment plan. Both the nature and the severity of a language problem, as well as the individual child's strengths and challenges in responding, can be considered in making a prognostic statement (option a). It follows, therefore, that the decision-making process for determining the need for intervention (e.g., for late talkers) is complex (option b), and the available research and individual speech and language profiles need to be considered. Young children often respond poorly to formal tests; therefore, because of the range of communication behaviors exhibited by young children, clinicians should not rely on a single assessment measure (option c). Objective criteria are important (option d) for ensuring consistency in the assessment of the severity of a child's language impairment.

7. c. The child has an adequate nonverbal intellectual quotient, does not have specific speech sound errors that are affecting the intelligibility of his speech, and does not make unusual language errors or have odd use of words, but he does have consistent difficulty formulating sentences, finding the right words to express his intent, and vocabulary challenges, all of which are influencing his ability to perform academically. These are characteristics of children with specific language impairment. Autism spectrum disorder (option a) is characterized by producing odd or unusual language or as having a particular focus on literal or concrete thinking. An intellectual disability (option b) is not a feature of this child's profile, inasmuch as he has adequate nonverbal intelligence. This child is clearly demonstrating more than a language delay (option d) inasmuch as he is 8 years of age and in second grade and his expressive language difficulties are now interfering with his ability to express his intent and to participate fully in the classroom. Speech sound disorder (option e) is not a sufficient explanation, because sound production is adequate but sentence formulation and word selection are particular challenges.

8. a. The mother's report of differences in reference to the child's linguistic influence and culture within which he was raised is an indication of likely impairment. The score on an articulation test that measures standard English productions (option b) fails to account for the sound structure difference of African American English. Frustration (option c) when he is asked to repeat himself may or may not be related to a language impairment. Some children are often frustrated when their messages are not heard or understood on the first attempt. Furthermore, if the listener is unfamiliar with a particular dialect, they probably would not understand initial productions. Damian's tendency to drop off ends of words (option d) is also not a differential language consideration for impairment. These types of pronunciations are common in African American English. Damian's hesitation to respond (option e) would not necessarily reflect a speech disorder; his past life and cultural experiences and his current situation, in an unfamiliar community and culture with adults he does not know, would certainly affect his comfort and ease with responding.

9. b. Damian and his mother probably share an African American English dialect, and the mother's confirmation that Damian is competent in all other aspects of his language development in comparison with his siblings is indicative of a language difference. His language difference can be explained by his experience with his previous community. Damian's ability to cooperate and respond (option a) during screening is not a differentiating feature of language difference or impairment; many children with language impairments are able to respond and cooperate during testing. Damian's scores on a formal vocabulary measure (option c) are also not useful in this situation because this measure is a biased assessment of his knowledge. Although Damian's mother has no trouble understanding him (option d), this is not sufficient to rule out a language impairment; many family members are able to understand their children with language impairments because of their familiarity with their children's talk and content of their talk. Also, knowing he is misunderstood (option e) and repeating what he has said is a strategy used frequently by children with a language impairment in their attempts to have their message understood.

10. a. An 18-month-old should begin to demonstrate some autosymbolic play in which he or she is able to pretend to go to sleep, drink from a cup, or eat from a spoon while at the same time beginning to develop true verbal communication-like agents, such as actions, objects, recurrence, and so forth. Young children often use gestures (option b), and therefore this is not a concern. They are beginning to use true verbal communication and require meaningful and conventional gestures to ensure their intent is understood. Attention to tasks (option c) is also not of great concern at this age because young children are highly engaged in movement and exploration of their environment, moving quickly from one exploration to the next. Use of facial expressions

(option d) is also not a significant concern at this point; Ethan is smiling and looking and should begin to develop additional expressions matched to the emotional situation he is experiencing. Ethan's preference to play with toys with sounds and those that require some means-ends thinking, such as pop-up toys, is not uncommon at this age; toddlers are continuing to explore the environment and trying to figure out how things work.

11. b. Ethan will slowly and progressively add new words to his lexicon, and as he approaches 50 words, he is likely to begin putting two words together. This is the expected trajectory for language development even if Ethan is responding with a slight delay or lateness in his verbal expression. It is unlikely for a late talker to engage in unusual repetitive behaviors (option a); this happens more frequently among children with or suspected of having autism. Distorted or poorly understood words (option c) are also unlikely to be a problem; children who are late talkers typically add words that are easily understood in context and often contain speech sounds that they are comfortable producing. Children who struggle with verbal expression can become frustrated (option d), but Ethan, as a late talker, is already using gestures to augment his communication to ensure that he is being understood. Although many children who are developing their language in a typical manner say words and then do not say them again until several months later (option e), this usually occurs before 18 months. If children are not saying some words used previously, they are usually trying new words to add to their repertoire and words that were lost are soon to return.

12. d. It is critical to acknowledge what you hear a parent saying, identify any concerns you share, and put a plan in place to ensure that these concerns can be addressed in a family-centered and meaningful way. You may suspect the child has autism (option a); however, it would be inappropriate to make such a statement without a careful assessment of the early markers of autism. Because the child has early medical complications, ongoing involvement of a team is important. It is inappropriate to suggest that the mother's stress (option b) is causally related to her daughter's joint attention and social communication challenges, because there is no evidence of this. The child's failure to respond as expected probably exacerbates the stress the mother is currently experiencing; furthermore, many families experience similar stresses and do not have children who present with Amelia's challenges. A child's prematurity (option c) should be considered in defining expected development; however, if Amelia's gestation age (i.e., 17 months) is taken into account, the current

observations would be as concerning as they are at 19 months. Providing personal care or respite support (option e) is reasonable, but it does not address a primary problem: the current social communication deficits being reported and observed for Amelia.

13. c. The interdisciplinary service model typically involves professionals from a variety of disciplines with formal communication challenges; their services are arranged by a case manager or assessment coordinator. Some disciplines are directly involved and others provide consultation. In a unidisciplinary approach (option a), individuals from the same discipline would be involved (e.g., a team of SLPs). In a multidisciplinary approach (option b), members of each discipline typically completes independent evaluations with separate recommendations that are reported to the team and family. In a transdisciplinary approach (option d), it is more likely that one individual would do all or most of the assessment through interactions with the child and family, whereas members of other disciplines would observe or provide suggestions to the primary individual. Although an interdisciplinary assessment approach is working toward coordinated services (option e), this term is not typically used to define assessment team approaches; instead, it is used to describe an effort to coordinate services for children with special needs.

14. c. Children with autism have difficulty interacting with another about shared actions or objects. Receptive (option a) and expressive language (option b) are often impaired in children with autism, receptive language deficits being more predictive of autism than expressive impairments; however, receptive and expressive language impairments are common in a range of conditions, and so they are not specifically predictive of autism. Pretend play (option d) and imitation (option e) are also areas of challenge for children with autism. As a cluster, these deficits are descriptive of children with autism; however, impairment in joint attention remains the best predictor.

15. e. Individuals with autism spectrum disorders have difficulty understanding a listener or character's cognitive state, recognizing character goals in stories, and inferring mental states; therefore, an assessment of narrative language and storytelling can provide some specific information about the ability to take on the perspective of another. Although each of the other assessments are important and the skills tested may be impaired in individuals with autism spectrum disorders, the assessments do not provide specific information about theory of mind. Assessment of figurative language (option a) and word knowledge (option b) provide specific information about an

individual's understanding of concrete versus more abstract language concepts. The number of quality social interactions (option c) is important for establishing social competence; because of the limited opportunities to engage in such interactions, individuals with autism spectrum disorders are at risk for further social isolation. However, these assessments does not necessarily provide specific information about deficits in theory of mind. Assessment of pitch, intensity, and intonation (option d) are critical paralinguistic features in the expression of language in social contexts but not in defining deficits of theory of mind.

16. d. The Test of Nonverbal Intelligence—3 is a language-free formal measure of cognitive ability that can be used by SLPs interested in determining a child's general nonverbal intelligence. It requires only a pointing response and is an appropriate tool for use with clients from age 5 through adulthood. The Leiter International Performance Scale—R (option a) is also a formal measure of nonverbal intelligence for children aged 2 to 18 years, but it requires pantomime when instructions are given; there are concerns about this child's ability to process and imitate oral and motor movements. The Merrill-Palmer Scales of Mental Tests (option b) is used for children aged 18 months to 4 years and examines a number of developmental domains, which include cognition, language, motor social emotional, and self help adaptive behavior. The Cognitive Abilities Scale (option c) is typically used for children aged 3 to 47 months, and it is an informal tool that would not provide the standard score required for this child's comprehensive evaluation. The Swanson Cognitive Abilities Scale (option e) is used primarily for children who are nonverbal, which is not the case in this situation.

17. b. Pivotal response training is a contemporary behavior approach that is backed by strong evidence for the support of social communication in natural settings. It enables shared control for teaching, reinforces attempts at responding, entails child-preferred activities and materials, and ensures choices to facilitate initiation throughout the day. Floor time (option a), although frequently used for children with challenges in affect and establishing attachment, is a relationship-based intervention that emphasizes following a child's lead; evidence of positive effects is limited, and it is most often used in the home setting or in one-on-one situations with an adult or peer. Discrete trial training (option c) is a more traditional behavioral approach that is highly prescribed and is focused on teaching isolated skills in a one-on-one situation with predetermined criteria for correct responses; it is not the best choice for facilitating

spontaneous communication and social interaction in natural contexts such as the classroom. Social story training (option d) helps decrease inappropriate behaviors and increase more appropriate thinking about social situations; it does not necessarily foster choice making, shared control of teaching opportunities, or the implementation of child-preferred activities and materials. Sensory integration training (option e) is often recommended for children with autism, but there is little evidence for its effects on social communication and would not be a priority intervention for implementation in Jack's current classroom situation.

18. e. Imitation does not require intentional communication, which is an ultimate goal in language intervention. Imitation is clinician or adult controlled (option a), but because clinicians are providing a language model, adult control is not a significant shortcoming of this strategy. Imitation is not contextualized speech (option b) and does not require semantic knowledge (option c); children can imitate sequences of sounds and words without necessarily knowing what they mean. Imitation can be used to model syntactic structure (option d).

19. a. Prelinguistic milieu teaching is an attempt to facilitate a child's need to communicate by employing several techniques that foster communication, such as placing desired object out of reach, using time delay or waiting expectantly for a child to indicate what he or she wants, changing a routine or protesting an event, and so forth. Showing, pointing, and commenting (option b) are strategies typically used to establish joint attention in a child. Although modeling a desired production (option c), reinforcing a child's communication attempts, and following a child's lead (option d) are important strategies to support engagement with a child, they would not necessarily lead to fostering a need to communicate. Differential reinforcement strategies and the use of prompting and fading (option e) are behavioral modification techniques not typically associated with prelinguistic milieu teaching.

20. c. Michael has a profile typically associated with nonverbal learning disability: He is verbal, is a good reader, and has responded to tutoring and accommodations to address his written language challenges, but he continues to have math difficulties, reading comprehension deficits, and social difficulty, being unable to interpret the nonverbal cues of his peers. Michael has more than just a specific language impairment (option a), inasmuch as his academic performance is also affected. Although Michael's social challenges are often reported for children with Asperger disorder (option b), this

condition does not explain Michael's current academic difficulties and does not fit with his reported history of language impairment. He also does not demonstrate the restricted or specific interests characteristic of children with Asperger disorder. Michael has no evidence of hyperactivity or attention problems (option d) that interfere with learning. Michael can read, so he does not have dyslexia (option e).

21. d. Young children who have experienced a period of otitis media are at risk for conductive hearing loss. This type of hearing loss is often associated with deficits in perceiving high-frequency consonants, such as sibilant sounds. Children with such a hearing loss may also not hear these high frequency sounds in their own speech. Cluster reduction (option a), nasalization (option b), velar fronting (option c), and gliding (option e) are not necessarily related to hearing loss or are not features of the speech of children who have a history of otitis media.

22. c. Children with language impairments demonstrate a number of problems. For example, they have less story complexity and fewer episodes (option a), more intrusions of irrelevant information and poorer use of cohesive devices (option b). Most distinctive is less use of conjunctions and of elaborated noun phrases. There is less frequent use of personal pronouns and of past-tense verbs (option d), shorter and less complex C-units, inadequate word use, and inadequate syntactic structure (option e).

23. b. Discrete trial teaching involves the use of differential reinforcement, modeling, and prompting as part of a traditional behavioral approach to intervention. In comparison, naturalistic teaching involves establishing meaningful and successful communication (option a), as well as more child-initiated interactions (option c). Although syntactic and semantic structures (option d) may be taught through the use of modeling and prompting, this is not an expectation of discrete trial teaching. More contemporary behavioral approaches entail the use of child choice and child-preferred activities and materials (option e).

24. e. Fey and colleagues (2003) suggested that the highest priority for setting intervention goals should be forms and functions that a child uses in 10% to 50% of required contexts. The forms and functions that a child is already using in required contexts (option a) and the forms that a child is not using (option b) or does not understand in receptive tasks (option c) are of lower priority. Although forms and functions used in only 1% to 10% of required contexts are a high priority, they would not be considered the highest priority for starting intervention.

25. b. There is a continuum of naturalness in language intervention from least natural (or clinician directed) to most natural (child-centered approaches). Hybrid approaches involve some clinician direction in addition to following the child's lead, and one of these approaches is focused stimulation, in which the clinician provides repeated models of targeted language production in natural play and communication contexts. Facilitated play (option a) is a more child-centered approach and is one of the most natural intervention approaches. Drill (option c), modeling (option d), and clinician-directed activities (option e) are considered to be the least natural contexts for intervention; they do not represent a balance between child- and clinician-directed activities.

26. c. Several goals and activities have been suggested to support prelinguistic milieu teaching (Warren et al., 2008). If a goal has been established to increase conventional gestures, then the clinician might first create a communication routine in which a child will look at an action or object and then the clinician provides the desired object or action when the child uses a gesture, such as pointing. Although waiting expectantly (option a) is an effective strategy, it is often used to encourage combinations of gaze, vocalizations, and gestures. The child should certainly look at a desired object (option b), but looking is a goal for establishing spontaneous and coordinated gaze; verbally prompting the child to gaze (option d) is a similar strategy. Communication is an ultimate goal of intervention; therefore, modeling a vocalization (option e) addresses a specific goal for increasing the frequency of vocalizations in a child who is already vocalizing.

27. c. Children with specific language impairment most often exhibit difficulty with producing well-formed sentences that include appropriate morphological endings and syntactic structures. Comprehension of word meanings (option a) and simple sentences (option b) are less likely to be impaired than are morphology and syntax. Furthermore, most children with specific language impairment have adequate nonverbal cognitive abilities (option d) and manage the motor requirements for writing (option e).

28. a. The most efficient and effective strategy would be to identify the phonological processes the child is using and begin to address production through a minimal-contrast approach. The rationale is to emphasize word meaning on the basis of the phonological combinations of words. Although sound discrimination training (option b) may be used in intervention to increase a child's recognition of approach sound patterns, it does not necessarily

correct the actual sound errors. Approaching the task developmentally and tackling one sound at a time on the basis of the developmental pattern (option c) is inefficient. There is no connection between the sounds the child can and cannot say (option d). Including sound practice in isolation, then nonsense syllables, and finally words (option e) is phonetic-based and inefficient for this patient.

29. e. The SLP should initiate a language-based phonological approach emphasizing final consonants. These sounds should be acquired before 4 years of age (option b) and should be used in meaningful word contexts. Although supporting the parents to facilitate language and communication through storybook reading (option c) is a general language support strategy, it does not necessarily foster sound production. There is no indication of a cognitive deficit (option a), nor is there evidence of difficulty producing nasal or plosive sounds (option d).

30. c. Pragmatics is the use of language in meaningful social contexts. It requires the child to take turns in play, both initiating and responding to discourse either verbally or nonverbally. Although storytelling is a pragmatic context, focusing on irregular past tense (option a) is a morphological and not pragmatic goal. Increasing the child's production of final consonants (option b) or clusters (option d) supports the child's learning to use sound patterns in conversation and play, but these are not skills directly related to pragmatics. Facilitating word combinations (option e) in nonfunctional contexts such as drill or adult-directed intervention does not enhance pragmatic language use in meaningful contexts.

31. d. Early language stimulation is best supported by parents or a child's primary caregivers and those who can foster an infant's language learning experiences on a daily basis. Creating readiness activities (option a), introducing storybook reading (option b), and teaching symbolic play (option c) are strategies that might be introduced at a later developmental stage; infants might not be responsive to these strategies. Communicating with physicians about the importance of screening for language impairment (option e) is essential, but it does not address strategies for early intervention.

32. c. Discourse involves extended utterance use in conversation and storytelling and requires an ability to use cohesive devices—references, conjunctions, and clausal elements—that help form a coherent message that makes sense to the listener. The other options refer to other aspects of language production that are not directly linked to discourse problems,

although a child with a language impairment may have difficulties in any of these areas. Morphology (option a) refers to the study of the smallest meaningful units of language; children with discourse problems do not typically have difficulty with word structure. Children with vocabulary deficits (option b) are unlikely to have connected language that is sufficient to evaluate discourse. Although gesture use (option d) can contribute to effective discourse, it is typically not an intervention goal. This is also true of phonology (option e), in that speech sound production is not a typical goal for supporting discourse production.

33. d. ADHD is a complex disorder that is not easily differentiated from a language disorder. It is however, a more behaviorally based disorder with implications for cognitive function, whereas a language disorder is a disorder of cognition that involves the form, content, and use of language. ADHD and language disorders frequently co-occur (option a). The diagnostic criteria for ADHD also includes several language criteria, such as not listening when spoken to, not following instructions, talking excessively, blurting out answers, difficulty waiting for turns and interrupting others; these issues complicate the diagnostic process (option b). The co-occurrence of learning disabilities and ADHD, as well as learning disabilities and language disorders, is frequent, another complication in the differential diagnostic process (option c). Tests developed to assess language (option e) often focus on attention to tasks and task completion; therefore, formal measures cannot reliably help differentiate attention and language deficits.

34. b. Phonological awareness has been identified as a stable and robust predictor of reading. It is one of the five factors that are predictive of reading disability (Catts et al., 2001; Hogan et al., 2005; Lonigan et al., 2000). The ability to think about and reflect on language (option a) is known as metalinguistic awareness, of which phonological awareness is one part. Letter-sound correspondence (option c), or phonics, is the linking of the written letter to the sound it makes. Phonological awareness is best assessed through rhyming, segmentation, and sound deletion tasks (option d). Phonological awareness intervention is often implemented in kindergarten through second grade; however, students with reading disabilities in later grades have also benefited (option e; e.g., see Swanson et al., 2005).

35. a. Reading is a language-based developmental skill that is affected by language deficits; therefore, because SLPs working with developmental language problems, their involvement in supporting students

with or at risk for reading disabilities is critical. SLPs typically work on supporting phonological awareness because of their knowledge and skill in the area of sound and language production and meaning, whereas reading specialists typically support word attack and word recognition (option b), phonics (option c), and alphabet knowledge (option d). Although SLPs offer individual assessment and intervention (option e), their value is enhanced when supporting children with reading disabilities if they collaborate with teachers and reading specialists to provide curriculum-relevant language intervention so that the children can access the general education curriculum.

36. d. Historically, children with learning disabilities have generally been viewed as less popular than their peers (option a) and as experiencing a hostile communication environment with peers. Children with learning disabilities have also been identified as different from their peers through ratings by teachers, peers (option b), and self-report (option c). Furthermore, peer relationship challenges in children with learning disabilities are often noted in childhood, and these social stresses affect later academic, vocational, and emotional deficits (option e).

37. b. Cognitive referencing is the practice of determining the presence of a learning disability primarily through a discrepancy between general aptitude, as measured by an IQ test, and academic achievement (Troia, 2005); it has also been used to identify specific language impairment (i.e., discrepancy between nonverbal IQ and performance on a spoken language measure). Neither use is appropriate for determining the level of deficit or the need for intervention. Need for services can be determined by whether the language a child has will help the child thrive personally, socially, academically, and vocationally. It is also not appropriate to deny services because language and developmental levels are commensurate. Low achievement scores (option a) are often a confounding variable in trying to differentiate children with a disability and those who are just underachieving for reasons that cannot be clearly explained. Response to intervention (option c) is a regular education initiative to enhance educational opportunities for all children, through the use of evidence-based and differentiated instruction for all students to prevent disabilities and to identify students who do have learning disabilities or require special educational services. In Maria's case, no evidence-based instruction is being provided, and a disability has already been identified. A wait-to-fail approach (option d) is often used to identify students who may not reach their expected achievement

in reading, math, and written language skills. It is an inefficient method to support the learning needs of students with or at risk for learning challenges. The former SLP failed to consider that verbal performance (option e) on a measure of intelligence does not indicate a student's ability or need to have a functional communication system.

38. b. Children in the early invented-spelling stage typically have alphabetic knowledge and can name some letters, but they usually omit vowels and encode only parts of words. At the nonspelling stage (option a), children have no letter-sound correspondence or concept of words, as Joshua does. At the phonetic spelling stage (option c), children typically have a strong understanding of letter-sound correspondence, segment letters at word boundaries, and provide letter names for long vowels, although they continue to omit unstressed vowels and nasals in their spelling. The stages of mixed phonetic and visual spelling (option d) and conventional spelling (option e) are later stages of spelling development in which children must attend to visual configurations of words, must possess knowledge of different conventions for the same sound, and demonstrate knowledge of conventional spelling rules and recognition of spelling errors.

39. c. Morphological errors and grammatical errors typically occur in the written language samples of students with LLD. Writing expository text or summaries is typically more challenging than narrative story writing (option a). Written language length is also typically reduced for children with LLD (option b). Furthermore, the use of cohesive ties (option d), which serve as the linguistic glue for storytelling, is reduced in the written narratives. Executive function skills (option e), like problem solving and organization, are problematic for children with LLD, in comparison with typical peers, when approaching writing tasks.

40. c. In focused stimulation, the clinician carefully arranges the interaction to increase the likelihood that the child produces an utterance with the obligatory context being targeted (in this case, teaching the copula *is*). Vertical restructuring (option a) is another hybrid intervention approach, but it is a particular form of expansion that is used to highlight a targeted linguistic structure. In vertical restructuring, a clinician usually takes pieces of information a child has produced and expands them into a more complete utterance. In parallel talk (option b), the clinician talks about the child's actions, providing a running commentary of what the child was doing. Although expansion (option d) may occur in a

focused stimulation approach, it is primarily a strategy of taking what a child has said and adding grammatical markers or more semantic details to the child's utterance so that it approaches an acceptable adult utterance (e.g., expanding "kitty ball" to "The kitty is playing with the ball" or "That is the kitty's ball"). Recasting (option e) increases a child's utterance, but in this case, the child's utterance is expanded into a different type or more elaborated version. For example, you might recast "kitty ball" to "Is the kitty playing with the ball?" or a negative sentence such as "The kitty does not have the ball."

41. e. In the expanding spontaneity phase of PECS, the child is learning to expand the contexts in which he or she is demonstrating the ability to exchange pictures with a communication partner. The increased distances between the picture stimuli and the communication partners requires the child to spontaneously seek out the stimuli and someone with whom to share his or her request. In the commenting phase (option a), the child would be learning to respond to questions such as "What do you see?" or "What do you have?" The physical exchange phase (option b) requires the child only to hand a picture card to a communication partner in exchange for a desired item. In the answering questions phase (option c), the child would be responding to the question, "What do you want?" In the picture discrimination phase (option d), the child is taught to choose a desired item from among several pictures.

42. b. Procedural knowledge involves knowing how to perform an action. Knowing that information fades over time (option a) is part of a theory of forgetting known as *decay theory*. Effective working memory enables one to retrieve information (option c), but failure to do so is part of what is known as *interference*. Knowing the extent and depth of information (option d) is related to storage strength in retrieving vocabulary. The ease with which a word is used (option e) is related to retrieval strength.

43. d. Clustering is a control process in short-term memory that allows a person to place information into meaningful categories, such as animals, foods, colors, and adjectives. Tagging information (option a) involves setting up retrieval paths to facilitate memory (e.g., remembering "ranid" means frog by connecting an image of a frog in the rain). Relating information to known material (option b) involves using analogies to already existing knowledge (e.g., understanding "cricket" because of its similarities to baseball). Using mnemonics (option c) involves organizing material that enhances recall, such as using the acronym *HOMES* to remember the five Great Lakes. Chunking (option e) involves grouping or recoding information into smaller units. For example, we can code a phone number by area code, second three digits, and final four digits (312-980-1234).

44. d. Tertiary prevention is used to reduce a disability by trying to restore more effective functioning. Services are provided for a child with an identified disorder in hopes of improving the child's communication, social interaction, and behavior. Primary prevention is the attempt to eliminate or inhibit the onset or development of a disorder by reducing susceptibility. Setting up a language stimulation class for teenaged mothers (option b), offering low-cost speech and hearing screenings at community events (option c), and offering language literacy workshops for parents of children at risk (option e) are all examples of primary prevention strategies. Secondary prevention involves early detection and treatment to eliminate a disorder or hinder its progress by preventing further complications. Neonatal hearing screening (option a) is an example of secondary prevention.

45. d. The description fits best with Williams syndrome. Affected children are characterized by an interstitial deletion from the long arm of chromosome 7 and an unusual pattern of language acquisition, with higher levels of growth in verbal than nonverbal cognitive skills. Down syndrome (option a) involves an extra copy of chromosome 21 and mild to moderate mental retardation, with notable deficits in speech, language, and hearing. Prader-Willi syndrome (option b) results from gene loss on chromosome 15 and manifests with characteristic facial features, short stature, obesity, and communication problems, with delays both in speech-sound production and in receptive and expressive language and with particular challenges in pragmatics. Vocabulary and reading decoding and comprehension are strengths, and mental retardation does not appear to be a significant area of deficit. Angelman syndrome (option c) is a neurogenetic disorder characterized by intellectual and developmental delay, sleep disturbance, seizures, and a generally happy demeanor. It is caused by deletion or inactivation of genes on the maternally inherited chromosome 15. Fragile X syndrome is an inherited form of mental retardation without obvious dysmorphic features; thus, it is often difficult to identify affected children in their early years. They usually have an uneven cognitive profile with relative strengths in verbal production but weaknesses in gesture use and symbolic play.

46. c. Opticon is an aided AAC intervention that changes print to a tactile representation and assists deafblind students who rely on Braille for academic

information. Finger spelling (option a), anticipatory cues (option b), Braille (option d), and communication boards (option e) are all unaided techniques for which assistive technology is not required.

47. e. Scaffolded instruction provides guidance for a student through verbal communication to support what the student cannot do. When a student identifies a reinforcer and self-rewards after a predetermined criterion is reached or exceeded, he or she is employing a self-reinforcement strategy (option a). Goal setting (option b) targets learning efforts, provides information on progress, and motivates performance. Self-instruction (option c) is self-talk used by students to help guide their behavior. Self-monitoring (option d) requires a student to self-assess whether a targeted behavior has occurred.

48. a. Jennifer will probably receive a diagnosis of Asperger disorder. Although she has a social impairment and a restricted interest, she does not exhibit a delay in cognitive or language development, which is a requirement for a diagnosis of autistic disorder (option c). Rett disorder (option b) usually manifests with a deceleration of head growth, loss of purposeful hand movements, loss of social engagement, and severe impairments in language and cognitive development. Childhood disintegrative disorder (option d) usually manifests with a significant loss of previously acquired skills before age 10 years, including communication, social or adaptive skills, bowel or bladder control, and play or motor skills. A child with PDD-NOS (option e) exhibits a severe and pervasive impairment in social interaction and communication or stereotyped behavior. Interests and activities are present, but criteria for autistic disorder or other PDD are not met.

49. b. Dynamic, intense behavior in public conversations is considered acceptable in children using AAVE whereas children using standard American English exhibit more restraint, less emotion, and less intensity in verbal arguments. Interruption (option a) is sometimes used in standard American English because it is considered helpful, whereas interruption in AAVE is considered rude. Narratives in AAVE are more associational and not topic-centered (option c), which is more common in standard American English. In AAVE, direct eye contact (option d) is used in the speaker role but not in the listener role, whereas children using standard American English may perceive lack of eye contact as "not listening." Wit and sarcasm (option e) are an important part of pragmatic dialogue in AAVE, whereas such interactions are often considered hostile by children using standard American English.

50. d. The test-teach-retest model is a dynamic assessment method in which clinicians assess a particular skill, provide selected intervention on the basis of principles of a task, and then reassess performance to determine whether the child has learned the targeted skill. In "testing the limits" (option a), traditional procedures are modified in that the child is asked to describe the test question and tell why they gave the answer they did. Interviewing on responses (option b) is a method in which questions are generated to help children understand their thinking about test problems so that they can become aware of targeted skills. In graduated prompting (option c), a child's zone of proximal development is identified by providing a hierarchy of prompts. In measure modifiability (option e), Likert scales are used to rate a child at the beginning and end of a dynamic assessment and intervention phase.

51. d. The role of school-based SLPs includes understanding a student's individual learning style and integrating development of linguistic skills that are necessary to support academic success. Making sure that all children serviced master all academic standards, (option a) is too inclusive as a goal. Conversely, addressing only linguistically based standards (option b) and identifying and working on only standards that cause academic difficulty (option c) limit SLPs to a narrow area of intervention. Facilitating the development of nonlinguistic standards (option e) is not a primary goal of practice.

52. c. Researchers have identified no direct relationship between cognitive levels and language development; that is, some language abilities may be better developed than general cognitive ability, whereas others may be either correlated with or less developed than such ability. Furthermore, researchers have questioned cognitive level as a meaningful predictor of whether a child will benefit from intervention; children with language skills commensurate with their intelligence benefit from intervention.

53. c. Responsiveness to intervention (RTI) was developed to retain more children in general education and reduce the time, paperwork, and caseloads of special educators, including SLPs (Montgomery, 2008). The three-tiered model used in RTI is a systemic approach with successive tiers that involve increasingly intensive levels of intervention. Tier 1 is a research-based core classroom curriculum. Tier 2 is a targeted strategic support offered in the classroom; the interventions may be delivered by SLPs. Tier 3 is an intensive, systematic intervention often provided specialists such as SLPs. Students who continue to have difficulties despite these levels of intervention

are then usually considered for evaluation by the special education team, often including the SLP. Identifying and practicing how to "look back" in the chapter for key information is a tier 2 activity. Rereading the chapter to students (option a), previewing the test with students (option b), and preteaching the vocabulary (option d) are examples not of strategic support but of tutoring. Enlarging the print (option e) is an accommodation, not a support.

54. c. The PLEP should not be a duplication of the standardized measures discussed in the evaluation or reevaluation (options a, b, and e). Instead, the PLEP should describe the skills or areas identified during the evaluation process that have the greatest impact on the child's educational performance. "Joe appears unaware of directions" (option d) is not specific to the child's education performance.

55. b. In education, accommodations offer different ways for a student to learn and to share what they have learned. A word bank simply changes the way knowledge is assessed and does not change the curriculum or expectations of learning. Modifications (option a) actually change the curriculum and expectations placed on a student. Inclusion (option c) is an educational philosophy and policy that supports every child with a disability to be educated, to the maximum extent appropriate, in the classroom that the child would otherwise attend. Objectives (option d) are easily measurable and often include specific skills required to achieve a goal; use of a word bank is not a specific skill being developed.

56. b. Chunking has been found to be an effective instructional strategy for coding complex and/or lengthy material. Although preteaching vocabulary words (option a) and repeating the words (option c) may be helpful in familiarizing a student with the vocabulary, they are not examples of strategic learning. Reducing the number of words to learn (option d) alters the expectations of learning and therefore is a modification, not a strategy.

57. c. Metalinguistic awareness (option c) refers to the consciousness of language; for example, as in this case, being able to recognize an incomplete direction. Pragmatics (option a) involves using language for different purposes, changing language according to the needs of a listener or situation, and following rules for conversations and storytelling. Although questioning directions is a pragmatic skill, it is more specifically an example of metalinguistic awareness. Phonological awareness (option b) is the recognition that words are composed of sounds; morphological

awareness (option d) is the awareness that words are composed of morphemes. Syntax (option e) is the grammatical structure of language.

58. c. A test-teach-retest method such as that described is dynamic assessment. Narrative assessment (option a), assessment of semantic development (option b), assessment of language processing capacity (option d), and norm-referenced assessment (option e) are formats of assessment that do not include a teaching component and thus do not measure a student's ability to learn or improve in a skill (unless given in a pretest-teach-posttest format).

59. a. When an individual is first introduced to a particular skill or concept, it may be advantageous for the clinician to establish the goals and control the materials and context. After that time, a naturalistic intervention is typically supported; it might be in a hybrid format during middle stages of therapy (option b) or during transition and generalization (option c). In the final stages of therapy (options d and e), clinician-directed intervention should be minimal.

60. d. Many children with Down syndrome have more difficulty with expressive language than they do with understanding speech and language; that is, receptive language skills are usually more advanced than expressive language skills. Furthermore, many children with Down syndrome have difficulties with intelligibility of speech and speech sound production.

61. a. This boy lacks social language skills such as turn-taking which is a pragmatic skill. Such skills would be targeted in discourse treatment. The other areas of language—syntax (option b), morphology (option c), semantics (option d), and phonology (option e)—are language components of form and content.

62. e. Poor academic performance is probably related to vocabulary weaknesses; therefore, it would be best to target word definitions and word retrieval skills. It is unlikely that improvement in auditory discrimination skills (option a), the use of complex sentences (option b), social language (option c), or ability to understand and use figurative language (option d) would have a large, direct effect on academic performance, inasmuch as these areas were not reported to be of concern.

63. d. Dynamic assessment is an interactive approach to assessments in which the ability of the learner to respond to intervention is the focus (option d). Thus

the SLP actively intervenes (option a) and the individual's ability to problem solve (option b) is monitored from before the time the intervention is introduced through and until the end of the intervention period (option e). The correct answer is (option c) in that such learning may in fact, be measured and monitored for progress.

64. a. It is not true that collaboration with teachers is unimportant. Classroom teachers can often provide insight into a child's language in a natural setting (in comparison with decontextualized testing sessions). Chronological age is not always the best predictor of appropriate treatment (option b). Some children with language difficulties also have difficulty with discourse skills (option c). Criterion-referenced assessment may indeed include teacher checklists (option d). A combination of standardized and criterion-referenced tests do provide baseline information (option e).

65. d. Argument text requires planning and revising one's stance according to the reader's expected response. Required length (option a), differences in grammar and punctuation (option b), and knowledge about the topic (option c) are not particular to argument text; they are applicable to almost all genres of writing. Story grammar (option e) is necessary for narrative writing, not for arguments.

66. b. Students demonstrate understanding of vocabulary and concepts by being able to discuss, summarize, and contrast these. Knowledge (option a) requires only the ability to list, identify, and name. Analysis of information (option c) is measured by tasks that require looking at individual parts of information. Synthesis (option d) is elicited in assignments that require integration of information. Evaluation of information (option e) is elicited in tasks that require an assessment or judging of that information.

67. b. Number of different words has been found to differentiate typically developing children from those with language impairments better than type-token ratio (option a). The Expressive Vocabulary Test (option c) is a standardized measure of vocabulary and not a measure of lexical diversity in narratives. Mean length of utterance (option d) and mean length of a C-unit (option e) are measures of grammatical complexity, not lexical diversity.

68. c. Standard deviations provide an estimate of how different a score is from the mean score on the test. A score that is 1.25 to 1.5 standard deviations below the mean is often considered to be statistically different enough to reflect a language disorder.

However, best practice includes the use of more than one measurement (option b). One standard deviation (option a) would overidentify 17% of the population as having a language disorder. Two standard deviations (options d and e) would underidentify (miss) those with language disorders, inasmuch as only 2% of population performs in this range.

69. b. In models of language production such as Bock and Levelt's (1994), the route begins with something that a person wants to convey (conceptual level). This is followed by selecting the appropriate words from one's internal lexicon (lexical-semantic level) before transforming them into sounds (phonological level) and then speaking them (utterance). Although this model is considered to be bidirectional—that is, in oral language, one hears sounds and then attaches meaning to these (i.e., comprehension)—the other options are not in the correct order.

70. e. Childhood aphasia (option e) is an older term that stems from the belief that affected children have a lesion in the brain, like an adult with aphasia. This term is no longer used unless the medical history (e.g., stroke) supports its use. Language impairment (option a), language disability (option b), language disorder (option c), and language delay (option d) are each accepted as typical ways to describe a child who performs poorly in a language assessment.

71. d. A descriptive-developmental model in assessment describes in detail a child's current level of language functioning, including form, content, and use. Comparing the results of the child's performance with the normal developmental sequence helps guide a language intervention program. A systems model (option a) focuses on communication problems and the environment; that is, in a systems model of language disorders, the problem is in the child's environment. Such a model is more appropriate for students learning English as a second language or for those with severe difficulties such as developmental disabilities. Although categorical (option b), specific disabilities (option c), and medical (option e) models do provide useful information about the possible cause of a language disorder, children with the same label are very different; thus, such models do not inform intervention specific to a child's needs.

72. a. Students demonstrate understanding of vocabulary and concepts by being able to discuss, summarize, and contrast these (option b) facilitate. Knowledge (option a) requires the ability to list, identify, name, define (e.g., define ocean, lake, pond etc.). Analysis of information (option c) is measured by tasks that require looking at individual parts of information

(e.g., what makes the Atlantic Ocean an ocean?). Synthesis (option d) is elicited in assignments that require integration of information (e.g., what evidence do we find in oceans for global warming?). Evaluation of information (option e) is elicited in tasks that require an assessment or judging of that information (e.g., what do you think is the most important issue in regard to oceans today?).

73. b. Working memory tasks require the temporary storage and manipulation of information. In tasks such as phonological blending ("What a word do you get when you blend the sounds /d/-/ɑ/-/g/?"), the child must maintain internal representations (in this example, the phonemes) to guide his or her action (blend these into a morpheme). Sharing a story about a childhood experience (option a) is an example of a long-term memory task. Listing animals that live in the forest (option c) is an example of a naming task in which the child must maintain and manipulate the information to generate names. Repeating a phone number (option d) and repeating sentences verbatim (option e) are examples of short-term memory with no need to manipulate information.

74. b. Phonological awareness is the ability to consciously attend to and manipulate the sound structure of language, both syllables and sounds. Phonics requires learning to connect letters and letter patterns with the sounds they represent.

75. b. Criterion-referenced procedures measure what specific skills the child has mastered or is capable of mastering with support. Eliciting imitation and production helps to identify how the child may perform if given specific support. Although classroom observation (option a), developmental scales (option c), child-centered activities (option d), and play-based assessment (option e) are often important in gathering information on a child's abilities and difficulties, these do not identify how a child may perform with or without supports. Vygotsky (1978) suggested that a child first follows the adult's example in a task and then gradually develops the ability to perform that task without help. The area between what a child can do with help and what can be done without support is the "zone of proximal development."

76. b. Sarcasm is defined as stating the opposite of the true meaning, usually in a harsh or ironic manner. Sarcasm can be difficult to grasp (to understand the purpose of the comment). Persuasion (option a) is defined as communication by which the speaker seeks to convince the listener to perform an act or accept a point of view. Negotiation (option c) is defined as communication by which the participants

seek to resolve conflicts. Conversation (option d) is a dialogue between people, whereas narration (option e) is a monologue in which an event, an experience, or a condition is described. Although each of the other choices may include sarcasm, sarcasm is neither a necessary nor a defining characteristic of each of these.

77. e. Traditionally accepted methods of word retrieval strategies include mnemonic cueing (option a), rehearsal (option b), pausing (option c), and attribute cueing (option d) (German, 2005). A word bank is a modification imposed by the communication partner and is not a strategy implemented by the individual with a word-finding disorder.

78. d. Both naming accuracy and speed have been found to be associated with age-related changes in vocabulary growth and processing time.

79. c. A word-finding difficulty is defined as a failure or significant delay in attempting to say a word, the meaning of which he or she comprehends and a word that may have been spoken before (German, 2005). In one type of error, the target word is substituted with a phonologically similar word, such as "ocupus" for "octopus." This is an example of a phonological substitution. Substitutions of words from the same lexical neighborhood are observed when the semantic aspects of a word are inaccessible (e.g., "heart checker" for "stethoscope"). The substitution of a similar-sounding word ("tethoscope" for "stethoscope") is not an example of receptive or expressive vocabulary weakness, inasmuch as the word is apparently known.

80. a. Naming words when given a target, such as a category, is a divergent naming task. A person searches his or her internal lexicon for words that fit that category. Labeling a picture or object (options b, d, and e) is a single-word expressive task, or a convergent naming task (producing a specific response). Using a given word in a sentence (option c) is a generative language task, not a divergent one.

81. a. According to the core phonological deficit hypothesis, dyslexia is rooted in difficulty identifying and manipulating sounds within speech. There are numerous possible causes for learning disabilities, these include but are not limited to a core phonological deficit. Other "causes" for example are cognitive weaknesses and visual perception difficulties. The Matthew effect is not a basis for dyslexia. The Matthew effect (option b) suggests that children who fall behind in reading will read less, which increases the reading gap between them and their peers. Although

possibly a result of dyslexia, reading less is not a cause of dyslexia, which has instead a neurological, not experiential, basis. According to the simple view (option c), reading is the product of both decoding and linguistic comprehension; the phonological core is only part of the decoding component of reading. Whole-language theory (option d) is a constructivist approach to reading that emphasizes that children should focus on meaning. This approach moderates explicit skill instruction such as phonological awareness, in contrast to the phonological core deficit theory.

82. d. Phonological processes (option e) is a theoretical framework used to clasify children's speech sound disorders. Identifying target phonemes helps the children develop phonemic awareness, and using these words in a sentence helps them develop vocabulary. Discussing the meaning of the words (option a) targets only vocabulary. Identifying words of three or more syllables (option b) targets only phonemic awareness. Using two words in one sentence (option c) targets only vocabulary. Reading along with the SLP (option e) targets reading fluency through guided repeated reading but does not address phonemic awareness.

83. c. Poor ability to sound out unrecognized words is an example of a phonological deficit, not a semantic-pragmatic deficit. In fact, some children with autism spectrum disorders are hyperlectic (i.e., "read" [decode] although without meaning). Literal interpretation of figurative language (option a), poor turn-taking and topic maintenance (option b), problems initiating or responding to questions (option d), and difficulty with verbal and nonverbal cues of conversational partners (option e) are typical of autism spectrum disorders.

84. b. Theory of mind seeks to provide an explanation of the difficulties experienced by people with autism. Characteristics include an inability to understand the intentions of others and a lack of self-awareness as a social communicator. Although those with language-learning disabilities (option a), hearing loss (option c), intellectual deficits (option d), and dyslexia (option e) may have weakly developed interpersonal mental representations to guide them in interactions with others, this characteristic is not definitive for any of these disabilities.

85. c. Action sequences contain events that are related chronologically but not causally. In this story, the dog's events are clearly chronological, but there is no further elaboration (e.g., cause). Heaps (option a) are stories with ideas that are not related temporally or causally but around a perception. Descriptive

sequences (option b) describe characters and settings but have no causal or temporal links. Reactive sequences (option d) are narratives in which actions are related chronically and causally, but they do not mention characters' goal-directed behavior. True narratives (option e) include all components of story grammar (characters and a theme).

86. b. Although the examiner's comments may be transcribed verbatim for any language sample, such transcription is necessary if these comments are part of dialogue or lead the child to respond in a certain way.

87. a. Spelling involves three processes: alphabetic knowledge (ability to associate sounds with letters and use these sounds to form words), orthographic knowledge (understanding of the symbols used in written language), and morphological knowledge (internal structure of words).

88. e. Clinician-directed activities such as drill play are the least natural. The most natural activities are provided in child-centered activities such as daily activities (option c) and facilitated play (option d). In the hybrid approach, the clinician directs the activity initiated by the child, such as providing focused stimulation during a child-chosen activity (option a) and script therapy (option b).

89. a. In self-talk and parallel talk, actions are used as the stimuli for talking. Imitations (option b), expansions and extensions (option c), buildups and breakdowns (option d), and recasts (option e) are contingent on the child's speaking; that is, these techniques first require the child to make some sort of verbal comment. Therefore, if a child is extremely limited in verbal expression, the most opportunities for modeling by the clinician would be in response to actions rather than the child's verbal utterances.

90. b. An advantage of criterion-referenced procedures is that communication behaviors may be analyzed against an absolute standard, not with reference to other children's achievement. This analysis provides information about the child's strengths and needs and thus allows for identification of baseline (option c), intervention targets (option d), and progress (option e). One of the ways that this is accomplished is through the ability to control the linguistic stimuli (e.g., vocabulary and length of sentences; option a) so that areas of need are clearly identified and not confused with other factors.

91. b. Functional outcomes enable assessment of the child's ability to perform in school or of the child's life skills after intervention. Scores on "high-stakes"

(option a) and standardized tests (option c) demonstrate how the child responds in a decontextualized task but not functionally (real world). Although objectives (option d) and academic goals (option e) are important, they do not offer complete pictures of the child's functional performance in the classroom or daily living skills.

92. a. Young children are capable of rhyming; in early elementary school, children can match sounds; and phoneme substitution is developed through the mid-elementary years (as in internal manipulation of sounds; e.g., "What nonsense word do you get when you change the /l/ sound in 'teld' to a /p/ sound?").

93. b. In view of the observations of the child's conversational speech, it would be important to analyze a language sample for word finding in discourse behaviors such as word reformulations and the use of fillers and generic words. This information would be used in an individualized intervention plan. Assessing rapid automatized naming skills (option a), using a criterion-referenced measure of lexical diversity (option c), and identifying the ability to formulate syntactically correct sentences (option d) might be important but do not specifically address the presenting concern (speech mazes in conversation). Measuring the rate of speech (option e) might also provide information important for intervention, but it, too, does not yield specific information about the kinds of disruptions in speech.

94. d. Joe is described as a child with a specific language impairment. As the demands of school increase, it is likely that his difficulties, although subtle, will affect his academic achievement. In view of the relationship between oral and written language, it is likely that Joe's reading and writing skills are indeed delayed (option a) and that he is slow to process auditory information (option b). Joe's difficulties with pragmatics are a result of confusion in auditory processing; thus, a behavioral approach to intervention (option c) and consideration of autism spectrum disorders (option e) are not warranted.

95. b. Joe is described as a child with a specific language impairment. Therefore, it is important to functionally target syntax development through the use of curriculum vocabulary. His comprehension weaknesses are the root of what appear to be pragmatic difficulties;

therefore, it would be inappropriate to include social skills objectives (options a and c). Simply looking for and finding target words (option d) is not an effective method of developing syntax; repeating words verbatim (option e) is not an effective way to increase vocabulary or improve articulation.

Bibliography

American Psychiatric Association. (2000). *Diagnostic and statistical manual of mental disorders* (4th ed., Text Revision) [*DSM-IV-TR*]. Washington, DC: Author.

American Speech-Language-Hearing Association. (1988). *Prevention of Communication Disorders (Position Statement)* available from www.asha.org/policy.

Bock, K., & Levelt, W. (1994). Language Production: Grammatical encoding. In M. A. Gesnsbacher (Ed.), *Handbook of Psycholinguistics* (pp. 945–983). San Diego: Academic Press.

Catts, H., Fey, M., Tomblin, J. B., & Zhang, X. (2001). Estimating the risk of future reading difficulties in kindergarden children: A research-based model and its clerical implementation. *Language, Speech and Hearing Services in Schools, 32*, 38–50.

Fey, M. E., Long, S. H., & Finestack, L. H. (2003). Ten principles of grammatical intervention for children with specific language impairment. *American Journal of Speech-Language Pathology, 12*, 3–15.

German, D. J. (2005). *Word-Finding Intervention Program. Second Edition (WFIP-2)*. Austin TX: ProEd.

Hogan, T. P., Catts, H. W., & Little, T. D. (2005). The relationship between phonological awareness and reading: Implications for the assessment of phonological awareness. *Language, Speech and Hearing Services in Schools, 36*, 285–293.

Lonigan, C. I., Burgess, S. R., & Anthony, J. L. (2000). Development of emergent literacy and early reading skills in preschool children: Evidence from a latent variable longitudinal study. *Developmental Psychology, 36*, 596–613.

Montgomery, J. K. (2008). Models of RTI for SLPs: To this what we have been waiting for? *Perspectives on Language Learning and Education, 15*, 13–21.

Report of the National Reading Panel: Teaching Children to Read National Institute of Child Health and Human Development (2006). www.nichd.nih.gov/publications/hrp/smallbook.cfm

Rapin, I., & Allen, D. (1987). Developmental dysphasia and autism in preschool children: Characteristics and subtypes. In J. Martin, P. Fletcher, R. Grunwell & D. Hall (Eds.), *Proceedings of the first international symposium on specific speech and language disorders in children* (pp. 20–35). London: Afasic.

Swanson, T. J., Hodson, B. W., & Schommer-Akins, M. (2005). An examination of phonological awareness treatment outcomes for seventh-grade poor readers from a bilingual community. *Language, Speech and Hearing Services in Schedule, 36*, 336–345.

Troia, S. A. (2005). Responsiveness to intervention: Roles for speech-language pathologists in the prevention and identification of learning disabilities. *Topics in Language Disorders*, 106–119.

Vygotsky, L. S. (1978). *Mind and Society: The development of higher psychological processes*. Cambridge, MA: Harvard University Press.

Warren, S., Fey, M. E., Finestack, L. H., Brady, N. L., Bredin-Oja, S. L., & Fleming, K. K. (2008). A randomized trial of longitudinal effects of low-intensity responsivity education/prelinguistic milieu teaching. *Journal Speech, Language, Hearing Research, 51*, 451–470.

PART III

Speech Disorders: Identification, Assessment, Treatment, and Prevention

CHAPTER 8

Fluency Disorders

Tommie L. Robinson

1. Stuttering tends to be more prevalent among which of the following groups?
   a. Boys
   b. Girls
   c. The same for each
   d. Twins
   e. There is no difference

2. Many preschoolers who begin to stutter stop within the first year or two of onset without having received any professional treatment. This is called:
   a. Spontaneous recovery
   b. Normal dysfluency
   c. Consistency effect
   d. Adaptation effect
   e. Spontaneous correction

3. A child exhibited five dysfluencies per 100 words. This indicates that this individual:
   a. Is speaking within normal limits
   b. Is speaking with a fluency rate above average
   c. Should be enrolled in treatment
   d. Is showing mild stuttering characteristics
   e. Is showing mild to moderate stuttering characteristics

4. Stuttering moments are more common in preschool children in which of the following circumstances?
   a. Giving their age, using unfamiliar words, and using content words
   b. On function words in phrases and in the initial sounds in a sentence
   c. The first time using a novel word and giving their address
   d. On the initial consonants and vowel in novel words
   e. At the end of the word in novel sentences

5. Of the following speech and language disorders, which have been associated with stuttering or dysfluent behaviors?
   a. Linguistic complexity, aphasia, syntax, and spastic dysphonia
   b. Pragmatics, spastic dysphonia, and apraxia of speech
   c. Language complexity, voicing, cluttering, and spastic dysphonia
   d. Aphasia, bradylalia, apraxia of speech, and spastic dysphonia
   e. Aphasia, learning disabilities, attention deficit/hyperactivity disorder (ADHD), and apraxia of speech

6. The parents of a 6-year-old are worried that he is going to stutter. On the basis of current data, the clinician can tell them that the risk that the patient will developing stuttering at this time is:
   a. 50%
   b. 25%
   c. 100%
   d. 1%
   e. 75%

7. Analysis of epidemiology research on stuttering indicates that _____ is the variable that affects the true understanding of the prevalence and incidence of stuttering.
   a. Duration
   b. The number of new cases
   c. Normal fluency development
   d. Child development
   e. None of the above

8. An interruption in the flow of speech that is considered to be based on disease, physiological processes, or organic processes is called:
   a. Dysfluency
   b. Repetitions
   c. Tachylalia
   d. Bradylalia
   e. Blocks

9. Of the following descriptions, which, according to Daly (1993), is *not* a quantitative symptom of cluttering?
   a. Acceleration of speech rate between and within multisyllabic words
   b. Appropriate attention span but poor concentration
   c. Vowel stops, or pauses, before vowel-initial words without fear or muscular tension
   d. Six to eight units of repetition of single syllables, short words, and phrases, without apparent concern
   e. Articulation errors, including /r/ and /l/ phonemes, reduction of consonant cluster, or signs of oral apraxia

10. Of the following descriptions, which, according to Daly (1993), is a qualitative characteristic of cluttering?
    a. Writing errors, including poor integration of ideas and motor incoordination
    b. Reading errors, including skipping small words, revising text, or poor concentration
    c. Vocal monotony (lack of speech melody or intonation)
    d. Short attention span and poor concentration
    e. Disorganized speech, including abrupt topic shifts, incomplete phrases, and deficient word retrieval skills

11. A 20-year-old patient presented repetitions and prolongations on final, initial, and medial syllables; poor response to the adaptation effect; annoyance but not anxiety; dysfluency on a variety of phonemes; and no secondary features. The patient probably has:
    a. Qualitative cluttering
    b. Quantitative cluttering
    c. Neurogenic stuttering
    d. Dementia
    e. Classic stuttering

12. During the evaluation process for stuttering, Mary Elizabeth was requested to read the *Rainbow Passage* several times. During an analysis, the clinician noted that every time Mary Elizabeth approached the words *grandfather, swiftly, thinks, minus, frock,* and *banana,* she became dysfluent. This behavior is an example of:
    a. Word-finding difficulties
    b. The consistency effect
    c. Language and psychological effects on stuttering
    d. A neurological condition
    e. The adaptation effect

13. Tameka is undergoing an evaluation, and the clinician has her read a prose passage five times during the evaluation. Each time, the number of her dysfluencies decreases. These diagnostic findings indicate:
    a. The adaptation effect
    b. The consistency effect
    c. Reading and the psychological effects on stuttering
    d. A neurological condition
    e. A psychological condition

14. When a person adapts easily to a communicative situation, this adaptation may in fact be:
    a. Psychological
    b. Environmental
    c. Physiological
    d. Neurological
    e. None of the above

15. When a person shows evidence of difficulty with adaptation, this difficulty may in fact be:
    a. Psychological
    b. Environmental
    c. Physiological
    d. Neurological
    e. None of the above

16. When consistency in dysfluent behaviors is elevated, the basis for this behavior may in fact be:
    a. Psychological
    b. Environmental
    c. Physiological
    d. Neurological
    e. None of the above

17. When there is very little consistency in dysfluent behaviors, the basis for this behavior may in fact be:
    a. Psychological
    b. Environmental
    c. Physiological
    d. Neurological
    e. None of the above

18. Stuttering syndrome involves all the following *except:*
    a. Attitudes and perceptions
    b. Cultural variations
    c. Dysfluencies
    d. Secondary mannerisms
    e. Poor self-concept

19. The mother of a dysfluent child says, "I think that we waited too long to bring our child in for therapy." The clinician responds with the statement, "Well, the important thing is that she is here now and we will work together to help her." The clinician's response is an example of which counseling technique?
    a. Content responds
    b. Affect response
    c. Sharing self
    d. Reframing
    e. Affirmation

20. Smooth transition between the first two sounds of a phrase or after each pause is called:
    a. Continuous phonation
    b. Easy relaxed approach–smooth movements
    c. Easy-onset phonation
    d. Slow and easy talking
    e. None of the above

21. Which treatment method should be used with children who do not show shame and avoidance about their stuttering and with children who have had previous treatment but have residual stuttering in transfer?

    a. Fluency shaping
    b. Stuttering modification
    c. Continuous phonation
    d. Easy relaxed approach–smooth movements
    e. None of the above

22. Of the following methods, which is *not* a fluency-shaping technique?
    a. Slow and gentle talking
    b. "Proprioceptive" awareness of speech movements
    c. Easy phonation
    d. "Play" with stutter before releasing
    e. Decreased rate of speech

23. Of the following methods, which is *not* a stuttering modification technique?
    a. Stuttering slowly, without hurry or tension
    b. Stuttering with slow, relaxed, fluent endings
    c. Stretching of vowels and consonants
    d. Using good eye contact and work for overall comfort and effective communication
    e. Using counseling to deal with stuttering

24. The easy relaxed approach–smooth movements is associated with which of the following individuals?
    a. Janis Costello
    b. Bruce Ryan
    c. Hugo Gregory
    d. Susan Meyers and Lee Woodford
    e. Edward Conture

25. If a bilingual and bicultural adult is dysfluent in only one language, it is likely that this person is:
    a. A monolingual individual who stutters
    b. A bilingual and bicultural individual who stutters
    c. Suffering from an adult language disorder
    d. Suffering from an adult language delay
    e. Suffering from a neurological condition

26. Speech fluency assessments of bilingual and bicultural school-aged children who stutter should include:
    a. Both languages
    b. The preferred language of the home
    c. The dominant language
    d. The language of instruction
    e. The child's preferred language

27. Van Riper's preparatory set technique is based on which theory?
    a. Repressed needs theory
    b. Breakdown theories
    c. Anticipatory struggle theories
    d. Multifactorial theories
    e. Dysphemia

28. Techniques such as slow articulatory rate, continuous phonation, and gentle voice are known as:
    a. Management of fluency
    b. Fluency shaping
    c. Fluency inducing
    d. Stuttering modification
    e. Fluency circling

29. In prevention, training parents to talk less often and with simpler language, to interrupt less often, and to ask fewer questions is best described as:
    a. Contingency management
    b. Fluency shaping
    c. Reduction of speech-associated anxiety
    d. Vocal control treatment approach
    e. An example of stuttering modification

30. A patient underwent evaluation for stuttering. The patient exhibited primarily articulatory groping behavior. The speech-language pathologist (SLP) diagnosed apraxia of speech. Because the patient demonstrated articulatory groping behavior, it is likely that the patient exhibited which of the following speech dysfluency characteristics?
    a. Prolongations
    b. Blocks
    c. Hesitations
    d. Revisions
    e. Interjections

31. Contemporary viewpoints about stuttering are represented by the following broad categories:
    a. Breakdown, repressed need, and anticipatory struggle hypotheses
    b. Breakdown, regressed need, and anticipatory struggle hypotheses
    c. Breakdown, disorganization, and disintegration hypotheses
    d. Breakdown, repressed need, and environmental hypotheses
    e. Breakdown, multifactorial, and anticipatory struggle hypotheses

32. Clinicians sometimes assist clients in coping with external and environmental pressures that presumably precipitate their speech disruptions, especially in relation to family dynamics and changes. The approach for such treatment is rooted in which theoretical belief?
    a. Breakdown theories
    b. Repressed need theories
    c. Anticipatory struggle theories
    d. Environmental theories
    e. Multifactorial theories

33. Of the following statements regarding stuttering and avoidance behaviors, which is generally true?

    a. All people who stutter exhibit avoidance behaviors
    b. Approximately 70% of individuals who stutter exhibit stuttering behaviors
    c. Revisions, circumlocutions, and hesitations are examples of avoidance behaviors
    d. Repetition of whole words, prolongations, and revisions are examples of avoidance behaviors
    e. Only individuals with language difficulties avoid stuttering moments

34. A patient presents with aspects of stuttering that are linguistically based. This patient would probably exhibit all the following dysfluency behaviors *except:*
    a. Whole word repetitions
    b. Blocks
    c. Phrase repetitions
    d. Interjections
    e. Revisions

35. A preschool-aged child exhibits speech fluency characteristics that include more repetitions and prolongations with a few revisions, dysfluencies that are very relaxed, more than 10 dysfluencies per 100 words and rare reaction to his dysfluencies. It is likely that for this child, the SLP will diagnose:
    a. Normal fluency behavior
    b. Borderline stuttering
    c. Intermediate stuttering
    d. Advanced stuttering
    e. Language difficulties

36. Of the following characteristics, which statement is true with regard to beginning stuttering?
    a. Rise in pitch rise may be present toward the end of a repetition or prolongation
    b. Fixed articulatory postures are not evident
    c. Escape behaviors and secondary mannerisms are never present
    d. Awareness of difficulty and feelings of frustration are present
    e. Muscle tension does not appear in stuttering

37. Of the following characteristics, which statement is true with regard to intermediate stuttering?
    a. Blocks, repetitions, and prolongations are seldom noted
    b. Escape and secondary behaviors are used to terminate blocks
    c. Individuals anticipate blocks and use control mechanisms to combat them
    d. There is little fear before stuttering, but there is some shame
    e. Rise in pitch may be present toward the end of a repetition or prolongation

38. Of the following characteristics, which statement is true with regard to advanced stuttering?

a. Most frequent core behaviors are short, and there are frequent blocks and little tremor of lips, tongue, or jaw
b. Avoidance behavior is minimal
c. Repetitions and prolongations are definitely evident
d. Emotions of fear, embarrassment, and shame are very strong
e. Rise in pitch may be present toward the end of a repetition or prolongation

39. A child produced the utterance "Tucker . . . Tucker is a good dog." This is an example of:
a. Part-word repetition
b. Single-syllable word repetition
c. Multisyllabic word repetition
d. Phrase repetition
e. Revision

40. The phrase "I want my . . . where is my mommy?" Is an example of which type of dysfluent behavior?
a. Prolongation
b. Revision-incomplete phrase
c. Tense pause
d. Interjection
e. Circumlocution

41. Martin is a 3-year-old African American boy who is highly verbal and speaks African American dialect. He exhibits 9 dysfluencies per 100 words, has typically one-unit repetitions, and is also exhibiting interjections, revisions, and word repetitions. It is likely that Martin's speech fluency is:
a. Mildly affected
b. Borderline affected
c. Not an issue, but he exhibits a language delay not difference
d. Within normal limits
e. Mild to moderate fluency disorder

42. Cultural implications may be important considerations in the assessment and treatment of stuttering. Of the following situations, which are potential concerns for the SLP?
a. Child-rearing practices
b. Rules for interaction
c. Nonverbal communication
d. All the above
e. None of the above

43. During the assessment of speech fluency, SLPs often measure the time of the longest block. This measurement is commonly referred to as:
a. Longevity
b. Severity rating
c. Duration
d. Calibration
e. Tension measurement

44. The most commonly used measure for assessing the severity of stuttering is:
a. Lidcombe Program's Severity Rating Scale (Onslow et al., 1990)
b. Stuttering Severity Instrument–3 (Riley, 1994)
c. Scale for Rating Severity of Stuttering (Johnson et al., 1952)
d. All the above
e. None of the above

45. During an assessment of speech fluency, a 5-year-old patient demonstrated a speaking rate of 175 syllables per minute. According to the work of Pindzola and colleagues (1989), this rate of speech is:
a. Within the range for the child's age group
b. Below the range for the child's age group
c. Above the range for the child's age group
d. Two standard deviations below the mean for his age group
e. None of the above

46. During an assessment of speech fluency, a 25-year-old man had a speaking rate of 235 syllables per minute. According to the work of Andrews and Ingham (1971), the patient's speaking rate is:
a. Within the range for his age group
b. Below the range for his age group
c. Above the range for his age group
d. 1.5 standard deviations below the mean for his age group
e. None of the above

47. Of the following statements, which is *not* true?
a. Feelings, emotions, beliefs, and attitudes about communication are all components of stuttering
b. The experience of stuttering and the reactions of other people to stuttering have a notable effect on the stuttering
c. Of importance is that feelings, emotions, beliefs, and attitudes can be addressed only in treatment
d. A number of researchers have indicated that a preschool-aged child's sensitivity or reactivity to a new situation may be a prediction of chronicity
e. Clinical reports and the results of some studies indicate that persons who stutter may have unusually sensitive temperaments

48. Of the following behaviors, which should *not* be considered a component of stuttering?
a. Revisions
b. Avoidance behaviors
c. Part-word repetitions
d. Blocks
e. Syllable repetitions

49. When assessing individuals who stutter, clinicians should determine the frequency of stuttered moments, types of stuttering, duration of stuttering, and:
    a. Secondary mannerisms
    b. Severity
    c. Escape behaviors
    d. Type of treatment
    e. None of the above

50. It is important in a diagnostic assessment to address speech naturalness, speech rate, and concomitant or associated behaviors. The importance is rooted in the patient's:
    a. Gender
    b. Cultural background
    c. Age
    d. Socioeconomic level
    e. All the above

51. A preschool child is exhibiting borderline stuttering characteristics. He is showing excellent to above receptive and expressive language skills, and his cognitive skills are well within normal limits. His mother is extremely anxious and worried and often cries when the child is dysfluent. There is no family history of stuttering, and there is great discord between the parents as to what the next steps should be. It is likely that the clinicians' recommendations for this family might be:
    a. To wait and see whether there is spontaneous recovery; therefore, no formal recommendations are made
    b. To place the family in treatment for incipient stuttering because there are some dysfluencies
    c. To develop a prevention plan that would involve the child and the parents
    d. To refer back to the pediatrician and recommend a family therapist
    e. To work directly with the child and ignore the parents

52. An 18-year-old male immigrant from Russia exhibits the following characteristics: He speaks Russian and English fluently; he is severely dysfluent during all conversations with the clinician while speaking English, conversations with the father in Russian, narrative discourse in Russian and English, and reading in Russian and English; he avoids conversational situations as much as possible; he has secondary mannerisms associated with dysfluent behaviors; and he has no concomitant speech-language difficulties. This patient is an example of an individual exhibiting:
    a. Monolingual stuttering
    b. Language-dominant stuttering
    c. Bilingual stuttering
    d. Linguistic stuttering
    e. Psychological stuttering

53. An 18-year-old male immigrant from Russia exhibits the following characteristics: He speaks Russian and English fluently; he is severely dysfluent during all conversations with the clinician while speaking English, conversations with the father in Russian, narrative discourse in Russian and English, and reading in Russian and English; he avoids conversational situations as much as possible; he has secondary mannerisms associated with dysfluent behaviors; and he has no concomitant speech-language difficulties. An appropriate treatment approach for a bilingual stutterer would probably include:
    a. Using an indirect treatment approach and conducting more counseling on dealing with the speech fluency issues and coping with the stuttering
    b. Using a technical approach to address speech fluency in English, because it will allow for automatic transfer to the other language
    c. Addressing the severe speech fluency issues in both languages and, at the same time, working on feelings, attitudes, and acceptance
    d. Using an approach in which the dysfluencies are addressed, and the secondary mannerisms and attitude issues will automatically disappear
    e. Using a fluency-shaping approach by asking him to respond to your model of slow and easy talking

54. A 3-year-old boy comes from a family with very high expectations. He is enrolled in private preschool and does very well in school. His pediatrician, parents, and teachers have expressed some concerns, however, and he was evaluated by an SLP. The boy's mother appears to be a very tense person. He exhibited the following characteristics: cognitive skills that were within normal limits; above-average receptive and expressive language skills; repetitions and prolongations at a rate of 15 per 100 words; two revisions; and one incomplete phrase. The diagnostic finding for the preschooler is:
    a. Within normal limits
    b. Borderline stuttering
    c. Mild stuttering
    d. Moderate stuttering
    e. Severe stuttering

55. A 3-year-old boy comes from a family with very high expectations. He is enrolled in private preschool and does very well in school. His pediatrician, parents, and teachers have expressed some concerns, however, and he was evaluated by an SLP. The boy's mother appears to be a very tense person. He exhibited the following characteristics: cognitive skills that were within normal limits; above-average receptive and expressive language skills; repetitions and prolongations at a rate of 15 per 100 words; two revisions; and one incomplete phrase. Of the following courses of treatment for a preschooler diagnosed with mild stuttering, which is appropriate at this time?

a. Do nothing at this time; these speech fluency characteristics are within normal limits

b. Enroll the child in a prevention and early intervention program to address parental concerns and the child's speech fluency

c. Use an indirect treatment approach

d. Wait and discuss information with the parents at later date and then retest the child to determine the extent of the speech fluency behaviors

e. Enroll the child in a direct treatment program

56. A 3-year-old boy comes from a family with very high expectations. He is enrolled in private preschool and does very well in school. His pediatrician, parents, and teachers have expressed some concerns, however, and he was evaluated by an SLP. The boy's mother appears to be a very tense person. He exhibited the following characteristics: cognitive skills that were within normal limits; above-average receptive and expressive language skills; repetitions and prolongations at a rate of 15 per 100 words; two revisions; and one incomplete phrase. If treatment is recommended for a preschooler with mild stuttering, the appropriate course of action would be:

a. No treatment at this time

b. Prescriptive counseling for the parents only

c. Prescriptive counseling for the parents and demonstrations of appropriate interaction with the preschooler

d. Treatment for the child only

e. Prescriptive counseling for the parents and stuttering modification for the child

57. A 3-year-old boy comes from a family with very high expectations. He is enrolled in private preschool and does very well in school. His pediatrician, parents, and teachers have expressed some concerns, however, and he was evaluated by an SLP. The boy's mother appears to be a very tense person. He exhibited the following characteristics: cognitive skills that were within normal limits; above-average receptive and expressive language skills; repetitions and prolongations at a rate of 15 per 100 words; two revisions; and one incomplete phrase. When making clinical decisions about preschoolers, clinicians should take under consideration indicators of the need for treatment. The following are clinical indicators for enrollment in treatment *except:*

a. A family history

b. Change in the speech disruptions and evidence of more tension

c. Appropriateness of the child's speech language skills

d. Emotional reactions by the child

e. The child's lack of concerns about his speech

58. Many researchers have examined the conversational rates of parents of children who stutter. They have concluded that although the results are inconsistent, there is no information to support the claim that mothers' communication behaviors contribute to the causes of stuttering. There is, however, information that supports the notion that parental communication behaviors can be manipulated to promote positive outcomes for children who stutter. These behaviors are reflected in speaking rate, as well as:

a. Length and complexity of utterances, interruptions, and turn-switching pauses

b. Length and complexity of utterances, interruptions, and turn-taking

c. Length and complexity of utterances, turn-switching pauses, and turn-taking

d. Length and complexity of utterances, interruptions, and silence

e. Interruptions and turn-taking strategies

59. Many authorities have discussed the role of temperament and personality in the development and course of childhood stuttering. According to Conture and Curlee (2007), temperament is rooted in basic psychological processes. From a neurological standpoint, these psychological processes are believed to be tied to the combined influences of all the following *except:*

a. The degree of reactivity

b. The number and degree of self-regulatory processes that the child exhibits

c. The weakness of emotional responses

d. The level of physical activity and regularity of biological cycles

e. The ability to facilitate or inhibit reactive and emotional responses

60. During the stuttering evaluation process, the SLP tries to elicit speech in a variety of speaking situations. An SLP collects several speech samples. In this task, the clinician asks the patient to describe how the SLP does his or her job. In addition, the patient is asked to discuss a movie he or she had just seen. This clinical interaction is an example of what type of communicative interaction?

a. Conversation

b. Monologue

c. Reading

d. Narrative discourse

e. Description

61. A preschool child is enrolled in stuttering treatment, and the SLP is using a direct treatment approach. The approach focuses on the child's speech, the parenting style, and the child's temperament. The SLP is focusing on teaching the parents how to conduct treatment, monitor progress, and measure stuttering in everyday settings. The program that the SLP is using is

a. The Lidcombe Program Onslow et al (2003)

b. The Gregory early intervention program Gregory (2003)

c. A stuttering prevention program

d. The indirect treatment approach to early intervention

e. The indirect treatment approach for early intervention and childhood stuttering

62. There is evidence to support the notion that with above-average mean length of utterance (MLU), preschool children who stutter display stuttering-like behaviors and children who do not stutter display nonstuttering-like dysfluent behaviors. When the children's MLUs are in the average range, dysfluent behavior is less evident. These findings lend support to the hypothesis that:

a. Utterance length and complexity are directly linked to stuttering

b. Utterance length and complexity indicate that language issues are the underlying factor associated with stuttering

c. Utterance length and complexity may change speech-language planning and production and may support the maintenance of speech fluency

d. Utterance length and complexity are the causes of stuttering

e. Utterance length and complexity have no direct relations to stuttering

63. A parent training group includes eight mothers, each with a preschooler who stutters or who is at risk for stuttering. All the parents are from middle-income backgrounds and are highly educated, stay-at-home mothers. The parents are eager to learn as much information as possible about stuttering. The appropriate treatment for the group of parents would be to:

a. Have the parents purchase information from the Stuttering Foundation of America, have the highly educated parents meet together, and find out whether they have questions

b. Have the parents meet together, have them share stories about their children, and guide them on the best possible way for dealing with the stuttering

c. Teach the parents to use normally slower talking and shorter utterances, to minimize questions, to use pauses during conversations, and to avoid corrections; parents are also encouraged to discuss issues that affect stuttering

d. Teach parents how to videotape speech at home, monitor behaviors, and avoid situations that cause stuttering, and discuss issues that affect stuttering

e. None of the above

64. A stuttering treatment program is designed for children in preschool and early elementary school who stutter. The program focuses on universal rules, primary rules when airflow and laryngeal difficulties are present, and secondary rules when concomitant behaviors are present. This program is described in which of the following publications?

a. *Clinical Management of Childhood Stuttering* (Wall and Myers, 1995)

b. *Symmetric Fluency Training for Young Children* (Shine, 1988)

c. "An Indirect Treatment Approach for Early Intervention for Childhood Stuttering" (Richels & Conture, 2007)

d. "The Fluency Rules Program for School-Age Children Who Stutter" (Runyan & Runyan, 2005)

e. *Working With People Who Stutter: A Lifespan Approach* (Bennett, 2006)

65. Counseling is a very important part of providing speech therapy to individuals who stutter. Counseling is a dynamic process that is everchanging. The role of the SLP is to help the patient or client manage change. Although many approaches have been used in managing stuttering, the current approach made popular by DiLollo, Manning, and Neimeyer (2005) focuses on the belief that humans create their own reality and construct personal meanings with the development of narratives. This broad area of counseling is known as:

a. Narrative therapy

b. Constructivist counseling

c. Psychotherapy

d. Self-actualization

e. Self-help

66. A school-based clinician uses a stuttering program that is an integrated treatment approach. It addresses overt stuttering and attitudinal-emotional consequences of stuttering and provides strategies for managing teasing and bullying. The program is ideal for patients aged 7 to 12 years; it is delivered in a 4-week intensive period. The basic treatment goals and components include speech-related, attitudinal-emotional, self-management, and environmental concerns. This program is described in:

a. "The Comprehensive Stuttering Program for School-Age Children with Strategies for Managing Teasing and Bullying" (Langevin et al, 2005)

b. "The Fluency Rules Program for School-Age Children Who Stutter" (Runyan & Runyan, 2005)

c. *Working With People Who Stutter: A Lifespan Approach* (Bennett, 2006)

d. *Assessment of Fluency in School-Age Children* (Thompson, 1983)

e. *Cooper Personalized Fluency Control Therapy–Revised* (Cooper & Cooper, 1985)

67. Byrd and associates (2005) indicated that one third of the children who exhibit fluency disorders also have a concomitant phonological impairment. Although data on treatment outcomes are limited, Wolk (1998) outlined six clinical principles that are based on which approach?

a. Modification of phonological errors but a direct approach for the modification of dysfluency
b. The concurrent application of phonology and fluency intervention strategies
c. Direct modification of dysfluency with allowing phonological errors to naturally correct themselves
d. Modification of the phonological errors and use of this approach to address the dysfluency
e. None of the above

68. There are many similarities and differences between adolescents and adults who stutter. It is well established that motoric, behavioral, emotional, and cognitive aspects of stuttering are important components. One aspect that is very important to the treatment process is attitudinal-emotional. From the following list, which secondary goal is directed to the attitudinal-emotional area of treatment?
a. Positive attitudes toward communication
b. Openness about stuttering and fluency-enhancing techniques
c. Reduced avoidance behaviors
d. Increased family understanding of the causes and development of stuttering
e. Improved communication and social skills

69. An SLP developed goals for a 20-year-old college student with a history of stuttering. His stuttering was considered moderate in nature. The SLP's goals focused on self-monitoring, self-evaluation, problem-solving, manipulating the environment, and sequencing practice activities. Of the following categories, which best describes the goals that the SLP is working on?
a. Speech-related goals
b. Attitudinal-emotional goals
c. Self-management goals
d. Environmental goals
e. Self-study

70. Working on cognitive-behavioral skills has long been thought to contribute to the maintenance of improved fluency in adolescents and adults. Ivey and colleagues (1987) identified some cognitive-behavioral tasks of therapy. Of the following tasks, which is *not* cognitive-behavioral?
a. Examining transfer of skills
b. Examining how one thinks and, if necessary, changing thinking and cognition
c. Ensuring that patients act on those cognitions through behavior in their daily lives
d. Engaging in decision making to determine how to act
e. None of the above

71. A patient exhibits subtle but salient features of stuttering. These include syllable repetitions, prolongations, and secondary mannerisms. Her speaking difficulties affect her socially, emotionally, educationally, and vocationally. The likely diagnosis for this patient will be:
a. Overt stuttering
b. Covert stuttering
c. Social stuttering
d. Psychological stuttering
e. Neurogenic stuttering

72. A patient exhibits subtle but salient features of stuttering. These include syllable repetitions, prolongations, and secondary mannerisms. Her speaking difficulties affect her socially, emotionally, educationally, and vocationally. Because the diagnosis is covert stuttering, the course of treatment for this patient would probably include:
a. A counseling approach in conjunction with a techniques approach
b. Techniques and strategies alone
c. Counseling alone
d. Fluency shaping
e. All the above

73. An adolescent with learning disabilities is having difficulties with dysfluent behaviors. He is often dysfluent when trying to retrieve a word during conversation, when storytelling, and when he is trying to organize what he wants to say. He exhibits primarily word and phrase repetitions, as well as hesitations. Also noted are articulatory gropings and interjections. His diagnosis is:
a. Dysarthric stuttering
b. Apraxic stuttering
c. Dysnomic stuttering
d. Language stuttering
e. Psychogenic stuttering

74. Transfer of skills is the biggest challenge that clinicians face when working with individuals who stutter. Of the following definitions, which is accurate for the main goal of transfer?
a. To generalize clinic-established behavior to representative everyday speaking situations
b. To promote sequential modification to promote fluency in progressively more difficult situations
c. To modify the antecedents or stimuli that trigger stuttering in situations beyond the clinic
d. To self-evaluate speech in all speaking situations
e. To self-educate so that one is ready to speak in all situations

75. An SLP completed a diagnostic protocol that included case history (medical, social, occupational, and personal information; onset and development of stuttering); testing of general functions (language [vocabulary, reading, naming] speech [motor speech examination], and cognition); speech fluency assessment (reading, spontaneous speech, automated speech, trial therapy and techniques, speaking situations, and stuttering severity); and self-assessment. This protocol is probably for:
a. Acquired stuttering
b. Apraxic stuttering
c. Dysarthric stuttering
d. Dysnomic stuttering
e. All the above

Answers

1. a. According to Bloodstein and Ratner (2008), stuttering is more prevalent among boys than among girls, by a ratio of 3:1.

2. a. It is believed that 20% to 80% of children who stutter recover normal speech without treatment (Bloodstein, 1995; Andrews, et al., 1983; Guitar, 2006); this phenomenon is known as *spontaneous recovery* (or *natural recovery*). However, it is very difficult to determine which of the children who stutter will spontaneously or naturally recover. This is why prevention and early intervention are very important.

3. a. Five dysfluencies per 100 words is considered within normal limits. A child who exhibits 10 or more dysfluencies per 100 words is considered to be at risk for difficulties. In that case, the child would also exhibit repetitions of whole words and phrases and exhibit interjections and revisions.

4. b. Stuttering moments in preschoolers are more common in function words and phrases and in the initial position of sounds in a sentence. Adults would probably have more difficulty with the content words and in giving information that is high in value content.

5. d. Aphasia, bradylalia, apraxia of speech, and spastic dysphonia are all speech and language disorders that have been associated with stuttering. Adults with aphasia often exhibit dysfluent speech behaviors or neurogenic stuttering symptoms. Bradylalia is a slow rate of speech. Apraxia of speech is often associated with stuttering in that the symptom of articulatory groping can be confused with stuttering characteristics. Spastic dysphonia is referred to as *laryngeal stuttering,* and the symptoms are very similar to those of stuttering. Linguistic complexity (option a), syntax (option a), pragmatics (option b), language complexity (option c), learning disabilities (option e), and ADHD (option e) are not speech and language disorders.

6. b. In general, by age 6, the risk of developing stuttering is minimized; that is, there is only a 25% chance that the individual will develop stuttering if his speech is currently normal.

7. a. In research on the epidemiology of stuttering, the most confusing variable is duration of stuttering. It seems that there is no universal measure by which parents and researchers define "duration." Therefore, a particular definition of duration truly influences

the interpretation of the research data and information about the development of stuttering.

8. a. Dysfluency is the pathological interruption of the flow of speech. The term *dysfluency* is used by some clinicians to refer to "stuttering." The terms *disfluency* and *dysfluency* are used synonymously by most clinicians. Repetitions and blocks (options b & e) are terms used to describe different dysfluent behavior. Option c refers to rapid speech rate, while option d refers to an abnormally slow rate of speech.

9. b. According to Daly (1993), individuals who clutter have an inappropriate (short) attention span and poor concentration. Quantitative symptoms are measurable symptoms that may be used to quantify different components of cluttering.

10. e. According to Daly (1993), individuals who clutter have been described as having disorganized speech, including abrupt topic shifts, incomplete phrases, and deficient word retrieval skills.

11. c. The particular symptoms are all characteristics of neurogenic stuttering. These characteristics are not similar to characteristics of quantitative or qualitative cluttering. The annoyance characteristic might be similar to that in dementia. There are a few similarities to classic stuttering in that repetitions and prolongations are evident. The biggest clues are dysfluencies on final and medial syllables and poor response to the adaptation effect.

12. b. The consistency effect is being dysfluent on the same words in a consistent manner. Mary Elizabeth demonstrates this because there is a core group of words for which she is consistently dysfluent. This illustrates the construct of high consistency, which lends support to the psychological nature of stuttering.

13. a. Clinicians and researchers have found that dysfluent behavior does decrease with multiple readings of a prose passage; this is a demonstration of the adaptation effect.

14. a. It is believed that being able to adapt easily ameliorates the psychological aspects of stuttering. In adapting easily, the individual reduces the fear of speaking and therefore increases fluent behavior.

15. d. When a person has difficulty with adaptation, there may be instability with behaviors, which reflects

the neurological aspects of stuttering. If the person behaves inconsistently or shows difficulties with adapting to a new reading up to five times, then further testing of neurological abilities is warranted.

16. a. Elevated consistency in this case means that the individual is consistently dysfluent on the words she or he uses and in the same situations. This would suggest that there is a psychological component arising from fears, environmental influences, and other factors.

17. d. It is well documented that with neurological conditions, there appears to be inconsistency in behaviors. Inconsistency is characteristic of speech behaviors as well. Therefore, low consistency is often indicative of neurological difficulties.

18. b. Although very important to the evaluation and treatment of stuttering, cultural variations are not included in the classic definition of stuttering.

19. d. Luterman (1996) describes this technique as "Pollyannaish" in that the clinician always finds the good in what the patient or client says in making clinical observations. This is a good example of a parent who blames herself for waiting too long to seek services for her child. The clinician reframed the mother's statement to help her move on and to use positive energy for dealing with her child's difficulties.

20. b. Easy relaxed approach–smooth movements is a treatment technique in which smooth transitions are used between the first two sounds of each phrase or breath group. It allows the patient or client to develop, easily and quickly, a "normal"-sounding voice.

21. b. Stuttering modification should be used in clinical situations such as these, so that clinicians not only are dealing with the dysfluencies but also are helping these children to speak more fluently and, therefore, control the stuttering more efficiently.

22. d. "Playing" with the stutter before releasing is a stuttering modification technique rather than a fluency-shaping technique. Fluency-shaping techniques are not so direct and are designed to alter stuttering and shape it into fluent speech.

23. c. Stretching of vowels and consonants is a fluency-shaping technique rather than a stuttering modification technique. Stuttering modification techniques are designed to assist the person to stutter more fluently.

24. c. Hugo Gregory at Northwestern University in Evanston, Illinois, promoted the use of this technique and encouraged patients, clients, and students to use it while maintaining normal rate, loudness, pitch, and expression.

25. b. This person is a bilingual and bicultural individual who stutters in one language. From the information given, nothing else can be determined. In order to examine language, testing would have to be performed in each language. The same holds true for neurological considerations. Although the problem could be a language disorder, no evidence of language disorder is given in this description.

26. a. When assessing the speech fluency of bilingual and bicultural individuals who stutter, considerations should be given to both languages. This is important because language must be ruled out or confirmed as a factor in the process. In addition to the speech fluency skills, other areas of the assessment (e.g., language, speech sound production) need to be addressed in both languages. In order to complete the differential diagnostic process, such testing must be done.

27. c. According to the anticipatory struggle theories, individuals who stutter believe that speaking is difficult. Van Riper's technique would therefore allow people who stutter to predict when stuttering moments will occur and to use techniques to handle those difficult moments.

28. b. Slow articulatory rate, continuous phonation, and gentle voice are all fluency-shaping techniques that are used to help patients and clients feel fluent. These techniques are used change the stuttering into fluent speech.

29. c. Each of these activities is used to reduce speech-associated anxiety. Parents are encouraged to talk less and to comment rather than badger the child with numerous questions. Parents are also encouraged to use simpler language and to avoid interrupting the child. These techniques constitute a model of communication for the child, and their use also lessens the stress associated with communication.

30. b. Articulatory groping behavior is a characteristic of apraxia of speech. It is often confused with, or looks similar to, blocks. It is very easy for clinicians to confuse this motor speech symptom with the blocking behavior that is noted in stuttering.

31. a. Bloodstein and Ratner (2008) identified the breakdown, repressed need, and anticipatory struggle hypotheses as the broad areas of theory development

concerning the cause of stuttering. Although there are many theories as to the cause of stuttering, they probably belong to one of these broad areas.

32. c. Communicative failure or pressure is thought to result from external or environmental changes, and stuttering under these circumstances is thought to arise from the notion that speaking is difficult. This theoretical position is consistent with the anticipatory struggle explanation. Temperament and certain personality traits can also influence fluency.

33. c. Revisions, circumlocutions, and hesitations are examples of avoidance behaviors. There are no data to identify the percentage of individuals who both stutter and exhibit avoidance behaviors. Clinicians should be alert for these dysfluency characteristics as indicators of avoidance behaviors.

34. b. Of the types of dysfluency listed, the only one that is not linguistically based is blocks. Blocks are, instead, instances when this person is unable to produce sounds.

35. b. The child is exhibiting borderline stuttering characteristics. There are too many dysfluencies for the child's speech to be considered normal, and there is not enough tension to indicate intermediate stuttering.

36. a. Rises in pitch at the end of a repetition or prolongation are often characteristic of beginning stuttering. This feature might be an indicator that overall tension is now present in the speech pattern as well.

37. b. Escape behaviors are used to terminate blocks in intermediate stuttering. Blocks are core to the behavior, and there may be repetitions and prolongations. Affected individuals avoid blocks as much as possible, and there is a great deal of fear before stuttering. Rises in pitch are noted more with beginning stuttering.

38. d. Emotions of fear, embarrassment, and shame are major characteristics of advanced stuttering. The other characteristics may include tense blocks, lip tremors, extensive avoidance behaviors, and complex escape behaviors.

39. c. Because the repeated word is a whole word with more than one syllable, this utterance is considered a multisyllabic word repetition.

40. b. The example cited above is a revision–incomplete phrase because the phrase was not completed and what was said was revised.

41. d. Martin's speech is within normal limits because he is exhibiting fewer than 10 dysfluencies per 100 words.

The interjections, revisions, and word repetitions are expected for his age group; regardless of dialect spoken.

42. d. Child-rearing practices, rules for interaction, and nonverbal communication are all potentially important considerations. In working with preschoolers, SLPs also work with families and observe and attempt to change how they interact. Child-rearing practices are evident in family settings, and they differ from culture to culture. How people culturally interact is also important and is rooted in their value systems. Nonverbal communication differs among cultural groups and influences how SLPs interact with patients or clients.

43. c. The time of the longest block is known as *duration*. This is an important variable for determining the severity of stuttering.

44. b. The Stuttering Severity Instrument–3 (Riley, 1994) is the assessment instrument most commonly used to evaluate severity of stuttering. There is a dearth of formal instruments for assessing speech fluency in adults and children. The data reported are the range, which consists of the highest and lowest scores obtained. There is no measure of central tendency or dispersion from the mean.

45. a. Pindzola and colleagues (1989) indicated that the average range of syllables per minute for a 3-year-old is 116 to 163; thus, the child's rate of syllables per minute is slightly above average. The data reported are the range, which consists of the highest and lowest scores obtained. There is no measure of central tendency or dispersion from the mean.

46. c. Andrews and Ingham (1971) indicated that the range of syllables per minute for this age group is 162 to 230. The estimated rate that was reported is above the expected normative values.

47. c. It is important to keep in mind that feelings, emotions, beliefs, and attitudes can be addressed in the evaluation, treatment, and any other environment. The statement that these components "can be addressed only in treatment" is therefore incorrect.

48. a. Revisions should not be considered a component of stuttering because they are really an indicator of language formulation. However, clinicians should take under consideration the effect of revisions on avoidance behaviors.

49. b. Severity is a component of the diagnostic assessment. Secondary mannerisms, escape behaviors, and type of treatment influence severity.

50. b. Speech naturalness, speech rate, and concomitant or associated behaviors are all rooted in cultural practices. Clinicians must be mindful of this fact and consider those variables in the clinical process.

51. c. The clinician needs to develop a prevention plan that would involve the child and the parents. Because this mother is anxious, it is obvious that she needs counseling. In addition, however, the child will need to be seen in counseling so that the mother learns how to interact with him. The prevention plan would also include talking with both parents.

52. c. The client demonstrates bilingual stuttering. He is equally dysfluent in both languages. It would be advantages if the patients SLP was fluent in both languages.

53. c. Treatment should address the severe speech fluency issues in both languages and, at the same time, work on feelings, attitudes, and acceptance. This plan is appropriate for him because he is dysfluent in both languages equally. In addition, the other treatment approaches do not address his need for stuttering modifications. They focus more on fluency shaping.

54. c. The diagnosis is that of mild stuttering. There is no mention of tension or secondary mannerisms, which would exacerbate the situation and result in a more severe degree of stuttering. The number of dysfluent words and the types of dysfluencies described are consistent with this severity rating.

55. b. He should be enrolled in a prevention and early intervention program to address parental concerns and the child's speech fluency. The parents need help with transitions and also will need help in developing strategies for interacting communicatively with their child.

56. c. Prescriptive counseling for the parents and demonstrations of appropriate interaction with the preschooler should be implemented. The parents need to have a better understanding of the communication disorder, and the clinician should demonstrate to the parents how to interact with the child.

57. e. Children do not need to show concern in order to be enrolled in treatment. Although this is a big issue for adolescents and adults, it is not as much of a concern for preschoolers and younger children.

58. a. Speaking rate, length and complexity of utterances, interruptions, and turn-switching pauses can be modified through parent education and training. During the treatment process, clinicians manipulate these variables, or help parents manipulate them, so that speech rate is modeled as slow and easy. Clinicians also teach strategies on reducing the length and complexity of utterances used with the child. Furthermore, clinicians teach parents how to avoid interruptions and to model appropriate turn-taking strategies for the child in order to maximize speech fluency.

59. c. The weakness of emotional responses is not a variable that is part of the psychological processes identified. The concern is actually, as Conture and Curlee (2007) would describe, about the strength of the emotional response associated with reactivity, that is important.

60. d. Both are narrative discourse tasks. They allow the clinician to obtain a sample of speech *and language* in spontaneous speaking tasks. This provides the clinician with information regarding linguistic organization and speech fluency.

61. a. The Lidcombe Program (Onslow et al., 2003) is a parent-centered process in which the parent serves as the clinician for his or her child. It is a highly regarded program that is gaining popularity because of its effectiveness with children.

62. c. Utterance length and complexity may influence speech-language planning and production and may support the maintenance of speech fluency. This is seen clinically when parents are taught to reduce the language demands on their child. In using this model, the child reduces sentence length and complexity, and dysfluencies decrease.

63. c. Parents are taught to use normally slower talking and shorter utterances, to minimize questions, to use pauses during conversations, and to avoid corrections. Parents are also encouraged to discuss issues that affect stuttering. Teaching parents to reduce language demands, reduce speech anxiety, and reduce time pressures is important in parent counseling. In addition, talking about the parents' needs is pertinent to issues that affect stuttering and is important for demystifying stuttering.

64. d. "The Fluency Rules Program for School-Age Children Who Stutter," by Runyan and Runyan (2005), focuses on universal rules; primary rules when airflow and laryngeal difficulties are present; and secondary rules when concomitant behaviors are present.

65. a. Narrative therapy is designed to help patients cope with the behaviors stuttering and to help them approach the problem of gaining fluency.

66. a. "The Comprehensive Stuttering Program for School-Age Children" (CSP-SC) by Langevin and colleagues, outlines a treatment that addresses the components discussed.

67. a. The six clinical principles are based on the modification of phonological errors but a direct approach for the modification of dysfluency. This approach allows clinicians to focus on what the child is saying, rather than how the child says it. It minimizes the emphasis on articulation and keeps speech fluency as the main focus.

68. d. Increased family understanding of the causes and development of stuttering is an appropriate secondary goal but is not germane to the treatment issues at hand. The primary focus should be on the attitudinal and emotional elements of the patient.

69. c. Self-management goals include self-monitoring, self-evaluation, problem-solving, manipulating the environment, and sequencing practice activities. This area is very important for increasing the patient's awareness of stuttering.

70. a. Transfer of skills is not a goal of cognitive-behavioral therapy; instead, it is a general goal for transferring and generalizing the skill set that is being taught.

71. b. The patient is trying to conceal her difficulties by engaging in covert stuttering behavior.

72. a. A counseling approach in combination with a techniques approach is the appropriate course of treatment. In order to deal with covert stuttering, its existence has to be brought to a conscious level through counseling; at the same time, fluency techniques need to be taught.

73. c. This adolescent is exhibiting neurogenic stuttering characteristics. Clinicians may be confused by the articulatory gropings and think of apraxic stuttering, but the other features are those of dysnomic (neurogenic) stuttering.

74. a. Generalizing clinic-established behavior to representative everyday speaking situations is the biggest challenge of speech fluency therapy. SLPs often teach patients to be fluent in the context of therapy, but they must also devise ways to make transfer and generalization an everyday skill.

75. e. This is a comprehensive protocol for stuttering to determine a differential diagnosis that encompasses all the disorders listed.

Bibliography

Anderson, J. D., Pellowski, M. W., Conture, E. G., & Kelly, E. M. (2003). Temperamental characteristics of young children who stutter. *Journal of Speech, Language, and Hearing Research*, *46*(5), 1221–1233.

Andrews, G., Craig, A., Feyer, A.-M., Hoddinott, S., Howie, P., & Neilson, M. (1983). Stuttering: A review of research findings and theories circa 1982. *Journal of Speech and Hearing Disorders*, *48*, 226–246.

Andrews, G., & Ingham, R. (1971). Stuttering: Considerations in the evaluation of treatment. *British Journal of Communication Disorders*, *6*, 129–138.

Bennett, E. M. (2006). *Working with people who stutter: A lifespan approach*. Pearson Merrill Prentice-Hall: Upper Saddle River, NJ.

Bloodstein, O. (1995). *A handbook on stuttering* (5th ed.). Thomson-Delmar: Clifton Park, NY.

Bloodstein, O., & Ratner, N. (2008). *A handbook on stuttering* (6th ed.). Thomson-Delmar: Clifton Park, NY.

Byrd, C., Wolk, L., & Davis, B. L. (2005). Moving towards an understanding of the phonological pieces of the stuttering puzzle. In R. Curlee & E. Conture (Eds.), *Stuttering and related disorders of fluency*. (3rd edition). Thieme Medical: Philadelphia, PA.

Conture, E. G., & Curlee, R. F. (2007). *Stuttering and related disorders of fluency* (3rd ed.). New York: Thieme.

Cooper, E., & Cooper, C. (1985). *Cooper personalized fluency control therapy-revised*. Allen, TX: DLM Teaching Resources.

Daly, D. A. (1993). Cluttering: Another fluency syndrome. In R. Curlee (Ed.), *Stuttering and Related Disorders of Fluency* (pp. 151–175). New York: Thieme Medical Publishers.

DiLollo, A., Manning, W. H., & Neimeyer, R. A. (2005). Cognitive complexity as a function of speaker role for adult persons who stutter. *Journal of Constructivist Psychology*, *18*, 215–236.

Gregory, H. H. (2003). *Stuttering therapy: rationale and procedures*. Boston: Pearson Education, Inc.

Guitar, B. (2006). *Stuttering: An integrated approach to its nature and treatment* (3rd ed.). Baltimore: Lippincott, Williams and Wilkins.

Ivey, A. E., Ivey, M. B., & Simek-Downing, L. (1987). *Counseling and psychotherapy* (2nd ed.). Prentice-Hall, Inc: Englewood Cliffs, NJ.

Johnson, W., Darley, F., & Spriestersbach, D. (1952). *Diagnostic Manual in Speech Correction: A Professional Training Workbook*. New York: Harper & Brothers.

Langevin, M., Kully, D. A., & Ross-Harold, B. (2005). The comprehensive stuttering program for school-age children with strategies for managing teasing and bullying. In Conture E. G. & Curlee R. F. (Eds.), *Stuttering and related disorders of fluency* (3rd ed pp. 131–150). New York: Thieme.

Langevin, M., Kully, D. A., & Ross-Harold, B. (2007). The comprehensive stuttering program for school-age children with strategies for managing teasing and bullying. In E. G. Conture & R. F. Curlee (3rd ed.), *Stuttering and related disorders of fluency*. New York: Thieme Medical Publishers, pp. 131–149.

Luterman, D. M. (1996). *Counseling persons with communication disorders and their families* (3rd ed.). Austin, TX: PRO-ED.

Manning, W. H. (2001). *Clinical decision-making in fluency disorders* (2nd ed.). San Diego, CA: Singular.

Onslow, M., Costa, L., & Rue, S. (1990). Direct early intervention with stuttering: Some preliminary data. *Journal of Speech and Hearing Disorders*, *55*, 405–416.

Onslow, M., Packman, A., & Harrison, E. (2003). *The lidcombe program of early stuttering intervention: a clinician's guide*. Austin, TX: PRO-ED.

Pindzola, R., Jenkins, M., & Lokken, K. (1989). Speaking rates of young children. *Language, Speech and Hearing Services in Schools*, *20*, 133–138.

Richels, C. G., & Conture, E. G. (2007). An indirect treatment approach for early intervention for childhood stuttering. In E. G. Conture & R. F. Curlee (3rd ed.), *Stuttering and Related Disorders of Fluency*. New York: Thieme Medical Publishers, pp. 77–99.

Riley, G. (1994). *Stuttering Severity Instrument for Children and Adults* (ed 3). Austin, TX: PRO-ED.

Robinson, T. L., Jr., & Crowe, T. A. (1998). Culture-based considerations in programming for stuttering intervention with African American clients and their families. *Language, Speech and Hearing Services in the Schools, 29*, 172–179.

Robinson, T. L., Jr., & Crowe, T. A. (2001). Fluency and voice. In D. M. Ruscell, *Tests and measurements in speech-language pathology*. Boston: Butterworth-Heinemann.

Runyan, C. M., & Runyan, S. E. (2005). Fluency Rules Program: For the Young Stutterer. In E. G. Conture & R. F. Curlee (3rd ed.), *Stuttering and related disorders of fluency*. New York: Thieme Medical Publishers.

Ruscello, D. M. (2001). *Tests and measurements in speech-language pathology*. Boston: Butterworth-Heinemann.

Shapiro, D. A. (1999). *Stuttering intervention: A collaborative journey to fluency freedom*. Austin, TX: PRO-ED.

Shine, R. E. (1988). *Symmetric fluency training for young children* (3rd ed.). Austin, TX: PRO-ED.

Thompson, J. (1983). *Assessment of fluency in school-aged children*. Interstate: Danville, IL.

Wall, M. J., & Myers, F. L. (1995). *Clinical Management of childhood stuttering* (2nd ed.). Austin, TX: PRO-ED.

Wolk, L. (1998). Intervention strategies for children who exhibit coexisting phonological and fluency disorders: A clinical note. *Child Language Teaching and Theories, 14*, 69–82.

CHAPTER 9

Resonance Disorders

David L. Jones

1. The primary goal of surgical repair of a cleft palate is to:
   a. Improve function of the eustachian tube
   b. Provide a hard-soft palatal mechanism that sufficiently separates the oral and nasal cavities during speech
   c. Give the parents a psychological lift
   d. Improve feeding
   e. Prevent dental malocclusion

2. The palatoplasty procedure that is designed to add length to the soft palate and minimize the contractile forces generated by palatal scar tissue is:
   a. The V-Y procedure
   b. Furlow Z-plasty procedure
   c. The intravelar veloplasty procedure
   d. Von Langenbeck procedure
   e. The pharyngeal flap procedure

3. What syndrome is characterized by macroglossia and macrostomia?
   a. Apert syndrome
   b. Crouzon syndrome
   c. Beckwith-Wiedemann syndrome
   d. Down syndrome
   e. Velocardiofacial syndrome

4. Which syndrome is characterized by cardiac problems, velopharyngeal inadequacy, and typical facies (e.g., long face, almond-shaped eyes, broad nasal base)?
   a. Treacher Collins syndrome
   b. Apert syndrome
   c. Prader-Willi syndrome
   d. Hemifacial microsomia
   e. Velocardiofacial syndrome

5. Facial asymmetry, microtia, preauricular tags, hypoplasia or atresia of the external auditory meatus, and conductive hearing loss are common in what disorder?
   a. Fetal alcohol syndrome
   b. Velocardiofacial syndrome
   c. Prader-Willi syndrome
   d. Hemifacial microsomia
   e. Pierre Robin sequence

6. In this syndrome, hypernasality resulting from muscle hypotonia is evident during childhood, but it resolves after puberty:
   a. Fetal alcohol syndrome
   b. Velocardiofacial syndrome
   c. Prader-Willi syndrome
   d. Hemifacial microsomia
   e. Treacher Collins syndrome

7. Which is *not* an identifying characteristic of the Pierre Robin sequence?
   a. Cleft lip
   b. Cleft palate
   c. Micrognathia
   d. Glossoptosis
   e. Airway obstruction

8. You are examining a child who has hypernasal speech. On oral mechanism examination, you see the zona pellucida, a bony notch in the posterior hard palate, and a bifid uvula. You would recommend the following:
   a. Initiate articulation therapy
   b. Initiate oral motor therapy
   c. Recommend orthodontic management
   d. Defer treatment until after the patient reaches puberty
   e. Refer the patient to an otorhinolaryngologist or plastic surgeon to consider a diagnosis of submucous cleft palate

9. What is the primary paired muscle of soft palatal movement and velopharyngeal closure?
   a. Palatoglossus
   b. Levator veli palatini
   c. Tensor veli palatini
   d. Superior pharyngeal constrictor
   e. Palatopharyngeus

10. A child exhibits normal resonance and adequate oral pressure with no audible nasal emission during the production of nearly all oral consonants. However, severe audible nasal emission is perceived during production of /s/ and /z/. It is likely that the patient has:
    a. Phoneme-specific nasal emission
    b. Velopharyngeal insufficiency
    c. An anterior palatal fistula
    d. A posterior palatal fistula
    e. A fistula at the juncture of the hard and soft palates

11. The compensatory articulation pattern most frequently observed in children with cleft palate is the:
    a. Glottal stop
    b. Pharyngeal fricative
    c. Velar stop
    d. Mid-dorsum palatal stop
    e. Epiglottal-pharyngeal fricative

12. Figure 9-1 shows the velopharyngeal port in the "rest" position (far left), then moving toward velopharyngeal closure (far right). The velopharyngeal closure pattern shown in this figure is:
    a. Adynamic
    b. Circular
    c. Circular with Passavant's ridge
    d. Sagittal
    e. Coronal

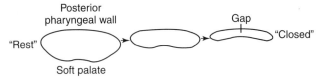

Figure 9-1

13. Figure 9-2 shows the velopharyngeal port in the "rest" position (far left), then moving toward velopharyngeal closure (far right). The velopharyngeal closure pattern shown in this figure is:
    a. Adynamic
    b. Circular
    c. Circular with Passavant's ridge
    d. Sagittal
    e. Coronal

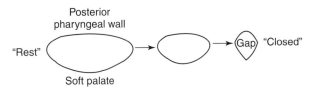

Figure 9-2

14. During speech, velar position is influenced primarily by what three muscles?
    a. Tensor veli palatini, levator veli palatini, and palatopharyngeus
    b. Tensor veli palatini, palatoglossus, and palatopharyngeus
    c. Levator veli palatini, palatopharyngeus, and salpingopharyngeus
    d. Levator veli palatini, palatoglossus, and palatopharyngeus
    e. Tensor veli palatine, palatopharyngeus, and musculus uvulae

15. Contraction of this muscle adds bulk to the nasal surface of the soft palate, resulting in the "velar eminence" or "velar knee":
    a. Tensor veli palatini
    b. Superior pharyngeal constrictor
    c. Musculus uvulae
    d. Stylopharyngeus
    e. Palatopharyngeus

16. What articulators are involved in producing a pharyngeal fricative?
    a. Posterior pharyngeal wall and tongue tip
    b. Posterior pharyngeal wall and soft palate
    c. Posterior pharyngeal wall and larynx
    d. Posterior pharyngeal wall and tongue base
    e. The vocal folds

17. In comparison with a speaker who does not have cleft palate, the levator muscle of an individual with a repaired cleft palate is active at what level in relation to its maximum output?
    a. The same level as in the individual without a cleft
    b. At a level higher than normal
    c. At a level lower than normal
    d. At a level higher than normal for vowels and lower than normal for consonants
    e. None of the above

18. If no oral-nasal fistula is present, which of these indirect methods of velopharyngeal assessment can provide evidence that the velopharyngeal port is open during speech?
    a. Nasometry
    b. Oral manometry
    c. Measurement of nasal airflow
    d. Electromyography
    e. Accelerometry

19. Which best allows for assessing the anatomical relationship between the adenoid pad and the vertical level of maximum velopharyngeal closure?
    a. Frontal view videofluoroscopy
    b. Lateral view videofluoroscopy
    c. Frontal view video-endoscopy
    d. Lateral view video-endoscopy
    e. Videostroboscopy

20. Of the following statements regarding nonspeech velopharyngeal muscle training exercises (e.g., blowing, sucking, and gagging), which is correct?
    a. In these exercises, the velopharyngeal musculature is not working against any type of resistive force
    b. With the appropriate therapy schedule, gagging exercises can improve velopharyngeal function
    c. These exercises provide muscle training during speech production

d. Increased levator muscle activity during blowing leads to increased muscle activity during speech
    e. The research evidence in regard to the effectiveness of muscle training is positive

21. The continuous positive airway pressure (CPAP) device:
    a. Exercises the velopharyngeal mechanism by resisting velopharyngeal port opening movements during speech
    b. Exercises the velopharyngeal mechanism by resisting velopharyngeal port closing movements during speech
    c. Improves tongue placement during speech
    d. Facilitates tighter lip closure during the production of labial consonants
    e. Improves respiratory support for speech

22. Which therapy approach has been successful in improving velopharyngeal function for speech?
    a. Electrical stimulation
    b. Blowing exercises
    c. Sucking exercises
    d. Mechanical stimulation of the faucial pillars
    e. None of the above

23. A 7-year-old patient with a repaired cleft palate has consistent hypernasality and audible nasal emission. Video-endoscopy reveals a short palate that demonstrates minimal mobility and lateral pharyngeal walls that are markedly mobile. What surgical procedure would be most appropriate?
    a. Sphincter pharyngoplasty
    b. Palatal lengthening
    c. Posterior pharyngeal wall augmentation
    d. Pharyngeal flap
    e. Defer surgical management until the patient is past puberty

24. A 44-year-old patient with a repaired cleft lip and palate demonstrates evidence of gross velopharyngeal incompetence. Video-endoscopy reveals a short soft palate and a large velopharyngeal gap. The patient cannot undergo stimulation for improved velopharyngeal function and is not interested in surgical management. Which approach would be best?
    a. Obturator (or speech bulb)
    b. Palatal lift
    c. Oral-motor therapy for velopharyngeal function
    d. Biofeedback therapy
    e. Palatal stimulation

25. The sphincter pharyngoplasty is most appropriate for which pattern of velopharyngeal closure?
    a. Coronal
    b. Sagittal
    c. Circular

d. Circular with Passavant's ridge
e. Adynamic

26. What is the major factor that influences the success of secondary management of velopharyngeal incompetence?
a. The presence of a repaired cleft palate
b. Type of cleft palate (unilateral versus bilateral)
c. Gender
d. Age at surgery
e. The degree of preoperative velopharyngeal movement

27. An 8-year-old with a repaired cleft palate is examined. His speech is dominated by glottal stop substitutions. What is the most appropriate short-term recommendation?
a. Prosthodontic management
b. Articulation therapy
c. Surgical management
d. Palatal expansion
e. Palatal stimulation

28. When and how should blowing tasks be performed by children who demonstrate perceptual evidence of velopharyngeal dysfunction?
a. Blowing tasks should never be used
b. Blowing tasks should be performed intensively for an extended period of time (for instance, 3 weeks)
c. Blowing tasks should be performed while the oral resistance to blowing is increased
d. Blowing tasks should be performed in conjunction with sucking tasks in order to alternate positive and negative oral pressures
e. Any blowing activity should be carried out with the intent of showing the child the concept of oral versus nasal airflow

29. A 47-year-old woman sustained traumatic brain injury 8 months ago. She exhibits moderate to severe hypernasality with weak pressure consonants. She has adequate articulatory placement and normal velopharyngeal anatomy but no velopharyngeal movement during speech. The most appropriate treatment option would be:
a. Pharyngeal flap
b. Sphincter pharyngoplasty
c. Speech bulb (obturator)
d. Palatal lift
e. Palatoplasty

30. If a child with a repaired unilateral cleft lip and palate exhibits normal resonance, and if nasal emission is audible during the production of all anterior consonants but not during productions of /k/ or /g/, you would suspect:
a. Velopharyngeal insufficiency
b. Phoneme-specific nasal emission

c. An anterior palatal fistula
d. A posterior palatal fistula
e. A failed pharyngeal flap procedure

31. Which of the following studies enable observation of lateral pharyngeal wall movement during speech?
a. Nasal video-endoscopy
b. Lateral view videofluoroscopy
c. Measurement of nasal airflow
d. Nasometer
e. Lateral stationary radiography

32. The degree of nasality that is perceived by a listener is caused by:
a. The size of the velopharyngeal opening
b. The size of the velopharyngeal opening and the ratio of the nasal-oral acoustic impedances
c. The ratio of the nasal-oral acoustic impedances
d. The thickness of the pharyngeal walls
e. The degree of mouth opening

33. Which muscle is affected by a complete cleft of the palate?
a. Orbicularis oris inferior
b. Orbicularis oris superior
c. Masseter
d. Levator anguli oris
e. Levator veli palatini

34. Hypernasality is perceived during the production of which of the following?
a. Voiceless fricative consonants
b. Voiceless plosive consonants
c. Vowels and vocalic consonants
d. Vowels and voiceless consonants
e. Denasalized nasal consonants

35. Audible nasal emission is perceived during the production of which of the following?
a. Voiceless fricative consonants
b. Vowels and voiced consonants
c. Vowels and voiceless consonants
d. Denasalized nasal consonants
e. Nasal consonants (/m/, /n/, /ng/)

36. A 9-year-old boy with Crouzon syndrome exhibits moderate hyponasality during articulation testing and during conversational speech. Which of the following structural abnormalities would *not* explain the presence of the hyponasality?
a. Enlarged adenoids
b. Bilateral nasal cavity obstruction
c. Restricted velopharyngeal opening
d. Mandibular protrusion
e. Midface hypoplasia (undergrowth of maxilla and nasal structures)

37. Which of the following statements is true?
    a. The degree of velopharyngeal closure is the same for all pressure consonants
    b. The degree of velopharyngeal closure is the same for all vowels
    c. The velopharyngeal port is typically closed during the production of nasal consonants
    d. The degree of velopharyngeal closure varies according to vowel height
    e. The velopharyngeal port is closed to the same degree for oral consonants and vowels, and it is open for nasal consonants

38. A 5-year-old boy exhibits a moderate degree of hypernasality. The sustained production of which phoneme would be perceived as *least* nasal?
    a. [i]
    b. [a]
    c. [u]
    d. [n]
    e. [m]

39. Anterior displacement of a distinct portion of the posterior pharyngeal wall during speech is known as:
    a. Pharyngeal wall constriction
    b. Passavant's ridge
    c. Pharyngeal frication
    d. Palatopharyngeal closure
    e. Zona pellucida

40. Hypernasality can be an early symptom of which neurological disease?
    a. Multiple sclerosis
    b. Huntington disease
    c. Spasmodic dysphonia
    d. Alzheimer disease
    e. Amyotrophic lateral sclerosis

41. For which of the following neurological conditions is hypernasal speech *not* a common characteristic?
    a. Multiple sclerosis
    b. Myasthenia gravis
    c. Amyotrophic lateral sclerosis

    d. Flaccid dysarthria
    e. Neurofibromatosis

42. The velopharyngeal musculature is innervated by:
    a. Oculomotor nerve (cranial nerve III)
    b. Pharyngeal plexus (branches of glossopharyngeal nerve [cranial nerve IX] and vagus nerve [cranial nerve X])
    c. Abducens nerve (cranial nerve VI)
    d. Hypoglossal nerve (cranial nerve XII)
    e. Trigeminal nerve (cranial nerve III)

43. The formation of Passavant's ridge is attributed to what muscle?
    a. Palatoglossus
    b. Palatopharyngeus
    c. Musculus uvulae
    d. Middle pharyngeal constrictor
    e. Superior pharyngeal constrictor

44. A 6-year-old boy undergoes pharyngeal flap surgery. Two months after surgery, he exhibits moderate to severe hyponasality and complains that he has difficulty breathing through his nose. On the basis of this information, the clinician can conclude that:
    a. The pharyngeal flap is too narrow
    b. The pharyngeal flap is too low
    c. The pharyngeal flap is too wide
    d. The boy has overlearned velopharyngeal closure
    e. The pharyngeal flap has dehisced completely

45. Which of the following is true with regard to perceived nasality?
    a. When speaking rate slows, perceived nasality increases
    b. When speaking rate is faster, perceived nasality increases
    c. Faster speaking rate at higher fundamental frequencies increases perceived nasality
    d. Perceived nasality is lowest at slower speaking rates, increases at normal speaking rates, then decreases at faster speaking rates
    e. Speaking rate has no affect on perceived nasality

1. b. Repair of the palate is primarily a procedure that allows for the development of normal speech. Although the procedure also improves function of the eustachian tube, gives the child's parents a psychological lift, improves feeding, and prevents dental malocclusion, these are all of secondary concern in the surgical repair of the palate.

2. b. The Furlow Z-plasty procedure adds length to the soft palate and minimizes the contractile forces generated by palatal scar tissue. The primary concern with the other choices is that the postoperative scar is in a straight line, which can lead to increased stiffness and shortening within the soft palate.

3. c. Crouzon's syndrome is characterized by macroglossia and macrostomia. None of the other syndromes mentioned are characterized by an enlarged tongue and abnormally large size of the mouth.

4. e. Cardiac problems, velopharyngeal inadequacy, and typical facies are the characteristic features of velocardiofacial syndrome. It is imperative that speech-language pathologists recognize these features, because speech-language pathologists are often the first professionals to identify children who have velocardiofacial syndrome.

5. d. Hemifacial microsomia, also known as oculo-auriculo-vertebral dysplasia, is the only disorder mentioned that involves significant malformation of the external ear, in addition to facial asymmetry and conductive hearing loss.

6. c. Spontaneous improvement in resonance is known to occur in individuals with Prader-Willi syndrome and not in the other disorders.

7. a. Cleft palate, micrognathia, glossoptosis, and airway obstruction are the classic characteristics of the Pierre Robin sequence. This syndrome is not characterized by cleft lip.

8. e. The observations noted from the oral mechanism examination are typical characteristics of a submucous cleft palate. Because a speech-language pathologist's scope of practice does not include making this diagnosis, it is necessary to refer the patient to a physician for diagnosis.

9. b. Although the other muscles are velopharyngeal muscles, only the levator veli palatini has been proved to displace the soft palate posteriorly and superiorly to affect velopharyngeal closure in speech.

10. a. A fistula (either anterior or posterior) or velopharyngeal insufficiency would result in audible nasal emission during the production of more speech sounds in addition to /s/ and /z/. Audible nasal emission on /s/ and /z/ is commonly found in cases of phoneme-specific nasal emission (along with /ʃ/, /ʒ/, /tʃ/, and /dʒ/).

11. a. Although the other patterns are also compensatory articulations that are observed in children with cleft palate, the glottal stop is the error that occurs most frequently.

12. e. By definition, a coronal pattern of closure is characterized by prominent displacement of the soft palate toward closure with little to no contribution by the other structures such as the lateral and posterior pharyngeal walls.

13. d. By definition, a sagittal pattern of closure is characterized by prominent displacement of the lateral pharyngeal walls toward the midline with little to no contribution by the other structures.

14. d. Several electromyographic studies have demonstrated that the levator veli palatini, palatoglossus, and palatopharyngeus muscles are coactivated during speech, which suggests that an agonist-antagonist relationship is present to control the open and closed velar positions.

15. c. Only the location of the musculus uvulae can explain the bulk that appears on the nasal surface of the soft palate during speech.

16. d. Both videofluoroscopic and nasal endoscopic studies have demonstrated that the tongue base and posterior pharyngeal wall articulate to produce the pharyngeal fricative.

17. b. Research has demonstrated that the cleft palate levator functions at a level higher than normal, which is close to its maximum output during speech.

18. c. The signals of the nasometer (option a) and accelerometer (option e) do not indicate the presence of velopharyngeal closure-opening; the oral manometer (option b) measures oral pressure only; and electromyography (option d) measures muscle activity.

The presence of nasal airflow during the production of oral pressure sounds indicates that the velopharyngeal port is open.

19. b. Frontal and lateral view video-endoscopy (options c and d) do not exist, and frontal view videofluoroscopy (option a) does not enable visualization of velar displacement or adenoid size and position. Videostroboscopy (option e) is an instrument for laryngeal examination.

20. a. There is no research evidence that nonspeech activities improve velopharyngeal function for speech.

21. b. The positive nasal airway pressure provided by the CPAP device works against the velopharyngeal mechanism as it attempts to close during speech. Thus, it provides a muscle resistance exercise during speech production.

22. e. No research has demonstrated that the approaches listed improve velopharyngeal function during speech.

23. d. The pharyngeal flap is indicated in individuals who have a short, immobile soft palate and good medial movement of the lateral pharyngeal walls.

24. a. This patient has what appears to be a gross structural inadequacy. The soft palate is too short for a palatal lift (option b) to be a viable option. A speech bulb will provide adequate obturation of the defect. Oral motor therapy is not as effective in improving muscle function for speech as is palatal stimulation. Biofeedback is not viable in this case because of gross structural inadequacy.

25. a. The structural augmentation provided by the sphincter pharyngoplasty "fills in" the velopharyngeal gap that occurs with a coronal pattern of closure.

26. e. The greater the amount of preoperative displacement of the velopharyngeal structures, the greater is the chance that surgical management will be successful.

27. b. Lack of oropharyngeal movement is inherent to the production of the glottal stop. Consequently, this child's potential for velopharyngeal function is unknown. When articulatory placement is improved, velopharyngeal movement can improve. When that occurs, the clinician can make a valid determination about velopharyngeal status.

28. e. Although there is no evidence that blowing tasks improve velopharyngeal function, these tasks can serve as a vehicle to demonstrate how air should flow through the vocal tract and to contrast oral airflow with nasal airflow. They should not serve as a therapeutic activity to directly improve velopharyngeal closure for speech.

29. d. In view of the neurological cause of this patient's velopharyngeal insufficiency (VPI) and the fact that she has no velopharyngeal movement, surgical management would probably be unsuccessful (options a and b). Apalatoplasty (option e) is inappropriate, and a speech bulb [option c] can be more difficult to fit because the soft palate is of normal length. A palatal lift is the most commonly employed approach to managing neurogenic VPI.

30. c. When nasal emission is audible during the production of anterior consonants but not posterior consonants, an anterior fistula is probably present. The class of phonemes listed (all anterior consonants; option b) is not consistent with a diagnosis of phoneme-specific nasal emission, and if the problem is velopharyngeal insufficiency (option a), nasal emission would probably be audible during all consonant production. /K/ and /g/ would be effected with a posterior palatal fistula (option d), and a failed pharyngeal flap would result in vasodepression for all possessive consonants.

31. a. Lateral view videofluoroscopy (option b) and stationary radiography (option e) provide a view of velar displacement but not lateral pharyngeal wall movement. Nasal airflow measurement (option c) and nasometry (option d) do not provide images of the velopharyngeal mechanism.

32. b. Perceived nasality is not determined by the size of the velopharyngeal port alone (option a) or by the ratio of the nasal-oral acoustic impedances alone (option c). Both size of the velopharyngeal port and the oral acoustic impedance (e.g., degree of mouth opening [option e], tongue height, thickness of pharyngeal walls [option d]) in relation to the nasal acoustic impedance (option c) have a profound affect on the degree of nasalization that is produced and perceived. Thickness of the pharyngeal walls is not a consideration in perceived degree of nasality (option d).

33. e. The orbicularis oris superior (option b) and, perhaps, the levator anguli oris (option d) would be affected by a cleft of the lip but not by a cleft palate. Only the levator veli palatini muscle is in the region where palatal clefting occurs. The other options (a and c) would not be affected by a cleft.

34. c. Because hypernasality is an acoustic phenomenon, voicing must occur in order for hypernasality to be perceived; therefore, it would not be perceived

during the production of voiceless consonants (options a, b, and d). A denasalized nasal consonant (option e) would be consistent with hyponasality, not hypernasality.

35. a. Although audible nasal emission can be perceived during voiced consonants (options b, d, and e), vocal tract airflow velocity is too low during vowel production for nasal airflow turbulence to occur (option c).

36. d. The size and position of the mandible would not have an influence on the presence or degree of hyponasality. Enlarged adenoids (option a), nasal cavity obstruction (option b), restricted velopharyngeal opening (option c), and midface hypoplasia (option e) pertain to some manner of obstruction of the nasal or nasopharyngeal airway.

37. d. Some of the earliest studies of velopharyngeal function (e.g., Kenneth L. Moll's work in the early 1960s) revealed that the degree of palatopharyngeal closure varies according to both vowel and consonant context.

38. b. During the production of [a], oral acoustic impedance is lower in comparison to [i], [u], [n], or [m] (options a, c, d, and e). With a lower oral impedance, vocal tract sound transmission is more likely to occur through the oral cavity rather than the nasal cavity. Thus, the resultant percept is more oral.

39. b. Anterior displacement of a distinct portion of the posterior pharyngeal wall during speech is the definition of Passavant's ridge.

40. e. When the bulbar system is the first system to be affected by amyotrophic lateral sclerosis, velopharyngeal dysfunction can occur before other subsystems of the speech production system are involved.

41. a. Myasthenia gravis, amyotrophic lateral sclerosis, flaccid dysarthria, and neurofibromatosis (options b, c, d, and e) involve conditions for which oropharyngeal muscle weakness can occur; this leads to decreased mobility of the soft palate and hypernasal speech.

42. b. Research studies have revealed that the pharyngeal plexus supplies the primary innervation to the velopharyngeal musculature.

43. e. Of the five choices, only the superior pharyngeal constrictor is in the anatomical position to form Passavant's ridge.

44. c. The child is showing signs of nasal obstruction, which can be caused only by a pharyngeal flap that is too wide.

45. a. Several studies have demonstrated that slowing speech rate or increasing speech production time results in an increase in perceived nasality. This is contrary to what had been assumed for many years.

Bibliography
Moll, K. L. (1960). Velopharyngeal closure on vowels. *Journal of Speech and Hearing Research*, 3, 227–238.

CHAPTER 10

Voice Disorders

Joseph Stemple

Ashwini Joshi

Anysia Ensslen

1. In which breathing pattern is thoracic enlargement achieved by expansion of the lower thoracic and abdominal cavities during inspiration?
   a. Diaphragmatic-abdominal breathing
   b. Clavicular breathing
   c. Thoracic breathing
   d. Speech breathing.
   e. None of the above

2. The maximum volume of air that can be exhaled after a maximum inhalation is:
   a. Inspiratory capacity
   b. Vital capacity
   c. Functional residual capacity
   d. Total lung capacity
   e. Tidal volume

3. Men have a vital capacity:
   a. In the range of 1 to 2 L
   b. In the range of 3 to 4 L
   c. In the range of 4 to 5 L
   d. Of variable range
   e. b and c

4. The function of the visceral and parietal pleura is which of the following?
   a. To prevent the lungs from collapsing
   b. To provide hydration to the lungs
   c. To aid in gaseous exchange
   d. To aid in upward motion of the rib cage
   e. All the above

5. What is the function of the interpleural space?
   a. To allow the lungs to contract and expand within the thoracic cavity without friction
   b. To provide hydration to the lungs

c. To aid in gaseous exchange
d. To aid in upward motion of the rib cage
e. All the above

6. The three passive forces of expiration are:
   a. Elastic recoil, torque, and gravity
   b. Elastic recoil, gravity, and vital capacity
   c. Gravity, vital capacity, and torque
   d. Gravity, elastic recoil, and exhalation
   e. Vital capacity, gravity, and exhalation

7. The primary muscles of inhalation are:
   a. External intercostal muscles
   b. Internal intercostal muscles
   c. Rectus abdominis muscles
   d. Transverse and oblique abdominal muscles
   e. Sternocleidomastoid muscle

8. Ms. Clarke, age 28, is currently in graduate school, studying to become an opera singer. Although she uses abdominal and diaphragmatic breathing adequately on inhalation, she complains of "running out of air" and is unable to completely sing a long phrase with adequate breath support. A voice specialist has concluded that Ms. Clarke requires better coordination of the muscles of controlled expiration. Which set of muscles is the voice specialist referring to?
   a. Internal intercostal muscles
   b. External intercostal muscles
   c. Internal intercostal muscles and abdominal muscles
   d. Sternocleidomastoid muscle
   e. All the above

9. On expiration, the diaphragm:
   a. Flattens
   b. Rises
   c. Extends
   d. Flattens or extends
   e. Rises and extends

10. The rate at which air is expelled per second through the glottis during sustained phonation is which of the following?
    a. Vital capacity
    b. Phonation quotient
    c. Maximum phonation time
    d. Tidal volume
    e. None of the above

11. The major function of the larynx is which of the following?
    a. Singing
    b. Swallowing
    c. Phonation
    d. Airway protection
    e. All the above

12. In relation to the vertebral column, the larynx is located from approximately the level of the:
    a. C1 to C3 vertebrae
    b. C3 to C6 vertebrae
    c. T3 to T6 vertebrae
    d. T1 to T3 vertebrae
    e. L1 to L4 vertebrae

13. The superior opening of the larynx is formed by the:
    a. Epiglottis
    b. Hyoid
    c. Aryepiglottic fold
    d. Thyroid cartilage
    e. Cricoid cartilage

14. Increase in intrathoracic pressure for coughing and sneezing is enabled by the approximation of:
    a. The ventricular folds
    b. The vocal folds
    c. The arytenoid cartilages
    d. The cricoid and thyroid
    e. All the above

15. The _____ is shaped like a signet ring.
    a. Thyroid cartilage
    b. Hyoid
    c. Arytenoid cartilage
    d. Cricoid cartilage
    e. None of the above

16. Elevation and lowering of the larynx for respiration and phonation is carried out by the:
    a. Intrinsic laryngeal muscles
    b. Extrinsic laryngeal muscles
    c. External intercostal muscles
    d. Internal intercostal muscles
    e. Diaphragm

17. The three major cartilages of the larynx related to phonation are:
    a. The cricoid, thyroid, and epiglottis
    b. The thyroid, arytenoid, and cuneiform
    c. The thyroid, arytenoid, and cricoid
    d. The corniculate, cuneiform, and epiglottis
    e. None of the above

18. The most anterior prominence of the arytenoid cartilage, where the vocal folds attach, is which of the following?
    a. The vocal process
    b. The muscular process
    c. The thyroid prominence
    d. The interarytenoid space
    e. None of the above

19. The prominence of the arytenoid cartilage that forms the attachment for the posterior and the lateral crico-arytenoid muscles is known as:
    a. The vocal process
    b. The muscular process
    c. The thyroid prominence
    d. The interarytenoid space
    e. None of the above

20. A 15-year-old boy who is undergoing a voice evaluation complains of a high-pitched voice, frequent pitch breaks, and an inability to project his voice. Videostroboscopic evaluation has demonstrated no mass lesions, paresis, or paralysis leading to a diagnosis of functional falsetto. The problems that this patient is experiencing with his voice may result from misuse of which intrinsic laryngeal muscles?
    a. Thyroarytenoid
    b. Cricothyroid
    c. Vocalis
    d. All the above
    e. a and c

21. The muscles responsible for elevation of the larynx in the neck are:
    a. The suprahyoid muscle
    b. The infrahyoid muscle
    c. The intrinsic laryngeal muscles
    d. The abductor muscles
    e. None of the above

22. Through videostroboscopic evaluation, a speech-language pathologist who specializes in voice has determined that a patient has sufficient glottal closure during phonation, but the patient is having difficulty abducting the vocal folds again after phonation. Which intrinsic laryngeal muscle is affected?
    a. Lateral cricoarytenoid
    b. Thyroarytenoid
    c. Posterior cricoarytenoid
    d. Cricothyroid
    e. Sternohyoid

23. Mr. Angelo has come to a speech language pathologist for a voice evaluation. His major complaint is difficulty altering the pitch of his voice. Which muscle and nerve are likely to be affected?
    a. Cricothyroid muscle and recurrent laryngeal nerve
    b. Cricothyroid muscle and external branch of the superior laryngeal nerve
    c. Thyroarytenoid muscle and recurrent laryngeal nerve
    d. Thyroarytenoid muscle and superior laryngeal nerve
    e. Lateral cricoarytenoid muscle and recurrent laryngeal nerve

24. Which muscles aid in more complete adduction of the posterior aspect of the vocal folds?
    a. Transverse and oblique interarytenoid muscles
    b. Thyroarytenoid muscle
    c. Posterior cricoarytenoid muscle
    d. Cricothyroid muscle
    e. All the above

25. The recurrent laryngeal branch of the vagus nerve innervates all of the intrinsic laryngeal muscle *except* the:
    a. Lateral cricoarytenoid muscle
    b. Thyroarytenoid muscle
    c. Posterior cricoarytenoid muscle
    d. Cricothyroid muscle
    e. Arytenoid muscle

26. This layer of the vocal fold helps to maintain the integrity of the vocal fold shape:
    a. Epithelium
    b. Superficial layer
    c. Intermediate layer
    d. Deep layer
    e. None of the above

27. The two layers of the vocal fold that form the vocal ligament are:
    a. Epithelium and superficial layer
    b. Superficial and intermediate layers
    c. Intermediate and deep layers
    d. Superficial and deep layers
    e. Epithelium and intermediate layer

28. Ms. Thomas complains of persistent diplophonia and breathy voice. A possible pathological process consistent with this vocal characteristic is which of the following?
    a. Vocal fold nodules
    b. Muscle tension dysphonia
    c. Unilateral vocal fold paralysis
    d. Bilateral vocal fold paralysis
    e. Polyp

29. Jenny is a 19-year-old high school student who is undergoing a voice evaluation. Jenny complains of a gradual onset of a hoarse vocal quality and also stated that her voice "is harder to produce" (requires more effort). Jenny is a cheerleader and sings in the school choir. Jenny also often baby-sits for her two younger brothers and must raise her voice to hold their attention. Which pathological process of the vocal folds has developed or is likely to develop?
    a. Vocal fold nodules
    b. Acute laryngitis
    c. Vocal fold polyp
    d. Vocal fold hemorrhage
    e. None of the above

30. The myoelastic-aerodynamic theory of phonation was proposed by:
    a. Titze
    b. Van den Berg
    c. Bernoulli
    d. Boyle
    e. Husson

31. The three steps necessary before normal glottal tone initiation are:
    a. Adduction of the vocal folds, tension and elongation of the vocal folds, and airflow from the lungs
    b. Abduction of the vocal folds, relaxing of the vocal folds, and airflow from the lungs
    c. Abduction of the vocal folds, tension and elongation of the vocal folds, and airflow from the lungs
    d. Adduction of the vocal folds, relaxing of the vocal folds, and airflow from the lungs
    e. a and d

32. An increase in pitch is brought about by increased contraction of the _____ muscle and a decreased contraction by the _____ muscle.
    a. Cricothyroid; thyroarytenoid
    b. Cricothyroid; posterior cricoarytenoid
    c. Posterior cricoarytenoid; thyroarytenoid
    d. Cricothyroid; cricothyroid
    e. Thyroarytenoid; thyroarytenoid

33. The fundamental frequency of the voice in healthy women ranges from:
    a. 100 to 150 Hz
    b. 180 to 220 Hz
    c. 75 to 100 Hz
    d. 250 to 300 Hz
    e. None of the above

34. Jitter is an acoustic measure of:
    a. Cycle-to-cycle variation in amplitude
    b. Cycle-to-cycle variation in frequency
    c. Fundamental frequency
    d. Intensity
    e. Duration

35. Shimmer is an acoustic measure of:
    a. Cycle-to-cycle variation in amplitude
    b. Cycle-to-cycle variation in frequency
    c. Fundamental frequency
    d. Intensity
    e. Duration

36. How long is a normal adult male's vocal fold?
    a. 5 to 10 mm
    b. 30 to 40 mm
    c. 17 to 21 mm
    d. 50 to 53 mm
    e. 55 to 60 mm

37. The main goal of _____ is to identify the primary vocal misuses and to modify or eliminate these behaviors.
    a. Hygienic voice therapy
    b. Physiological voice therapy
    c. Symptomatic voice therapy
    d. Psychogenic voice therapy
    e. b and c

38. The main goal of _____ is to use facilitating techniques to directly modify vocal components such as pitch, loudness, and laryngeal tension.
    a. Hygienic voice therapy
    b. Physiological voice therapy
    c. Symptomatic voice therapy
    d. Psychogenic voice therapy
    e. All the above

39. The main goal of _____ is to evaluate the subsystems responsible for voice production (respiration, phonation, resonance) and develop direct therapy exercises to improve that relative balance.
    a. Hygienic voice therapy
    b. Physiological voice therapy
    c. Symptomatic voice therapy
    d. Psychogenic voice therapy
    e. Lee Silverman Voice Treatment

40. The main goal of _____ is to explore the psychodynamics of the voice.
    a. Hygienic voice therapy
    b. Physiological voice therapy
    c. Symptomatic voice therapy
    d. Psychogenic voice therapy
    e. All the above

41. Spasmodic dysphonia is thought to be a pathological process of the:
    a. Central nervous system
    b. Vocal fold cover
    c. Vocal fold vibration
    d. Peripheral nervous system
    e. a and d

42. Mr. Pitt was recently intubated in an acute care facility. After extubation, he exhibited a dysphonic voice quality. What vocal pathological process probably occurred as a result of extubation?
    a. Vocal nodules
    b. Spasmodic dysphonia
    c. Granuloma
    d. Papillomas
    e. Polyps

43. "Think loud" or "be loud" is the primary goal of what voice therapy program?
    a. Vocal function exercises
    b. Lee Silverman Voice Treatment
    c. Resonant voice therapy
    d. Yawn-sigh technique
    e. Pushing method

44. Ms. Qin is 45 years old and has been smoking two packs of cigarettes per day for 25 years. She now complains of hoarseness and decreased pitch. What is the likely disease process?
    a. Vocal hemorrhage
    b. Spasmodic dysphonia
    c. Reinke edema
    d. Papillomas
    e. None of the above

45. Both maximum phonation time and s/z ratio (measures of breath support and glottal efficiency) are methods of evaluating:
    a. Respiration and phonation
    b. Pitch
    c. Loudness
    d. Resonance
    e. General voice quality

46. _____ demonstrates the characteristics of vocal fold vibration and the integrity of the mucous membrane of the vocal folds.
    a. Acoustic evaluation
    b. Aerodynamic measures
    c. Laryngeal videostroboscopy
    d. Laryngeal endoscopy
    e. Perceptual voice assessment

47. A spectrogram represents _____ on the horizontal axis and _____ on the vertical axis.
    a. Time; frequency
    b. Frequency; time
    c. Time; intensity
    d. Frequency; intensity
    e. None of the above

48. Gray scale (darkness) on the spectrogram represents:
    a. Frequency
    b. Intensity
    c. Resonance
    d. Poor data
    e. Duration

49. On a spectrogram, which of the following acoustic features is indicative of a stop-plosive?
    a. Noise burst at the moment of release
    b. Slow formant transition

c. Transient noise
d. First formant frequency
e. All the above

50. The relative timing of stop-release and the initiation of phonation is known as:
    a. Rise time
    b. Fall time
    c. Formant transitions
    d. Voice onset time
    e. a and b

51. Nasal sounds are weak sounds because of:
    a. Creation of resonance in the vocal tract
    b. Smaller vocal tract
    c. Creation of antiresonances within the vocal tract
    d. Complete opening of the oral cavity
    e. Velopharyngeal closure during the production of nasal sounds

52. A patient has bilateral vocal nodules that are adding mass to the vibratory tissues. What would be expected to occur at the first harmonic on a spectrogram?
    a. Rises
    b. Falls
    c. No change
    d. Variation
    e. Findings that cannot be predicted

53. What is the phenomenon in which two articulators are moving at the same time to produce different phonemes?
    a. Coarticulation
    b. Assimilation
    c. Phonation
    d. Formant transition
    e. All the above

54. Subglottal pressure is which of the following?
    a. The measure of air pressure beneath the vocal folds necessary to initiate and maintain phonation
    b. The measure of air pressure behind the lips necessary to initiate and maintain phonation
    c. The measure of air pressure above the vocal folds necessary to initiate and maintain phonation
    d. The measure of air pressure at the diaphragm necessary to initiate and maintain phonation
    e. None of the above

55. Instrumental measurement of vocal function is beneficial because:
    a. It aids in increased reliability and validity of perceptual judgments
    b. The averaged performance of a target group can be more clearly defined

c. Progress in therapy sessions may be more effectively gauged

d. Objective acoustic and physiological data are obtained

e. All the above

56. In a(n) _____, the total phonatory capabilities of the voice with regard to frequency (in hertz) and intensity (in decibels) are plotted.
a. Phonetogram
b. Spectrogram
c. Visual analog scale
d. Audiogram
e. None of the above

57. Phonation threshold pressure is which of the following?
a. A measure of air pressure behind the lips necessary to initiate and maintain phonation
b. Measure of air pressure at the diaphragm necessary to initiate and maintain phonation
c. A measure of minimal subglottal air pressure required to initiate phonation
d. All the above
e. a and c

58. Talbot's law—that images linger on the retina for 0.2 seconds after exposure—is the basic principle of:
a. Stroboscopy
b. Endoscopy
c. Inverse filtering
d. Phonetography
e. Pressure/flow technique

59. Stroboscopy yields laryngeal images in:
a. Slow motion
b. Simulated slow motion
c. Real time
d. Both slow motion and real time
e. None of the above

60. _____ is a method by which nonlaryngeal acoustic features added by the resonators are subtracted from the radiated acoustic signal, which restores the signal to a simpler form that represents what the vocal folds produced.
a. Stroboscopy
b. Electroglottography
c. Inverse filtering
d. Spectral analysis
e. Fourier analysis

61. The focus of _____ is to produce voice with slightly abducted vocal folds and minimal subglottic pressure.
a. Symptomatic voice therapy
b. Resonant voice therapy
c. Physiological voice therapy

d. Hygienic voice therapy
e. All the above

62. The ratio of abductor to adductor duration in the larynx is called:
a. Open quotient
b. Closed quotient
c. Speed quotient
d. Phonation quotient
e. None of the above

63. _____ can be defined as aperiodic noise caused by rapidly flowing air through the glottis.
a. Whisper
b. Confidential voice
c. Vibrato
d. Tremor
e. Vocal fry

64. Of the following, which is the only direct physiological measure of laryngeal muscle function?
a. Electroglottography
b. Electromyography
c. Subglottal pressure
d. Acoustic analysis
e. None of the above

65. Recommendations for good vocal hygiene may include:
a. Hydration
b. Decreased throat clearing
c. Smoking cessation
d. All the above
e. a and c

66. If environmental stressors become so severe, a patient may develop maladaptive voice production in the presence of a structurally normal laryngeal mechanism. This maladaptive vocal behavior is known as:
a. Vocal fold paresis
b. Muscle tension dysphonia
c. Diplophonia
d. Granuloma
e. None of the above

67. What is the major disadvantage of using an electrolarynx?
a. Mechanical-sounding voice
b. External device
c. Used in the early postoperative stages
d. All the above
e. None of the above

68. A _____ is created from the back wall of the trachea into the esophagus, allowing placement of a valved tube that enables speech in persons who undergo a total laryngectomy.

a. Passy-Muir valve
b. Tracheostomy
c. Intubation
d. Tracheoesophageal puncture
e. Pharyngoplasty

69. Which type of speech is produced by taking air in through the mouth, trapping it in the upper esophagus, and releasing it?
a. Esophageal speech
b. Electromechanical speech
c. Tracheoesophageal speech
d. Confidential speech
e. None of the above

70. A 53-year-old man comes to your office with a note from his physician that reads: "Unilateral true vocal fold paralysis after cardiac surgery 2 weeks ago." Is the paralysis probably on the left or right side, and what branch of the vagus has been damaged?
a. Left side; recurrent laryngeal nerve
b. Right side; recurrent laryngeal nerve
c. Left side; superior laryngeal nerve
d. Right side; superior laryngeal nerve
e. None of the above

71. A 37-year-old woman comes to you with complaints of chronic hoarseness and difficulty breathing in conjunction with voice use. The patient reports having asthma and gastroesophageal reflux. A likely diagnosis may be which of the following?
a. Muscle tension dysphonia
b. Vocal cord dysfunction
c. Vocal nodules
d. Unilateral vocal fold paralysis
e. Granuloma

72. A 15-year-old high school singer, heavily involved with choir, has received a diagnosis of bilateral vocal nodules. What should the primary intervention be?
a. Surgical removal of nodules
b. Medication for gastroesophageal reflux
c. Physiological voice therapy approaches
d. Complete voice rest
e. All the above

73. On laryngeal videostroboscopy, lesions were found bilaterally at the junction of the anterior one third and posterior two thirds of the vocal folds. These lesions most likely are which of the following?
a. Cysts
b. Polyps
c. Granuloma
d. Nodules
e. a and b

74. A 34-year-old woman complains of sudden onset of severe hoarseness during attendance at a sporting event. The likely diagnosis is which of the following?
a. Vocal fold hemorrhage
b. Granuloma
c. Laryngopharyngeal reflux
d. Vocal fold polyps
e. None of the above

75. A 25-year-old man complains of muscular pain of the neck muscles, hoarseness, and vocal fatigue. He has no significant medical or surgical history. Stroboscopic findings revealed strong medial compression of the ventricular folds and erythema. The likely diagnosis is which of the following?
a. Myasthenia gravis
b. Muscle tension dysphonia
c. Unilateral vocal fold paralysis
d. Conversion aphonia
e. Damage to the right recurrent laryngeal nerve

1. a. In diaphragmatic-abdominal breathing, the diaphragm flattens, expanding the lower thoracic and abdominal cavities during inspiration. In clavicular breathing (option b), the two clavicles pull up slightly at the end of maximum inhalation, expanding the very top of the thoracic cavity. In thoracic breathing (option c), the chest wall moves upward and outward, and more work is required than for diaphragmatic-abdominal breathing. During speech breathing (option d), a greater volume of air is taken into the lungs than during quiet breathing, and more timing and control is required than those provided by diaphragmatic-abdominal breathing.

2. b. Vital capacity is the maximum volume of air that can be exhaled after a maximum inhalation. Inspiratory capacity (option a) is the maximum amount of air that can be inhaled. Functional residual capacity (option c) is the volume of air left in the lungs at the end of a normal breath. Total lung capacity (option d) is the entire volume of air that the lungs are able to hold. Tidal volume (option e) is the amount of air that is generally inspired and expired in a normal respiratory cycle.

3. c. On average, men have a vital capacity of 4 to 5 L; it is not variable (option d). On average, women have a vital capacity of 3 to 4 L (option b). On average, nether men or women have a vital capacity as small as 1 to 2 L (option a).

4. a. The visceral and parietal pleura aid in preventing the lungs from collapsing. They do not provide hydration to the lungs (option b). The alveoli are responsible for gas exchange in the lungs (option c). The external intercostal muscles contract to aid in elevation of the rib cage (option d).

5. a. The interpleural space ensures that the lungs can contract and expand within the thoracic cavity without friction. The interpleural space does not provide hydration to the lungs (option b). The alveoli are responsible for gas exchange in the lungs (option c). The external intercostal muscles contract to aid in elevation of the rib cage (option d).

6. a. Elastic recoil, torque, and gravity are the three passive forces of expiration. Elastic recoil is the natural tendency of the lungs and rib cage to return to their original shape. Torque is the force produced by the untwisting of the cartilages next to the sternum. Gravity aids somewhat in the lowering of the rib cage. Vital capacity (options b and c) is the maximum volume of air that can be exhaled after a maximum inhalation and is not a passive force of expiration. Exhalation (options d and e) is also not a passive force of expiration.

7. a. The external intercostal muscles are the primary muscles of inhalation. The internal intercostal muscles (option b) are muscles of controlled expiration. The rectus abdominis muscles (option c) and the transverse and oblique abdominal muscles (option d) aid in extended expiration during speech or singing. The sternocleidomastoid muscles (option e) are paired muscles coursing in a diagonal direction across the neck; they are not a muscles of respiration.

8. a. The internal intercostal muscles are the primary muscles of controlled expiration. The external intercostal muscles (option b) are the primary muscles of inhalation. The abdominal muscles (option c) aid in extended expiration during speech or singing. The paired sternocleidomastoid muscles (option d) are not associated with respiration.

9. a. On expiration, the diaphragm flattens. This helps expand volume in the thoracic cavity and lungs, causing the air pressure inside the lungs to be less than the pressure of the atmosphere. Air from the atmosphere then flows into the lungs. On expiration, the diaphragm does not rise (option b) or extend (option c), nor does it both flatten and extend (option d) or rise and extend (option e).

10. b. Phonation quotient is the rate at which air is expelled through the glottis per second during sustained phonation. Vital capacity (option a) is the maximum volume of air that can be exhaled after a maximum inhalation. Maximum phonation time (option c) is the amount of a time that phonation can be sustained on a single breath. Tidal volume (option d) is the amount of air exchanged during inspirations and expirations of normal quiet breathing.

11. d. The vocal folds adduct, especially during swallowing, helping prevent foreign materials from entering the airway. Although the larynx does play a part in the acts of singing (option a), swallowing (option b), and phonation (option c), the primary function of the larynx is airway protection.

12. b. The larynx is located at approximately the level of the third cervical vertebrae to the sixth cervical

vertebrae. The larynx is not close to the upper cervical (option a), thoracic (options b and c), or lumbar vertebrae (option d).

13. c. The aryepiglottic fold forms the superior opening of the larynx. The epiglottis (option a) folds back over the superior opening of the larynx to protect the airway during a normal swallow. The hyoid (option b) is the bone from which the larynx is suspended. The thyroid cartilage (option d) is shaped like a shield and protects the larynx anteriorly. The cricoid cartilage (option e) is shaped like a signet ring and articulates with the three cartilages (thyroid cartilage and arytenoid cartilages) that support the vocal folds.

14. a. An increase in intrathoracic pressure is required for coughing and sneezing. This increase in pressure is enabled by the ventricular folds, not the vocal folds (option b). The arytenoid cartilages (option c) aid in more complete closure of the vocal folds during phonation. The cricoid and thyroid cartilages (option d) do not aid in pressure increase during coughing and sneezing.

15. d. The cricoid cartilage is shaped like a signet ring. The hyoid (option b) is the bone from which the larynx is suspended. The thyroid (option a) and arytenoid cartilages (option c) are not shaped like a signet ring. The thyroid cartilage (option a) protects the larynx anteriorly. The arytenoid cartilages (option c) aid in more complete closure of the vocal folds during phonation.

16. b. The elevation and lowering of the larynx is carried out by the extrinsic laryngeal muscles. The intrinsic laryngeal muscles (option a) aid in the tensing and lengthening of the vocal folds. The external intercostal muscles (option c) are muscles of inspiration. The internal intercostal muscles (option d) are muscles of expiration. The diaphragm (option e) is a muscular and tendinous respiratory structure that separates the abdomen and thorax.

17. c. The three major cartilages of the larynx are the thyroid, arytenoid, and cricoid cartilages. The cuneiform and corniculate cartilages (options b and d) are not considered major cartilages of the larynx. The epiglottis (options a and d) is an important structure that aids in airway protection during swallowing; the epiglottis is not a cartilage.

18. a. The vocal process is the most anterior prominence of the arytenoid cartilages, where the vocal folds attach. The muscular process (option b) provides insertion for the posterior cricoarytenoid and lateral cricoarytenoid muscles. The thyroid prominence (option c) is a protruding area of the thyroid

cartilage. The interarytenoid space (option d) is the space between the arytenoid cartilages.

19. b. The muscular process forms the attachment for the posterior and the lateral cricoarytenoid muscles. The vocal process (option a) is the most anterior prominence of the arytenoid cartilages, where the vocal folds attach. The thyroid prominence (option c) is a protruding area of the thyroid cartilage. The interarytenoid space (option d) is the space between the arytenoid cartilages.

20. d. In falsetto, the cricothyroid muscles (option b) lengthen and tense the vocal folds along the medial edge of the vocalis muscles (option c), and the more lateral thyroarytenoid muscles (option a) disengage.

21. a. The suprahyoid muscles are responsible for elevation of the larynx in the neck. The infrahyoid muscles (option b) are responsible for depression of the larynx in the neck. The intrinsic laryngeal muscles (option c) work to tense and elongate the vocal folds. The abductor muscles (option d) work to abduct the vocal folds.

22. c. The posterior cricoarytenoid is the only muscle of vocal fold abduction; it opens the vocal folds after phonation. The lateral cricoarytenoid (option a), the thyroarytenoid (option b), and the cricothyroid (option d) are all muscles of vocal fold adduction. The sternohyoid (option e) is an extrinsic muscle of the larynx.

23. b. The cricothyroid muscle works to lengthen and tense the vocal folds, thus altering the pitch of the voice. The cricothyroid muscle is innervated by the external branch of the superior laryngeal nerve, not the recurrent laryngeal nerve (option a). The thyroarytenoid muscle (options c and d) is an intrinsic laryngeal muscle that makes up the body of the vocal fold. The lateral cricoarytenoid muscle (option e) is an intrinsic laryngeal adductor muscle.

24. a. The transverse and oblique interarytenoid muscles aid in more complete adduction of the vocal folds. The thyroarytenoid muscle (option b) is an intrinsic laryngeal muscle that makes up the body of the vocal fold. The posterior cricoarytenoid muscle (option c) is the only muscle of vocal fold abduction. The cricothyroid muscle (option d) works to lengthen and tense the vocal folds.

25. d. The cricothyroid muscle is innervated by the superior laryngeal branch of the vagus nerve. The lateral cricoarytenoid (option a), the thyroarytenoid (option b), the posterior cricoarytenoid (option c)

and arytenoid muscles are innervated by the recurrent laryngeal branch of the vagus nerve.

26. a. The epithelial layer of the vocal folds helps maintain the vocal fold shape. The superficial layer (option b) does not help maintain the shape of the vocal folds. The superficial layer is composed primarily of loosely organized elastin fibres surrounded by interstitial fibres. On post of the mucosa it is thought to furnish a cushion for actions of the vocal ligament. The intermediate (option c) and deep layers (option d) help form the vocal ligament.

27. c. The intermediate and deep layers of the vocal fold help form the vocal ligament. The epithelium (options a and e) helps maintain the vocal fold shape. The superficial layer (options b and d) does not help form the vocal ligament.

28. c. Consistent diplophonia is most commonly caused by unilateral vocal fold paralysis. Diplophonia is not usually caused by vocal fold nodules (option a), muscle tension dysphonia (option b), or polyps (option e). Diplophonia is not caused by bilateral vocal fold paralysis (option d).

29. a. Consistent phonotrauma over time (excessive and loud singing, shouting, cheering) probably leads to vocal fold nodules. Acute laryngitis (option b) is an inflammation of the vocal folds and larynx caused by allergens, infections, reflux, and disease. Vocal fold polyps (option c) are the result of a period of abuse. Vocal fold hemorrhage (option d) is caused by acute trauma to the vocal folds.

30. b. The myoelastic-aerodynamic theory of phonation was proposed by Janwillem Van den Berg. Ingo Titze (option a) proposed the phonation theory. Daniel Bernoulli (option c) proposed the Bernoulli effect, stating that air speed increases air pressure decreases. Robert Boyle (option d) proposed Boyle's law, which describes the inversely proportional relationship between the absolute pressure and volume of a gas. Raoul Husson (option e) developed the neurochronaxic theory of voice production.

31. a. For normal glottal tone initiation, three steps are required: adduction of the vocal folds, tension and elongation of the vocal folds, and sufficient airflow from the lungs. The vocal folds do not abduct (options b and c) and do not relax (options b and d) for normal glottal tone initiation.

32. a. Upon contraction of the cricothyroid muscle, the vocal folds tense and elongate, which causes an increase in pitch. Upon relaxation (decreased contraction) of the thyroarytenoid muscle, the vocal folds more easily tense and elongate, which also causes an increase in pitch. The posterior cricoarytenoid muscle (options b and c) is the only muscle of vocal fold abduction. For pitch to increase, both an increased contraction of the cricothyroid muscle and a decreased contraction of the thyroarytenoid muscle is needed.

33. b. On average, the fundamental frequency of the voices of healthy women ranges from 180 to 220 Hz. On average, that in healthy men ranges from 100 to 150 Hz (option a). On average, that in healthy children (boys and girls) ranges from 250 to 300 Hz (option d).

34. b. Jitter is a measure of cycle-to-cycle variation in frequency. Shimmer is a measure of cycle-to-cycle variation in amplitude (option a). Fundamental frequency (option c) is the lowest frequency in a periodic waveform and is typically measured in hertz, intensity (option d) is a measure of power per unit area and is typically measured in decibels, and duration (option e) is a measure of time and is typically measured in milliseconds.

35. a. Shimmer is a measure of cycle-to-cycle variation in amplitude. Jitter is a measure of cycle-to-cycle variation in frequency (option b). Fundamental frequency (option c) is typically measured in hertz, intensity (option d) is typically measured in decibels, and duration or time (option e) is typically measured in milliseconds.

36. c. On average, a vocal fold of a normal adult male measures approximately 17 to 21 mm in length.

37. a. The main goal of hygienic voice therapy is to identify the primary vocal misuses and to modify or eliminate these behaviors. The main goal of physiological voice therapy (option b) is to evaluate the current physiological condition of the patient's voice production and develop direct therapy exercises to improve that condition. The main goal of symptomatic voice therapy (option c) is to use facilitating techniques to directly modify vocal components such as pitch, loudness, and laryngeal tension. The main goal of psychogenic voice therapy (option d) is to explore the psychodynamics of the voice.

38. c. The main goal of symptomatic voice therapy is to use facilitating techniques to directly modify vocal components such as pitch, loudness, and laryngeal tension. The main goal of hygienic voice therapy (option a) is to identify the primary vocal misuses and to modify or eliminate these behaviors. The

main goal of physiological voice therapy (option b) is to evaluate the present physiological condition of the patient's voice production and develop direct therapy exercises to improve that condition. The main goal of psychogenic voice therapy (option d) is to explore the psychodynamics of the voice.

39. b. The main goal of physiological voice therapy is to evaluate the current physiological condition of the patient's voice production and developing direct therapy exercises to improve that condition. The main goal of hygienic voice therapy (option a) is to identify the primary vocal misuses and to modify or eliminate these behaviors. The main goal of symptomatic voice therapy (option c) is to use facilitating techniques to directly modify vocal components such as pitch, loudness, and laryngeal tension. The main goal of psychogenic voice therapy (option d) is to explore the psychodynamics of the voice. The Lee Silverman Voice Treatment (option e) manipulates vocal loudness to effect the speech subsystems of respiration, phonation, resonation, and articulation.

40. d. The main goal of psychogenic voice therapy is to explore the psychodynamics of the voice. The main goal of hygienic voice therapy (option a) is to identify the primary vocal misuses and to modify or eliminate these behaviors. The main goal of physiological voice therapy (option b) is to evaluate the present physiological condition of the patient's voice production and developing direct therapy exercises to improve that condition. The main goal of symptomatic voice therapy (option c) is to use facilitating techniques to directly modify vocal components such as pitch, loudness, and laryngeal tension.

41. a. Spasmodic dysphonia is a laryngeal dystonia thought to be mediated in the brainstem, which is part of the central nervous system. Vocal fold cover (option b) disease includes Reinke edema and vocal nodules. Vocal fold vibration (option c) is disrupted in most laryngeal diseases and is only one characteristic of disease. Peripheral nervous system (option d) disease includes vocal fold paralysis and paresis.

42. c. A granuloma may result from injury to the mucosa in the cartilaginous portion of the posterior vocal fold during intubation. Vocal fold nodules (option a) result most often from misuse or abuse of the voice. Spasmodic dysphonia (option b) is a motor control disorder; papillomas (option d) result from the human papillomavirus. Polyps (option e) are common benign tumors of the larynx that occur as the result of vocal abuse.

43. b. Lee Silverman Voice Treatment, used for persons with Parkinson's disease, focuses on vocal loudness to effect change in the subsystems of respiration, phonation, resonance, and articulation. Vocal function exercises (option a) focus on enhancing the relationship between the three of those subsystems (resonance, phonation, and respiration). Resonant voice therapy (option c) focuses on building a continuum between oral sensations and easy phonation builds from basic speech to conversation. The yawn-sigh technique (option d) is used as a method for relaxation. The pushing method (option e) is used in cases of vocal hypofunction.

44. c. Reinke edema is an inflammatory process caused by chronic irritation, such as that produced by smoking. The swelling interferes with vocal fold vibration thus producing hoarse voice quality and decreased pitch. Vocal hemorrhage (option a) is sudden in onset and is caused by vascular problems. Spasmodic dysphonia (option b) is a motor control disorder. Papillomas (option d) result from the human papillomavirus.

45. a. Maximum phonation time and s/z ratio provide information related to respiratory support and glottal efficiency during phonation. Pitch (option b), loudness (option c), resonance (option d), and general voice quality (option e) are not related to these vocal features.

46. c. Laryngeal videostroboscopy provides simulated slow-motion images of vocal fold motion and the integrity of the mucous membrane of the vocal folds. Acoustic evaluation (option a) is a noninvasive measure of vocal function. Aerodynamic measures (option b) provide measures of airflows and air pressures required for phonation. Laryngeal endoscopy (option d) provides an image of the vocal folds that useful for identification of disease but does not provide any information about vocal fold vibration. A perceptual voice assessment (option e) is a subjective measure of the perceptual variables of pitch, loudness, and quality.

47. a. On the spectrogram, time is represented on the horizontal axis and frequency on the vertical axis. Intensity is depicted by the gray scale.

48. b. On the spectrogram, intensity is depicted by the gray scale. The frequency (option a) is represented on the vertical axis, and time or duration (option e) is represented on the horizontal axis.

49. a. The noise burst at the moment of release is caused by simultaneous oral and velopharyngeal closures and thus a momentary cessation of airflow

emission. The transition between formants is rapid, not slow (option b), and there is no transient noise (option c). The first formant frequency (option e) is not characteristic in this type of consonant.

50. d. Voice onset time is the time segment between the release of a stop and the onset of voicing for the vowel that follows. Rise time (option a) is the speed with which the acoustic signal attains maximum intensity, whereas the fall time (option b) is the speed with which the signal attains minimum intensity. Rapid movement of the articulators causes sudden changes in the resonance peaks of the vocal tract and occurs during transition from one speech sound to another. These are known as formant transitions (option c).

51. c. A major production feature is that Nasal sounds create antiresonances in the vocal tract: these are, frequency regions in which amplitudes of the source components are severely attenuated. Nasal sounds are produced with a larger vocal tract (option b) than do oral sounds because velopharyngeal opening (option e) occurs. There is also reduced opening (option d) of the oral cavity.

52. b. Vocal nodules add mass to the vocal folds while limiting the mucosal wave and amplitude of vibration. Because the vocal folds cannot stretch as easily to phonate at higher frequencies, the harmonics are reduced in comparison with the fundamental frequency.

53. a. In coarticulation, two articulators move at the same time to produce different phonemes. In assimilation (option b), one articulator modifies its movements because of context. Phonation (option c) occurs at the level of the vocal cords. Rapid movement of the articulators causes sudden changes in the resonance peaks of the vocal tract and occurs during transition from one speech sound to another. These are known as formant transitions (option d).

54. a. For phonation, air pressure is created under the abducted vocal folds. This air is released when the vocal folds adduct, which leads to phonation. It is not measured at the lips (option b), above the vocal folds (option c), or at the diaphragm (option d).

55. e. Instrumental assessment is a beneficial tool in the diagnosis and intervention of voice disorders. It provides objective evidence (option d) for the perceptual judgment of the voice (option a), and the database can be used to measure average performance and deviation from average for the same population (option b). Finally, it provides tangible evidence of success in therapy (option c).

56. a. A phonetogram provides an "envelope" of the intensity at the various frequencies in a person's vocal range. In a spectrogram (option b), frequency is plotted in relation to time. The visual analog scale (option c) is a 10-mm scale in which each millimeter represents 10 units. The audiogram (option d) is a plot of the auditory response with regard to frequency and intensity.

57. c. Phonation threshold pressure is the minimum subglottal pressure necessary to initiate phonation. It does not represent air pressure at the lips (option a) or diaphragm (option b).

58. a. In stroboscopy, Talbot's law is used to create simulated slow-motion images of vocal fold motion by means of a strobe light. Endoscopy (option b) is used to observe vocal fold structure. Inverse filtering (option c), phonetography (option d), and pressure/flow technique (option e) are not instrumental procedures used for visualization.

59. b. Stroboscopy yields laryngeal images in simulated slow motion; Talbot's law—that an image lingers on the retina for 0.2 seconds—is used to create these images. Each pulse of the strobe light illuminates a point on the vibratory cycle, which is visually fused with successive cycles, which produces the perception of apparent motion. Thus, it is not truly slow motion (option a), real time (option c), or both slow motion and real time (option d).

60. c. Inverse filtering is a method by which nonlaryngeal acoustic features added by the resonators are subtracted from the radiated acoustic signal. Stroboscopy (option a) involves visualization of the vocal folds. Electroglottography (option b) measures vocal fold contact across time. Spectral analysis (option d) displays the glottal sound source and filtering characteristics across time. Fourier analysis (option e) is the analysis of a complex wave into its sine wave components.

61. b. The focus of resonant voice therapy is to produce voice with slightly abducted vocal folds and minimal subglottic pressure. Symptomatic voice therapy (option a) involves modification of deviant vocal symptoms. In physiological voice therapy (option c), the goal is to improve the balance among voice respiratory support, laryngeal muscle strength, control and stamina, and supraglottic modification of the laryngeal tone. Hygienic voice therapy (option d) focuses on identifying the primary and secondary behavioral causes of the voice disorder and then modifying or eliminating these causes.

62. c. Speed quotient is the ratio of abductor to adductor duration in the larynx. Open quotient (option a) is the ratio of the duration of the open period of the vocal folds to the total period of the cycle. Closed quotient (option b) is the ratio of the duration of the closed period of the vocal folds to the total period of the cycle. Phonation quotient (option d) is the ratio of vital capacity to the maximum phonation time.

63. a. Confidential voice involves vibrating vocal folds with a voice in a reduced intensity (option b); it is defined as aperiodic noise caused by rapidly flowing air through the glottis. Vibrato (option c) is produced by a regular pulsating change in pitch, whereas a tremor (option d) is rhythmic and caused by involuntary contractions of the muscle. Vocal fry (option e) occurs when the vocal folds are vibrating at the lowest voice register.

64. b. Electromyography is an instrumental procedure for measuring the electrical potential of muscle activity; of the options listed, it is the only direct measure of laryngeal muscle function. Electroglottography (option a) measures vocal fold contact across time by placing electrodes on the neck. Subglottal pressure (option c) measures the air pressure built up below the vocal folds. Acoustic analysis (option d) provides information about the acoustic waveform of the voice.

65. d. Hydration (option a), decreased throat clearing (option b), and smoking cessation (option c) are all vital for a healthy laryngeal mechanism.

66. b. This description is consistent with muscle tension dysphonia. Vocal fold paresis (option a) is caused by a disruption of the peripheral nervous system. Diplophonia (option c) is a symptom of disease, whereas a granuloma (option d) is a structural abnormality.

67. a. The major disadvantage of the electrolarynx is the perception by listeners of a mechanical-sounding voice. The advantages are that it can be used externally (option b) and in the early postoperative stages (option c).

68. d. The tracheoesophageal puncture is a surgical procedure to enable placement of a speaking valve. A Passy-Muir valve (option a) is a type of prosthesis placed in the tracheoesophageal puncture. A tracheostomy (option b) is a stoma created in the trachea without the placement of a tube into the esophagus. Intubation (option c) is performed orally. A pharyngoplasty (option e) is a surgical procedure used to improve velopharyngeal function for speech.

69. a. Esophageal speech is produced by taking air in through the mouth, trapping it in the upper esophagus, and releasing it. Electromechanical speech (option b) is produced by the use of an artificial larynx. Tracheoesophageal speech (option c) is produced with the use of a speaking valve or prosthesis fitted over the tracheoesophageal puncture. Confidential speech (option d) is achieved by soft phonation.

70. a. The left recurrent laryngeal nerve loops around the aorta before innervating the laryngeal muscles. This nerve is sometimes damaged during cardiac surgery as a result of its proximity to the cardiac structures. Because innervation is ipsilateral, the left vocal cord would be paralyzed.

71. b. Difficulty breathing is the most common symptom of vocal cord dysfunction as a result of the paradoxical movement of the vocal cords. This condition is often misdiagnosed as asthma. Laryngopharyngeal reflux is a common trigger of the paradoxical vocal fold motion.

72. c. Vocal nodules are caused by vocal misuse or abuse, and behavioral management is required. For long-term benefits, physiological voice therapy, which would improve the relationship between the subsystems of respiration, phonation, and resonance would be the treatment of choice. Surgical removal of the nodules (option a) is not necessary because nodules result from improper use of the laryngeal muscles and reappear if the technique is not corrected. Gastroesophageal reflux is not indicated as a problem, and so medication (option b) is unnecessary. Complete voice rest (option d) will only temporarily resolve the hoarseness.

73. d. Nodules are characteristic at the location of this junction, occurring bilaterally and at the point of maximum contact at the vocal folds. Vocal fold cysts (option a) and polyps (option b) are most often unilateral. Granulomas (option c) are also most often unilateral, although some postsurgical granulomas occur bilaterally.

74. a. Vocal fold hemorrhage is a pathological process of sudden onset. Granuloma (option b), Gastroesophageal reflux (option c), and vocal fold polyps (option d) are typically gradual in onset and do not result from vocal misuse.

75. b. Compression of the ventricular folds and erythema are consistent with vocal hyperfunction. The diagnosis of muscle tension dysphonia is consistent with the history of muscular pain, often associated with pain of the styloglossus muscle, and with lack of medical or surgical history.

PART IV

Neurogenic Disorders

CHAPTER 11

Neurological Disorders

Carl Coelho
Mary R.T. Kennedy
Nidhi Mahendra
Monica McHenry
Edythe A. Strand
Linda I. Shuster

1. The potential implications of a single unilateral lesion in the temporal-parietal region of the left hemisphere include:
   a. Difficulty with naming
   b. Difficulty understanding what is said
   c. Difficulty with reading
   d. Difficulty with writing
   e. All of the above

2. What are the potential implications of a single unilateral lesion in right hemisphere?
   a. Left-sided neglect
   b. Right-sided hemiplegia
   c. Aphasia
   d. Dementia
   e. a and b

3. Why does hemiplegia rarely accompany Wernicke aphasia?
   a. The lesion is too small
   b. The basal ganglia is typically spared
   c. The lesion involves the thalamus
   d. The lesion occurs in the prefrontal region
   e. None of the above

4. *Aphasia* is defined as an acquired impairment of the cognitive system specialized for comprehending and formulating language. In a person with aphasia, other cognitive capacities are relatively intact. Which of the following etiological factors would be excluded as a cause of aphasia?
   a. Stroke
   b. Traumatic brain injury

c. Genetic syndrome
d. Gunshot wound
e. None of the above

5. Which of the following deficits would not be expected to be compromised in aphasia?
   a. Reading
   b. Written language
   c. Producing and understanding American Sign Language
   d. Comprehension of spoken commands
   e. None of the above

6. The circle of Willis is a ring-shaped set of arteries that connects the basilar artery and the internal carotid arteries to the _____, which supply blood to the brain hemispheres.
   a. Vertebral arteries
   b. Anterior communicating arteries
   c. Cerebral arteries
   d. Common carotid arteries
   e. All of the above

7. The circle of Willis may help to mitigate the effects of occlusion of one of the feeder arteries _____ the circle of Willis.
   a. Above
   b. Below
   c. Within
   d. All of the above
   e. None of the above

8. Occlusions of the main branch of a cerebral artery are more serious than occlusions in _____.
   a. Watershed regions
   b. Peripheral branches
   c. Internal carotid arteries
   d. Vertebral arteries
   e. None of the above

9. The arcuate fasciculus connects regions in the temporal lobes with regions in the frontal lobes and is one type of _____ fiber tract.
   a. Commissural
   b. Association
   c. Projection
   d. Descending
   e. None of the above

10. The sylvian fissure (lateral fissure) divides the _____ and _____ lobes _____ and extends partially between the _____ and _____ lobes _____.
    a. Frontal, occipital, posteriorly, temporal, parietal, anteriorly

b. Frontal, parietal, anteriorly, parietal, occipital, posteriorly
c. Frontal, limbic, anteriorly, parietal, temporal, posteriorly
d. Frontal, temporal, anteriorly, temporal, parietal, posteriorly
e. None of the above

11. Brodmann area 44, or the _____ area, is an important area in spoken language.
    a. Wernicke
    b. Association
    c. Broca
    d. Prefrontal cortical
    e. None of the above

12. The Wernicke area is also known as:
    a. The auditory association cortex
    b. The primary auditory cortex
    c. Brodmann area 27
    d. The insular cortex
    e. All of the above

13. Broca aphasia is characterized by:
    a. Nonfluent spontaneous speech and intact auditory comprehension
    b. Nonfluent spontaneous speech, mildly impaired auditory comprehension, and intact reading and writing
    c. Nonfluent spontaneous speech, mildly impaired auditory comprehension, impaired reading and writing, and intact repetition
    d. Nonfluent spontaneous speech, mildly impaired auditory comprehension, impaired reading and writing, impaired repetition, and intact naming
    e. None of the above

14. Wernicke aphasia is characterized by:
    a. Fluent spontaneous speech, mildly impaired auditory comprehension, and impaired reading and writing
    b. Fluent spontaneous speech, poor auditory comprehension, impaired naming, and intact reading, writing, and repetition
    c. Fluent spontaneous speech, intact auditory comprehension, and impaired reading, writing, naming, and repetition
    d. Nonfluent spontaneous speech and impaired auditory comprehension, naming, and repetition
    e. None of the above

15. When a person is suspected of having a stroke, one of the first procedures ordered by the attending physician is a brain scan. Why?
    a. To determine the appropriate medical intervention
    b. To confirm or rule out a hemorrhagic event
    c. To document brain swelling
    d. To identify a potential source of neurological changes
    e. All of the above

16. Repetition of responses when they are no longer appropriate—for example, in a naming task, after naming an apple, labeling all subsequent pictures "apple"—is referred to as:
    a. Egocentrism
    b. Emotional lability
    c. Decreased self-monitoring
    d. Perseveration
    e. None of the above

17. When assessing a patient with aphasia, standardized tests are particularly useful when the clinician wants to:
    a. Compare a patient's test performance with that of other patients or with that of non–brain-injured adults
    b. Compare a patient's performance across several test occasions
    c. Communicate with other professionals about the patient's performance
    d. All of the above
    e. None of the above

18. The behavioral, cognitive, and emotional consequences of brain injury may affect the patient's performance in testing and treatment activities. These consequences include:
    a. Slowed responding
    b. Difficulty initiating purposeful behavior
    c. Impulsivity
    d. Self-doubt or extreme cautiousness
    e. All of the above

19. The purposes of communication testing for a brain-injured patient include:
    a. Diagnose communication impairments, including nature and severity
    b. Arrive at a prognosis
    c. Assist in planning specific medical interventions
    d. a and b
    e. None of the above

20. The observations of Paul Broca and Karl Wernicke were the basis of contemporary _____ models of aphasia.
    a. Localizationist
    b. Phrenological
    c. Connectionist
    d. a and c
    e. None of the above

21. Strokes are a loss of blood supply to the brain. Strokes are classified as either:
    a. Permanent or transient
    b. Ischemic or hemorrhagic
    c. Atherosclerotic or occlusive
    d. Hypoperfusional or reversible
    e. None of the above

22. In diaschisis, brain function is disrupted in regions distant from the _____ but _____ to it by neuronal pathways.
    a. Infarcted area; connected
    b. Occlusion; unconnected
    c. Artery; connected
    d. Lesion; unconnected
    e. None of the above

23. Aneurysms are pouches formed in weakened arterial walls. The stretched arterial walls within aneurysms are susceptible to rupture; when this occurs, it is referred to as:
    a. Collateral sprouting
    b. Hemorrhagic stroke
    c. Extracerebral hemorrhage
    d. Ischemic stroke
    e. None of the above

24. _____ are collections of dilated, thin-walled veins connected to a tangled mass of thin-walled arteries.
    a. Microaneurysms
    b. Primary intracranial tumors
    c. Arteriovenous malformations
    d. Thromboses
    e. None of the above

25. Why are strokes that result in Broca aphasia also associated with right-sided hemiplegia?
    a. The lesion is close to the postcentral gyrus
    b. The lesion is close to the precentral gyrus
    c. The lesion disrupts the angular gyrus
    d. The lesion extends deeply to the basal ganglia
    e. All of the above

26. Destruction of the left optic tract (posterior to the optic chiasm) causes blindness in the visual field contralateral to the side of injury; this condition is known as:
    a. Bitemporal hemianopsia
    b. Right-sided homonymous hemianopia
    c. Left quadrantanopia
    d. Left-sided homonymous hemianopia
    e. None of the above

27. Disconnection syndromes are caused by damage to the _____.
    a. Arcuate fasciculus
    b. Corpus callosum
    c. Angular gyrus
    d. All of the above
    e. None of the above

28. Right-handed patients with _____ disconnection syndrome cannot name, describe, write about, or talk about objects placed in their left hand and out of sight.

a. Anterior
b. Posterior
c. Complete
d. a and b
e. None of the above

29. Right-handed patients with _____ disconnection syndrome cannot verbally respond to visual information that is presented only to the right hemisphere.
a. Anterior
b. Posterior
c. Complete
d. a and b
e. None of the above

30. If basic perception in a sensory modality is intact, then failure to recognize familiar stimuli in that modality is known as_____.
a. Apraxia
b. Aphasia
c. Agnosia
d. Alexia
e. None of the above

31. Brain imaging technology has called into question the classic concepts of the relationships between brain damage and aphasia syndromes. Two of the most important findings are:
a. Chronic Broca or Wernicke aphasia includes brain damage beyond those cortical areas.
b. Aphasia may be the result of large tumors or traumatic brain injury.
c. Aphasia can be caused by damage deep in the brain, below the perisylvian cortex and its association areas.
d. a and c
e. b and c

32. In the testing of sentence comprehension, what are "garden path" sentences?
a. Sentences that create expectations in the listener's mind and then confirm the expectations
b. Sentences that create expectations in the listener's mind and then violate the expectations
c. Sentences that are long and distracting
d. Sentences that skip from topic to topic
e. None of the above

33. An example of a standardized test for aphasia is:
a. Discourse Comprehension Test
b. Western Aphasia Battery
c. Peabody Picture Vocabulary Test-Revised
d. Revised Token Test
e. All of the above

34. Several variables may affect the single-word comprehension of persons with aphasia, including:
a. Frequency of occurrence
b. Semantic or acoustic similarity
c. Dialect
d. Referent ambiguity
e. a, b, and d

35. The Rating Scale of Speech Characteristics from the Boston Diagnostic Aphasia Examination is a subjective scale that can be used to construct a speech profile, which may be compared with profiles of major aphasia syndromes. The rating scale includes:
a. Phrase length
b. Melodic line
c. Grammatical form
d. Articulatory agility
e. All of the above

36. Scores from the Western Aphasia Battery can be used to generate the following quotients:
a. Aphasia
b. Language
c. Cortical
d. All of the above
e. None of the above

37. The speech-language pathologist (SLP) first sees many brain-injured patients at bedside, where the SLP conducts a brief interview and may administer a communication screening test. The purpose of this interview is to give the clinician a sense of:
a. The patient's background, problems, and concerns
b. The nature and severity of the speech, language, and communicative problems
c. The need for more comprehensive testing to follow
d. All of the above
e. None of the above

38. Reading tests for non–brain-damaged children and adults:
a. Are inappropriate for persons with aphasia
b. Are no more useful than the reading subtests from aphasia tests
c. Provide for more comprehensive assessment of aphasic adults' reading than is possible with aphasia tests
d. May have childish content that aphasic adults find offensive
e. None of the above

39. When a clinician examines the speech production of adults with aphasia, it is important to rule out:
a. Apraxia of speech
b. Dysarthria
c. Neurological stuttering

d. All of the above

e. None of the above

40. The FAS test is an example of:
    a. Tests of generative naming
    b. Spelling tests
    c. Tests of written language
    d. All of the above
    e. None of the above

41. The form of the stimuli to be named (drawings, photographs, real objects) has _____ effect on most aphasic adults' naming performance.
    a. A major
    b. A minimal
    c. A differential
    d. A neutral
    e. None of the above

42. Variables that may affect the probability that an aphasic adult will benefit from therapy include:
    a. Nature and severity of brain injury
    b. Patient's medical and physical condition
    c. Patient's age
    d. a and b
    e. a and c

43. Frequency and duration of treatment sessions are influenced by:
    a. Patient's medical and physical condition
    b. Patient's insurance coverage
    c. Complexity of the treatment program
    d. All of the above
    e. None of the above

44. Resource-allocation models of cognition suggest that humans have a finite amount of cognitive resources for carrying out mental operations. If the resources needed exceed the supply available, performance _____.
    a. Stops
    b. Speeds up
    c. Deteriorates
    d. All of the above
    e. None of the above

45. Clinicians may control the difficulty of treatment tasks by manipulating characteristics of the stimuli, such as:
    a. Intensity and salience
    b. Clarity and intelligibility
    c. Novelty and interest value
    d. a and b
    e. a, b, and c

46. Decisions regarding what a clinician will treat are based on the clinician's conclusion about the nature of the patient's communicative impairment. General approaches to treating persons with aphasia include consideration of:
    a. Relative level of impairment
    b. Fundamental processes
    c. Functional abilities
    d. a, b, and c
    e. b and c

47. Measuring a patient's performance across time enables clinicians to establish baselines against which effects of the treatment can be measured. Several methods are available for accomplishing this goal, including:
    a. Baseline-treatment design
    b. Criterion-treatments design
    c. Multiple-baseline design
    d. a and c
    e. None of the above

48. Clinicians may promote generalization of treatments by:
    a. Training in settings to which generalization is desired
    b. Targeting behaviors that will be rewarded only in the treatment setting
    c. Altering the training environment, task stimuli, or response contingencies to make them increasingly similar to daily life
    d. a and b
    e. a and c

49. Early studies of the efficacy of aphasia therapy yielded equivocal findings. More recent studies have been better designed, and the findings suggest that treatment for adults with aphasia is efficacious if:
    a. Treatment is delivered by qualified personnel
    b. Intensity, content, duration, and timing are appropriate for the recipients
    c. Sensitive and reliable measures are used to document the effects of treatment
    d. All of the above
    e. a and b

50. Early intervention for overall communication development (within a few weeks of onset of aphasia) is more efficacious than:
    a. Melodic intonation therapy
    b. Direct attention training
    c. Late intervention
    d. All of the above
    e. None of the above

51. The primary objective of aphasia treatment is:
    a. To improve test scores
    b. Improve word retrieval
    c. To improve real-world communication
    d. All of the above
    e. None of the above

52. Not all patients with aphasia are candidates for treatment. Those who are not are:
    a. Too ill or too weak
    b. Too severely aphasic
    c. Poorly motivated to participate
    d. b and c
    e. a, b, and c

53. Patients who remain globally aphasic 1 month or longer after onset of disability are likely to:
    a. Demonstrate dramatic improvement
    b. Demonstrate steady but slow improvement
    c. Remain globally aphasic
    d. Develop cognitive deficits
    e. None of the above

54. *Neurological recovery* refers to the point at which spontaneous physiological recovery is essentially complete. For patients with _____, this occurs faster, and for patients with _____, this recovery may last longer.
    a. Large strokes; small strokes
    b. Ischemic or occlusive strokes; hemorrhagic strokes
    c. Transient ischemic accidents; thromboses
    d. Multiple strokes; single strokes
    e. None of the above

55. In contemporary philosophies of aphasia treatment, the following treatment activities would be a priority:
    a. Reading and writing of lists of individual words
    b. Oral reading of the grandfather passage
    c. Sorting colored plastic chips
    d. Composing e-mail messages to grandchildren or other relatives
    e. None of the above

56. Most persons with aphasia have impairments of short-term memory that compromise their auditory comprehension of:
    a. Familiar utterances
    b. Highly redundant messages
    c. Noncontextual sentences
    d. a and b
    e. None of the above

57. Non–brain-injured listeners rely on top-down processes to comprehend language and rely on _____ processes when the top-down processes fail.
    a. Rote
    b. Problem-solving
    c. Attention
    d. Text-based
    e. All of the above

58. Treatment involving single-word comprehension drills are best suited for patients who:
    a. Do not comprehend phrases or sentences
    b. Can comprehend sentences but not individual words
    c. Also have apraxia
    d. All of the above
    e. None of the above

59. Clinicians can manipulate the difficulty of discourse comprehension tasks by adjusting:
    a. Familiarity
    b. Length
    c. Redundancy
    d. All of the above
    e. a and b

60. Persons with aphasia who have severe impairments in written language may benefit from treatment focused on:
    a. American Sign Language
    b. Increasing manual strength
    c. Survival writing skills
    d. Syntax training
    e. None of the above

61. Several studies have shown that aphasia treatment groups improve communicative abilities of patients with:
    a. Acute aphasia
    b. Chronic aphasia
    c. Fluent aphasia
    d. Nonfluent aphasia
    e. All of the above

62. The first step in designing a program to treat an acquired reading deficit is:
    a. Assessing reading skills
    b. Examining spelling ability
    c. Obtaining a literary history
    d. All of the above
    e. None of the above

63. Adults with aphasia who cannot return to recreational reading often benefit from acquiring:
    a. Rudimentary written language skills
    b. Books on tape
    c. Training with Braille
    d. Survival reading skills
    e. All of the above

64. Reading comprehension of text-level materials can be manipulated through the adjustment of:
    a. Familiarity
    b. Length
    c. Vocabulary
    d. Syntactic complexity
    e. All of the above

65. Confrontation naming drills are popular with some clinicians; however, in work on oral verbal expression, such activities:
    a. May not have lasting effects
    b. May not improve functional communication skills
    c. May facilitate single-word written responses
    d. a and b
    e. All of the above

66. An example of connected-speech drill activities is:
    a. Picture description
    b. Prompted story telling
    c. Procedural discourse
    d. All of the above
    e. None of the above

67. Right hemisphere damage may affect overall communicative skills without disrupting:
    a. Cognition
    b. Memory
    c. Language
    d. Attention
    e. All of the above

68. Patients with right hemisphere damage and communicative deficits may appear:
    a. Abstract
    b. Disconnected
    c. Verbose
    d. Efficient
    e. b and c

69. With regard to right hemisphere damage, there is little information about:
    a. Predictions of recovery
    b. Linguistic impairments
    c. Lesion localization
    d. All of the above
    e. None of the above

70. In left-sided neglect, responsivity toward _____ is reduced:
    a. Right-sided information
    b. Visual information
    c. Left-sided information
    d. All visual and auditory information
    e. All of the above

71. Left-sided neglect can occur in the following modalities:
    a. Auditory
    b. Olfactory
    c. Visual
    d. Tactile
    e. All of the above

72. Left-sided neglect is a negative predictor of the recovery of:
    a. Functional communication
    b. Memory skills
    c. Independence in daily living
    d. All of the above
    e. None of the above

73. Anosognosia is a disorder in which patients may:
    a. Fail to notice contralesional limbs
    b. Deny hemiplegia
    c. Fail to claim ownership of contralesional limbs
    d. All of the above
    e. None of the above

74. Focal damage anywhere in the brain can interfere with attention; however:
    a. In contrast to the left hemisphere, the right hemisphere orients attention across spatial boundaries
    b. Frontal areas in the right hemisphere are more active than comparable areas in the left hemisphere for selective attention and vigilance
    c. The left hemisphere plays a role in maintaining attention in states of vigilance
    d. All of the above
    e. a and b

75. The most fundamental attentional deficit that can occur after right hemisphere damage is:
    a. Hyperarousal
    b. Hypoarousal
    c. Left-sided neglect
    d. Anosognosia
    e. None of the above

76. Emotional prosodic comprehension deficits often observed in patients with right hemisphere damage appear to be related to:
    a. Reduced responsivity to paralinguistic information
    b. Decreased attention
    c. Left-sided neglect
    d. Problems in pitch perception
    e. a and d

77. Discourse problems in patients with right hemisphere damage arise from specific cognitive impairments that affect:
    a. The capacity for integrating information
    b. Responding to alternative meanings
    c. Forming and revising inferences
    d. All of the above
    e. None of the above

78. Depression can occur after a stroke with either right hemisphere or left hemisphere lesions. In patients with right hemisphere damage, it is important not to confuse depression with:

a. Flat affect
b. Reduced use of prosody
c. Confabulation
d. a and b
e. None of the above

79. Right hemisphere damage may disturb:
   a. Appreciation of humor
   b. Sensitivity to and understanding of the emotions conveyed verbally
   c. Ability to verbally convey emotional information
   d. All of the above
   e. None of the above

80. Sites of lesions associated with left-sided neglect include:
   a. Frontal and parietal cortex
   b. Basal ganglia, internal capsule, and thalamus
   c. Temporal and occipital cortex
   d. All of the above
   e. a and b

81. Which statement accurately distinguishes between a traumatic brain injury (TBI) and an acquired brain injury (ABI)?
   a. A TBI is caused by a direct blow to the head and brain or by sudden acceleration or deceleration of the head, whereas ABI represents a broader term that refers to brain injury that occurs after birth with any neurological basis (e.g., stroke or tumor)
   b. TBI occurs before or after birth, whereas ABI occurs after the age of 18
   c. TBI occurs after birth, whereas ABI occurs before birth
   d. TBI and ABI mean the same thing; they are indistinguishable
   e. TBI includes psychological or emotional trauma that may be linked to brain damage, whereas ABI has a neurological basis

82. Which group makes up the largest segment of the population who sustain TBI?
   a. The male population from adolescence to middle age
   b. Boys and girls
   c. Physically abused women
   d. Infants
   e. TBI is equally prevalent in all groups of the population

83. Approximately _____ traumatic brain injuries (TBIs) occur in the United States each year.
   a. 500,000
   b. 250,000
   c. 3 million
   d. 1.4 million
   e. 5 million

84. The _____ are the areas of the brain most directly responsible for forming new memories; impairment in short-term memory is the most common impairment associated with a TBI.
   a. Temporal lobes
   b. Parietal lobes
   c. Hippocampi
   d. Occipital lobes
   e. Cerebellar lobes

85. With regard to an open TBI, which of the following statements is true?
   a. There is diffuse damage to many areas of the brain
   b. Facial bones have been penetrated
   c. The person loses consciousness
   d. The scalp has been penetrated and skull has been fractured
   e. The skull has been penetrated or depressed into brain tissue, which results in focal or "localized" brain damage

86. With regard to shaken-baby syndrome, which of the following statements is true?
   a. It can result in TBI
   b. It is a form of child abuse
   c. It can result in permanent cognitive impairments
   d. It can result in death
   e. All of the above

87. In describing brain damage from a TBI, clinicians refer to *coup* and *contracoup* injuries. What do these terms mean?
   a. Diffuse brain damage
   b. Brain damage that has occurred in an area of brain that is opposite from where the initial blow occurred
   c. Brain damage that is close in vicinity to where the initial blow to the head occurred
   d. Brain damage that is close in vicinity to where the initial blow to the head occurred and brain damage that has occurred in an area of brain that is opposite from where the initial blow occurred
   e. Brain damage that has extended into regions of the brain that are close to where the initial blow occurred

88. Which two lobes of the brain are most commonly injured in association with a closed TBI?
   a. Occipital and frontal lobes
   b. Cerebellar lobes
   c. Occipital and parietal lobes
   d. Temporal and parietal lobes
   e. Temporal and frontal lobes

89. When emerging from a coma, most patients with TBI:
   a. Are aware of their abilities and disabilities
   b. Remember the accident

c. Do not remember the accident

d. Are oriented to person, place, and time

e. Remember everything up to the accident

90. When a patient is emerging from a coma with difficulty sustaining attention after a TBI, which of the following communication goals would be important initially?
    a. To recall the events that led up to the accident
    b. To establish consistent and reliable means for communicating (e.g., thumbs up or down)
    c. To maintain a daily planner to compensate for poor memory for daily events
    d. To be able to understand jokes and sarcasm
    e. To practice appropriate pragmatics

91. TBI most commonly results in which communication impairment?
    a. Dysarthria
    b. Apraxia of speech
    c. Aphasia
    d. Cognitive-communication disorders
    e. Alexia

92. The most common linguistic or language impairment associated with closed TBI is:
    a. Impaired word-finding or word-fluency skills
    b. Reduced auditory comprehension
    c. Syntactic errors
    d. Impairment in written expression
    e. Impaired reading comprehension

93. When dysarthria is the result of a closed TBI, which type is the most likely to be present?
    a. Flaccid
    b. Hypokinetic
    c. Mixed
    d. Spastic
    e. Hyperkinetic

94. Memory impairment is a common consequence of TBI. Which type of memory is most likely to be preserved?
    a. Explicit memory
    b. Implicit memory
    c. Episodic memory
    d. Memory for future events or plans
    e. Word retrieval, especially names

95. Which type of attention is most likely to remain impaired in someone who has made sufficient recovery from a TBI that they are able to return to school or work?
    a. Divided attention
    b. Sustained attention
    c. Alertness
    d. Focused attention
    e. Selective attention

96. Which standardized test is typically administered to adults with TBI by SLPs and occupational therapists and provides information about functional memory abilities?
    a. Ross Information Processing Assessment (Ross, 1986)
    b. California Verbal Learning Test, 2nd Edition (Delis et al., 2000)
    c. Wechsler Memory Scales-III (The Psychological Corporation, 1997)
    d. Rivermead Behavioral Memory Test (Wilson et al., 2003)
    e. Scales of the Assessment for Traumatic Brain Injury (Adamovich & Henderson, 1992)

97. With regard to using and interpreting standardized cognitive and language assessment tools that identify underlying processing impairments with patients with TBI, which of following statements is the most accurate?
    a. Impairments in performance on these tests are transferable or generalize to everyday cognitive and communication problems
    b. Impairments in performance on these tests help clinicians identify the patients' own goals
    c. Processing strengths and weaknesses identified in standardized impairment tests do not necessarily reflect everyday cognitive and communication problems
    d. Functional goals are easy to generate once the clinician knows the patient's processing impairments
    e. Most standardized tests of impairments are psychometrically weak

98. Which of the following statements best describes the natural course of cognitive and communication recovery for a child who sustained a moderate or severe TBI at the age of 8?
    a. Cognitive and communication disorders that are initially severe improve within 6 months and become subtle later in childhood, but then become much more noticeable in adolescence because of the increasing demands of social skills and academics
    b. There is little to no recovery from a moderate or severe TBI through adolescence
    c. The brain completely reorganizes in such a way that these children recover cognitive and communication skills to such a degree that those skills are equivalent to those of their peers
    d. The most recovery of cognitive and communication disorders occurs shortly after the injury (within 6 months), but beyond this point the child's skills decline steadily until about 20 years of age

e. The most recovery of cognitive and communication disorders occurs shortly after the injury (within 6 months), but beyond this point there is little to no further recovery

99. Confabulation is a communication problem after TBI:
    a. In which the patient unintentionally expands or elaborates on the truth to the point that the patient is inaccurate
    b. In which the patient is intentionally lying
    c. And is very uncommon in the early phases of cognitive recovery from TBI
    d. And is considered a serious underlying psychiatric disorder
    e. And is responsive to medication

100. An adult has sustained a TBI that has resulted in a number of cognitive impairments. She interrupts people in conversation and keeps talking long after conversation partners want to end the conversation. Her family reports that this was *not* her style of communication before the injury. What combination of cognitive impairments most likely explains this communication behavior?
    a. Organizational difficulty
    b. Memory loss
    c. Impaired impulse control and divided attention
    d. Impaired problem solving
    e. Inability to maintain attention

101. In using an aphasia test battery to evaluate someone who is highly confused and agitated after sustaining a severe TBI, you find that he has difficulty following simple commands, naming common objects, repeating sentences, and generating items from a given category. How would you interpret these results?
    a. These results cannot be interpreted
    b. It is likely that this person has aphasia
    c. It is likely that this person has anomia
    d. It is likely that this person's confusional state is affecting his language comprehension and expression
    e. It is likely that this person will develop dementia

102. Which assessment tool is the most commonly used to evaluate someone who is in a coma?
    a. Scales of Cognitive Ability for Traumatic Brain Injury
    b. Glasgow Coma Scale
    c. Disability Rating Scale
    d. Communicative Effective Index
    e. Levels of Cognitive Functioning

103. Self-awareness of disability is reduced in patients with TBI. Which statement accurately reflects how self-awareness recovers in various domains?

    a. Awareness of physical, cognitive, memory, and communication disabilities recovers at the same rate and in the same manner
    b. Awareness of cognitive and communication disabilities recovers first, followed by awareness of physical and memory disabilities
    c. Patients rarely become aware of physical, cognitive, memory, and communication disabilities
    d. Patients are aware of their abilities and disabilities while in the hospital but lose this awareness once they reenter the community, home, and school
    e. Patients become aware of physical disabilities first, followed later by awareness of cognitive, memory, and communication disabilities; some never gain "full" awareness of the latter disabilities

104. Process-specific attention training is based on the assumption that attention processes are hierarchical, from the most basic or sustained attention to the most complex or divided attention. With regard to the use of this approach for adults with TBI, which of the following statements is true?
    a. All patients should begin training with sustained attention
    b. Patients should proceed through all levels of attention training
    c. There is strong evidence that once patients reach criterion at each level, attention skills will transfer automatically into everyday, functional activities without direct instruction
    d. There is little evidence that once patients have reached criterion at each level, attention skills will automatically transfer into everyday, functional activities without direct instruction
    e. There is no evidence that process-specific attention training improves performance in decontextualized attention activities or in everyday, functional activities

105. Which of the following instructional techniques should be considered in training or teaching the use of compensatory cognitive or memory strategies to patients with TBI?
    a. Method of vanishing cues
    b. Metacognitive strategy instruction
    c. Spaced retrieval
    d. Errorless learning
    e. All of the above

106. An outpatient with cognitive and communication disorders resulting from a TBI comes to you for therapy. His employer is holding his job for him. There are specific tasks that he must be able to do to be successful at this job. On the basis of your cognitive and communication assessment, you determine that it *is* possible

for him to return to work successfully. What approach would you take in therapy?
a. Teach him to use reading, writing-texting, and communication strategies that will allow him to compensate for his impairments and practice using these in role-playing with the materials he will have at work
b. Directly train specific, decontextualized cognitive processes
c. Tell him to purchase a daily planner or a personal digital assistant (PDA)
d. Refer him to a vocational counselor because this is not within your scope of practice
e. Teach him internal memory strategies such as visual imagery

107. The rehabilitation team may provide coma stimulation to patients with TBI. Which of the following statements best describes the current state of evidence on the efficacy or effectiveness of coma stimulation?
a. Few carefully controlled investigations have demonstrated the efficacy or effectiveness of coma stimulation (i.e., the evidence is weak)
b. Many carefully controlled investigations have demonstrated the efficacy or effectiveness of coma stimulation (i.e., the evidence is strong)
c. Many carefully controlled investigations on the efficacy or effectiveness of coma stimulation have been performed, but the results of these investigations are inconclusive (i.e., the evidence is weak)
d. No carefully controlled investigations of the efficacy or effectiveness of coma stimulation have been performed
e. There is strong evidence from animal models that coma stimulation would be effective in humans

108. Which form of memory is most closely related to executive functions and is frequently impaired after a TBI?
a. Retrieval
b. Long-term memory
c. Prospective memory
d. Short-term memory
e. Recognition memory

109. Which of the following pragmatic problems are you most likely to observe in someone with TBI who does not have aphasia or dysarthria?
a. Inability to maintain eye contact
b. Difficulty with topic maintenance and coherence
c. Nonuse of social greetings
d. Nonuse of gestures
e. Trouble using intonation and prosodic features of speech

110. Patients with TBI typically have some kind of difficulty with metacognition (thinking about their thinking). Which is the best description of metacognition?
a. Self-monitoring and self-control
b. Autobiographical beliefs about oneself, often called self-monitoring and self-control
c. Self-monitoring
d. Self-control
e. Autobiographical beliefs about oneself, often called *self-awareness*

111. For patients with TBI who are receiving acute care or are in acute rehabilitation units, cognitive rehabilitation that trains isolated cognitive processes is:
a. Not strongly supported by evidence, inasmuch as improvement is confounded by the effects of spontaneous recovery
b. Strongly supported by evidence, inasmuch as improvement is not influenced by the effects of spontaneous recovery
c. Not possible, inasmuch as most patients at these levels of care remain in minimally conscious states
d. Supported by the evidence in cases in which clinicians directly teach the transfer of these skills to functional activities
e. Is supported by evidence in patients who have sustained strokes

112. A patient has sustained a TBI that includes skull fracture, which extends to the internal auditory meatus. As an SLP, you should:
a. Expect the individual to have a spastic dysarthria
b. Perform an assessment of cranial nerves III, IV, and VI (nerves that control eye movement)
c. Perform an assessment of cranial nerve I (the nerve that provides visual information to the brain)
d. Ensure that the patient receives a complete audiological assessment of the integrity of the acoustic-vestibular nerve (cranial nerve VIII), and check for the patient's sense of taste and for muscle weakness in the face (facial nerve VII)
e. Perform assessment of cranial nerve XII (the nerve that innervates muscles of the tongue)

113. The conflicts in Iraq and Afghanistan have resulted in record numbers of blast injuries to the head and limbs. Which of the following is frequently observed in returning soldiers with TBI?
a. Polytrauma (trauma to multiple body systems)
b. Post-traumatic stress disorder
c. Hearing loss
d. Mild, moderate, or severe brain injury
e. All of the above

114. Various rehabilitation professionals work together to provide comprehensive, best-practice care to patients with TBI. In which disciplines is cognitive rehabilitation part of the scope of practice?
    a. Social work and neuropsychology
    b. Speech-language pathology, occupational therapy, and neuropsychology
    c. Physical therapy
    d. Recreational therapy
    e. Nursing and social work

115. A good approach to keep up to date with the research evidence and practice recommendations on the effectiveness of cognitive and communication rehabilitation for patients with TBI is to:
    a. Read systematic reviews posted on the American Speech-Language Hearing Association's (ASHA's) Web site
    b. Visit Web sites of other organizations that are dedicated to the review of evidence and the creation of practice recommendations
    c. Attend workshops or conferences in which leaders in evidence-based practice are presenting their reviews and recommendations
    d. Form discussion groups at work
    e. All of the above

116. The most common cause of irreversible dementia in adults older than 65 is:
    a. Vascular dementia
    b. Vitamin B_{12} deficiency
    c. Depression
    d. Alzheimer disease
    e. Drug side effects

117. The most pervasive feature of the syndrome of dementia is:
    a. Positive family history of dementia
    b. Episodic memory impairments
    c. Depression
    d. Coronary artery disease
    e. None of the above

118. Long-term memory is thought to consist of two distinct memory systems. These are:
    a. Declarative memory and nondeclarative memory
    b. Lexical memory and semantic memory
    c. Working memory and episodic memory
    d. Sensory memory and nondeclarative memory
    e. None of the above

119. The two memory systems that are affected earliest and most severely in persons with dementia of the Alzheimer type are:
    a. Sensory memory and procedural memory
    b. Working memory and episodic memory
    c. Semantic memory and procedural memory
    d. Procedural memory and episodic memory
    e. Working memory and sensory memory

120. Working memory consists of four component systems: the central executive, the articulatory-phonological loop, the visuospatial sketchpad, and the episodic buffer. Which of the working memory components is subserved by the dorsolateral prefrontal cortex?
    a. The visuospatial sketchpad
    b. The episodic buffer
    c. The central executive
    d. The articulatory-phonological loop
    e. a and d

121. Working memory consists of four component systems: the central executive, the articulatory-phonological loop, the visuospatial sketchpad, and the episodic buffer. Of these four component systems, which one is thought to be subserved by Broca area and the cortex surrounding it?
    a. The episodic buffer
    b. The articulatory-phonological loop
    c. The visuospatial sketchpad
    d. The central executive
    e. None of the above

122. The following is a risk factor that increases the likelihood that a person will develop irreversible dementia:
    a. A nonvegetarian diet
    b. Inability to speak English fluently
    c. History of TBI
    d. Deterioration in driving performance
    e. Nutritional deficiency

123. There is strong empirical evidence that which of the following factors increases risk for developing Alzheimer disease?
    a. Being left-handed
    b. Having two copies of the type 4 allele of apolipoprotein E
    c. Having low blood pressure (hypotension)
    d. Having poor hand-eye coordination
    e. Hearing loss

124. The most common cause of irreversible dementia for persons younger than 65 years is:
    a. Dementia associated with Huntington disease
    b. Frontotemporal dementia
    c. Vascular dementia
    d. Dementia of the Alzheimer type
    e. a and c

125. With regard to primary progressive aphasia (PPA), which of the following statements is false?
    a. PPA is characterized by language and cognitive deficits
    b. PPA is a distinct type of frontotemporal dementia

c. SLPs work to teach compensatory communicative strategies to patients with PPA

d. PPA has the same symptom profile as Alzheimer dementia

e. b and c

126. For an SLP working with a patient who has dementia, it is not within the scope of practice to:
    a. Screen and comprehensively assess cognitive status in persons with dementia
    b. Counsel family caregivers about the nature of dementia and its progression
    c. Establish a medical diagnosis of the type of dementia
    d. Implement direct and indirect interventions to manage a patient's dementia
    e. Involve the family in treatment of the patient

127. You are an SLP working in a Medicare-certified skilled nursing facility. By law, what must happen for every newly admitted resident within 14 days of admission?
    a. Residents must be assessed for the possibility of swallowing impairments
    b. Residents must be administered a federally mandated assessment instrument called the Minimum Data Set
    c. Residents' Medicare status and secondary insurance (if any) must be verified
    d. Residents' need for rehabilitation services must be determined by an interdisciplinary rehabilitation team
    e. All of the above

128. The neuropathological process of Alzheimer disease is characterized chiefly by progressive loss of neuronal cells in which area of the brain?
    a. Basal ganglia
    b. Cerebellum
    c. Hippocampus and the entorhinal cortex
    d. Corpus callosum
    e. All of the above

129. With regard to language impairments in persons with Alzheimer disease, which of the following statements is generally true?
    a. Persons with Alzheimer disease tend to experience breakdowns in phonological and syntactical awareness early on in the disease
    b. Persons with Alzheimer disease almost never exhibit impaired discourse (spontaneous speech)
    c. Word retrieval impairments are among the earliest linguistic deficits in Alzheimer disease
    d. Persons with Alzheimer disease often perform poorly on working memory tasks
    e. a and b

130. On the Mini-Mental State Examination (Folstein et al, 1975), scores in which range would suggest that a patient has no impairment in cognitive status?
    a. 16 to 24
    b. 30 to 40
    c. 27 to 30
    d. 20 to 30
    e. a and d

131. On the Mini-Mental State Examination (Folstein et al, 1975), scores in which range would suggest that a patient has cognitive impairments corresponding to moderate severity of dementia?
    a. 8 to 15
    b. 16 to 24
    c. 25 to 33
    d. 27 to 30
    e. None of the above

132. Which of the following tests may *not* be used as a standardized test to assess communicative functioning in persons with dementia?
    a. Mini-Mental State Examination (MMSE)
    b. Arizona Battery for Communication Disorders of Dementia (ABCD)
    c. Communicative Activities of Daily Living (CADL-2)
    d. Functional Linguistic Communication Inventory (FLCI)
    e. Western Aphasia Battery (WAB)

133. For a patient with dementia, semantic memory functioning may be appropriately assessed by which of the following tasks?
    a. Retelling a short story
    b. Describing features of a common object
    c. Reading short sentences
    d. Repeating a sequence of numbers in the right order
    e. None of the above

134. According to current published evidence, one of the most sensitive tasks for differentiating between healthy aging and early Alzheimer disease is:
    a. Providing accurate biographical information
    b. Demonstrating immediate and delayed recall of a short story
    c. Naming black and white line drawings of common objects
    d. Copying a complex figure
    e. All of the above

135. To assess the communicative abilities of a patient with moderately severe dementia, which of the following standardized tests of linguistic communication is most appropriate?
    a. Boston Diagnostic Aphasia Examination (BDAE)
    b. Arizona Battery for Communication Disorders of Dementia (ABCD)

   c. Functional Linguistic Communication Inventory (FLCI)

   d. Repeatable Battery for Assessment of Neuropsychological Status (RBANS)

   e. Western Aphasia Battery (WAB)

136. To rule out the presence of depression in a patient with suspected dementia, one instrument to use is the _____.

   a. Clinical Dementia Rating (CDR) Scale

   b. Dementia Mood Assessment Scale

   c. Mattis Dementia Rating Scale

   d. Arizona Battery for Communication Disorders of Dementia (ABCD)

   e. Functional Linguistic Communication Inventory (FLCI)

137. For an SLP working with a patient who has suspected dementia, it is not within the scope of practice to:

   a. Administer the Communicative Abilities of Daily Living–2 to characterize the functional communication of a person diagnosed with dementia

   b. Develop and administer a therapy plan employing spaced retrieval training

   c. Conduct otoscopy and cerumen management for a patient with dementia

   d. Conducting a modified barium swallow (MBS) examination for a patient with dementia and dysphagia

   e. Counseling the patient's caregivers

138. With regard to verbal communication abilities of patients in the late stages of Alzheimer disease, which of the following statements is true?

   a. Functional communication is impossible for persons with late-stage Alzheimer disease

   b. Most patients in the late stages of Alzheimer disease are still able to produce language

   c. Most patients in late stages of Alzheimer disease are nonverbal

   d. Limited episodic memory abilities are spared in persons with late-stage Alzheimer disease

   e. a and b

139. With regard to the naming abilities of persons with Alzheimer disease, which of the following statements is false?

   a. Performance on generative naming tasks is more impaired than on confrontation naming tasks

   b. Performance on confrontation naming tasks is significantly more impaired than on generative naming tasks

   c. Performance on semantic fluency tasks is more impaired than on letter fluency tasks

   d. Performance on naming high-frequency items is better than on naming low-frequency items

   e. None of the above are false

140. The SLP is about to conduct an assessment of cognitive-linguistic functioning for a patient with mild dementia who resides in a skilled nursing facility. As the SLP prepares for testing and explains test instructions to a patient with dementia, it becomes apparent that the patient is having significant difficulty in hearing the SLP comfortably. If testing proceeds, the results of the evaluation will not be valid because of the confounding presence of hearing loss. Which of the following represents a solution to this situation?

   a. Referring the patient to an audiologist for a comprehensive evaluation

   b. Canceling the scheduled evaluation for that day

   c. Raising the SLP's vocal loudness substantially and completing the assessment

   d. Conducting otoscopy and hearing screening and using an assistive listening device

   e. Carry out testing as planned

141. The term *direct interventions* for patients with dementia refers to:

   a. An SLP's training of professional and personal caregivers of persons with dementia

   b. An SLP's provision of individual or group therapy to persons with dementia

   c. An SLP's provision of continuing education training for dementia management to other professionals

   d. An SLP's modification of the physical environment to support communication with patients who have dementia

   e. An SLP's training of caregivers in the use of prospective memory aids

142. A technique in which patients with dementia are trained to recall information over gradually increasing time intervals is called:

   a. Errorless learning

   b. Spaced retrieval training

   c. Simulated presence therapy

   d. Semantic feature analysis

   e. Reminiscence therapy

143. The conceptual principle of "reminiscence therapy" for persons with dementia is that:

   a. Reducing the number of errors during new learning improves retention of information

   b. Informal conversation stimulates recall of specific information about a theme

   c. Physical and cognitive exercise improves functional performance

   d. Tangible stimuli and sharing thematic memories stimulates recall

   e. Memory training results in the learning of new information

144. An SLP is making a home visit to a 70-year-old patient who has had Parkinson disease for the past 3 years. Which finding has the greatest significance for this patient's care?
    a. The patient's speech is less intelligible now than during the SLP's previous visit
    b. The patient uses a walker and walks slowly with very short steps
    c. The patient has lost considerable weight since the SLP's last visit
    d. The patient reports that his grandchildren visited with him for 2 days
    e. The patient and caregiver have been engaging in various indirect treatment activities

145. Mrs. A received a diagnosis of Parkinson disease nearly 5 years ago, now lives in a skilled nursing facility, and is taking medications for managing the symptoms of Parkinson disease. She has resting state tremors and a soft, monotonous voice, and her speech is often slurred and unintelligible, which makes it difficult for staff to understand her. Her episodic memory is mildly impaired, and she is known to become confused on occasion, but she responds well when cued or given a tangible stimulus to facilitate recall. Her gait is rather unsteady, and although she has been given a walker, she keeps forgetting to take it with her and has had multiple falls as a result. Which of the following is an appropriate therapy goal for an SLP?
    a. Using the Brain Fitness Software to work on her cognitive skills
    b. Conducting nonspeech oromotor movement drills to improve her speech intelligibility
    c. Conducting dysphagia therapy to improve her feeding and swallowing
    d. Using spaced retrieval training to work on remembering to take her walker
    e. Training staff to implement postural feeding techniques

146. Mr. B, 78 years old, has a long history of diabetes mellitus (type II) and chronic hypertension. His hypertension is often exacerbated because he sometimes forgets to take his blood pressure medication. His medical history reveals two transient ischemic attacks in the past 3 years, documented on magnetic resonance imaging (MRI). Recently, Mr. B's cognitive skills have declined considerably. He is often confused, is easily fatigued, and has become very forgetful. During verbal interactions, he forgets what he is saying midsentence and struggles to retrieve names of common objects. He also has difficulty reading and correctly interpreting short, simple documents on which his signature is needed. Which of the following causes is the best explanation for Mr. B's cognitive impairment?
    a. Pseudodementia
    b. Late-onset Alzheimer disease
    c. Vascular dementia
    d. Frontotemporal dementia
    e. Semantic dementia

147. In a long-term care setting, when a patient with dementia demonstrates limited restorative potential in response to direct interventions, an SLP can discontinue restorative therapy and develop a plan of care specifically called the _____.
    a. Functional maintenance plan
    b. Caregiver training plan
    c. Minimum data set
    d. Reevaluation plan
    e. Restorative therapy plan

148. With regard to swallowing disorders or dysphagia in persons with dementia, which of the following statements is false?
    a. In patients with dementia, dysphagia may be treated only with indirect interventions
    b. Patients with dementia can have oral, pharyngeal, or esophageal swallowing impairments
    c. In patients with dementia who have dysphagia, the degree of dementia is often moderate or severe
    d. Patients with dementia in long-term care settings are considered at high risk for malnutrition and dehydration
    e. Dysphagia is commonly found in elderly patients with dementia

149. With regard to treating cognitive-communicative impairments in persons with dementia, which of the following statements is generally false?
    a. Medicare does not reimburse SLPs for providing direct interventions to patients with dementia
    b. Medicare reimburses SLPs for developing functional maintenance plans (FMPs) to provide care for patients with dementia
    c. Medicare regulations require that SLPs document evidence of restorative potential in a patient with dementia in order to be reimbursed for providing therapy services
    d. Medicare regulations require that SLPs document the need for skilled services before providing therapy services to a patient with dementia
    e. None of the above

150. Researchers have demonstrated that for patients with dementia, tangible sensory stimuli facilitate recall of personal biographical information. A specific example of such stimuli, documented in the literature to enhance recall of biographical information, is:
    a. Dance movements
    b. Memory wallets and memory books
    c. Laptop computers
    d. Arts and crafts activities
    e. Checklists for reminder of scheduled activities

DYSARTHRIA

151. Your patient demonstrates rapid speech rate, fleeting dysfluencies, and reduced loudness. She reports feeling as if she speaks loudly, but everyone asks her to speak up. What type of dysarthria do you diagnose?
    a. Flaccid
    b. Spastic
    c. Hypokinetic
    d. Hyperkinetic
    e. Ataxic

152. You read in your patient's medical chart that he was in a coma for several months. What type of dysarthria do you expect to see?
    a. Flaccid
    b. Spastic
    c. Hypokinetic
    d. Hyperkinetic
    e. Ataxic

153. You conduct a motor speech evaluation and notice frequently perfect articulation, with inconsistent imprecision. The most notable characteristic of the patient's diadochokinetic rates is irregular timing. What type of dysarthria do you diagnose?
    a. Flaccid
    b. Spastic
    c. Hypokinetic
    d. Hyperkinetic
    e. Ataxic

154. What condition is the most likely to result in a mixed flaccid-spastic dysarthria?
    a. Cardiovascular accident (CVA)
    b. Parkinson disease
    c. Repeated head trauma (such as that experienced by boxers)
    d. TBI
    e. Huntington chorea

155. Your patient demonstrates overall good intelligibility with occasional disruptions and imprecision caused by involuntary movements. Loudness is typically within normal limits but is intermittently too loud or too soft. What type of dysarthria do you diagnose?
    a. Flaccid
    b. Spastic
    c. Hypokinetic
    d. Hyperkinetic
    e. Ataxic

156. Why does spastic dysarthria rarely co-occur with apraxia of speech?
    a. Spastic dysarthria is caused by damage to the brainstem

    b. Apraxia of speech is caused by lesions in the basal ganglia
    c. Spastic dysarthria is caused by bilateral upper motor neuron lesions
    d. Apraxia of speech is typically caused by a right-sided CVA
    e. Apraxia of speech is caused by a cerebellar lesion

157. You are working in an amyotrophic lateral sclerosis (ALS) clinic, where you monitor patients every 3 months. Of the following situations, which would you expect?
    a. Individuals with bulbar onset require motor speech intervention later than those with spinal onset
    b. Advanced audio coding (AAC) is not needed
    c. Patients demonstrate primarily hypokinetic dysarthria
    d. Individuals with spinal onset require motor speech intervention later than those with bulbar onset
    e. Patients exhibit no cognitive deficits

158. You are working in a Parkinson disease clinic in which the neurologist specializes in early diagnosis and intervention. Your treatment regimen is as follows:
    a. Begin the Lee Silverman Voice Treatment (LSVT) when the patient demonstrates or reports that the disease is affecting his or her speech, even if the effect is mild
    b. Begin LSVT when the patient demonstrates or reports that the disease affects speech moderately to severely
    c. Begin LSVT only when intelligibility is less than 80%
    d. Begin articulatory intervention to maintain intelligibility when changes to speech are apparent
    e. Begin respiratory intervention to provide an adequate driving force for voice production when changes in speech are apparent

159. Beukelman and colleagues (2004) recommended an AAC assessment for individuals with ALS when their speaking rate approaches 125 wpm. Why?
    a. Slow speech reduces intelligibility
    b. Listeners do not tolerate speaking rates less than 125 wpm
    c. Rapid deterioration in intelligibility often occurs when speaking rate reaches roughly 50% of habitual speed
    d. Cognitive decline parallels speaking rate decline
    e. Emotional deterioration parallels speaking rate decline

160. At your monthly rounds, you are discussing a patient with ALS. You recommended a palatal lift prosthesis, but other team members saw no reason for this intervention because of the degenerative nature of the

disease. To make your case, you recall that Esposito and associates (2000) recommended considering a palatal lift prosthesis for individuals with ALS. What was their rationale?
a. Reducing hypernasality increased intelligibility about 30%
b. Wearing a palatal lift prosthesis improved swallowing
c. A palatal lift reduced the need for an AAC device
d. Speaking was less effortful with the lift in place
e. Conversational partners reported less listener burden

161. You are counseling a patient with Parkinson disease who is considering neurosurgical intervention (e.g., pallidotomy, thalamotomy). On the basis of the available literature, what can you tell her about the likely benefit of such procedures on her speech production?
a. There will probably be significant postoperative improvements in ratings of general motor function and disease severity, but not in speech production
b. There will probably be significant postoperative improvements in speech production, but not in ratings of general motor function
c. Any improvements in speech production will probably not be maintained
d. Multiple surgical procedures are necessary to effect improvement in speech and motor function
e. The risks associated with surgery outweigh the benefits

162. A candidate for intervention at the level of the respiratory system should demonstrate all the following *except:*
a. Estimated subglottal pressure of less than 5 cm H_2O
b. Subglottal pressure of 5 cm H_2O sustained for less than 5 seconds
c. Moderate to severe breathiness
d. Inadequate subglottal pressure for phonation
e. Ability to say only one word at a time

163. What is the typical limitation of studies in which instrumentation-based biofeedback (such as a Respitrace) is used to improve speech breathing patterns?
a. Participants show improvement in the clinic but are unable to generalize the target behaviors
b. Speech breathing patterns do not change
c. Participants develop exaggerated speech breathing patterns in the clinic
d. Participants move too quickly through the training task hierarchy
e. It is not possible to set objective criteria to move through the training task hierarchy

164. One of the most basic abilities required for adequate speech breathing is inspiratory checking. Why?
a. It encourages laryngeal valving to control expiratory airflow
b. It promotes increased prephonatory inspiration
c. It regulates expiratory airflow by controlling the descent of the rib cage
d. It strengthens the muscles of expiration
e. It reduces the likelihood of inspiratory stridor

165. Of the following, which is *not* a critical component of the LSVT?
a. Intensive practice
b. "Think loud"
c. Daily home practice
d. "Big breaths"
e. Increasing pitch range

166. An individual with isolated damage to the pharyngeal branch of the vagus nerve will most likely benefit from:
a. An obturator
b. A palatal lift prosthesis
c. Sucking and blowing exercises
d. Palatal icing
e. Biofeedback through the use of the Nasometer

167. A patient would be an appropriate candidate for a palatal lift prosthesis if he or she:
a. Sustained subglottal pressure of 5 cm H_2O for 1 second
b. Demonstrated a velopharyngeal orifice area of 3 mm^2 as measured by the pressure-flow procedure (Warren & DuBois, 1964)
c. Produced 15% nasalance on the Zoo passage, as measured by the Nasometer
d. Demonstrated occasional velopharyngeal closure during nonnasal sounds
e. Demonstrated fair to good articulation

168. How does the continuous positive air pressure (CPAP) program developed by Kuehn (1997) follow the principles of motor learning and strength training?
a. The patient is encouraged to practice three times a week
b. It incorporates nonspeech tasks in the therapy program
c. The velum is closing against resistance during speech
d. It stimulates the velum in a manner comparable with icing
e. The practice stimuli are blocked by phonemes

169. The most useful tasks for differential diagnosis of dysarthria in a motor speech evaluation are:
a. Assessment of conversational speech and alternating motion rates (AMRs)

b. Articulation testing in all positions of words

c. Intelligibility testing in words and sentences

d. Assessment of sustained phonation and an examination of speech mechanism

e. Assessment of production of words with plosives and nasals

170. A comparison of single word and sentence intelligibility can guide treatment by demonstrating:
a. Whether a pacing strategy would be a viable option
b. Whether the patient has adequate subglottal pressure for voicing
c. Whether improving articulation of individual phonemes will increase intelligibility
d. Whether oromotor exercises would benefit the patient
e. How many words a patient can say in one breath

171. Increased vocal effort is considered to be a holistic intervention strategy because:
a. Respiratory effort decreases
b. Articulatory precision is typically not affected
c. It affects more than one physiological system
d. It improves comprehensibility
e. It is typically accompanied by increased speaking rate

172. Comprehensibility may be improved by any of the following *except:*
a. Oromotor exercises
b. Alphabet board supplementation
c. Training the listener
d. Instructing partners in resolving communication breakdowns
e. Being aware of contextual cues

173. An example of signal-independent information is:
a. Precise articulation
b. Normal voice quality
c. Resonance within normal limits
d. Awareness of topic
e. Appropriate speaking rate

174. Of the following, which is *not* an effect of alphabet board supplementation?
a. Increased articulatory precision
b. Longer listening processing time
c. Syntactic information
d. Reduced speaking rate
e. Improved vocal quality

175. What internal evidence makes it difficult to recommend rate-control strategies?
a. Few studies have demonstrated their efficacy
b. Individuals dislike speaking slowly
c. Research is typically based on a small number of participants

d. Randomized control trials are lacking

e. Participants in the available studies may not resemble your patient

176. Of the following, which is the strongest argument against the use of oromotor exercises to treat dysarthria in adults?
a. Patients may not perform them correctly
b. Families may not understand why clinicians are not working directly on speech production
c. Insurance companies will not pay for them
d. Motor programming for speech tasks is different than motor programming for nonspeech tasks
e. They are too tiring for the patients

177. What is the benefit of increasing speaking rate in an individual with reduced articulatory precision who speaks slowly?
a. It reduces listener burden
b. Articulatory precision increases
c. It increases comprehensibility
d. It makes the speaker feel more "normal"
e. There is no benefit

178. You instruct your patient with moderate spastic dysarthria to put breaks between words. Listeners report understanding more of his speech with this strategy. Why?
a. Breaks provide linguistic boundaries for the listener
b. Breaks allow the articulators to relax between words
c. Breaks reduce laryngeal tension
d. Breaks increase articulatory precision
e. All the above

179. You are screening a patient in acute care. You note that all speaking attempts are unintelligible, the patient does not initiate language, and comprehension appears poor. Your first priority is:
a. Establish consistent "yes"/"no" responses
b. Conduct a complete speech and language assessment
c. Instruct the family to begin oromotor exercises
d. Provide an electrolarynx for voicing
e. Begin articulation therapy

180. For clinical purposes, why are treatment effectiveness studies more relevant than treatment efficacy studies?
a. They are based on a larger number of participants
b. They are conducted under ideal clinical conditions
c. They have an untreated control group
d. They are conducted under typical clinical conditions
e. Treatment is administered intensively

181. You are conducting a complete motor speech assessment to determine the most appropriate course of

treatment for an individual with severe flaccid dysarthria. What test is the most useful?
a. Single word and sentence intelligibility
b. Articulation
c. Articulatory force generation
d. Oromotor strength
e. Range of tongue movement

182. According to Ramig and colleagues (1995), "The LSVT group did not deteriorate to levels below pre-treatment in vocal intensity over the 12-month [follow-up] period. The placebo group had statistically significant deterioration of vocal intensity levels from before to 12 months after treatment in conversational monologues." How would you interpret this statement?
a. Across groups, gains apparent immediately after treatment were maintained 12 months after treatment
b. Individuals who received LSVT maintained skills higher than pretreatment abilities
c. Individuals who received LSVT did not achieve improvement with treatment
d. Individuals who received LSVT performed better in conversational monologues than in structured practiced phrases
e. Pretreatment baselines were inconsistent for conversational monologues

183. You completed an evaluation of a 25-year-old man 2 years post TBI, with a complaint of hypernasality and nasal emission and the findings are as follows:
a. Nasalance during a nonnasal passage without nose clips = 45%
b. Intelligibility without nose clips = 30%
c. Intelligibility with nose clips = 30%
d. Ability to sustain "ah" for 30 seconds
e. Pressure sounds are produced with weak oral pressure

184. You are evaluating a patient who appears very anxious and complains frequently of pain. Speech is completely intelligible, but voice quality is harsh and excessively soft, as though he is holding his breath. Speaking rate is somewhat fast. Your most appropriate immediate course of action is:
a. Refer for a laryngeal videostroboscopic evaluation
b. Initiate the LSVT
c. Confer with his physician and neuropsychologist to obtain information regarding his pain
d. Introduce a pacing strategy to reduce speaking rate
e. Refer for psychological counseling

185. Your patient demonstrates 98% intelligibility, nasal emission on plosives, nasalance of 35%, adequate subglottal pressure for speech, absence of gag reflex,

normal voice quality, and appropriate loudness. He wants to return to his former job as a radio broadcaster. The most appropriate intervention is:
a. Drills to improve articulatory precision
b. Fitting for a palatal lift prosthesis
c. Palatal desensitization
d. LSVT
e. Drills to improve inspiratory checking

186. Your patient sustained a TBI 3 years ago and has had extensive therapy. He wishes to return to work as a telemarketer. He demonstrates mildly reduced articulatory precision, with intelligibility around 95%, slightly breathy voice quality, somewhat reduced loudness, 15% nasalance, normal gag reflex, and adequate subglottal pressure for speech. What is the most appropriate intervention?
a. Drills on the specific sounds that are imprecise
b. Fitting for a palatal lift prosthesis
c. LSVT
d. Amplification
e. None, because his speech is adequate for functional communication

187. You are working with a college student who is majoring in business with a specialty in sales. He has spastic cerebral palsy. He is most intelligible when he puts breaks between words, but he states that his sales personality does not come through when he does so. What would you suggest?
a. To use a pacing strategy all the time because that is when he is most intelligible
b. To attempt stretching words out without breaks between them
c. To speak naturally in his first attempt but use a pacing strategy if his speech is not understood
d. To use a pacing strategy in his first attempt but proceed to natural conversational style if his speech is understood
e. To have a backup AAC device with him at all times

188. You are evaluating a 13-year-old girl who demonstrates idiopathic hypernasality. Its onset reportedly occurred after a fall off a horse, although her mother also mentioned a growth spurt. Her nasalance score during connected speech at typical loudness (about 70 dB SPL at 30 cm mouth-to-microphone distance) was 33%. It decreased to 27% with increased vocal effort (about 75 dB SPL). Her gag reflex was present. When discussing the evaluation results, you mention increased vocal effort as a possible therapy option. The girl's immediate response is, "Oh, I could never talk that loud!" What strategy seems most appropriate?
a. Convince her and her parents that increasing loudness is an effective way to improve velopharyngeal closure

b. Recommend a pharyngeal flap
c. Recommend a palatal lift
d. Reassess her in 6 months
e. Begin trial therapy with CPAP

189. You are working with a 21-year-old individual who is fluent in both English and Spanish. She speaks English at work and Spanish with her parents at home. You conduct the motor speech evaluation in English. You notice left facial weakness, tongue deviation to the left, and the velum pulling toward the right on phonation. Intelligibility is 95%. There is no evidence of aphasia. What is the most reasonable conclusion regarding her intelligibility in both languages?
   a. English will be more intelligible because she speaks it more frequently
   b. Spanish will be more intelligible because it was her first language
   c. Intelligibility will be equal in both English and Spanish
   d. Her parents will have difficulty understanding her Spanish
   e. Her co-workers will have difficulty understanding her English

190. Why is it inappropriate to work on increasing vital capacity to improve speech breathing strategies in a person with flaccid dysarthria?
   a. Only a relatively small percentage of vital capacity is needed for speech production
   b. Individuals with flaccid dysarthria typically do not have speech breathing difficulties
   c. Vital capacity will increase spontaneously and dramatically as the patient begins to walk
   d. Increasing expiratory reserve volume is more beneficial
   e. Teaching the patient to speak on "residual air" will help them extend utterance length effectively

191. Which is the most appropriate three-word phrase for assessing nasal air emission?
   a. "Never on Sunday"
   b. "Pop the top"
   c. "Use the rule"
   d. "Mom made marmalade"
   e. "Pinpoint the problem"

192. The use of Permax to facilitate the uptake of dopamine in a person with hypokinetic dysarthria represents management at what level of the chronic condition model?
   a. Pathophysiology
   b. Impairment
   c. Functional limitation
   d. Disability
   e. Societal

193. The most appropriate motor learning paradigm for speech generalization is:
   a. Therapy twice a week, single-sound drills, 100% feedback
   b. Therapy twice a week, randomized drills, 100% feedback
   c. Therapy five times a week, randomized drills, feedback every five productions
   d. Therapy five times a week therapy, single-sound drills, feedback every five productions
   e. Therapy five times a week therapy, single-sound drills, 100% feedback

194. The patient asks, "Will wearing my palatal lift make my soft palate work on its own?" You respond:
   a. "Yes, if you wear it consistently."
   b. "Yes, it will stimulate the muscles of the soft palate."
   c. "No, there is no evidence to show that wearing the lift stimulates the muscles."
   d. "I don't know. Everyone responds differently to it."
   e. "Yes, if you continue your blow up a balloon every day."

195. If an individual has difficulty lifting the tip of his or her tongue to make a /t/, an appropriate intervention could be:
   a. Tongue strengthening exercises
   b. Swallowing exercises
   c. Deliberate omission of /t/
   d. The substitution of /p/ for /t/
   e. Any compensatory strategy that minimizes the distance between the tongue and alveolar ridge

CHILDHOOD APRAXIA OF SPEECH

196. Childhood apraxia of speech (CAS) is:
   a. A language disorder reflected in a delay in expressive language
   b. A speech disorder reflecting a disorder of neuromuscular innervation
   c. A cognitive disorder reflecting neurological impairment
   d. A speech disorder reflecting inefficiency in planning and programming movement gestures for volitional speech production
   e. A phonological impairment caused by difficulty with acquisition of the sounds in the child's language

197. For making a differential diagnosis between CAS and a severe phonological impairment, which of the following would provide the most important diagnostic information?
   a. A standardized articulation test

b. A language sample

c. An oral structural-functional examination

d. A motor speech examination

e. Evaluation of respiratory and phonatory adequacy

198. Of the following, which would *not* be indicative of the presence of CAS?

a. Vowel distortions

b. Inconsistent performance over repeated trials

c. Difficulty achieving articulatory configurations

d. Low tone

e. Voicing errors

199. CAS is frequently associated with:

a. Dysarthria

b. Weakness

c. Phonological impairment

d. Stuttering

e. Receptive language deficits

200. ASHA has a position statement regarding a definition and the characteristics of CAS. According to that position statement, the following are true of CAS except:

a. Apraxia of speech exists as a distinct diagnostic type of childhood (pediatric) speech-sound disorder

b. Use of the term *apraxia of speech* implies a shared core of speech and prosody features, regardless of the time of onset, whether the condition is congenital or acquired, or the specific etiology

c. CAS has been associated causally with known neurological entities (e.g., intrauterine stroke, infections, trauma), as one sign of complex neurobehavioral disorders (e.g., genetic, metabolic), or as an idiopathic neurogenic speech-sound disorder

d. The developmental pediatrician or the pediatric neurologist has primary responsibility for the diagnosis of CAS

e. Research literature indicates that, at present, there is no validated list of diagnostic features of CAS that differentiates this symptom complex from other types of childhood speech-sound disorders, including those primarily resulting from phonological-level delay or neuromuscular disorder (dysarthria)

201. A 3-year-old child is referred to you. He enters the room easily, establishes eye contact, gestures that he wants you to play with him with the toys, begins to pretend he is filling the car with gas, and then engages you in racing the cars around a track. He laughs appropriately, with good respiratory support and normal phonation. He says "ma" when he wants his mother to see that he is winning. He occasionally produces /ba/, /ba ba/, /da/, /da da/, and /ta/. He occasionally exhibits a neutral vowel with varied intonation but has little vowel differentiation. He uses

numerous gestures to indicate when it is his turn, that he wants a different car, and so forth. His mother reports that her pregnancy and delivery were normal, the child's gross motor development has been normal, and the child has no difficulty with chewing or swallowing. There is no history of otitis media, seizures, head injuries, or serious illness. Your initial clinical hypothesis, which focuses the rest of your assessment tasks, would best be:

a. This child has dysarthria

b. This child has autism

c. This child has a phonological impairment

d. This child has CAS

e. This child has a phonological impairment and CAS

202. A 3-year-old child is referred to you. He enters the room easily, establishes eye contact, gestures that he wants you to play with him with the toys, begins to pretend he is filling the car with gas, and then engages you in racing the cars around a track. He laughs appropriately, with good respiratory support and normal phonation. He says "ma" when he wants his mother to see that he is winning. He occasionally produces /ba/, /ba ba/, /da/, /da da/, and /ta/. He occasionally exhibits a neutral vowel with varied intonation but has little vowel differentiation. He uses numerous gestures to indicate when it is his turn, that he wants a different car, and so forth. His mother reports that her pregnancy and delivery were normal, the child's gross motor development has been normal, and the child has no difficulty with chewing or swallowing. There is no history of otitis media, seizures, head injuries, or serious illness. Your initial assessment tasks would include all the following *except:*

a. A motor speech examination

b. A structured language sample

c. Examination of respiratory and phonatory coordination

d. A receptive language test

e. An oral structural-functional examination

203. Of the following, which is *not* true about CAS?

a. CAS typically occurs without concomitant language problems

b. In children who have difficulty with speech acquisition, the degree to which motor planning impairment may be contributing varies

c. CAS is dynamic with regard to neural maturation and treatment effects

d. Diagnostic markers may vary with age, with neural maturation, and as a result of treatment

e. Children with CAS are at higher risk for literacy problems

204. Of the following, which is most important in the treatment of CAS?

a. Working on auditory discrimination and auditory perception

b. Improving phonological awareness

c. Maximizing the number of practice trials per session

d. Beginning early to work on pragmatic language

e. Working on the three earliest developing sounds in isolation and then in words

205. You determine a diagnosis of severe phonological impairment in a child. The parent reports that a previous speech pathologist diagnosed apraxia. She wants to know why you do not think the child is apraxic. One plausible short answer would be:

a. "The child has some tongue and lip weakness, as well as hypernasality, which is not the case in CAS."

b. "The child is exhibiting predictable substitution errors, consistency over repeated trials, and several phonological processes such as stopping and final consonant deletion, which are more associated with phonological impairment, but he does not exhibit vowel distortions or lexical stress, which are errors commonly seen in CAS."

c. "The child has no difficulty with blowing, lip smacking, or moving the tongue laterally."

d. "The child has no dysfluencies, and so CAS is not the correct diagnosis."

e. "The child has difficulty with articulation, and so phonological impairment is the best term to use."

206. Oral apraxia is:

a. Always present with CAS

b. Best diagnosed through the motor speech examination

c. Best diagnosed through the oral structural-functional examination

d. Best diagnosed through examination of neuromuscular function

e. Seen only in children with apraxia acquired through stroke or brain injury

207. Implementation of the principles of motor learning is often noted to be important to treatment in CAS. According to those principles, which of the following suggestions would *not* be recommended in the treatment of CAS?

a. Practicing movement in nonspeech activities

b. Choosing the set size on the basis of the severity of the apraxia

c. Practicing the stimuli in blocks, moving to more random practice as the child's performance improves

d. Relying initially on extrinsic feedback and gradually more on intrinsic feedback

e. Avoiding games and activities that take time and attention away from practice of producing the stimuli

208. For a child with CAS, what is the best way to improve the child's proprioception during speech therapy?

a. Provide thermal stimulation and brushing

b. Have the child practice blowing with and without feedback

c. Use a mirror during the sessions so that the child can watch both himself or herself and the clinician in the mirror

d. Use a bite block first during nonspeech tongue movements and then in speech drills

e. Have the child stay in an articulatory position longer and then make the movement transition into the vowel shape and throughout the word slowly

209. In addition to working on accurate movement gestures for consonant and vowel accuracy in words in CAS treatment, it is common to include a treatment goal related to what skill? (Choose the answer most specific to CAS.)

a. Increased expressive vocabulary

b. Increased receptive vocabulary

c. Improved comprehension and production of grammatical forms

d. Improved lexical and sentential stress

e. Improved strength and range of motion of the tongue and lips

210. Of the following treatment approaches, which would be the best (but not only) choice for a child with severe apraxia of speech characterized by a small phonemic inventory, numerous vowel distortions, and fewer than 10 intelligible words?

a. Phonological awareness intervention

b. Cycles approach

c. Fast ForWord Language

d. Enhanced milieu teaching

e. Dynamic temporal and tactile cueing (DTTC)

ADULT APRAXIA OF SPEECH

211. Adult apraxia of speech is a disorder of:

a. Language

b. Cognition

c. Attention

d. Motor planning and programming

e. Motor execution

212. According to the Academy of Neurologic Communication Disorders and Sciences' treatment guidelines for acquired apraxia of speech, a speech characteristic that is considered nonspecific for this disorder is:

a. Slow rate of speech

b. Articulatory groping

c. Sound distortion errors

d. Prosodic disturbances

e. Difficulty initiating utterances

213. According to Duffy (2005), the type of dysarthria that is most likely to be confused with apraxia of speech is:
    a. Hypokinetic dysarthria
    b. Spastic dysarthria
    c. Ataxic dysarthria
    d. Hyperkinetic dysarthria
    e. Flaccid dysarthria

214. You have diagnosed apraxia of speech in an adult patient. On the basis of the current evidence, which treatment would be most likely to benefit this patient?
    a. CPAP
    b. A palatal lift prosthesis
    c. A metronome pacing approach
    d. The eight-step continuum/integral stimulation
    e. Sound amplification

215. You have a patient who has a diagnosis of aphasia and apraxia of speech. He is trying to name a picture of a cat. If he produced an error, which of the following errors would be most likely to reflect the apraxia, rather than the aphasia?
    a. /dɔ:g/
    b. /blætnoʊ/
    c. /ðæt/
    d. /taigɜːʳ/
    e. lion

216. In sound production treatment for apraxia of speech (Wambaugh, 2004), the type of stimuli used in treatment are:
    a. Sounds in isolation
    b. Minimal pairs
    c. Sounds in syllables
    d. Multisyllabic words
    e. Sounds in phrases

217. According to Duffy (2005), you should suspect apraxia of speech if the patient demonstrates a mismatch between the ability to produce complex voluntary speech and the ability to produce:
    a. Sentences
    b. /pʌtʌkʌ/
    c. Simple "automatic" speech tasks
    d. Short phrases
    e. Conversation

218. The sites of cortical brain lesions most commonly proposed to produce apraxia of speech are the left inferior frontal cortex (Broca area), the left parietal cortex, and:
    a. The left superior temporal cortex
    b. The left anterior insula
    c. The left side of the cerebellum
    d. The left supplementary motor area
    e. Vermis

219. There has been considerable controversy regarding whether apraxia of speech can be distinguished from:
    a. Aphasia
    b. Spastic dysarthria
    c. Dementia
    d. Cluttering
    e. Flaccid dysarthria

220. In your clinical practice, you would expect a pure apraxia of speech to occur:
    a. Frequently after a left hemisphere stroke
    b. Only after a right hemisphere stroke
    c. Rarely after a left hemisphere stroke
    d. Frequently in patients younger than 50 years who have sustained a left hemisphere stroke
    e. Rarely after a right hemisphere stroke

221. A patient who has sustained a left hemisphere cerebrovascular accident presents with difficulties producing speech. Prosody is impaired. She produces speech-sound errors, including distortions and distorted substitutions, and her rate of speech is slow. Your testing has revealed no evidence of problems in auditory comprehension, reading, or writing. Although articulation difficulties are evident, the patient demonstrates no impairment in naming and no agrammatism. Evaluation of oral structure and function reveals no evidence of significant weakness or incoordination. In view of these findings, the most likely diagnosis is:
    a. Aphasia
    b. Dysarthria
    c. Apraxia of speech
    d. Alzheimer disease
    e. Depression

222. According to some theories about apraxia of speech, there are subtypes of this disorder as a result of differences in:
    a. Site of lesion
    b. Etiology (stroke versus TBI)
    c. Gender
    d. Handedness
    e. Education

223. In contrast to a patient who has aphasia alone, a patient who has both apraxia of speech and aphasia may make the following complaint:
    a. "I can't think of the words I want to say."
    b. "People talk too fast for me."
    c. "I know the words I want to say, but I can't say them."
    d. "I can't read as well as I used to."
    e. " I now slur my words"

224. For the treatment of acquired apraxia of speech, which approach is supported by evidence of its efficacy?
    a. Prompts for restructuring oral muscular phonetic targets (PROMPT)
    b. Metronome pacing
    c. Nonspeech oromotor training
    d. The use of prosthetic devices
    e. Biofeedback

225. According to Duffy (2005), one way that severe acquired apraxia of speech may be different from the milder form is that the severe form may be accompanied by:
    a. Dementia
    b. Aphasia
    c. Nonverbal oral apraxia
    d. Spastic dysarthria
    e. Ataxic dysarthria

1. e. This lesion occurs within the distribution of left middle cerebral artery and thus potentially results in aphasia. Aphasia can lead to difficulties with all the problems suggested: naming, comprehension, reading, and writing.

2. a. A lesion to the right hemisphere could potentially result in left-sided neglect but not right-sided hemiplegia, which would result from a left hemisphere lesion (option b). Aphasia (option c) typically does not result from right-sided brain damage (nearly 100% of right-handed adults have left-hemisphere dominance for speech and language, in comparison with 85% of left-handed adults). Dementia (option d) also would not result exclusively from a lesion in the right hemisphere; instead, it is associated with diffuse brain disease.

3. e. Wernicke aphasia is typically associated with a lesion to the Wernicke area in the left temporal lobe. The locale of this lesion is posterior to the motor strip, which is implicated in hemiplegia.

4. c. Stroke, traumatic brain injury, and gunshot wounds are considered acquired brain injuries. A genetic syndrome would be classified as congenital in nature and would not be consistent with the definition of aphasia.

5. e. Reading, written language, proficiency in American Sign Language, and comprehension of speech all involve the processing of symbols (verbal and manual signs) and thus would be compromised to varying degrees as a result of aphasia.

6. c. The vertebral arteries merge to form the basilar artery, which, with the internal carotid arteries, connects at the circle of Willis to the cerebral arteries. Three pairs of cerebral arteries—right and left anterior, a middle, and a posterior—branch off the circle of Willis. The left middle cerebral artery, which supplies blood to the "language zone," is also known as the "artery of aphasia."

7. b. Because the circle of Willis is supplied by two vertebral arteries (which merge to form the basilar artery) and two internal carotid arteries, an occlusion below the circle in one of the feeder arteries does not result in a decrease in blood to the cerebral arteries.

8. b. The distributions of the cerebral arteries overlap slightly at their boundaries; therefore, occlusions at the periphery of an artery's distribution may not lead to as much serious brain damage because of the collateral blood supply.

9. b. The arcuate fasciculus is one type of association fiber tract connecting regions within a brain hemisphere. Commissural fiber tracts, such as the corpus callosum, cross between the brain hemispheres. Projection fibers carry information from motor neurons in the brain to neurons in the brain stem or spinal cord (descending pathways) or from sensory neurons in the peripheral nervous system to the brain (ascending pathways).

10. d. The sylvian fissure divides the frontal and temporal lobes anteriorly and the temporal and parietal lobes posteriorly. This fissure is sometimes referred to as the frontotemporoparietal fissure after the parts of the brain that surround it.

11. c. Brodmann area 44, located in the posterior inferior frontal lobe of the left hemisphere, just anterior to the premotor cortex, is also known as the Broca area and is important in the organization of movement sequences for the muscles of speech.

12. a. The Wernicke area, located in the midtemporal lobe of the left hemisphere, is important for auditory comprehension and is also known as a auditory association cortex.

13. e. Persons with Broca aphasia are nonfluent. Words are produced slowly and with great effort. The utterances are short and consist predominantly of content words (nouns, verbs, a few adjectives); function words (conjunctions, articles, prepositions) are missing. Patients with Broca aphasia write as they talk. Their comprehension of spoken and printed messages is better than their speech or writing, but careful testing reveals subtle difficulties even with this comprehension.

14. b. The speech of patients with Wernicke aphasia is fluent: that is, produced without effort, smoothly, and copiously. Utterances may be long, syntactically well-formed sentences with normal intonation; however, they may be filled with paraphasic errors and lacking in meaningful content. Written language resembles their speech. The predominant feature of Wernicke aphasia is impaired comprehension of spoken or printed materials. In some affected patients, comprehension of printed language is better than that of spoken materials.

15. b. A common early intervention for patients suspected of having a stroke is to administer a blood thinner. If the individual has suffered a hemorrhagic stroke, the blood thinner would exacerbate the condition. Therefore, a brain scan is ordered to confirm or rule out hemorrhage.

16. d. The frequency and persistence of perseverative responses are related to severity of brain damage. Perseveration is often apparent during the first few days and weeks after injury, but it decreases with ongoing recovery.

17. d. Standardized tests often do not provide the detail needed to describe a particular patient's pattern of performance. Clinicians may need to supplement standard test procedures to follow-up on a patient's performance or to improvise and examine variables that may affect performance. However, standardized tests are useful for comparing the performance of a patient with that of a comparison group (option a), for establishing a baseline of performance on a fixed set of language tasks (option b), and to have a basis for discussing a patient with other professionals (option c).

18. e. Behavioral, cognitive, and emotional consequences of brain injury compromise patient's performance in clinical and everyday activities. The patient's personality, intellect, social skills, interests, and coping strategies must also be considered in the performance profile.

19. d. The severity and nature of a patient's communication disorder have implications for the diagnosis, the prognosis, and decisions about treatment. The initial evaluation is directed toward this end.

20. c. The localizationist models of aphasia first described in the mid-1800s by Broca, and Wernicke laid the foundation for contemporary connectionist models. Connectionist descriptions of aphasia emphasize the importance of the perisylvian region in the left hemisphere.

21. b. Strokes can be ischemic (deprived of blood) or hemorrhagic (caused by bleeding). Eighty percent of all strokes are ischemic (also known as *occlusive*) and occur when an artery is blocked, which prevents blood from reaching an area of the central nervous system. Hemorrhagic strokes are caused by a rupture of a cerebral blood vessel.

22. a. Diaschisis plays a role in the impairments seen immediately after a stroke. Brain function is disrupted in regions that are distant from the injury site but connected to it by neuronal pathways.

23. b. An extracerebral hemorrhage (option c) is caused by bleeding from a blood vessel of the meninges or on the surface of the brain because the bleeding is outside the brain. Hemorrhages within the brain or brain stem are called *intracerebral hemorrhages.* Hemorrhagic stroke occurs when the stretched arterial area within an aneurysm ruptures.

24. c. Arteriovenous malformations are tangled masses of arteries and veins that gradually increase in size over time. For patients with arteriovenous malformations, the greatest danger is a rupture and resultant hemorrhage.

25. b. Broca aphasia is caused by damage to the Broca area, which is situated at the lower end of the premotor cortex, a strip in front of the primary motor cortex. The premotor cortex is important in the sensory monitoring of movement and control of certain muscle groups of the body. The primary motor cortex is responsible for the execution of movement. The Broca area is adjacent to the primary motor cortex for the face, hand, and arm, and because descending pyramidal tract fibers pass beneath the Broca area, persons with Broca aphasia usually have right-sided hemiplegia.

26. b. Generally, involvement of the optic tract posterior to the optic chiasm will result in contralateral visual field blindness known as homonymous hemianopia. Homonomous is the same part of the visual field affected in each eye. Hemianopia is damage in half of the visual field of one or both eyes.

27. b. Disconnection syndromes are created when nerve fiber tracts in the corpus callosum are damaged or destroyed. Complete disconnection syndrome is usually the result of a commissurotomy when a neurosurgeon cuts the connections between the hemispheres to prevent seizures originating in one hemisphere from traveling to the other. Partial disconnection syndromes are caused by strokes or tumors.

28. a. The symptoms represent anterior disconnection syndrome and are caused by isolation of the somatosensory and motor cortex in the right hemisphere from the language-dominant left hemisphere.

29. b. The most common impairments of patients with posterior disconnection syndrome are visual impairments attributable to isolation of the visual cortex from the language-dominant left hemisphere. This

isolation is caused by destruction of visual fibers crossing in the posterior corpus callosum.

30. c. An agnosia is a perceptual impairment that results in a failure to perceive stimuli in a specific sensory modality despite the fact that sensory transmission is damaged. However, true modality-specific agnosia is rare. Many cases reported in the literature may not be true agnosia but rather the result of sensory deficits, comprehension disorders, expressive disorders, or unfamiliarity with test stimuli.

31. d. Research findings suggest that persisting Broca aphasia and Wernicke aphasia are the result of lesions that extend beyond the Broca and Wernicke areas, respectively. In addition, numerous reports indicate that patients with lesions deep in subcortical regions of the left hemisphere are often aphasic. Connectionist models predict global symptoms such as speech fluency rather than specific impairments such as failure of word retrieval.

32. b. Several variables may affect a brain-injured individual's sentence comprehension, such as length and syntactic complexity or predictability. Some sentences are predictable—that is, they create expectations in the listener's mind—but then violate the expectations ("garden path" sentences). In the sentence "The boy whistling tunes guitars," the listener may initially assume that "whistling" is the sentence's main verb, only to discover that "tunes" is actually the main verb.

33. b. The Western Aphasia Battery is the only standardized test for aphasia listed. The other tests were not developed specifically for aphasia and are intended to assess single modalities versus language reception and expression as a whole. The Discourse Comprehension Test, the Revised Token Test, and the Peabody Picture Vocabulary Test examine comprehension of discourse-length texts, sentences, and single words, respectively.

34. e. Patients with aphasia have difficulty with infrequently occurring words (option a); however, impaired performance with words that rarely occur in everyday communicative interactions may not translate to a significant functional handicap. Both semantic and acoustic similarity (option b) may influence single-word comprehension; semantic confusions ("sister" for "brother") are more frequent than acoustic confusions ("fog" for "dog"). If pictured stimuli are ambiguous (option d), patients may experience difficulty not because they do not understand the words but because they cannot determine what the pictures represent.

35. e. In addition to the rating variables listed, other dimensions included in the rating scale are paraphasias in running speech, word finding relative to fluency, sentence repetition, and auditory comprehension.

36. d. There are a number of test quotients that are part of the Western Aphasia Battery. The aphasia quotient is derived from the subtests of spontaneous speech and auditory comprehension subtests. The language quotient is based on results of the same subtests as the aphasia quotient, with the addition of reading and writing subtests. The cortical quotient is a combination of the language quotient with the scores on the subtests of praxis and construction (drawing, block design, calculation, and Raven's Progressive Matrices).

37. d. This initial interaction helps the SLP prepare for a more formal subsequent evaluation. This assists the clinician in including selection of the most appropriate test materials, the need for obtaining additional background information from a family member, the assistance of an interpreter (if needed), and identification of an optimal time to perform the assessment (when patient is most awake and alert).

38. c. Aphasia tests are designed to sample a broad array of language abilities, and few involve comprehensive testing of any language modality. Many typical standard reading tests permit assessment of reading vocabulary and paragraph comprehension and, furthermore, allow for determination of reading grade level.

39. d. Because nonfluent aphasia (particularly Broca aphasia) is associated with a lesion in the premotor cortex, it is not unusual for patients with Broca aphasia to also exhibit apraxia of speech (also linked to lesions of the motor association cortex), dysarthria (unilateral upper motor neuron lesion), or other neurological impairments of speech production (neurological stuttering). Thus, the presence or absence of these concomitant disorders should be determined.

40. a. Such tests are also referred to as *word fluency tasks* and may involve naming words beginning with the letter *F, A,* or *S* (FAS test) or naming animals or foods. Although performance on such tests appears to reveal brain injury, they are not useful for discriminating among aphasic syndromes or distinguishing aphasic patients from other brain-injured groups. Such tasks also have little value in predicting everyday functional communication.

41. c. For most patients with aphasia, naming performance is not influenced by the form of the stimuli. However, for patients with severe impairments complicated by perceptual deficits, real objects may facilitate naming performance.

42. d. The type and severity of the brain injury and the patient's mental and physical states are important variables in establishing prognosis. Other factors that also contribute to this judgment are the patient's motivation and enthusiasm. Age alone is not a reliable predictor of benefit of therapy. In general, a brief trial period of therapy often helps determine response to treatment.

43. d. The patient's ability to withstand a course of aggressive therapy may be compromised by a complex medical condition. The complexity of the treatment plan—that is, a single treatment objective versus several—also dictates frequency and duration of treatment. Factors external to the patient, such as availability of transportation and insurance coverage, also play a role in frequency and duration planning and can also influence the course of therapy.

44. c. In resource-allocation models, the mental operations are called *cognitive processes,* and the mental energy, which is contained in a central pool, is referred to as *processing resources.* Activation of any cognitive process depends on the transfer of processing resources from the pool to the process. More complex processes require more resources than do simple processes. If several cognitive processes are active simultaneously, each draws from the pool. If demand for resources exceeds the amount available in the pool, some processes are shut down or shortchanged. It is not known whether brain damage reduces the amount of resources in the pool or compromises access to the pool while the amount of resources in the pool remains constant. In either case, the effect is reduced performance for that cognitive process.

45. e. In addition to the variables named, other manipulations include redundancy and contextual support, and they affect the workload associated with perception, discrimination, and comprehension of the stimuli presented within the task. The options listed for the question such as intensity, salience, clarity, intelligibility, novelty, and interest value can all be varied in treatment. Manipulations of stimuli are designed to alter the task demands along the continuum of difficulty.

46. d. In terms of relative level of impairment, the clinician may treat areas of strengths or weaknesses. The fundamental processes approach involves treatment of the disabilities that the clinician believes underlie the various linguistic impairments observed in the person with aphasia. The functional abilities approach consists of targeting skills that will be important to the individual in the daily life.

47. d. In the baseline-treatment design, the behavior to be treated is measured several times in succession before treatment begins. Changes in the rate or accuracy of behavior from baseline to after treatment begins provide evidence regarding effectiveness of treatment. The multiple-baseline design involves two or more behaviors measured under baseline conditions, followed by treatment of one of the behaviors. If the treated behavior changes and the other behaviors do not change, the effect of treatment is assumed.

48. e. The rationale is to foster response generalization so that the patient uses the taught behavior in functional contents. The treatment variations described in options a & c are designed to facilitate generalization. Other techniques for facilitating generalization include targeting behaviors that will be naturally rewarded in daily life, allowing training conditions to vary within limits, using easy responses to elicit difficult responses, and rewarding patients' spontaneous generalization of clinic-acquired skills to daily life.

49. d. Research designs to study the efficacy of aphasia treatment have improved as different variables have been studied. Research indicates that the variables listed in options a, b, and c are important in determining treatment efficacy. In summary, when the issues of treatment efficacy (does treatment result in a significant change in test scores?) and effectiveness (does treatment translate to meaningful changes in functional communication?) are examined, it is clear that most of the studies have focused on treatment efficacy and documented positive results. Future research should focus on treatments which are both efficacious as well as effective.

50. c. Various researchers have concluded that, according to scores on aphasia tests, delaying language therapy for persons with aphasia has no major effects on outcome. Others have argued that clinicians do more in the first few weeks after stroke than treating specific speech and language behaviors: Clinicians are also actively engaged in patient and family education, identifying community resources for the family, and advising clinical team members about the best way to communicate with the patient. Therefore, delaying or eliminating counseling, education, and support early on could result in irreversible negative effects on outcome.

51. c. In most instances, what patients with aphasia desire most is to regain sufficient language skills to get on with their lives. The clinician's responsibility is to

ensure that treatment goals are functionally oriented and that clinical tasks generalize to the real world.

52. e. For each patient with aphasia, clinicians must judge whether treatment will yield improvements in the patient's functional communication and that those improvements justify the cost. Patients with aphasia who are too sick, in whom the aphasia is too severe, or who refuse therapy are poor candidates for treatment.

53. c. Only about one in five patients with global aphasia achieve any functional use of language, and most who do nonetheless remain profoundly aphasic.

54. b. Neurological recovery from ischemic strokes is typically complete within 4 to 6 weeks, and from hemorrhagic strokes, within 3 to 6 months.

55. d. Current treatment techniques are emphasizing functionality and generalization of treatment activities to the patient's everyday life. The answer is an example of an activity directed to both functionality and generalization to everyday life.

56. c. The comprehension of noncontextual sentences can be a difficult task for persons with aphasia. In treatment tasks focused on improving sentence and discourse comprehension, redundancy and familiarity should be considered one index of task difficulty.

57. d. Normal listeners use knowledge-based (top-down) processes to comprehend auditory or printed language. Lexical and syntactic analyses (text-based) processes are used only when the top-down processing strategies fail to produce unambiguous meanings.

58. a. Single-word comprehension drills are used for patients with severe comprehension deficits. These drills are used as starting point for drills in which length, information load, and message complexity are gradually increased.

59. d. Research shows that there are a number of effective ways to manipulate discourse comprehension tasks for brain-injured persons. Options a, b, and c are three ways that can be utilized by the clinician. Other variable manipulations that modify message complexity may include salience (degree to which main ideas are easily identified), directness (information is stated versus implied), and speech rate.

60. c. With functionality and generalization as guiding therapeutic principles in mind, survival writing skills might include such skills as writing checks, making grocery lists, or generating e-mail messages. All are geared to facilitate communicative interactions.

61. b. Communicative functions are very limited in this patient group. Group treatment emphasizes functional communication skills such as discourse interaction and communicating with others by any available means. Treatment groups also serve other important purposes, including family support, psychosocial support, treatment, and community reentry.

62. c. Obtaining a literary history will include determining how much reading the patient engaged in before the onset of the disability, as well as what types of reading materials (e.g., mystery novels, newspapers, sports magazines) the patient enjoyed.

63. d. Survival reading skills might include recognition of street signs, traffic signs, warning signs, and door signs (restrooms, exits, entrances) and reading grocery lists, bus schedules, newspaper headlines, or names and phone numbers.

64. e. Patients with aphasia should be reading printed texts that challenge but do not exceed their reading abilities. Difficulty of reading materials can be adjusted by manipulating variables that affect comprehension of spoken discourse (familiarity, length, and redundancy), as well as variables that have a wider range in reading materials (vocabulary and syntactical complexity).

65. d. Confrontation naming drills have patients identify pictures or objects designated by the clinician. Research indicates that the activity may not have lasting effects (option a) or significantly influence functional communication skills (option b). Confrontation naming drills are useful for helping patients progress from automatic responses of words and phrases toward spontaneous production of more purposeful words and phrases. Confrontation naming drills should be considered a step along the way but not the final step in the treatment process.

66. d. Connected-speech drills consist of different activities and often proceed from tasks in which patients' responses are constrained (picture description) to less constrained tasks (prompted story telling, procedural discourse).

67. c. Right hemisphere damage may affect overall communicative skills without disrupting language. Patients with right hemisphere damage may appear disconnected, abrupt, verbose, less sensitive to situational cues, less insightful, less efficient, and less animated. Communicative deficits observed after right hemisphere damage are also associated with problems in attention, left-sided neglect, visual-perceptual deficits, cognitive impairments, and affective and emotional deficits.

68. e. Patients with right hemisphere damage may appear abrupt, less sensitive to situational cues, less insightful, less efficient, and less animated. Patients with right hemisphere damage may also appear disconnected, verbose, or both.

69. c. Only since the 1990s have researchers begun to identify lesions sites within the right hemisphere and attempted to correlate the findings with specific right hemisphere damage cognitive and communicative deficits.

70. c. Treatment of right-hemisphere damaged patients cognitive and communication deficits may be difficult due to cognitive and behavioral problems such as attention problems, impulsivity and impaired problem solving. Neglect is also seen in this population patients will exhibit left hemispatial neglect for different forms of sensory stimuli. In some patients, neglect can masquerade as or further reduce movement in hemiplegia.

71. e. Left-sided neglect can be manifested in any sensory modality. It is, however, most commonly observed in visual perception.

72. d. Neglect is an important consideration in treatment because of its negative effect on communication such as reading and the comprehension of print. These are a number of treatments that have been developed for neglect but the data are mostly anecdotal. In addition, left-sided neglect can also interfere with writing, self-care activities, safely navigating through space, and attention to significant information in ipsilesional as well as contralesional space. The potential degree of involvement suggests that neglect is a negative factor.

73. d. Anosognosia may occur independently of neglect, but it usually occurs in concert with other signs of neglect. Patients with anosognosia may experience unconscious perception in that they are aware of body parts on an intellectual level but fail to acknowledge them on an emotional level.

74. e. The right hemisphere appears to play a particular role in attentional operations. Findings of numerous studies suggest that arousal is somewhat lateralized to the right hemisphere. The right hemisphere is particularly engaged in orienting attention. Frontal areas in the right hemisphere are more active than comparable left hemisphere areas when selective attention and vigilance are required.

75. b. Reduced arousal (hypoarousal) inhibits environmental awareness, restricts focus of attention, and affects spatial and nonspatial attentional operations.

76. e. Results of prosodic perception studies suggest that individual parameters of prosody can be selectively impaired in patients with left- and right-hemisphere damage. The left hemisphere appears to be dominant for time-dependent features, such as temporal order and duration. The right hemisphere appears dominant for time-independent features, such as spectral information. Right hemisphere damage appears to disrupt the ability to perceive spectral information. Also, in right hemisphere damage, perception of pitch may be more impaired than perception of duration and timing; pitch perception may be more important for patients in distinguishing type of emotions.

77. d. Right hemisphere damage may leave patients linguistically intact but impaired in the ability to manage complex discourse. Patients may be less sensitive to shades of meaning, speaker intentions, conversational rules, overall themes, inferences, and internal motivations of others.

78. d. Depression might seem to be a natural reaction to the physical and cognitive impairments that can accompany stroke, but it is not always correlated with degree of physical disability or functional impairment. Flat affect and reduced use of prosody may result from stroke, but they are not necessarily signs of depression. Actual signs of depression include feelings of sadness, hopelessness, sleep disturbance, reduced concentration, psychomotor slowing, and agitation.

79. d. All these deficits can result from right hemisphere damage. They may be related to cognitive and attentional impairments, to deficits in theory of mind, and to problems in retrieving lexical-semantic representations of emotion.

80. e. The most common cortical site is the parietal lobe, although the frontal lobe has also been implicated. The most common subcortical site is the thalamus. Lesions of the basal ganglia and internal capsule have also been linked to neglect.

81. a. *Acquired brain injury,* a broadly used term, refers to several kinds of brain injury, including "traumatic" brain injury. A TBI occurs after birth and is caused by the head's striking an object or structure or by the sudden acceleration or deceleration of the head (e.g., as in whiplash).

82. a. Young adult men and adolescent boys are most likely to sustain a TBI; it is reasoned that this segment of the population is more likely than other segments of the population to engage in "at risk" activity that could result in accidents.

83. d. The Centers for Disease Control and Prevention (CDC) report that 1.4 million persons sustain a TBI each year in the United States (http://www.cdc.gov/ncipc/factsheets/tbi.htm; accessed June 16, 2009).

84. c. Hippocampi are housed just medial to the temporal lobes and are actively involved in storing short-term memories.

85. e. Unlike a closed TBI, an open TBI occurs when the skull is penetrated or depressed. Typically, this results in damage to the part of the brain that is close to point of penetration (i.e., localized brain damage).

86. e. Shaken-baby syndrome is an example of TBI that results from an indirect blow to the brain as the infant is shaken. This is similar to a whiplash injury in an adult. Whether intentional or unintentional, it is considered a form of child abuse and as with any TBI can result in lasting, permanent effects and death.

87. d. *Coup* refers to brain damage close to where the blow to the head occurred, whereas *contracoup* refers to the opposite, meaning that brain damage occurred on the side opposite to where the blow to head occurred. Patients with TBI can have both coup and contracoup injuries.

88. e. The frontal and temporal lobes of the brain rest on the bony surfaces of the inside base of the skull. These surfaces are not smooth; instead, they have ridges. When the brain is suddenly accelerated and decelerated, the ventral portion of the frontal lobes and the anterior tips of the temporal lobes are most likely to be damaged.

89. c. Patients who emerge from coma do not simply "wake up," as typically portrayed in the popular media. They are very confused, have difficulty staying awake, and lapse in and out of sleep. They do not have immediate access to memories of being injured.

90. b. Patients who emerge from coma have trouble communicating their basic wants and needs. Although some such patients may attempt to speak, many do not until further cognitive gains are made. Thus, it is most appropriate for clinicians to target a reliable means for communicating first and work on other communication problems later after basic communication is established.

91. d. Cognitive-communication disorders are the cognitive-based language, speech, and pragmatic disorders displayed by patients with TBI. Although dysarthria, aphasia, and apraxia of speech may also be present in patients with TBI, these other communication disorders are much less likely to occur: Researchers have reported a prevalence of 10% to 40%.

92. a. It is not too surprising that word-finding skills are the most commonly reported "language" impairment associated with TBI. Patients with closed TBI have sustained diffuse injury to multiple regions in the brain; likewise, generating words from given categories, or searching for the right word in conversation, also requires multiple regions of the brain. The evidence of this is very strong; this finding has been documented over 40 years of research.

93. c. Closed TBI causes shearing and stretching of axons, which connect various regions of the brain and cerebellum. A "mixed" form of dysarthria is more likely to be associated with a closed TBI, because multiple regions of the brain and cerebellum are injured, as are axons connecting those regions. Other types of dysarthria result from damage to more specific regions; for example, hypokinetic dysarthria is caused by damage to the basal ganglia.

94. b. Implicit memory is preserved after a TBI, whereas the other forms of memory listed are all typically impaired, in relation to the individual's preinjury memory abilities. Implicit memory is unconscious learning that is based on procedures and sequences and often includes motor skills. Explicit, episodic memory occurs at a conscious level and is sensitive to fluctuations in attention and the use of learning strategies, whereas remembering what needs to be done in the future is a special form of memory that interacts with executive functions, called *prospective memory*. Difficulty with word retrieval is a very common consequence of TBI.

95. a. Patients who have recovered cognitive and communication abilities such that they might return to school or work continue to find that divided attention—paying attention to two or more things at once—continues to be challenging for them. These are patients whose more basic attention processes of alertness, sustained attention, and focused attention have improved dramatically since their injury and may be at preinjury levels.

96. d. The Rivermead Behavioral Memory Test is the only test listed that identifies functional memory impairments. The Ross Information Processing Assessment includes questions that tap memory processes, but these tasks are not functional and do not generalize to functional, daily activities and communication. The Wechsler Memory Scales–III and the California Verbal Learning Test, Second Edition, are standardized tests that tap a variety of memory processes; both are typically administered by neuropsychologists, although SLPs may administer them. The scales of the Assessment for Traumatic Brain Injury test

many cognitive and memory processes and are administered by SLPs but do not test functional skills.

97. c. The World Health Organization created a framework for describing impairments, limitations, and restrictions. Most standardized tests for cognitive and communication disorders after TBI provide clinicians with "impairment" information (i.e., underlying cognitive or language processes such as auditory processing impairment, memory interference, or reduced word fluency). These tests tend to be psychometrically strong. The impairments out of context, however, are not necessarily reflected in how a person performs in everyday, contextualized activities. For example, someone with TBI may perform well in a structured task of following complex instructions of increasing length in the clinic room but may have great difficulty performing the same tasks in a noisy shopping mall.

98. a. Like adults with TBI, children with TBI may demonstrate the most improvement during spontaneous neurological recovery shortly after the injury, within 6 months. Many such children return to elementary school with special education support and may even rejoin back the regular mainstream classroom. However, longitudinal studies have shown that when these children enter adolescence, additional executive function and social communication disabilities become more obvious. A possible reason for this is the new, additional requirements of this phase of development, including inhibition, verbal reasoning, and social skills.

99. a. Research and clinical evidence supports the view that confabulation is not intentional and does not reflect some underlying psychiatric disorder that would be responsive to medication. Some patients go through an early period of confusion in which they confabulate. It is assumed that patients confabulate to make sense of their surroundings and to provide answers to questions that, under other circumstances, they would easily answer correctly. Although some patients make up elaborate stories, most simply elaborate on what could be a plausible statement.

100. c. Patients with poor impulse control and difficulty paying attention to two or more things at a time are likely not to notice subtle changes in conversation, including the verbal and nonverbal cues that conversants give to notify the other that they are ready (or not ready) to relinquish their turn or to end the conversation.

101. d. SLPs may use an aphasia test battery with patients who are still confused as they recover from TBI.

Indeed, confusional states can result in poor performance across virtually all domains of language, speech, and pragmatics. Until environmental and other forms of confusion (e.g., disorientation) subside, however, it is not possible to diagnose the presence of aphasia reliably. Until then, the SLP can only assume that the confusional state is interfering with the patient's language skills.

102. b. Glasgow Coma Scale is used throughout acute care to identify "levels" of consciousness of patients in coma. Three domains are described: verbal, motor, and visual. The other assessment tools are all useful for identifying cognitive impairments, disabilities, and functional communication in patients with TBI, but someone in a coma would be unable to participate in these assessments. The Levels of Cognitive Functioning includes a level described as "coma," but it is not used widely by trauma centers and does not differentiate between types of responses during coma in the way that the Glasgow Coma Scale does.

103. e. It was once believed that all patients with TBI overestimated their ability or underestimated their disability. There is now strong evidence that self-awareness emerges first for physical impairments and later for more subtle and less tangible impairments in cognitive, memory, and communication domains. Not all patients with TBI become "fully" self-aware of how their cognitive, memory, and communication abilities differ after injury from before injury.

104. d. Direct training of specific attention processes has been controversial for many years. Systematic reviews of the evidence reveal that although improvement at each discrete level of attention is documented, there is little to no evidence that this improvement generalizes or transfers to everyday activities that require these attention processes. In fact, there *is* evidence that clinicians must explicitly teach the use of self-regulated attention strategies in functional activities.

105. e. There is evidence that each of the instructional techniques listed is effective when patients with TBI are taught to use compensatory strategies. Spaced retrieval and method of vanishing cues are useful for getting patients to effortlessly and automatically use strategies. Metacognitive strategy instruction involves explicitly training the patient to self-predict, make a strategy decision, carry out the strategy, compare performance with prediction, and so forth; it is useful during effortful studying and learning. There is also strong evidence that

for patients with cognitive disorders after TBI, errorless or nearly errorless levels of practice provide sufficient practice.

106. a. Best practice is to use a functional, individualized approach with this patient. Because you believe that it *is* possible that he could successfully return to work, with sufficient compensatory support for his cognitive and communication impairments, it would be wise to form a "partnership" with the patient, inasmuch as he knows his job better than you do. On the other hand, make sure that his description of his job activities is accurate. Contact the employer to verify that these are the activities and tasks that he must be able to perform. Also, find out whether any part of his job has changed since his injury; then incorporate these changes or "new" tasks into therapy. The use of internal memory strategies such as visual imagery are unlikely to be transferred to specific tasks needed at work; these are more useful in studying specific text-based material.

107. a. Unfortunately, few carefully controlled studies have documented the efficacy or effectiveness of coma stimulation in patients with TBI, whereas some evidence of benefit has been obtained from animal studies.

108. c. Prospective memory includes both "memory" and several executive functions. It is the memory for future events. This kind of memory requires that the person encodes the need to recall the future event (e.g., a doctor's appointment at 2 PM tomorrow) and reminds himself or herself the following day. Prospective memory may also include taking action to ensure that the event will be remembered (e.g., writing it down in a daily planner), alerting oneself the following day to review the planner, or to use retrieval mechanisms to "remind" oneself of the appointment. Although short- and long-term memory are inherent in this unique form of memory, executive functions of considering the use of a strategy ("I'd better write this down because I may forget it") and then implementing the strategy (writing it down) would be needed to compensate for prospective memory impairment.

109. b. The most likely pragmatic problem to be observed in the TBI population as a whole is in topic management or coherence. Patients have difficulty maintaining, expanding, and shifting topics, which requires subtle attention skills, memory for details, inhibition of one's own thoughts, and logical internal organization of subtopics; any combination of these difficulties could result in problems with topic

management or topic coherence. The other pragmatic domains that are listed are more automatic than topic management, and they rely on implicit learning, which is often preserved after a TBI.

110. e. Self-awareness about one's cognition or thinking is a belief that people acquire during a lifetime and therefore are considered "autobiographical." These beliefs are constructs separate from the self-monitoring (self-assessment) and self-control (decision to change what one is doing in response to one's self-assessment) that occur during activities. This perspective of metacognition in patients with TBI has been demonstrated: for example, they may be accurate at self-monitoring but may not make good self-control decisions about how to change what they are doing to enhance their memory, such as pay closer attention, write things down, and remove distractions.

111. a. Spontaneous recovery in the early weeks or months after a TBI provides an inherent confound when treatment efficacy is examined. Researchers in a few studies have attempted to control experimentally for this effect when examining the treatment effects of comprehensive, transdisciplinary intervention; however, none have done so while examining the effects of working on isolated cognitive processes (e.g., selective attention, working memory span, reaction time).

112. d. The internal auditory meatus is the hole opening where cranial nerves VII (facial nerve) and VIII (auditory-vestibular nerve) exit and enter the periphery on their way to and from the brainstem, in which they synapse with cranial nuclei. A skull fracture that extends to the internal auditory meatus has the potential for damaging either of these cranial nerves, resulting in hearing loss (VIII), facial paralysis (VII), or loss of taste (VII).

113. e. Blast-related injuries are the "signature" injury from these military conflicts. Blast injuries cause not only brain injury but also trauma to multiple bodily systems that results in blindness, hearing loss, and post-traumatic stress disorder, among other injuries.

114. b. Cognitive rehabilitation is defined within the scope of practice of speech-language pathology, occupational therapy, and neuropsychology. Across these disciplines, there is some overlap in the assessment and treatment of patients with cognitive and communication disorders from TBI; this overlap depends on the work setting, historical practice, and training. Best practice occurs with when all

three are working together and complementing each other for the good of the patient.

115. e. Any of these activities could provide "current" best-practice recommendations. The activities that a clinician chooses are probably dependent on the work setting, the clinician's access to peer-reviewed journals, and the availability of funds to attend workshops and conferences.

116. d. The "most common" cause of dementia is Alzheimer disease. Vascular dementia is a major form of irreversible dementia, but it is not the most common; instead, vascular or multi-infarct dementia is thought to be the second most common form of dementia. Vitamin B_{12} deficiency and depression are reversible (not irreversible) causes of dementia.

117. b. A positive family history of dementia is a risk factor that increases the probability that a person may develop dementia, but it is not a pervasive feature of the syndrome of dementia. Depression may result from a diagnosis of dementia or may be the cause of cognitive impairments. However, depression does not occur in all persons with dementia. Coronary artery disease may co-occur with dementia but is not a feature of the dementia syndrome. Episodic memory impairment is the most common and earliest reported symptom of dementia.

118. a. Lexical memory and semantic memory are two subsystems of declarative memory. Working memory is one aspect of short-term memory, and episodic memory is one aspect of declarative memory. Sensory memory is a very brief register of sensory information that operates at the earliest stage of information processing.

119. b. Working memory and episodic memory are the two human memory systems that are most vulnerable to the effects of Alzheimer disease. Impairments in these memory systems manifest early and are pervasive even in persons with mild dementia of the Alzheimer type. Semantic memory is eventually affected in more moderate stages of dementia but is relatively spared early during the onset of the disease. Procedural memory, an aspect of nondeclarative memory, is well preserved into moderate stages of dementia.

120. c. The central executive system is subserved by the dorsolateral prefrontal cortex. The visuospatial sketchpad is supported by the occipitoparietal cortex. The articulatory-phonological loop is thought to be subserved by the Broca area and the cortex surrounding it, as well as by the inferior temporal and inferior parietal cortices. The episodic buffer

component of working memory has not been conclusively linked to a single identifiable neurological or cortical substrate.

121. b. Evidence from multiple neuroimaging studies reveal that the articulatory-phonological loop is subserved by the Broca area and the cortex surrounding the Broca area, as well as by the inferior temporal and inferior parietal cortices. The visuospatial sketchpad is supported by the occipitoparietal cortex, whereas the central executive system is subserved by the prefrontal cortex, specifically the dorsolateral prefrontal cortex. The episodic buffer has not been conclusively linked to a single identifiable neurological or cortical substrate.

122. c. To answer this question, you must identify risk factors for developing dementia. A nonvegetarian diet (option a) and inability to speak English fluently (option b) are not risk factors for developing dementia. Deteriorated driving performance (option d) results from dementia but is not a risk factor for developing dementia. Driving performance is affected significantly because it is a cognitively demanding task that requires complex executive function ability. If a patient suffers from one or more TBIs, the probability that this person will develop dementia is significantly increased.

123. b. The presence of two copies of the type 4 allele of apolipoprotein E has been conclusively shown to significantly enhance the risk of developing Alzheimer disease. In fact, patients who have two copies of this allele are eight times more likely to develop late-onset Alzheimer disease than is someone who has no copies. Being left-handed (option a), hypotension (option c), and poor hand-eye coordination (option d) have not been demonstrated to increase the likelihood of developing Alzheimer disease.

124. b. Dementia associated with Huntington disease (option a) is indeed associated with younger age at onset than is Alzheimer disease because Huntington disease is diagnosed much earlier in life than is Alzheimer disease. However, dementia associated with Huntington disease is not the most common cause of dementia before age 65; frontotemporal dementia is. Vascular dementia (option c) and dementia of the Alzheimer type (option d) refer to other causes of irreversible dementia but are not causes that account for the largest number of diagnoses before age 65.

125. d. PPA is characterized by language and cognitive deficits (option a) and is a distinct type of frontotemporal dementia (option b), and SLPs work to

teach PPA patients compensatory communicative strategies (option c). PPA manifests rather differently than Alzheimer disease in terms of presenting symptoms, neuroanatomical regions involved, and progression of symptoms over time. PPA almost always begins with a progressive decline of language and communicative abilities.

126. c. When working with patients who have dementia, SLPs can screen and assess cognitive status (option a), counsel family caregivers about the nature and progression of dementia (option b), and implement interventions for management of the dementia. These activities in accordance with the current position of the American Speech-Language Hearing Association about the role of SLPs working with patients who have dementia. Making a medical diagnosis of the type of dementia requires an interdisciplinary team that is often led by a physician (to integrate the patient's symptoms, clinical findings, and results of laboratory work), a radiologist (to interpret brain imaging data), and a neuropsychologist or SLP (who assesses cognitive status and activities of daily living) in order to arrive at a final diagnosis. An SLP alone cannot make a medical diagnosis of the type of dementia.

127. b. Determinations of swallowing impairments (option a), insurance status (option c), and need for rehabilitation services (option d) are not legally mandated. Administration of the Minimum Data Set—part of the Resident Assessment Instrument (RAI)—is federally mandated by the Omnibus Budget Reconciliation Act (OBRA) for all patients residing in Medicare-certified facilities. Per law, this assessment must be administered and results documented within 14 days of a resident's admission to a skilled nursing facility and must be repeated quarterly thereafter.

128. c. The medial temporal lobe region, specifically the hippocampus and the entorhinal cortex, are affected earliest in the neuropathological process of Alzheimer disease. The basal ganglia (option a), cerebellum (option c), and corpus callosum (option d) are not typically involved in Alzheimer disease, but they are often involved in subcortical dementias.

129. c. Persons with Alzheimer disease do not experience phonology and syntax problems (option a) early on. Discourse measures are rather sensitive to dementia because most persons with dementia do present discourse-level impairments (option b). Working memory problems (option d) do not necessarily reflect language impairments. People with Alzheimer disease do exhibit impairment in word retrieval early in the course of the disease.

130. c. The Mini-Mental State Examination is an 11-item, 30-point screening and assessment measure that is used to coarsely quantify cognitive impairments in older adults and in persons with dementia. Scores in the range of 27 to 30 are indicative of the absence of a cognitive impairment. Scores between 15 and 20 on the MMSE suggest the presence of cognitive impairment and are associated with mild dementia. It is not possible to score between 31 and 40 (option a), because the maximum possible score on the MMSE is 30 points. Scores ranging from 20 to 30 (option d) reflect both no demonstrated cognitive impairment (scores between 27 and 30) and mild dementia (scores below 27). Scores of 16 to 24 (option a) do reflect cognitive impairment.

131. a. Scores of 8 to 15 are indicative of moderate severity of dementia. Scores of 16 to 24 (option b) suggest the presence of cognitive impairment and are associated with mild dementia. It is not possible to score in the range of 25 to 33 (option c) because the maximum possible score on the MMSE is 30 points. Scores ranging from 27 to 30 (option d) indicate that a person has no cognitive impairment.

132. a. The ABCD (option b), CADL-2 (option c), and FLCI (option d) are all tests that are appropriate for use with persons who have dementia when attempting to document performance on communication and language measures. The MMSE, however, is not designed to assess communicative performance; instead, it is best used as a screening measure of cognitive status and must be interpreted in accordance with age- and education-corrected norms.

133. b. Semantic memory is an aspect of declarative memory that stores conceptual knowledge or information. Thus, it can be assessed by having the patient describe features of a common object. Retelling a short story (option a) is a common task used for assessing episodic memory, not semantic memory described in Choices C and D Reading short sentences (options c) and repeating a sequence of numbers correctly (option d) are not semantic memory tasks but tasks that assess reading mechanics and digit span (a component of working memory), respectively.

134. b. On a short story recall task, healthy older adults perform similarly on immediate and delayed recall, whereas persons with early Alzheimer disease perform significantly worse on delayed recall than on immediate recall. Providing accurate biographical information (option a), naming line drawings of

common objects (option c), and copying a complex figure (option d) do not enable clinicians to distinguish reliably between healthy older adults and persons with Alzheimer disease.

135. c. The FLCI was specifically developed to assess patients with moderate and severe dementia. The BDAE (option a) is a test of aphasia and has not been standardized for persons with dementia; also, because its tasks are complex, the BDAE is not a logical choice for patients with moderate to severe dementia. The ABCD is targeted to patients with mild dementia; it is too complex and time consuming for a person with moderate to severe dementia to complete. The RBANS (option d) is a test not of linguistic communication but of overall neuropsychological functioning.

136. b. The Dementia Mood Assessment Scale enables a clinician to evaluate mood on the basis of direct observations of the patient and an interview. The CDR Scale (option a) and the Mattis Dementia Rating Scale provide information about the overall severity of dementia, and the ABCD provides information about the linguistic communication impairments of persons with dementia.

137. c. Administering the CADL-2 (option a), developing and administering a therapy plan (option b), and conducting a MBS examination (option d) fall squarely within the stated scope of practice of an SLP working with a person who has dementia. It is within the scope of practice to conduct otoscopy by itself. However, cerumen management, or ear wax removal, is not within the SLP's scope of practice and must be performed by a licensed nursing professional or a certified audiologist.

138. b. Contrary to what was thought in the 1980s and 1990s about the language abilities of patients with late-stage Alzheimer disease, a landmark study by Bayles and colleagues (2000) revealed that of a sample of 49 such patients, the majority remained able to produce language during an evaluation and were, in fact, typically not completely mute or nonverbal (option c). This study also revealed that participants retained some limited functional communication into the late stages of Alzheimer disease (option a). Episodic memory (option d) is earliest memory system affected in Alzheimer disease and is devastated in the late stages.

139. b. Generative naming tasks are those in which a person is given a semantic category (e.g., "animals") or a letter (e.g., the letter *F*) and is asked to generate as many exemplars as he or she can.

Confrontation naming tasks are those in which a person is shown real objects or pictures and asked to name them. According to multiple published research studies done by neuropsychologists, SLPs, and dementia researchers, there is evidence to support the statements that performances on generative naming (option a), semantic fluency (option c), and naming low-frequency items (option d) are more impaired. In general, patients with dementia perform better on confrontation naming tasks (in which there is a tangible stimulus to name) than on generative naming tasks (in which there is no tangible stimulus to be named).

140. d. Hearing loss is the third most common chronic health condition affecting older adults and is very common in older adults with dementia. In this situation, referring the patient to an audiologist (option a) may not resolve the situation because the patient may already have hearing aids that he or she chooses not to wear. Delaying the assessment for a referral to an audiologist, who is not situated within a skilled nursing facility, is inadvisable. Furthermore, referring to an audiologist without conducting otoscopy or a hearing screening independently is inefficient. Canceling the scheduled evaluation (option b) does not resolve this situation in any way. Raising the voice (option c) is inappropriate and can cause vocal strain if raised loudness is maintained for a full assessment; furthermore, the patient with dementia may not respond well to this modification. Conducting otoscopy and hearing screening and using an assistive listening device is within the SLP's scope of practice and helps the patient hear the examiner satisfactorily during the assessment.

141. b. *Direct intervention* refers to interventions in which the SLP provides individual or group therapy to persons with dementia. SLPs' training of caregivers (option a) and modification of a patient's physical environment (option d) refer to examples or types of indirect interventions. An SLP's provision of continuing education for other professionals (option c) is an example of a professional activity that is not a patient intervention.

142. b. In spaced retrieval training, recall attempts are spaced over increasing lengths of time. Errorless learning (option a) is a technique for constraining response sets in order to reduce the number of errors made during learning by persons with dementia. Simulated presence therapy (option c) is a therapy technique in which a familiar caregiver's speech or voice is recorded and played back as a cue to reduce agitation and negative behaviors in patients with moderate and greater severity of

dementia. Semantic feature analysis is a technique used in aphasia therapy to facilitate semantic activation and word retrieval skills.

143. d. Reminiscence therapy is the use of tangible stimuli (e.g., photos, keepsakes, newspaper articles) structured around a theme, in order to stimulate recall of personally relevant information. Reducing the number of errors during new learning (option a) refers to "errorless learning," a teaching technique that is used for persons with dementia but is not related to reminiscence therapy. Informal conversation (option b) does not stimulate specific recall of information related to a theme. Physical and cognitive exercise is not related to reminiscence therapy.

144. c. From the perspective of the speech language pathologist's scope of practice, the most significant finding the loss of considerable weight. This may be suggestive of a feeding or swallowing impairment that must be assessed and treated by the SLP to optimize the patient's nutritional status and to ensure that the patient can swallow safely. Reduced speech intelligibility (option a) is characteristic of hypokinetic dysarthria associated with Parkinson disease and is noteworthy here but not the finding of greatest significance for this patient. Use of a walker and presentation of a festinating gait (short, shuffling steps; option b) are symptomatic of motor impairments associated with Parkinson disease. A visit from the patient's grandchildren does not reveal a finding of the greatest significance for this patient's care.

145. d. Using Brain Fitness Software (option a) is not appropriate because there is no evidence that this therapy, when used by SLPs, is reimbursable, and there is no eminent rationale for using this software for this patient. There is little to no systematic evidence that nonspeech oromotor training (option b) generalizes to spontaneous speech. No information is provided to suggest that Mrs. A has dysphagia (option c). Spaced retrieval training may indeed effectively train this patient to remember a safety strategy such as using her walker.

146. c. Hypertension, diabetes, and a history of cerebrovascular disease (multiple transient ischemic attacks in this case) are strongly suggestive of the presence of vascular dementia. Pseudodementia (option a) is reversible dementia attributed to the presence of clinical depression in a patient; however, there is no information on whether Mr. B is depressed. Because of the history of cerebrovascular disease, Alzheimer disease is not the most likely diagnosis, although it is possible that he may have a

combination of Alzheimer disease and vascular disease. However, he would not have late-onset Alzheimer disease (option b). Frontotemporal dementia (option d) is associated with early age (before age 60 years) at onset.

147. a. A functional maintenance plan is a plan of care that is designed to maintain patients at a particular level of functioning. The intent of an FMP is to instruct support personnel to carry out a plan of care, for which the SLP provides oversight. A caregiver training plan (option b) and a reevaluation plan (option d) are not specific plans of care. The minimum data set (option c) is not a plan of care but part of a federally mandated assessment instrument for all residents of Medicare-certified long-term care facilities.

148. a. It is true that patients with dementia may present with impairments at any stage (oral, pharyngeal, esophageal) of swallowing (option b). Dysphagia is indeed more common in patients with moderate, moderately severe, and severe dementia (option c), although it can also occur in mild dementia, and patients with dementia are indeed at high risk for malnutrition and dehydration (option d) because of coexisting swallowing and cognitive impairments. Patients with dementia can benefit from direct interventions for swallowing impairments (e.g., compensatory strategies, safe swallow techniques, cuing, and prompting), from indirect interventions (e.g., diet modifications, participation in a restorative dining program, caregiver training), or from both.

149. a. Many clinicians erroneously believe that Medicare will not reimburse for appropriate and necessary interventions for persons with dementia. In fact, Medicare does reimburse SLPs for direct interventions as long as there is a justification of skilled services and evidence of restorative potential. The other options are all true statements.

150. b. Memory wallets and books have been repeatedly documented to facilitate recall and retention of personal biographical information by persons with dementia. Dance movements (option a), laptop computers (option c), and arts and crafts activities (option d) have all been successfully used in various therapeutic interventions with persons with dementia but have not been demonstrated to specifically facilitate recall of biographical information.

151. c. In establishing a differential diagnosis for the dysarthrias, it is best to focus on salient features: that

is, those that are present exclusively in one type of dysarthria (Duffy, 2005). Hypokinetic dysarthria has several salient features. It is the only dysarthria characterized by a rapid speech rate. Individuals with flaccid dysarthria (option a) typically speak at a normal rate, whereas the speech of individuals with spastic dysarthria (option b) is noticeably slow. Conversational speaking rate is not a key distinguishing characteristic of ataxic (option e) or hyperkinetic dysarthria (option d). Another key feature of hypokinetic dysarthria is an inability to accurately self-perceive loudness. Individuals with other types of dysarthria are aware of the appropriateness of their loudness levels, but hypokinetic dysarthria is characterized by a lack of internal "calibration" (Ramig et al, 1995). Finally, although fleeting dysfluencies are not consistently present in hypokinetic dysarthria, they are not present in any other dysarthria type.

152. a. The reticular formation is a complex network of cells that extends throughout the medulla, pons, and midbrain (Duffy, 2005). Although it has many roles, one of its primary functions is the regulation of consciousness. Damage to the brainstem can affect the cranial nerves housed there, as well as the reticular formation. Thus, it is not unusual to find flaccid dysarthria in association with long coma durations.

153. e. The hallmark of ataxic dysarthria is temporal dysregulation (Kent et al, 1997). Diadochokinetic (alternating motion) rates have been shown to be particularly sensitive to these timing irregularities. Irregular articulatory breakdowns are also common. Ataxic dysarthria is associated with damage to the cerebellar control circuit, whose primary function is coordinating timing within and among components of movement.

154. d. TBI causes diffuse lesions by means of any combination of axonal shearing, twisting of the brain in the skull, impact damage, and contracoup injuries. Although it may be possible to determine which dysarthria will result from a specific type of TBI, mixed dysarthrias are the most common. In contrast, many other disorders are associated with discrete lesions or chemical imbalances in the brain. For example, a bilateral CVA (option a) may cause spastic dysarthria. Repeated head trauma (option c) causes damage to deep cortical structures, particularly the basal ganglia, which leads most often to hypokinetic dysarthria. Finally, Parkinson disease (option b) and Huntington chorea (option e) are caused by imbalances between acetylcholine and dopamine.

155. d. The salient characteristic of hyperkinetic dysarthria is involuntary movement. The effect of hyperkinetic dysarthria on speech is unpredictable, however, and depends when involuntary movements occur. Involuntary movements can result in overshooting or undershooting articulatory targets, as well as over-adduction or underadduction of the vocal folds. The speech of an individual with hyperkinetic dysarthria can be distinguished from the irregular productions of an individual with ataxic dysarthria (option e), primarily because the cause of the irregular breakdowns has observable, physical manifestations. Furthermore, in the absence of involuntary movements, speech production is normal.

156. c. Apraxia of speech is caused by a unilateral lesion in the left cerebral hemisphere, particularly the parieto-frontal area. Apraxia of speech may be present in isolation, with no concomitant aphasia or dysarthria. In contrast, spastic dysarthria is caused by bilateral damage to upper motor neurons. Upper motor neurons constitute the corticobulbar tract, or the direct activation pathway, which travels from the motor cortex to innervation of the cranial nerves.

157. d. ALS can manifest with either bulbar or spinal onset. With bulbar onset, the damage begins in the corticobulbar tract and has rapid negative effects on speech production. In contrast, with a spinal onset, the damage begins in the spinal cord, first affecting gross motor movements. Yorkston and associates (1993) conducted a study to document disease progression in individuals with ALS. Their findings verified that speech is affected earlier with bulbar onset than with spinal onset. They also found differences in the progression of disease onset between men and women: Disease progression in women with bulbar onset is more rapid than in men with bulbar onset.

158. a. There is documented evidence that LSVT improves speech production in individuals with Parkinson disease (Spielman et al, 2007). The majority of the participants in the research to date have demonstrated mild dysarthria in association with the disease. There is no documentation of successful intervention with more severe dysarthria. An advantage of LSVT is that it is a whole-body approach, affecting multiple physiological systems simultaneously (Ramig & Dromey, 1996). For example, LVST has been shown to improve articulatory precision (Dromey et al, 1995). Thus, it would be inappropriate to target a single physiological system, such as articulation or respiration, when LSVT is most likely to effect changes in these, as well as in the phonatory system.

159. c. The timing of intervention is difficult for any individual with a degenerative disease. It is particularly hard to determine the ideal time to introduce an AAC device, inasmuch as many individuals may be reluctant to use one before it is absolutely necessary. Although it is generally accepted that an earlier introduction of an AAC device is preferable than a later or last-minute one, Beukelman and colleagues (2004) were the first investigators to provide an objective measure for guiding the timing of intervention. By combining data across several studies, they found that when speaking rate is reduced by roughly half, a rapid decline in intelligibility often occurs. The authors encouraged monitoring speaking rate at regular intervals and recommended an AAC assessment when speaking rate approaches 125 words per minute, regardless of relatively preserved intelligibility.

160. d. It is often controversial to recommend a complex or time-consuming intervention strategy for an individual with a rapidly progressing degenerative disease. The recommendation needs to be justified in terms of potential ability to maintain functional communication, as well as its effect on quality of life. In a retrospective study of 25 individuals with ALS, Esposito and associates (2000) found that a palatal lift prosthesis had been fitted for 21 individuals. According to chart reports, 76% benefitted from the palatal lift for at least 6 months. Of most importance, however, was that the majority of individuals who were fitted for a lift indicated that it was easier and less effortful to speak with the lift in place. In view of the detrimental effect of fatigue on the speech symptoms of ALS, a strategy to minimize vocal effort is worthy of consideration.

161. a. The majority of neurosurgical interventions for individuals with Parkinson disease are targeted toward debilitating physical limitations. There is no documentation that surgery improves their speech production. Farrell and colleagues (2005) studied the effects of pallidotomy, thalamotomy, and deep-brain stimulation on 22 patients, in comparison with a control group of 16 persons with Parkinson disease who did not undergo surgery. Although there were significant improvements in motor function after surgery, there was no perceptible effect on the patients' speech.

162. c. It may be difficult to determine whether respiratory intervention is appropriate for a patient, particularly one who may demonstrate breathiness, short phrases, reduced loudness, and seemingly reduced respiratory support. It is useful to keep in mind that the primary function of the respiratory system during speech production is to provide adequate

(options a and d) and constant (options b and e) subglottal pressure for phonation (option d). There are strategies that can be used to distinguish respiratory from laryngeal involvement. The most useful involve the indirect assessment of the ability to generate subglottal pressure. This can be done through the use of a home-made device developed by Hixon and co-workers (1982). The presence or absence of breathiness reflects laryngeal function, and does not enter into the decision to intervene at the respiratory level. ASHA provides guidelines and decision making suggestions for respiratory intervention (Helm-Estabrooks et al, 2003; Spencer et al, 2003).

163. a. One of the most difficult aspects of any treatment is generalization to real-life, nonclinical situations. This is particularly challenging with instrumentation-based biofeedback because of a potential reliance on online feedback for the production of target speech behaviors. There are few studies on the use of biofeedback to improve speech breathing patterns, and it is necessary to read and interpret them carefully to draw the correct conclusion. Murdoch and colleagues (1999) conducted a case study with Respitrace biofeedback and concluded that biofeedback techniques were superior to traditional therapy in establishing physiological change. They did not, however, note successful generalization of the improved speech breathing patterns when biofeedback was discontinued. Hodge and Hall (1994) highlighted this problem in another case study, in which, again, it was possible to establish but not generalize improved speech breathing patterns. Even with carefully designed studies involving systematic fading of biofeedback, generalization remains problematic.

164. c. *Inspiratory checking* can be a confusing term because it really refers to muscular activity during the expiratory phase of speech breathing. Inspiratory checking involves controlling the descent of the rib cage during expiration by using inspiratory muscles. The inspiratory muscle forces counteract the passive relaxation forces, which are in an expiratory direction above resting expiratory level (Hixon et al, 2008). A common problem in individuals with dysarthria, particularly flaccid dysarthria, can be air wastage that results from poor respiratory control or inadequate laryngeal valving at the onset of phonation. Teaching inspiratory checking can help the patient learn to conserve expiratory airflow, thus increasing the number of syllables produced per breath group.

165. d. LSVT is thoroughly grounded in key principles of motor learning, which include intensive training

(option a) and practice outside the clinic (option c) to facilitate generalization. The single external cue "Think loud" (option b) makes the program ideal for individuals with cognitive or memory deficits. The component of increasing pitch range (option e) is based on the concept of increasing the range of motion in the cricothyroid muscle. This is designed to address the limited range of motion found across physiological systems in Parkinson disease. The program is most effective when the focus is exclusively on the laryngeal system (Ramig & Dromey, 1996). Thus, a cue of "big breaths" would not be appropriate.

166. b. The pharyngeal branch of the vagus nerve innervates the all the muscles of the pharynx and soft palate except the stylopharyngeus (cranial nerve IX) and the tensor veli palatine (mandibular branch of cranial nerve V). It is responsible for pharyngeal constriction and for retraction and elevation of the velum during velopharyngeal closure for speech. When the pharyngeal branch is damaged, the muscular tissue involved in velopharyngeal closure is present but nonfunctional. An obturator (option a) is designed to fill space in the velopharyngeal port caused by velopharyngeal insufficiency (not enough tissue) and may be used in cases of cleft palate. It is not an appropriate intervention for velopharyngeal incompetence (tissue present but not working). No evidence supports the use of sucking and blowing exercises (option c) or palatal icing (option d) to stimulate palatal function for speech production (McWilliams & Bradley, 1965). It may be appropriate to use the Nasometer (option e) for biofeedback for individuals with mild velopharyngeal closure problems, although there is no evidence to support its use. Karnell and associates (2004) demonstrated in 19 patients that a palatal lift prosthesis can reduce hypernasality from an average of 35% to 17% nasalance (<28% is considered within normal limits).

167. e. A palatal lift prosthesis should not be recommended automatically. Fitting a lift is typically a time-consuming and expensive process. Netsell and Rosenbek (1985) and Yorkston and associates (2001) established very useful guidelines to determine the appropriateness of a palatal lift. The patient must be able to generate adequate subglottal pressure for speech; thus, an individual who sustains only 5 cm H_2O for 1 second (option a) would not be a candidate. The patient should demonstrate large and consistent velopharyngeal opening during nonnasal sounds. A velopharyngeal orifice area of less than 5 mm^2 (option b) or nasalance of less than 28% (option c) is considered within normal limits. Consistency is a critical concern. For example, occasional velopharyngeal closure during nonnasal sounds (option d) indicates that behavioral changes may help the patient obtain closure. One of the most critical criteria for establishing appropriateness for a palatal lift is at least fair to good articulation. If the individual has very reduced intelligibility as a result of an inability to reach articulatory contacts, a palatal lift will not functionally improve speech.

168. c. The concept behind CPAP is borrowed from sleep research to help individuals who have sleep apnea. When sleeping, an individual wears a mask over the nose. Air from an external pump travels into the nose and over the soft palate. This continuous positive airflow keeps the velopharyngeal port open, thus preventing a cessation of breathing (apnea) during sleep. Kuehn (1997) incorporated CPAP into a speech production program designed to improve velopharyngeal closure. With constant airflow across the velopharyngeal port, making closure during a nonnasal sound requires moving against resistance. Resistance is systematically increased as the pressure from the CPAP device is increased. This is a fundamental principle of strength training. A key element of Kuehn's program is the construction of speech stimulus, so that the closure against the resistance is performed in the context of speech. In addition, several principles of motor learning facilitate the acquisition and generalization of skills. Motor learning requires intensive practice; therefore, three times a week (option a) would be inadequate. Daily practice, at least twice a day, is recommended. Finally, the speech stimuli are randomly presented. Randomized stimuli, rather than blocked (e.g., all initial /t/ words practiced together) stimuli, have also been shown to facilitate generalization of learned behaviors.

169. a. This is a subjective judgment, and you may find different tasks to be useful as you gain clinical experience. Conversational speech is the most crucial portion of a motor speech evaluation because it will provide you will a number of diagnostic features. Fast speaking rate is only associated with hypokinetic dysarthria, while flaccid dysarthria is typically associated with a normal rate. AMRs are also particularly useful in distinguishing among dysarthria types. An arrhythmic, irregular, or syncopated pace distinguishes ataxic dysarthria from all others. Flaccid dysarthria AMRs may be produced imprecisely but with typically normal rates. Hypokinetic dysarthria AMRs are often characterized by very rapid, blurred productions in which articulatory targets are barely, if at all,

approximated. AMRs associated with spastic dysarthria, in contrast, are typically very slow and effortful. If you have difficulty judging the appropriateness of AMRs, it is useful to compare a tape recording of the patient's production with the sound of normal productions.

170. a. The effectiveness of pacing strategies (i.e., either stretching out words or putting breaks between words in order to slow speaking rate) is a well-documented, effective intervention strategy. Members of the Academy of Neurologic Communication Disorders and Sciences reviewed supplemented speech and pacing strategies (Helm-Estabrooks et al, 2004). In addition, Hustad (2001, 2007); Hustad & Beukelman (2002); and Hustad & Garcia (2002) conducted a series of studies investigating various aspects of both pacing and supplemented speech strategies. In a motor speech evaluation, it is useful to obtain a sample of both single word and sentence productions. A listener—ideally, someone unfamiliar with the patient—transcribes them; then you can compare intelligibility scores (number of words correctly conveyed divided by the total number of words spoken). If an individual is much more (e. g., at least 20%) intelligible in single words than in sentences, a strategy of word-by-word production or reduced speaking rate will probably be effective in increasing intelligibility.

171. c. A holistic intervention strategy is one that affects more than one physiological system. Increased vocal effort simply involves an individual speaking more loudly. The extensive work by Ramig and colleagues (2001) on the LSVT provides documentation that increased vocal effort has positive effects on respiration, phonation, and articulation. Other investigators have shown that increased vocal effort can result in improved velopharyngeal closure as well (McHenry & Liss, 2006). Increased vocal effort has a differential effect on sound production in different types of dysarthria. For example, with increased vocal effort, individuals with flaccid dysarthria tended to reduce hypernasality, whereas individuals with spastic dysarthria tended to increase hypernasality (McHenry & Liss, 2006). During a motor speech evaluation or trial therapy, it is often useful to explore holistic intervention strategies such as increased vocal effort and rate reduction.

172. a. According to Yorkston and associates (1999), comprehensibility strategies encourage communication partners to use all available modalities to convey a message. Although much of motor speech intervention focuses on increasing an individual's intelligibility, much is lost by not training the speaker and

potential conversational partners to take advantage of comprehensibility strategies, such as use of an alphabet board (option b). Hustad and colleagues' line of investigation highlights the usefulness of different types of comprehensibility strategies (Hustad, 2001, 2007; Hustad & Beukelman, 2002; Hustad & Garcia, 2002). Signal-independent information (i.e., information not conveyed solely by speech) takes advantage of more naturalistic communicative environments. Although many people may employ these strategies automatically, specifically training conversational partners (option c) and the speaker can result in much more effective communication. For individuals with cognitive or memory deficits, the speaker may have to rely on external cues (option e) by the conversational partner to facilitate communicative interactions. For example, "Are we still talking about..." may help quickly resolve a potential communicative breakdown (option d).

173. d. Signal-independent information is conveyed to the listener without reliance on the speech signal. When an individual has very reduced intelligibility, the listener must rely on information that is not conveyed in the speech signal to decipher the intended message. Signal-independent information can be conveyed in many forms and contributes to the comprehensibility of the message (Yorkston et al, 1999x). Examples of signal-independent information include providing the listener with knowledge of the topic, using contextual cues (e.g., expectations for a conversation at home versus in a class), use of an alphabet board (e.g., pointing to the first letter of each word as it is spoken), and semantic predictability.

174. e. When an individual uses an alphabet board to supplement speech, signal-independent information is provided to the listener. Typically, a speaker points to the first letter of each word as it is spoken. If used properly, this has the effect of putting breaks between words (providing word boundaries, a syntactic cue) and reducing speaking rate (giving the listener more processing time). Beukelman and Yorkston (1977) also showed that even when the listener could not see the alphabet board, perceived intelligibility was improved. This implies that the speaker's articulation improves with pacing strategies. It is unlikely, however, that vocal quality would be affected by these factors.

175. b. External evidence refers to available data-based literature and is extremely important for making clinical decisions. Equally important, however, is internal evidence. Internal evidence includes more

personal elements, such as the clinician's expertise and, of most importance, the patient's personal preferences. The greatest difficulty with rate-control strategies is that most patients (like most people) dislike speaking slowly. Of the human physiological systems (i.e., respiratory, phonatory, velopharyngeal, and articulatory), the only one working to its maximum capability is articulation (Tiffany, 1980). Basically, humans talk as fast as they are able. Because of this natural human tendency, it is extremely difficult to encourage people to slow down. Most patients would rather repeat an utterance than say it slowly the first time. It is up to the clinician to highlight the external evidence in the hopes that the patient will consider a rate-control strategy.

176. d. Clark (2003) provided an elegant, thorough, and clear explanation of the neuromuscular basis for treating speech production deficits. She highlighted the requirements for a strength-training program and the inherent inappropriateness of nonspeech tasks such as oromotor exercises as they are typically performed. Several other investigators have contributed to the arguments against such intervention. For example, McWilliams and Bradley (1965) demonstrated that although velopharyngeal closure improved during blowing and sucking tasks, the closure remained incomplete during speech. Moore and colleagues (1988; Moore, 1993) demonstrated different patterns of muscle activation patterns for chewing and repetitive babbling, even though the same muscles are used in these activities. These findings suggest that speech and nonspeech tasks are programmed differently in the brain. Finally, Forrest (2002) highlighted the relatively small amount of muscle strength necessary to generate the articulatory force produced during speech.

177. e. A very common presenting complaint of patients is that they speak too slowly. In view of the importance of internal evidence (i.e., considering a patient's preferences in determining an intervention), it is tempting to make increased speaking rate a therapy goal. Although this appears intuitively appropriate, this strategy can reduce intelligibility across all types of dysarthria. First, most individuals with dysarthria, particularly before speech intervention, are speaking naturally as fast as they physiologically are able. Second, rate reduction strategies are useful across many types of dysarthria, even those characterized by slow speech. If an individual with flaccid dysarthria increases speaking rate, he or she is more likely to undershoot articulatory targets, reducing precision. For

an individual with spastic dysarthria, increased speaking rate is likely to be associated with increased effort. As muscle activation increases, the effects of spasticity also increase, making speech even more effortful and slow. Hypokinetic dysarthria is the only type associated with an excessively rapid rate, which is typically produced in short bursts characterized by markedly reduced articulatory precision (sometimes called "blurred" speech). For individuals with ataxic dysarthria, who may demonstrate a slow rate, maintenance of the slow rate may facilitate coordination across and within physiological systems. Although increased speaking rate will improve naturalness, there is little clinical evidence to suggest that it will also improve articulatory precision (Yorkston et al, 1990).

178. e. For an individual with at least moderately reduced intelligibility, putting breaks between words has very noticeable advantages. Individuals with spastic dysarthria particularly benefit from this strategy. One of the most obvious gains is that listeners know where words begin and end (option a). Individuals with spastic dysarthria often sound as though phonation is continuous, and it becomes more strained as the utterance progresses. There is a tendency for tension to increase continuously. Thus, putting breaks between words, particularly if the articulators and vocal folds return to a resting or neutral position, can counteract the trend toward rising tension (option c). This may have the additional benefit of increasing articulatory precision (option d), because more relaxed articulators (option b) are not fighting internal tension to reach their targets.

179. a. Patients in acute care have needs that are very different and more urgent than those of individuals later in recovery. One of the most basic communicative functions for any human is to be able to communicate needs and preferences. This is particularly important in an acute care environment, in which communication is crucial and abilities may be markedly compromised. Although family members may be involved in critical decisions regarding care, particularly if the patient's comprehension is negatively affected, all attempts should be made to inform the patient of his or her situation and obtain consent for procedures if at all possible. Yorkston and associates (1995) provided an excellent protocol for assessing the ability to respond to "yes"/"no" questions. It is an invaluable tool in an intensive care or acute care setting.

180. d. Professionals in the field of speech and language have embraced evidence-based practice. This

implies that the assessments and treatments that they provide are grounded in research. There are different types of treatment studies, and they typically follow a hierarchy. Treatment outcome studies document a natural result and do not have a component of control to strengthen internal validity. The researchers simply document change, or lack of it, that may occur as a result of time, treatment, or both. The first attempt by ASHA to document the effectiveness of speech and language intervention (National Outcomes Measurement System) was this type of study. Clinicians simply documented change before and after therapy. There were no controls for issues such as spontaneous recovery or therapy intensity, nor was there documentation of change in individuals who did not receive treatment. In contrast, treatment efficiency studies are designed to determine the probability of benefit to individuals in a clearly defined population (e.g., patients with ataxic dysarthria) and are conducted under ideal conditions. Often, ideal conditions encompass daily treatment, a condition not easily met in a clinical setting. Treatment effectiveness studies, on the other hand, assess the effectiveness of treatment for a clearly defined population under average conditions. Finally, once a treatment has been established to be efficacious and effective, treatment efficiency studies determine whether a treatment can be performed with a minimum of expense or unnecessary effort. Few treatment regimens in this field have progressed though all types of studies. A good example of research in treatment development is the work of Ramig and colleagues (1995, 2001; Ramig & Dromey, 1996) on the LSVT. Their work progressed from treatment efficacy studies through treatment efficiency studies.

181. a. Flaccid dysarthria involves damage to the peripheral nervous system, from the cranial nerves to the muscles. It has a variety of causes, including TBI, tumors impinging on the cranial nerves, and surgical trauma (Duffy, 2005). Often, more than one cranial nerve is affected, and the damage can be unilateral or bilateral. In cases in which multiple physiological systems may be affected, isolated articulation tests are of little value. If a motor speech evaluation is viewed not only as a diagnostic tool but also as an opportunity for diagnostic therapy, a comparison of single word and sentence intelligibility will yield the most useful information. In this manner, the contribution of all physiological systems to intelligibility is considered, rather than focusing solely on articulation. The comparison of single word intelligibility with sentence intelligibility can indicate the appropriateness of a pacing or rate reduction strategy.

182. b. A critical feature of a well-designed treatment study is follow-up after treatment. In this investigation, data were collected before treatment, immediately after treatment, 6 months after treatment, and 12 months after treatment. Although immediate post-treatment scores would be expected to be higher than pretreatment scores, the ability to maintain such improvement over time is crucial for functional outcomes. In this example, the groups were compared 12 months after treatment. The placebo recipients' vocal intensity deteriorated significantly in comparison with pretreatment performance, whereas that of the LSVT recipients did not. However, the LSVT recipients did demonstrate deterioration in vocal intensity in comparison with their performance immediately after treatment.

183. c. An assessment would need to include an examination of velopharyneal closure for speech because of the complaint. In some cases a speech prosthesis such as a palatal lift may be beneficial for the client. A good way to determine whether a palatal lift prosthesis will be effective is to simulate its presence. This can be done by occluding the nasal passage with nose clips. The impact of nasal occlusion on intelligibility is of particular interest. If intelligibility improves with nose clips, the individual may be able to produce high-pressure phonemes (such as plosives and fricatives) more effectively, because air is not escaping through the nose. If, however, intelligibility does not improve during a speech sample with nose clips in place, it is unlikely that a palatal lift will provide a clinically significant improvement in speech production. Good to fair articulation is a recommended prerequisite for palatal lift fitting (Netsell & Rosenbek, 1985; Yorkston et al, 2001). In this case, intelligibility as low as 30% warrants the introduction of an AAC system. The individual needs a strategy for functional communication. Option d would provide information concerning phonation time (phonation) and hypernasality (resonation). Weak oral pressure sounds (option e) is a symptom of velopharyngeal inadequacy.

184. c. An ideal rehabilitation setting involves a multidisciplinary approach in which a number of professionals work closely in both the assessment and treatment of individuals with motor speech disorders. When conducting an evaluation, an impression of a patient's best performance is very valuable. Whenever possible, optimizing the environment and timing of testing can facilitate this goal. For example, young adults often perform better in the afternoon than early in the morning because they are

more alert later in the day. In this example, the patient is in pain, and it appears that his discomfort is affecting motor speech production. It is unlikely that you will obtain a valid indication of his performance if you continue the evaluation. With a multidisciplinary approach, you can confer with the physician and neuropsychologist to determine the nature of the patient's pain. Furthermore, it is always useful to ask the patient whether his physical state and speech during your evaluation are typical. Finally, it is constructive to determine the individual's best time of day and to obtain a conversational speech sample at that time.

185. b. A key consideration in a treatment plan is the individual's post-treatment goals. Speaking demands and expectations vary widely according to an individual's typical social interactions and vocational demands. For example, an individual who is elderly, retired, and socializes primarily with his or her spouse has different communication needs than someone returning to the workforce, particularly in a vocally demanding occupation. In this example, the patient's vocational goals require near-perfect speech production. He has many advantages, with nearly all physiological systems functioning within normal limits. Only velopharyngeal closure is in need of intervention. This individual also meets all the recommendations for candidacy for a palatal lift: good intelligibility, adequate subglottal pressure for speech, and no gag reflex. He would be an ideal candidate for palatal lift fitting.

186. c. Although LSVT was developed for individuals with hypokinetic dysarthria secondary to Parkinson disease, it is appropriate to consider in this example. The patient probably demonstrates mild flaccid dysarthria, but its effect is significant because of the individual's desire to resume telemarketing. There are many documented benefits of the LSVT program, all of which may help this patient. LSVT has been shown to improve articulatory precision, reduce breathiness, and increase loudness (Dromey et al, 1995; Ramig & Dromey, 1996; Ramig et al, 2001). The respiratory and velopharyngeal systems are not contributing to this patient's speech problem. Although the effectiveness of LSVT has not yet been documented for individuals with mild flaccid dysarthria, it makes physiological sense to consider it. For many therapy approaches, there is no direct evidence of their effectiveness. It is up to the clinician to logically speculate on the likely benefit of these approaches for the patient and change the treatment if periodic assessment indicates no change in speech production.

187. c. This is a case in which internal evidence (i.e., the patient's preference) is of paramount importance. If an individual does not believe in the recommended compensatory strategy, he or she is unlikely to implement it outside the clinic. A compromise is warranted in this example. Because the individual's chosen profession requires his personality to come through when he makes a sales pitch, it is reasonable to endorse natural speech as the first attempt. It is also crucial to minimize communication breakdowns and listener burden during sales pitches. Therefore, an immediate backup plan should be a pacing strategy, ideally with alphabet board supplementation to maximize the likelihood that his listeners will understand him.

188. e. Although it is known that increasing vocal effort may improve velopharyngeal closure in individuals with mild resonance problems (McHenry & Liss, 2006), internal evidence, or considering the patient's preferences, is key. Trying to convince someone (option a) of a strategy that is incompatible with his or her personality is counterproductive. A pharyngeal flap (option b) and a palatal lift (option c) are inappropriate because they are rather extreme solutions to a mild problem. It would be reasonable to reassess her in 6 months to see whether the growth spurt hypothesis is legitimate, but it would be more useful to use that time to begin trial therapy with CPAP (Cahill et al, 2004; Kuehn et al, 2002).

189. c. On the basis of the findings of the motor speech evaluation, a likely differential diagnosis is flaccid dysarthria. Although literature suggests differential effects of aphasia on first and second languages, it is not relevant to motor speech disorders. Unilateral flaccid dysarthria will affect both languages equally, and intelligibility should be roughly equivalent in both.

190. a. Approximately 20% of vital capacity is used for conversational speech production, which is about twice the size of an inhalation during quiet breathing (Hixon et al, 2008). Depending on the site of cranial nerve damage, individuals with flaccid dysarthria may demonstrate problems with speech breathing (option b), such as inadequate inspiration for speech or poor expiratory control. Although some improvement in vital capacity may occur as the patient becomes reconditioned, it is unlikely to be dramatic (option c). Vital capacity is determined largely by physiological variables. Expiratory reserve volume (option d) is the volume of air that can be breathed out after a quiet breathing exhalation. Although it is possible to increase utterance duration by

entering expiratory reserve volume, focusing on increasing the magnitude of prephonatory inspiration (combined with good expiratory control) is probably more effective. It is not possible to speak on "residual air" (option e). This is a misconception that comes from the term "residual volume." Residual volume air cannot be exchanged during a maximal exhalation. It remains in the lungs because of the pleural linkage, which prevents the lungs from completely collapsing.

191. b. It is important to distinguish among the terms *nasalization, hypernasality, denasality,* and *nasal air emission. Nasalization* simply refers to communication between the vocal tract and the nasal passageway. It is appropriate for the nasal sounds in English (i.e., /m/, /n/, /ŋ/). *Hypernasality* refers to the presence of nasal resonance during the production of nonnasal voiced sounds, particularly vowels and dipthongs. To assess hypernasality, a completely nonnasal phrase loaded with voiced sounds (option c) is required. In contrast, *denasality* is the lack of nasal resonance on sounds that should be nasalized and, as such, can occur only on /m/, /n/, and /ŋ/. For evaluation of denasality, a phrase loaded with nasal sounds (option d) is ideal. *Nasal air emission* refers to the addition of turbulent, audible nasal energy during phoneme production and most frequently occurs with high-pressure sounds (plosives, fricatives, and affricates). To assess nasal air emission, a phrase loaded with high-pressure sounds is essential such as the example above (option b).

192. a. The chronic condition model is a useful framework for conceptualizing motor speech problems. Yorkston and associates (1999) adapted the model from the World Health Organization (WHO; Wood, 1980). The chronic condition model has five levels. The pathophysiological level refers to the underlying neurological or cellular disorder. Pharmacological intervention (e.g., dopamine for individuals with Parkinson disease) is an example of intervention at this level. The impairment, or subsystem, level encompasses physiological changes caused by impairments in the respiratory, phonatory, articulatory, and velopharyngeal systems. An example of intervention at this level would be the use of a palatal lift prosthesis. The functional limitation level reflects the effect of the motor impairment on an individual's communicative function. Interventions to improve intelligibility target this level. The disability, or contextual, level refers to an individual's functioning in real-world social contexts. Because interaction with communicative partners is involved, intervention involving comprehensibility strategies targets this level. The societal level refers to the effect of the motor speech disorder on an individual's functioning in society. Intervention requires societal changes, such as the hiring and retention of individuals with motor speech problems.

193. c. Motor learning theory has become an important component of effective motor speech intervention. There are several issues to consider, including frequency of intervention, stimulus presentation, and frequency of feedback. In general, a combination of intensive treatment, randomized rather than blocked stimuli, and less frequent feedback is optimal for generalization. These concepts are illustrated in studies of apraxia of speech treatment (Knock et al, 2000; Wambaugh, 2002), as well as in work by Adams and Page (2000) on individuals without speech problems who are learning rate-control strategies.

194. c. The purpose of a palatal lift prosthesis is to keep airflow and acoustic sound energy from entering the nasal passageway. It does so by lifting the soft palate, forming a mechanical impedance to the flow of air and acoustic sound energy. The palate is elevated to create a bridge to the posterior pharyngeal wall. It is used for individuals who have adequate velopharyngeal tissue that is not functioning because of lack of innervation. Typically, the patient can still breathe through the nose, inasmuch as the lift does not completely close off the velopharyngeal port. There is no evidence that wearing a palatal lift will stimulate velopharyngeal function. If a patient develops normal velopharyngeal closure after wearing a palatal lift, it is probably attributable to spontaneous recovery.

195. e. The basis for the majority of motor speech intervention involves teaching compensatory strategies. Rarely is intervention at the pathophysiological or impairment level of the WHO model. Instead, the individual is taught to work around the deficit, progressing toward intelligible speech. Tongue strengthening exercises (option a) have no documented effectiveness in treating motor speech problems. Similarly, swallowing exercises (option b) are inappropriate. It is difficult for a patient to learn specific strategies of omission or substitution (options c and d), and so these strategies are inappropriate as well. Compensatory strategies, however, help minimize the distance between the tongue and alveolar ridge. If the patient has damage to the trigeminal nerve and has difficulty maintaining a stable and close jaw position, it is possible to simply prop up the jaw with the hand. If the problem is primarily in lingual function, the clinician may consider a palatal lift with a dropped palate. Filling in the palatal section of the lift can facilitate lingual contact by

reducing the distance required to reach the articulatory target. Often, clinical solutions require basic problem-solving skills, combined with a good understanding of the underlying physiology of the motor speech deficit.

196. d. The term *apraxia* relates to the difficulty with planning and programming movement gestures for volitional speech production and does not include the language disorder (option a) that often accompanies or coexists with apraxia. The correct term for a communication disorder caused by neuromuscular impairment (option b) is *dysarthria.* Although some children with CAS also have cognitive deficits (option c), the apraxia is not a feature of such deficits; some children even with severe CAS have normal cognition. Phonological impairment (option e) occurs with CAS, but either it occurs concomitantly or the child's planning and programming difficulties influences the acquisition of phonemes.

197. d. A motor speech examination is the best task in which to elicit speech from which judgments can be made about behavioral characteristics associated with CAS. A child with a phonological impairment and a child with CAS may produce very similar errors in a standardized articulation test (option a), with one-word responses and no cueing. Both the language sample (option b) and standardized articulation tests will allow the formation of clinical hypotheses, inasmuch as the clinician can observe speech characteristics that may be indicative of CAS, but forming hypotheses is not the most important task. Oral structural-functional examinations (option c) are nonspeech tasks and do not allow judgments about speech performance. Respiratory and phonatory functions (option e) are typically normal in CAS.

198. d. Vowel distortions (option a), inconsistent performance (option b), difficulty with articulation (option c), and voicing errors (option e) are all characteristics frequently associated with CAS. CAS is not associated with low tone, weakness, or decreased range of motion (although any of these may be present, in which case they are concomitant).

199. c. Although the term *apraxia* denotes the specific difficulty with planning and programming movement gestures, the child's motoric difficulties undermine his or her ability to practice and learn the rule governed phonological system; therefore, children with CAS typically have concomitant phonological impairment. Weakness (option b) and resulting dysarthria (option a) are not associated with CAS,

although they may co-occur in some children. Many children with CAS go through typical periods of developmental dysfluency; however, stuttering (option d) is not part of, nor does it typically co-occur with, CAS. Children with CAS often do have a receptive-expressive gap, whereby expressive language is much more impaired than receptive language (option e). Of course, children with CAS as part of more comprehensive cognitive impairment also have receptive language impairment, but this is not a frequent association.

200. d. The position statement includes this sentence: "It is the certified speech-language pathologist who is responsible for making the primary diagnosis of CAS, for designing and implementing the individualized and intensive speech-language treatment programs needed to make optimum improvement, and for closely monitoring progress." All other statements are included in the position statement and therefore are true.

201. e. This child has a very limited phonetic and phonemic inventory. You would hypothesize CAS because of the lack of vowel differentiation and because of the discrepancy between receptive and expressive language. If he has apraxia, he likely also has a phonologic impairment; CAS (option d) and phonological impairments (option c) are usually concomitant. The child shows no evidence of dysarthria (option a): he has no respiratory or phonatory problems and no difficulty with chewing or swallowing, and shows good tongue and lip strength during bilabial and lingual alveolar plosives. If he were autistic (option b), he would not show such good social interaction or imaginative play, and he would not initiate verbal and nonverbal communication. Of course, your assessment tasks will allow you to test your hypothesis.

202. c. An examination of respiratory and phonatory coordination enables you to measure one aspect of the child's performance that appears to be within normal limits. A motor speech examination (option a) is the most important task for determining the presence of an apraxia of speech. A structured language sample (option b) would be obtained to get a sense of all modalities the child uses to attempt to convey communicative intent, as well as to get a vowel and consonant inventory. A receptive language test (option d) would help document your impression of normal receptive language. An oral structural-functional examination (option e) would help determine or rule out an oral nonverbal apraxia.

203. a. CAS often occurs with concomitant expressive language problems. Although receptive language may

be normal, the difficulty with planning and programming movement gestures undermines the ability of the child to develop expressive vocabulary and syntax.

204. c. The motor learning literature has shown that in order to improve movement accuracy, the learner must practice the movements in the context for which it will be used (hence speech, or the chosen stimuli). Although an affected child may have deficits in auditory discrimination and auditory perceptual (option a) or phonological processing deficits (option b), which may need to be addressed, these are not the primary issues in CAS. Children with CAS do not necessarily have pragmatic language issues (option d). If the child with CAS does also have pervasive developmental disorder or autism, he or she may also have some pragmatic language issues that will need to be addressed, but it is not the important parameter to treat for CAS. Sounds are not worked on in isolation (option e) with CAS because the nature of the deficit is in planning the movement gesture; therefore, the syllable is the smallest unit to be targeted, usually through the use of real words.

205. b. The explanation of substitution errors, performance consistency, and phonological processes best describes the difference between characteristics of the CAS and those of phonological impairment. The explanation of weakness and hypernasality (option a) characterizes possible dysarthria and does not explain why you did not diagnose CAS. The absence of oral nonverbal apraxia (option c) does not rule out CAS. The absence of stuttering (option d) does not rule out CAS. Both CAS and phonological impairment imply difficulty with articulation (option e).

206. c. Many children with CAS, even severe CAS, have no oral nonverbal apraxia (option a). Oral nonverbal apraxia is tested in nonspeech contexts (option b). A test of speech skill would not elicit information about volitional nonspeech movement planning. Oral nonverbal apraxia is not related to neuromuscular impairment (option d). Oral nonverbal apraxia may be present with acquired CAS, CAS associated with complex neurobehavioral disorders, or idiopathic CAS (option e). In the oral structural-functional examination, the clinician can examine the child's ability to follow commands or imitate volitional nonspeech movement of the articulators.

207. a. Practicing movement in nonspeech activities would not be recommended (according to the principles of motor learning) for treating CAS. The motor learning literature has shown that in order to learn motor skill, people must practice the movement in the context for which it will be used (i.e., for improved speech production, the movements are practiced in the context of speech). Choosing the set size (option b) would be recommended because of the principle of mass versus distributed practice. *Massed practice* refers to the practice of a set of movements (such as consonant-vowel or consonant-vowel-consonant) many times without intervening stimuli. *Distributed practice* refers to practicing a number of movements (different syllables or words) within a session. Massed practice facilitates motor performance, which is accuracy of movement within the session during training, but hinders motor learning, which is retention and generalization of the movement. This issue is important to the choice of how large a stimulus set size to use. In general, the more severe the CAS, the smaller the set size the clinician would use. Practicing stimuli in blocks (option c) would also be recommended in the treatment of CAS. Blocked practice means that one stimulus would be practiced repeatedly; then practice would begin on the next stimulus, so that each one is practiced separately. In random practice, the stimuli are mixed up throughout the session. The cognitive motor literature has shown that random practice is better at facilitating the development of motor learning. It is therefore important that clinicians take this advantage into account when implementing treatment programs. For children who exhibit severe apraxia, random practice may be too difficult to allow rapid change in accuracy, which is motivational early in therapy. Relying first on extrinsic feedback and then intrinsic feedback would be recommended because research has shown that providing feedback on every trial actually inhibits motor learning. For children who are beginning therapy or who have severe CAS, however, early therapy requires frequent extrinsic (from the therapist) specific feedback to facilitate accurate movement. Afterwards, feedback should be less frequent and less specific (i.e., having the child rely more on intrinsic feedback: what they feel) to facilitate motor learning (generalization). Avoiding games and activities that take time and attention away from practice of producing the stimuli (option e) helps maximize the number of times a child practices the carefully selected stimuli, which helps the child improve motor skill.

208. e. If the child stays in an articulatory position longer and then makes the movement transition into the vowel shape and throughout the word more slowly, the child has more time to perform the proprioceptive processing to facilitate movement accuracy. A

great deal of research since the 1980s has demonstrated the important role of afferent proprioceptive information during the production of speech movements. Although thermal stimulation and brushing (option a) provide sensory stimulation, they do not give the child practice with the proprioceptive processing involved in ongoing speech motor control. Feedback about the success of generating air pressure and pushing the air out through rounded lips (option b) does not provide proprioception of movement gestures during speech. Although the mirror (option c) may provide visual feedback, it does not provide proprioceptive feedback. Bite blocks (option d) change the proprioception of jaw-tongue interactions as they occur during speech.

209. d. Children with CAS frequently exhibit lexical and sentential stress errors. Therapy goals focused on vocabulary (options a and b) and grammar (option c) may occur at some point in therapy, but they are not specific to CAS. Decreased strength and range of motion are not characteristics of CAS.

210. e. DTTC is a motor approach focused on improving the planning and programming of accurate movement gestures for volitional speech production. It incorporates visual and tactile cueing, varying rate and prosody, and implementing the principles of motor learning. Phonological awareness (option a) is not the core deficit in CAS. The cycles approach (option b) emphasizes the acquisition of phonological patterns and stems from a linguistic perspective of phonological behavior, rather than motor deficits. Fast ForWord Language (option c) was designed to address oral language skills with specific language impairment and auditory perceptual deficits, as opposed to motor planning and programming deficits. Enhanced milieu teaching is a naturalistic conversation-based strategy for teaching language and communication skills, rather than accurate movement gestures for correct syllable production.

211. d. Adult apraxia of speech is an acquired disorder of motor planning and programming. It is not a language (option a) or cognitive-based disorder (option b). Attention is the ability to attend to stimuli in the environment and not a speech disorder (option c). A disorder of motor execution is a dysarthria (option e).

212. b. The committee that developed the treatment guidelines argued that articulatory groping may be found in other disorders, such as phonemic paraphasias; therefore, it is nonspecific for acquired apraxia of speech. Options a and d are suprasegmental characteristics found in this population. Sound distortion errors (option c) is an articulatory

characteristic, and difficulty initiating utterances (option e) is also a characteristic found in the speech of persons with acquired apraxia of speech.

213. c. Ataxic dysarthria is most likely to be confused with apraxia of speech because of some overlap in the speech characteristics of the two disorders. Motor speech disorders are neurologically based impairments of motor planning, programming, neuromuscular control, or execution of speech. Apraxia is a disorder of motor planning and programming, while dysarthria manifests in problems of neuromuscular control or execution of speech. The different types of dysarthria are associated with different lesions of the central and peripheral nervous systems.

214. d. Of all these treatments, the eight-step continuum/integral stimulation is the only one for which there is evidence of its efficacy in treating apraxia of speech. Options a and b are methods for improving velopharyngeal closure for speech and used with patients who present with dysarthria. Metronome pacing (option c) is used to slow speech rate and increase syllable stress. Amplification (option e) might be used in conjunction with apraxia treatment if the person had a hearing loss that would benefit from amplification.

215. c. A sound distortion would be characteristic of apraxia of speech. Distortions are variations of intended target sounds that are nonallophonic and not other phonemes.

216. b. In sound production treatment, the clinician targets minimal pairs. Minimal pairs contrast an error production with a target sound in order to eliminate homonymy. In the treatment of apraxia the treatment involves the production of words or phrases wherein target contrasts are minimally different (e.g., shot-sought). The other options (a, c, d, e) are levels of treatment used in phonetic practice.

217. c. Duffy (2005) suggested that if it is easier for the patient to produce automatic reactive utterances than to produce more complex, voluntary speech, an apraxia of speech should be suspected. Sequential motion rate (SMR) is assessed via repetition of the syllable string in option b. Options a, d, and e are levels of linguistic complexity that may be used in the assessment of motor speech disorders.

218. b. In addition to lesions of the cortical areas listed above, lesions to the left anterior insula can produce apraxia of speech. The other options are not anatomical sites where lesions have been associated with apraxia of speech.

219. a. Because apraxia of speech usually co-occurs with aphasia, some authorities have argued that it is not a different disorder but is one manifestation of the aphasia. Options b and e are motor speech disorders that reflect different sites of lesion. Dementia (option c) is a static or degenerative cognitive disorder that can affect attention, memory, language, and problem solving. Cluttering (option d) is a fluency disorder that consists of rapid and irregular speaking rate, excesses disfluencies, and frequent additional symptoms such as language or phonological errors and attention problems.

220. c. Apraxia of speech rarely occurs in isolation. When it does occur, it is most frequently accompanied by aphasia, a language disorder. The sites of cortical brain lesions most commonly thought to produce apraxia of speech are the left inferior frontal cortex (Broca area), the left parietal cortex, and the left anterior insula.

221. c. Speech-sound errors, slow speech, and no problems with comprehension, reading, writing, naming, and grammatism indicate a diagnosis of apraxia of speech. Option a is not correct since there is no language problem. Similarly option b may be excluded since there is no evidence of weakness or incoordination of movement. The symptoms are not consistent with Alzheimer disease (option d), a cognitive disorder, or depression (option e), which is an affective disorder of mood. However, depression is often found in association with neurologic disease.

222. a. It has been suggested that different sites of lesion produce different apraxic characteristics. The sites of cortical brain lesions most commonly thought to produce apraxia of speech are the left inferior frontal cortex (Broca area), the left parietal cortex, and the left anterior insula. Etiology (option b), gender (option c), handedness (option d), and education (option e) have not been associated with different subtypes of apraxia of speech.

223. c. Patients with apraxia of speech often complain that they cannot pronounce words correctly. Options a, b, and d are symptoms of language-based problems (aphasia), while option e is sometimes a complaint of a person with a dysarthria.

224. a. PROMPT is the only one of these treatments for which there is some evidence to support its use. It is an approach that uses tactile cues to furnish touch pressure, kinesthetic, and proprioceptive cues to facilitate speech production skills. The sensory input is generally paired with additional auditory and visual information for the patient. Option b, metronome pacing, is used to manipulate a speaker's rate, and prosthetic devices (option d), such as a voice amplifier, are designed to improve speech. Option e provides the speaker with some type of physiologic signal that is typically not available in an effort to improve speech production. Nonspeech oromotor training has been used, but no documented change in speech production skills has been forthcoming.

225. c. Duffy (2005) suggested that in more severe cases of acquired apraxia of speech, a nonverbal oral apraxia usually accompanies the disorder. Dementia (option a) is a static or degenerative cognitive disorder that can effect attention, memory, language, and problem solving. Aphasia (option b) is an acquired language disorder that may manifest in difficulty producing or comprehending spoken or written language. Aphasia may co-occur with the motor speech disorders apraxia and dysarthria. Options d and e are types of dysarthria that reflect different sites of lesion.

Bibliography

Adamovich, B. B., & Henderson, J. (1992). *Scales of Cognitive Ability for Traumatic Brain Injury.* Austin, TX: Pro-Ed.

Adams, S. G., & Page, A. D. (2000). Effects of selected practice and feedback variables on speech motor learning. *Journal of Medical Speech-Language Pathology, 4,* 215–220.

Bayles, K. A., Tomoeda, C. K., Cruz, R. F., et al. (2000). Functional communication skills of late-stage individuals with Alzheimer's disease. *Alzheimer Disease and Associated Disorders, 14,* 176–181.

Beukelman, D. R., Ball, L. J., & Pattee, G. L. (2004). Intervention decision making for persons with amyotrophic lateral sclerosis. *Asha Leader, 14,* 4–5.

Beukelman, D. R., & Yorkston, K. M. (1977). A communication system for the severely dysarthric speaker with an intact language system. *Journal of Speech and Hearing Disorders, 42,* 265–270.

Cahill, L. M., Turner, A. B., Stabler, P. A., et al. (2004). An evaluation of continuous positive airway pressure therapy (CPAP) in the treatment of hypernasality following traumatic brain injury. *Journal of Head Trauma Rehabilitation, 19,* 241–253.

Clark, H. M. (2003). Neuromuscular treatments for speech and swallowing: A tutorial. *American Journal of Speech-Language Pathology, 12,* 400–415.

Dromey, C., Ramig, L. O., & Johnson, A. B. (1995). Phonatory and articulatory changes associated with increased vocal intensity in Parkinson disease: A case study. *Journal of Speech and Hearing Research, 38,* 751–764.

Duffy, J. R. (2005). *Motor speech disorders: Substrates, differential diagnosis, and management.* (2nd ed.). St. Louis: Elsevier Mosby.

Delis, D. C., Kramer, J. H., Kaplan, E., et al. (2000). *California Verbal Learning Test* (2nd ed.). San Antonio, TX: Psychological Corporation.

Folstein, M., Folstein, S., & McHugh, P. R. (1975). Mini-Mental State: A practical method of grading the cognitive state of patients for the clinician. *Journal of Psychiatric Research, 12,* 189–198.

Ross, D. (1986). *Ross Information Processing Assessment.* Austin, TX: Pro-Ed.

The Psychological Corporation. (1997). *WAIS-III-WMS-III Technical Manual.* San Antonio, TX: Author.

Wilson, B. A., Cockburn, J., & Baddeley, A. D. (2003). *The Rivermead Behavioural Memory Test–Second Edition.* London: Pearson Assessment.

Esposito, S. J., Mitsumoto, H., & Shanks, M. (2000). Use of palatal lift and palatal augmentation prosthesis to improve dysarthria in patients with amyotrophic lateral sclerosis: A case series. *Journal of Prosthetic Dentistry, 83,* 90–98.

Farrell, A., Theodoros, D., Ward, E., et al. (2005). Effects of neurosurgical management of Parkinson's disease on speech characteristics and oromotor function. *Journal of Speech, Language, and Hearing Research, 48,* 5–20.

Forrest, K. (2002). Are oral-motor exercises useful in the treatment of phonological/articulatory disorders? *Seminars in Speech and Language, 25,* 15–25.

Helm-Estabrooks, N., Hanson, E. K., Yorkston, K. M., et al. (2004). Speech supplementation techniques for dysarthria: a systematic review. (ANCDS Bulletin Board). *Journal of Medical Speech-Language Pathology, 12,* 9–29.

Helm-Estabrooks, N., Yorkston, K., Spencer, K., et al. (2003). Behavioral management of respiratory/phonatory dysfunction from dysarthria: A systematic review of the evidence. *Journal of Medical Speech-Language Pathology, 11*(2), 13–38.

Hixon, T. J., Hawley, J. L., & Wilson, K. J. (1982). An around-the-house device for the clinical determination of respiratory driving pressure: A note on making simple even simpler. *Journal of Speech and Hearing Disorders, 47,* 413–415.

Hixon, T. J., Weismer, G., & Hoit, J. D. (2008). *Preclinical speech science.* San Diego, CA: Plural Publishing.

Hodge, M., & Hall, S. (1994). Effects of syllable characteristics and training on speaking rate in a child with dysarthria secondary to near-drowning. In J. Till, K. Yorkston & D. Beukelman (Eds.), *Motor Speech Disorders.* Baltimore: Paul H. Brookes.

Hustad, K. C. (2001). Unfamiliar listeners' evaluation of speech supplementation strategies for improving the effectiveness of severely dysarthric speech. *Augmentative and Alternative Communication, 17,* 213–220.

Hustad, K. C. (2007). Contribution of two sources of listener knowledge to intelligibility of speakers with cerebral palsy. *Journal of Speech, Language, and Hearing Research, 50,* 1228–1240.

Hustad, K. C., & Beukelman, D. (2002). Listener comprehension of severely dysarthric speech: Effects of linguistic cues and stimulus cohesion. *Journal of Speech, Language, and Hearing Research, 45,* 545–558.

Hustad, K. C., & Garcia, J. M. (2002). The influences of alphabet supplementation, iconic gestures, and predictive messages on intelligibility of speakers with cerebral palsy. *Journal of Medical Speech-Language Pathology, 10,* 279–286.

Karnell, M. P., Hansen, J., Hardy, J. C., et al. (2004). Nasalance measurements as outcome indices for palatal lift management: Lift in versus lift out. *Journal of Medical Speech-Language Pathology, 21,* 21–30.

Kent, R. D., Kent, J. F., Rosenbek, J. C., et al. (1997). A speaking task analysis of the dysarthria in cerebellar disease. *Folia Phoniatrica et Logopaedica, 49,* 63–82.

Knock, T. R., Ballard, K., Robin, D., et al. (2000). Influence of order of stimulus presentation on speech motor learning: A principled approach to treatment for apraxia of speech. *Aphasiology, 14,* 653–668.

Kuehn, D. P. (1997). The development of a new technique for treating hypernasality: CPAP. *American Journal of Speech Language Pathology, 6,* 5–8.

Kuehn, D. P., Imrey, P. B., Tomes, L., et al. (2002). Efficacy of continuous positive airway pressure for treatment of hypernasality. *Cleft Palate± Craniofacial Journal, 39,* 267–276.

McHenry, M. A., & Liss, J. (2006). The impact of stimulated vocal loudness on nasalance in dysarthria. *Journal of Medical Speech-Language Pathology, 14,* 197–205.

Moore, C. A. (1993). Symmetry of mandibular muscle activity as an index of coordinative strategy. *Journal of Speech and Hearing Research, 36,* 1145–1157.

Moore, C. A., Smith, A., & Ringel, R. L. (1988). Task-specific organization of activity in human jaw muscles. *Journal of Speech and Hearing Research, 31,* 670–680.

McWilliams, B. J., & Bradley, D. P. (1965). Ratings of velopharyngeal closure during blowing and speech. *Cleft Palate Journal, 2,* 46–55.

Murdoch, B. E., Pitt, G., Theodoros, D. G., et al. (1999). Real-time continuous visual biofeedback in the treatment of speech breathing disorders following childhood traumatic brain injury: Report of one case. *Pediatric Rehabilitation, 3,* 5–20.

Netsell, R., & Rosenbek, J. C. (1985). Treating the dysarthrias. In J. K. Darby (Ed.), *Speech and Language Evaluation in Neurology: Adult Disorders.* New York: Grune & Stratton.

Ramig, L. O., Countryman, S., Thompson, L. L., et al. (1995). Comparison of two forms of intensive speech treatment for Parkinson disease. *Journal of Speech and Hearing Research, 38,* 1232–1251.

Ramig, L. O., & Dromey, C. (1996). Aerodynamic mechanisms underlying treatment related changes in vocal intensity in patients with Parkinson disease. *Journal of Speech and Hearing Research, 39,* 798–807.

Ramig, L. O., Sapir, S. S., Fox, C., et al. (2001). Changes in vocal loudness following intensive voice treatment (LSVT) in individuals with Parkinson's disease: A comparison with untreated patients and normal age-matched controls. *Movement Disorders, 16,* 79–83.

Spencer, K., Yorkston, K., & Duffy, J. R. (2003). Behavioral management of respiratory/phonatory dysfunction from dysarthria: A flowchart for guidance in clinical decision making. *Journal of Medical Speech-Language Pathology, 2,* 39–61.

Spielman, J., Ramig, L. O., Mahler, L., et al. (2007). Effects of an extended version of the Lee Silverman Voice Treatment on voice and speech in Parkinson's disease. *American Journal of Speech-Language Pathology, 16,* 95–107.

Tiffany, W. R. (1980). The effects of syllable structure on diadochokinetic and reading rates. *Journal of Speech and Hearing Research, 23,* 894–908.

Wambaugh, J. (2002). A summary of treatments for apraxia of speech and review of replicated approaches. *Seminars in Speech and Language, 23,* 293–308.

Wambaugh, J. (2004). Stimulus generalization effects of sound production treatment for apraxia of speech. *Journal of Medical Speech-Language Pathology, 12,* 77–92.

Warren, D. W., & DuBois, A. B. (1964). A pressure-flow technique for measuring velopharyngeal orifice area during continuous speech. *Cleft Palate Journal, 16,* 52–71.

Wood, P. H. N. (1980). Appreciating the consequences of disease: The classification of impairments, disability and handicaps. *The WHO Chronicle, 43,* 376–380.

Yorkston, K. M., Beukelman, D. R., Strand, E. A., et al. (1999). *Management of Motor Speech Disorders in Adults and Children.* (2nd ed.). Austin, TX: Pro-Ed.

Yorkston, K. M., Hammen, V. L., Beukelman, D. R., et al. (1990). The effect of rate control on the intelligibility and naturalness of dysarthric speech. *Journal of Speech and Hearing Disorders, 55,* 550–560.

Yorkston, K. M., Miller, R. M., & Strand, E. A. (1995). *Management of speech and swallowing in degenerative diseases.* San Antonio, TX: Communication Skill Builders.

Yorkston, K. M., Strand, E., Miller, R., et al. (1993). Speech deterioration in amyotrophic lateral sclerosis. Implications for the timing of intervention. *Journal of Medical Speech-Language Pathology, 1,* 35–46.

Yorkston, K. M., Spencer, K. A., Duffy, J. R., et al. (2001). Evidence-based practice guidelines for dysarthria: Management of velopharyngeal function. *Journal of Medical Speech-Language Pathology, 9,* 257–273.

CHAPTER 12

Dysphagia

JoAnne Robbins
Jacqueline Hind
Georgia Malandraki
Michelle Ciucci

ADULT DYSPHAGIA

1. Which laryngeal muscle is tested for motor function because its function (or lack thereof) will provide an understanding of swallowing sensory integrity?
   a. Thyrocricoid
   b. Cricothyroid
   c. Arytenoids
   d. Cricoarytenoid
   e. None of the above

2. The duration of swallowing apnea is longest in:
   a. Premature infants
   b. Full-term infants
   c. Young children
   d. Healthy young adults
   e. Healthy elderly people

3. Assessing pitch elevation provides information regarding:
   a. Upper esophageal sphincter opening
   b. Epiglottal inversion
   c. Potential for silent aspiration
   d. Base-of-tongue retraction
   e. Velopharngeal closure

4. Which of the following is not an immediate cause of swallowing difficulty in patients undergoing radiation treatment for head and neck cancer?
   a. Mucositis
   b. Taste changes
   c. Fibrosis
   d. Oral or pharyngeal dryness or both
   e. None of the above

5. When a patient with head and neck cancer is evaluated after surgery, it is most important to know:
   a. Current anatomy as described in the operative report
   b. How much radiation treatment was administered
   c. Type of chemotherapy
   d. Smoking history
   e. mucositis

6. Swallowing problems after intubation are:
   a. Unusual
   b. Often transient
   c. Predictable
   d. Always permanent
   e. Age related

7. A Zenker diverticulum is found in:
   a. The nasopharynx
   b. The stomach
   c. The thoracic esophagus
   d. Proximity to the upper esophageal sphincter
   e. The oropharynx

8. In a videofluoroscopic examination of swallowing function, a patient exhibits premature spillover and delayed initiation of the pharyngeal phase of the swallow. Of the following techniques, which would be the first to evaluate during the fluoroscopic examination?
   a. Chin tuck
   b. Turn head toward the weak side
   c. Mendelsohn maneuver
   d. Tilt head toward the strong side
   e. Supraglottic swallow

9. An adult patient in whom a pharyngeal tumor was diagnosed is referred for a swallowing evaluation. The patient is currently on a regular diet but reports some difficulty with solid foods and frequent coughing with thin liquids. During the videofluoroscopic examination, pharyngeal residue is observed with solids and semisolids, which is cleared with secondary swallows and no signs of penetration. The patient is scheduled to have pharyngeal surgery in 2 weeks. What would be the most likely recommendation for this patient?
   a. The patient's status should be NPO (*nil per os* [Latin], meaning "nothing by mouth") until the surgery is performed
   b. The patient should use a chin tuck technique while eating semisolids and solids
   c. The patient should remain on a regular diet and be reevaluated after the surgery
   d. The patient should remain on a regular diet before and after the surgery
   e. None of the above

10. A 73-year-old man is in a hospital after a stroke. He has been receiving all nutrition through a nasogastric tube tube for the past few weeks. During the clinical and bedside examination, you observe that the patient drools, has a very gurgly voice quality, and has a weak cough. What would be the next most appropriate step in the diagnosis for this patient?
    a. Test trial swallows with liquid and paste consistencies to determine the need for referral for a videofluoroscopic swallowing examination
    b. Directly refer the patient for a videofluoroscopic examination of his swallowing function
    c. Advise the patient to remain on nasogastric tube for a few more weeks until his swallow function improves, and reevaluate him at that time
    d. Directly refer the patient for an ultrasound examination of his swallowing function
    e. Recommend use of the chin-tuck position

11. On videofluoroscopic examination, a patient exhibits vallecular residue after the swallow. What would be the likely cause of this?
    a. Reduced cricopharyngeal opening
    b. Reduced velopharyngeal closure
    c. Lingual dysfunction
    d. a and c
    e. Labial spillage

12. During a videofluoroscopic examination, a patient exhibits markedly reduced anterior and superior hyolaryngeal complex movement. Some of the consequences of this event might include:
    a. Reduced opening of the upper esophageal sphincter
    b. Reduced epiglottic inversion
    c. Nasal regurgitation
    d. a and b
    e. All of the above

13. A patient has a tumor at the right trigeminal motor nuclei in the brainstem. Some symptoms would include:
    a. Reduced strength of the muscles of mastication in the contralateral (opposite) side
    b. Reduced strength of the muscles of mastication bilaterally
    c. Reduced strength of the muscles of mastication in the ipsilateral (same) side
    d. Reduced production of saliva in the ipsilateral side
    e. Reduced production of saliva in the contralateral side

14. A patient appears to have difficulty with obtaining good laryngeal elevation when he attempts to swallow his saliva. What muscle or muscles should be considered as possible contributors to the failure of this elevation?
    a. Mylohyoid
    b. Geniohyoid

c. Thyrohyoid
d. a and b
e. All of the above

15. When a patient is asked to stick out the tongue, the tongue deviates to the right. That means that the patient probably has a lesion in:
   a. The right cranial nerve XII
   b. The left cranial nerve XII
   c. The medulla bilaterally
   d. The pons bilaterally
   e. None of the above

16. In a male patient, food residue is noted in his left buccal cavity. His left lower face has very limited movement, but he can wrinkle his forehead bilaterally. This is suggestive of a:
   a. Left cortical lesion
   b. Right cortical lesion
   c. Left peripheral lesion
   d. Right peripheral lesion
   e. Bilateral cortical lesion

17. A 38-year-old patient who has had a recent stroke is undergoing videofluoroscopic swallowing examination. During the examination, the patient is observed using serial swallows to swallow even small amounts of liquid. Which of the following is *not* a possible cause of this symptom?
   a. Tongue weakness
   b. Pharyngeal weakness
   c. Fear of choking
   d. Anterior loss of food
   e. All are possible causes

18. Of the following characteristics of dysphagia, which is *not* commonly observed in patients with Parkinson disease?
   a. Excessive lingual rocking
   b. Drooling
   c. Inappropriate laughter while swallowing
   d. Delay in initiation of the pharyngeal response
   e. a and b

19. A 35-year-old woman is referred for a dysphagia evaluation with complaints of food sticking at the level of the sternal notch and extremely bad breath upon waking. A videofluoroscopic examination shows that her oropharyngeal swallowing mechanism is intact. The appropriate plan for this client is:
   a. Refer her for an evaluation of esophageal functioning
   b. Refer her to pulmonologists
   c. Have the patient begin lingual exercises to increase intrabolus pressure and facilitate esophageal transit

d. Send a report to her physician indicating that her condition is normal
   e. Modify diet viscosity

20. During a videofluoroscopic examination, recording images in the anteroposterior position allows for:
   a. Optimal visualization of epiglottic inversion
   b. Optimal visualization of bilateral pharyngeal movement and stasis
   c. Optimal visualization of aspiration
   d. Optimal visualization of the base of the tongue and posterior pharyngeal wall contact
   e. All of the above

21. In the dining room of a long-term care facility, you are evaluating the safety of oral intake for a patient with a diagnosis of Alzheimer disease. Which of the following should you consider during the examination?
   a. How the patient is positioned in the chair
   b. How much supervision the patient receives at mealtime
   c. The amount of outside distractions (i.e., TV, other people talking)
   d. Level of communication skills
   e. All of the above

22. A 62-year-old man with a recent right-sided cortical cerebral vascular accident is referred for a dysphagia evaluation because his nurses have observed him coughing when drinking. A videofluoroscopic examination reveals aspiration when he drinks thin liquids from a cup, occurring before the pharyngeal response is initiated. Which of the following is *not* a logical compensatory behavior to evaluate during the radiographic evaluation:
   a. Drinking with his chin tucked
   b. Taking a smaller sip of liquid
   c. Drinking liquid that is nectar-thick
   d. Turning his head to the right while drinking
   e. Drinking liquid that is milkshake consistency

23. Which of the following is *not* used to diagnose dysphagia?
   a. Videofluoroscopic swallowing assessment
   b. Fiberoptic endoscopic evaluation of swallowing (FEES)
   c. Digital laryngeal manipulation
   d. Bedside swallowing evaluation
   e. Ultrasonography

24. Isometric lingual exercises as a rehabilitative treatment for dysphagia would be appropriate for which of the following observations during a videofluoroscopic swallowing assessment?
   a. Excessive vallecular residue
   b. Nasal reflux

c. Reduced labial closure

d. Stasis in the mid-esophagus

e. All of the above

25. A 75–year-old patient with normal esophageal function is referred for a videofluoroscopic swallowing assessment because of weight loss. His medical history includes a respiratory infection 6 months ago. The fluoroscopic examination indicates no aspiration but does demonstrate trace penetration with one large bolus from a cup of thin liquid. Semisolids and solids are swallowed without difficulty. His diet is normal, and his appetite is good. His oral mechanism examination in within normal limits. The appropriate plan for this client is:

a. Referral to a neurologist

b. Beginning oromotor exercises to prevent penetration during swallowing

c. No therapy, because his oropharyngeal swallowing mechanism is age appropriate

d. Recommendation that he tuck his chin whenever he drinks

e. Thicken liquids to nectar consistency

26. Which of the following is *not* reliably determined during a noninstrumental bedside screening assessment of swallowing?

a. Patient's attention to the task of eating

b. Aspiration

c. Efficiency of mastication

d. Adequacy of labial seal

e. Ability to follow directions

27. Which of the following physiological processes is facilitated by hyolaryngeal excursion during swallowing?

a. Opening of the lower esophageal sphincter

b. Opening of the upper esophageal sphincter

c. Velar elevation

d. Vocal fold abduction

e. Labial closure

28. A 49-year-old man underwent a partial glossectomy surgery 6 months ago for lingual cancer. What is most likely to be clinically observed during a videofluoroscopic evaluation?

a. Difficulty propelling liquids through the oral cavity

b. Reduced labial seal

c. Aspiration during the swallow

d. Difficulty propelling solids through the oral cavity

e. All of the above

29. Which of the following is *not* an approach used to stimulate swallowing sensory awareness?

a. Texture

b. Temperature

c. Auditory

d. Taste

e. Touch pressure cues

30. The primary feature of lateral medullary syndrome (LMS), also called *Wallenberg syndrome*, is:

a. Oral stasis

b. Incomplete opening of the upper esophageal sphincter

c. Nasal regurgitation

d. Silent aspiration

e. Labial spill

31. Which of the following is *not* a phase of swallowing?

a. Oral

b. Pharyngeal

c. Esophageal

d. Laryngeal

e. Oral preparatory phase

32. Which of the following is commonly identified as a normal, healthy change in swallowing function with old age?

a. Nasal regurgitation

b. Slower initiation of the pharyngeal response

c. Stasis in the vallecula

d. Premature opening of the upper esophageal sphincter

e. None of the above

33. Maximum lingual pressure generation decreases with healthy aging as a function of:

a. Sarcopenia

b. Increased lingual rigidity

c. Lingual hemiparesis

d. None of the above: that concept is inaccurate

e. All of the above contribute to decreased lingual pressure generation

34. Diet modification as a compensatory strategy for dysphagia:

a. Is usually appropriate only in long-term care settings

b. Refers only to the texture of liquids and solid food

c. Is the first strategy to use

d. Is useful when behavioral or postural strategies, or both, are ineffective

e. Is used only for adult patients

35. Which of the following is *not* a risk factor for developing pneumonia?

a. Dysphagia

b. Poor oral hygiene

c. Being edentulous

d. Dependence for feeding

e. Motor speech disorder

36. A 78-year-old man with a diagnosis of amyotrophic lateral sclerosis (ALS) undergoes an outpatient evaluation of swallowing function. He currently lives at home with his family and has a diet of pureed solids and thin liquids. During the evaluation, he is noted to aspirate with all consistencies. Postural, dietary, and behavioral strategies do not eliminate aspiration. What is the logical next step?
    a. Refer the patient to a gastroenterologist so that a nasogastric tube can be placed before the patient leaves the hospital, to provide nutrition in the interim while waiting to have a permanent gastrostomy tube placed
    b. Discuss the options of continuing oral intake versus tube feeding with the patient and his family to develop a treatment plan
    c. Send the patient home with the recommendation to eat minimal amounts of food until a gastrostomy tube can be placed
    d. Explain to the patient that receiving nutrition from a gastrostomy tube will prevent him from getting pneumonia
    e. None of the above

37. Which of the following interventions is not effective for improving the opening of the upper esophageal sphincter?
    a. Mendelsohn maneuver
    b. Shaker exercise
    c. Lingual protrusion exercise
    d. Botulinum toxin injection
    e. None of the above are effective

38. Which of the following professionals is not a critical member of the dysphagia treatment team in the acute poststroke period?
    a. Speech-language pathologist (SLP)
    b. Dietitian
    c. Neurologist
    d. Oncologist
    e. Nursing staff

PEDIATRIC DYSPHAGIA

39. You are assessing an infant who was born at 30 weeks' gestation. If there are no severe postnatal complications, at what postnatal week would you expect the infant to be able to sustain nutritional needs by mouth without supplementation?
    a. Immediately after birth
    b. 2 weeks after birth
    c. 4 weeks after birth
    d. 6 weeks after birth
    e. 8 weeks after birth

40. At which age would a child be ready to transition to solid foods?
    a. 2 to 4 months
    b. 4 to 6 months
    c. 6 to 8 months
    d. 8 to 10 months
    e. 10 to 12 months

41. Which of the following does not contribute to increased protection of the airway in a 3-month-old infant?
    a. Flexibility of the thyroid and cricoid cartilages
    b. Close approximation of the velum to the epiglottis
    c. Positioning of larynx higher in the neck
    d. Larynx's remaining elevated and adducted for sequential swallows
    e. None of the above contribute to airway protection

42. A 5-month-old infant is taking soft cereal from a spoon but demonstrates involuntary protrusion of the tongue during oropharyngeal transit. What is the best course of action?
    a. Change texture to a thinner solid
    b. Place the food on the hard palate
    c. Train the parent in oral motor exercises to reduce tongue thrust
    d. Wait to see if this behavior disappears by 7 months of age
    e. Wait to see if this behavior disappears by 12 months of age

43. Which is the most common medical intervention for sialorrhea associated with cerebral palsy in children?
    a. Therapy to increase swallowing frequency
    b. Labial and lingual strengthening exercises
    c. Botulinum toxin injection
    d. Removal of the salivary glands
    e. Biofeedback treatment

44. At what anatomical level can the pharyngeal swallow be triggered and still be considered timely for a healthy person?
    a. Anterior faucial pillar
    b. Valleculae
    c. Pyriform sinuses
    d. a and b
    e. All of the above

45. A patient demonstrates decreased sensation in the oral cavity, although taste appears to be intact. Which cranial nerve do you suspect to be impaired?
    a. Cranial nerve V: trigeminal
    b. Cranial nerve VII: facial
    c. Cranial nerve IX: glossopharyngeal
    d. Cranial nerve XII: hypoglossal
    e. a and b

46. Which of the following is considered the most commonly recommended long-term alternative to nutrition and hydration by mouth?
    a. Feeding through Dobhoff tube
    b. Feeding through nasogastric tube
    c. Total parenteral nutrition
    d. Percutaneous gastrostomy
    e. None of the above

47. You note that a patient's velum deviates to the right during a sustained vowel. You suspect deficits in:
    a. Left cranial nerve X
    b. Right cranial nerve X
    c. Left cranial nerve XII
    d. Right cranial nerve XII
    e. Right cranial nerve VII

48. The "gold standard" for ruling out aspiration is considered:
    a. The clinical or bedside swallowing evaluation
    b. FEES
    c. Videofluoroscopy
    d. Ultrasonography
    e. Scintigraphy

49. A patient has a total laryngectomy. Of the following complications, which would be of the least concern?
    a. Aspiration of the bolus
    b. Stricture of the upper esophageal sphincter
    c. Abnormal tissue pockets in the pharynx
    d. Development of a fistula
    e. All of the above

50. Which of the following types of sensation is the most effective for eliciting the pharyngeal swallow?
    a. Taste
    b. Temperature
    c. Pain
    d. Touch
    e. Smell

51. An 18-month-old boy is seen by a speech pathologist for a speech and language evaluation. During the initial interview, the parents report that the boy started taking spoon feedings at 15 months of age; he frequently gags, especially on new textures; he easily becomes lethargic during feedings; and his feeding periods last longer than 50 minutes. The parents have also noticed that the boy has not gained any significant weight during the past 2 months. On the basis of this information, what should the SLP do?
    a. Tell the parents that these feeding behaviors are typical of their son's age and that they should not worry
    b. Refer the child for a complete swallowing and feeding evaluation

    c. Counsel the parents regarding spoon feeding and cup drinking techniques; a complete evaluation and treatment plan are not necessary at this point
    d. Suggest that the boy come back in 6 months for a complete evaluation
    e. Implement a home feeding plan to be carried out by the parents

52. A clinician is called into the neonatal intensive care unit to evaluate the oral feeding skills of a premature infant. During careful bedside examination, the clinician observes that the infant has a resting respiratory rate of 60 breaths per minute, and during feeding, the respiratory rate increases to more than 90 breaths per minute. The next step of the clinician is to:
    a. Stop oral feeding immediately
    b. Continue oral feeding but provide more breaks
    c. Stop feeding until the respiratory rate returns to normal levels and then continue
    d. Suggest nonnutritive sucking on a pacifier and continue oral feedings with frequent breaks
    e. None of the above

53. The swallowing function is being examined in a 2½-year-old child with spastic cerebral palsy, a hyperactive gag reflex, frequent coughing during feedings, and reduced oral sensation. What instrumental technique would be preferable to use in the evaluation of this child?
    a. Videofluoroscopy
    b. FEES
    c. Ultrasonography
    d. Auscultation
    e. Scintigraphy

54. A school-based SLP is performing a clinical bedside evaluation of Jenny, a 9-year-old girl with a diagnosis of cerebral palsy. Her condition is characterized by athetoid movements and low muscle tone. She is also severely dysarthric but has normal cognitive and intellectual skills. Her parents are insisting on her being orally fed, although you notice that she has severe difficulties to form and keep a bolus in her mouth and that her mealtimes last more than an hour. The parents also report that she exhibits frequent coughing with liquids, and they have noticed that Jenny has not gained weight in the past few months. What should the school SLP recommend for Jenny?
    a. Because her parents insist on oral feedings, the SLP should continue oral feedings at school and have Jenny perform oral-motor exercises to enable better bolus formation and reduction of anterior loss
    b. Jenny should be referred for a videofluoroscopic examination of her swallowing function, the results of which would determine whether she can continue oral feedings

c. If, because of the findings of the clinical evaluation, the SLP feels uncomfortable continuing oral feedings at school, the SLP should have the parents come to school and feed the child

d. The SLP should perform FEES to determine whether the child should be further referred for a videofluoroscopic evaluation

e. None of the above

55. A 9-month-old boy is seen for a feeding assessment. The infant was full-term and did not exhibit any feeding difficulties in the first months of life. The parents now report that they are worried because the child frequently gags, ejects food involuntarily with his tongue, sucks on the spoon during spoon feeding, and drools when teething. According to this information, which of the following is *not* correct?

a. Most of these behaviors are typical of the developmental feeding age of 5 months

b. The infant is healthy, and all his behaviors are typical of his age

c. The infant is mildly delayed in his feeding development

d. Drooling when teething is a typical behavior for his age

e. Hand and mouth feeding is common at this age

56. A mother is breastfeeding her 3-month-old infant. During feeding, she observes certain behavior that makes her stop the oral feeding and become concerned about her child's feeding. Which of the following behaviors (stress signal[s]) could she have noticed during the oral feeding?

a. The infant started breathing irregularly

b. The infant became lethargic during feeding

c. The infant started pushing the nipple away 5 minutes after the initiation of feeding

d. Both a and b

e. a, b, a and c

57. You are examining a 7-month-old girl who was born with trisomy 21 (Down syndrome). You observe generalized orofacial hypotonia and hyposensitivity focused on the facial muscles. On the basis of this information, what would be an appropriate treatment technique to increase orofacial sensitivity?

a. Apply deep, sustained pressure in and around the mouth

b. Apply firm but gentle stroking around the mouth and on the tongue

c. Mouth play with soft toys

d. Drinking through straws with a large diameter

e. Apply touch pressure to the tongue

58. The parents of a 5-month-old infant are about to start spoon feedings with the child. They are worried about this transition and decide to get some help from an SLP. Of the following strategies regarding spoon feedings, which would the SLP recommend?

a. The parents should use a long, round spoon at midtongue and slight downward pressure

b. The parents should use a flat spoon at the lateral portion of the tongue and slight downward pressure

c. The parents should use a flat spoon at midtongue and slight downward pressure

d. The parents should use a flat spoon at midtongue and no pressure

e. a and b

59. You are observing a 16-month-old child while the child is being fed by his mother. Whenever the spoon contacts the child's teeth, the child exhibits a tonic bite reflex. In this case, which of the following statements is true?

a. The tonic bite reflex disappears at 16 to 18 months of age, thus, this is a normal response

b. Pulling against the bite reflex will enable release of the bite

c. Dimming of the lights and quiet voices during feeding can reduce the frequency of occurrence of the reflex

d. Sensory stimulation of the faucial pillars will reduce the tonic bite reflex

e. None of the above are true

60. Mary is a newborn with a diagnosis of Pierre Robin sequence, characterized by micrognathia, a U-shaped cleft palate, and glossoptosis. You evaluate her oral-motor feeding skills when she is 2 days old. During the examination, what is the one clinical sign or symptom that you would *not* expect to see in this infant?

a. Ineffective suck

b. Nasal regurgitation

c. Anterior loss of liquid

d. Frequent gagging or choking

e. None of the above are expected

1. b. The cricothyroid muscle is the only laryngeal muscle innervated by the external branch of the superior laryngeal nerve. The external branch of this nerve also transmits sensory information from the supraglottic and glottic areas to the central nervous system. Thus, testing the motor function of the cricothyroid muscle (by asking the patient to raise the vocal pitch and evaluating the pitch range) yields an indication of the sensory integrity of the glottic and supraglottic areas. The term *thyrocricoid* (option a) is usually associated with the thyrocricoid membrane, and the arytenoids (option c) are small paired cartilages that constitute the posterior attachment of the vocal folds. The cricoarytenoid muscles (option d) are pairs of muscles that connect the cricoid and the arytenoid cartilages and receive their innervation from the recurrent laryngeal nerve of cranial nerve X (vagus nerve). Testing the motor function of the cricoarytenoid muscles is difficult, requires use of instrumental techniques, and can provide only sensory information regarding the subglottic laryngeal area.

2. e. In normal people, the functions of swallowing and respiration are well coordinated. Hence, every time a person swallows, complex hyolaryngeal actions close the laryngeal vestibule in order for respiration to cease during the swallow and for the airway to be protected from ingested material. Although swallowing apnea is longer in premature infants option a (4 seconds) than in full-term infants (0.67 to 0.87 seconds; option b), current research on the coordination between swallowing and respiration by evaluating the duration of swallowing apnea has revealed a significant age effect. As people age, the duration of swallowing apnea increases from 1 second in healthy young adults (option d) to 7.8 to 10.0 seconds in healthy elderly people. Many physiological parameters of deglutition apparently decline with age, and a longer swallowing apnea might reflect compensatory mechanisms to overcome these declines in other swallowing events.

3. c. Pitch elevation is a function achieved by the contraction of the cricothyroid muscle. The cricothyroid muscle is a laryngeal muscle and is not involved in functions such as the upper esophageal sphincter opening (option a), epiglottal inversion (option b) or base-of-tongue retraction (option d). Velopharyngeal closure separates the oropharynx and nasopharynx during swallowing and speech (option e). The cricothyroid muscle is innervated by the external branch of the superior laryngeal nerve. The external branch of this nerve also transmits sensory information from the supraglottic and glottic

areas to the central nervous system. Thus, assessing pitch elevation is a means of testing the motor function of the cricothyroid muscle and, indirectly, the sensory innervation of the upper laryngeal aditus. This means that inability to raise vocal pitch may be a sign of compromised laryngeal sensation and therefore a sign of silent aspiration.

4. c. Mucositis (option a) and oral dryness, oropharyngeal dryness, or both (option d) are symptoms that might appear as immediate consequences of radiation therapy in patients with head and neck cancer. Such types of symptoms can cause oral pain and result in diet alterations or even non-oral nutrition. Altered taste (option b) is most commonly a late consequence of radiation treatment in these patients but is not known to significantly alter the swallowing physiology. Fibrosis (option c) is the result of reduced capillary flow in the radiated area and is a late consequence of radiation treatment and a more significant problem than altered taste. It has been associated with significant swallowing difficulties in patients with head and neck cancer.

5. a. For a patient with head and neck cancer, it is important to have information on all the factors listed. After surgery, however, the most important information is the anatomy of the head and neck area. It is crucial to know which oral, pharyngeal, or laryngeal structures were resected during the surgery, because the swallowing physiology can be differentially altered, depending on which structures or muscles are missing. Recommendations and treatment are influenced by the current anatomy of the patient. Not every such patient is treated with radiation or chemotherapy. There is no information in the question regarding radiation (option b), or chemotherapy (option c); even if this patient also had these types of treatment, it would not be as important as knowing the current anatomy. Smoking history (option d) would not dictate a therapeutic approach for such a patient. Mucositis, which is inflammation and ulceration of the mucous membranes may present if the patient also had chemotherapy and/or radiation treatment.

6. b. Swallowing problems that occur after intubation are often transient. It is not unusual for intubation to have an effect on the swallowing physiology (option a). Effects of intubation on the swallowing mechanism might include local tissue damage, edema, or paresis as a result of infection or pressure in the nasal, oral, laryngeal, or tracheal areas that might affect swallowing integrity. Clinical evidence has showed that such

effects are not always predictable (option c). Prolonged intubation can lead to permanent problems, but short-term intubation would rarely cause permanent damage. Age is not a predictive factor in terms of potential for swallowing problems (option e).

7. d. A Zenker diverticulum, also known as *pharyngoesophageal diverticulum*, is an outpouching of the mucosa of the pharynx, found just above the upper esophageal sphincter. It was named after the German physician Friedrich Albert von Zenker.

8. a. Premature spillover of the material into the pharynx is a delayed initiation of the pharyngeal phase. Such a delay puts the patient at high risk for aspiration before the swallow occurs. Chin tuck is a posturing technique that physiologically increases the vallecular spaces, prevents the bolus from prematurely entering the pharynx, and reduces the risk for aspiration before the swallow occurs. Turning the head to the weak side (option b) and to the strong side (option d) are posturing techniques suggested for cases of unilateral pharyngeal weakness or paralysis, which are not mentioned in this question. The Mendelsohn maneuver (option c) is a technique that prolongs the hyolaryngeal superior and anterior movement in order to keep the airway protected and the cricopharyngeal sphincter open for a longer duration during the swallow, which are not necessary in this case. The supraglottic swallow (option e) is a breath-holding technique designed to voluntarily close the vocal folds.

9. c. This patient's swallowing function was functional or only minimally compromised. There is definitely no indication that the patient is at risk that would justify NPO until the surgery is performed (option a). Furthermore, no information about swallowing ability will be available until after the surgery. Therefore, the physician cannot conclude that the patient should be on a regular diet after his surgery (option d) until after a reevaluation. Secondary swallows were adequate for clearing the residue, and there is no mention of a posturing technique, such as chin tuck, that was effective with solids and semisolids (option b). Thus, the patient should remain on a regular diet until his pharyngeal surgery is performed and then a reevaluation should be considered. Secondary swallows and control of bolus size could also be suggested while the patient is on a regular diet.

10. b. The patient's symptoms indicate that he is probably aspirating and may not have an effective protective cough. If you choose to do multiple trial swallows with him (option a) using liquid and paste consistencies, there would be a significant aspiration risk. An ultrasound swallowing examination (option d)

provides clinical information regarding the oral phase of swallowing but not in the pharyngeal phase. Advising the patient to remain on a nasogastric tube until his swallow improves (option c) or use of the chin-tuck (option e) are not diagnostic steps but treatment recommendations; to make such recommendations a complete diagnostic profile of this patient, through videofluoroscopic swallowing examination (option b), is necessary. A videofluoroscopic examination will provide you with the most useful clinical information and will allow you to decide appropriate treatments.

11. c. Normally, after the pharyngeal swallow is triggered, and as the bolus is directed toward the pharynx, the base of the tongue makes complete contact with the posterior pharyngeal wall. This generates enough pharyngeal pressure so that the bolus can be directed inferiorly. Lingual dysfunction, which is usually associated with reduced lingual strength, would cause decreased pharyngeal pressure and inadequate inferior bolus propulsion, leading to vallecular residue. Reduced cricopharyngeal opening (option a) during the pharyngeal phase of the swallow could cause residue above the upper esophageal sphincter and in the pyriform sinuses, but not in the vallecular spaces. The major symptom that could be caused by reduced velopharyngeal closure during the swallow (option b) would be nasal penetration and not residue in the valleculae. Labial spillage (option e) is a symptom generally found with problems of lip closure during swallowing.

12. d. During the pharyngeal phase of a swallow, as the pharyngeal response is triggered, the geniohyoid, thyrohyoid, and mylohyoid muscles contribute to the anterior and superior movement of the hyoid. This movement causes a mechanical pull of multiple structures, including the larynx, the epiglottis and the upper esophageal sphincter. As the hyoid moves anteriorly and superiorly, it enables the larynx to elevate and the epiglottis to invert, allowing for protection of the airway. It also facilitates the wider opening of the upper esophageal sphincter. Thus, reduced hyolaryngeal complex movement would lead to reduced laryngeal elevation and protection and to reductions both in the opening of the upper esophageal sphincter (option a) and in epiglottic inversion (option b). Nasal regurgitation (option c) is usually a result of reduced velopharyngeal closure or pharyngeal obstruction and is not connected with the hyolaryngeal complex movement.

13. c. The motor nuclei of the trigeminal nerve (cranial nerve V) innervate the muscles of mastication. Branches, located at both sides of the brainstem, each innervate the ipsilateral muscles of mastication.

Thus, a disruption (in this case, a tumor) at the right trigeminal motor nuclei would cause reduced strength of the muscles of mastication on the ipsilateral side of the face.

14. e. Laryngeal elevation during the pharyngeal phase of the swallow is achieved through anterior and superior movement of the hyoid, once the pharyngeal response has been triggered. The major muscles that contribute to this forward and superior movement of the hyoid include all three muscles listed.

15. a. The cranial nerve responsible for the motor innervation of the tongue is the hypoglossal nerve, or cranial nerve XII. A bilateral lesion at the level of the medulla (option c) would create tongue weakness or paralysis of the tongue. A bilateral lesion at the level of the pons (option d) would not affect the hypoglossal nerve; however, higher motor fibers traveling to the hypoglossal nuclei in the medulla could be affected. If this was the case, the symptoms would be obvious in both sides of the tongue. During midline tongue protrusion, the genioglossus muscle is the main muscle of action. With a right cranial nerve XII lesion, the action of the ipsilateral (the right) genioglossus muscle is compromised; thus, during tongue protrusion, only the left genioglossus muscle pushes the tongue in protrusion, causing it to deviate towards the weak (right) side. A lesion at the left cranial nerve XII (option b) would cause the tongue to deviate toward the left side.

16. b. The symptoms described in this question are indicative of a lesion involving the facial nerve (cranial nerve VII). If the lesion was peripheral (involving the right [option d] or the left [option c] facial nerve), the entire right or left side of the face, respectively, would be affected. This patient has paralysis of the lower face but normal function of the upper facial muscles at the left side. Facial muscles below the forehead receive contralateral cortical innervation, but the frontalis muscle (forehead muscle) receives bilateral cortical innervation. Therefore, if the lesion is in one motor cortex (cortical), or its descending pathway, the forehead is not paralyzed, but the lower face on the side contralateral to the lesion exhibits weakness or paralysis. Because the symptoms of weakness for this patient are on the left side, the cortical lesion is on the right side. The case in question is not symptomatic of a bilateral lesion (option e).

17. d. Serial swallows of small boluses can be the result of many conditions. Tongue weakness (option a) could potentially cause poor bolus formation that leads to oral residue after the swallow, and serial swallows are used to clear that residue. Pharyngeal weakness

(option b) can also result in pharyngeal residue after the swallow, and serial swallows, again, are used to clear the residue. Frequent episodes of prior aspiration or penetration may make a patient fearful of choking (option c), so that the patient would swallow only small portions of a bolus at a time. Anterior loss of food is not related to serial swallows.

18. c. Cardinal motor disturbances of Parkinson disease secondary to a loss of dopamine (tremor, rigidity, akinesia or bradykinesia) can affect the facial muscles and result in an expressionless, "mask-like" appearance. Oral dysmotility characterized by lingual rocking (option a), drooling (option b), and delayed initiation of the pharyngeal response (option d) reflect the disintegration of volitional and automatic movements caused by Parkinson disease–related akinesia, bradykinesia, and rigidity.

19. a. Food sticking at the sternal notch and extremely bad breath upon waking are characteristic of esophageal stasis and gastroesophageal reflux; thus, further assessment of esophageal function is warranted. Referral to a pulmonologist (option b) would not be appropriate because respiratory involvement is not present. Lingual exercises (option c) would be appropriate only if oropharyngeal dysfunction were observed during the videofluoroscopic evaluation. Because the complaints are consistent with esophageal dysfunction, it would be negligent to do nothing (option d). Diet modification (option e) is a treatment and would not be appropriate since further diagnostic study is necessary.

20. b. The anteroposterior view allows for optimal visualization of bilateral movements and assessment of stasis. For example, effectiveness of a head turn for unilateral stasis is best evaluated in this view. Biomechanical movements, such as epiglottic inversion (option a) and base of tongue retraction (option d), and aspiration (option c), determined through imaging of the larynx, occur at midline and are often difficult to visualize with anteroposterior imaging because of the overlapping position of the spinal column.

21. d. Positioning (option a), supervision (option b), and environment (option c) and level of communication skills (option d) have all been shown to significantly affect the safety and success of oral intake in patients with dementia.

22. d. Turning his head to the right would not be logical because head turn is generally effective for unilateral postswallow pharyngeal stasis, which was not observed. Chin tuck (option a) is an appropriate response because of the potential to increase

vallecular space and containment of the bolus anteriorly in the oral cavity. Reduced bolus size (option b) is also an appropriate response because the smaller bolus may be better contained within the vallecular space. Drinking nectar-thick liquids (option c). Milkshake consistency liquids (option e) are appropriate responses because the bolus stays more cohesive and moves more slowly through the oropharynx, which provides additional time for adequate airway protection.

23. c. Digital laryngeal manipulation is a treatment for vocal hyperfunction and not an assessment tool for dysphagia. Videofluoroscopy (option a) is the instrumental radiographic examination most commonly used to diagnose dysphagia. FEES (option b) is also a commonly used instrumental tool in which a fiberoptic laryngoscope is passed transnasally to the hypopharynx, where the larynx and surrounding structures are directly visualized. Ultrasound (option e) is an imaging method used for oral recording. A bedside evaluation (option d) is a noninstrumental screening procedure usually used to determine whether instrumental evaluation is warranted.

24. a. Isometric lingual exercises have been show to increase intraoral pressure during swallowing, thereby decreasing stasis of material in the vallecula. Increased tongue force would be contraindicated for patients who have nasal reflux (option b) because increased contact of the tongue to the hard palate may facilitate bolus passage into the nasopharynx. Poor labial closure (option c) results from dysfunction of the buccinator or orbicularis oris muscles and not of intrinsic or extrinsic lingual muscles. Although pharyngeal stasis (option d) may be decreased with increased intrabolus pressure, lingual exercises have not been shown to be effective in esophageal clearance, particularly as far downstream as the mid-esophagus.

25. c. Although a recent respiratory infection can be an indication of aspiration, the patient's videofluoroscopic results were within normal limits for his age. Referral to a neurologist (option a) and beginning oromotor exercises (option b) would therefore be inappropriate. Chin tuck (option d) and thickened liquids (option e) would not be indicated because his swallowing function is age appropriate, and thus intervention, postural or otherwise, is not required. Although weight loss can be an indicator of dysphagia, the fact that his diet is unchanged should lead the health care team to look for other causes.

26. b. Aspiration is missed in as many as 60% of patients who undergo a noninstrumental assessment of swallowing. In patients who have a diagnosis of dementia, it is particularly important to evaluate attention to eating (option a) during a noninstrumental evaluation to assess the need for environmental management and cuing (option e). Efficiency of mastication (option c) and adequacy of labial seal (option d) are directly observable during a noninstrumental evaluation and are useful in identifying postural needs (neutral head posture in the case of poor labial seal) or behavioral needs (lingual sweep of the oral cavity).

27. b. Anterior and superior movement of the hyoid and larynx pull on the cricoid cartilage and facilitate opening of the upper esophageal sphincter. Relaxation of the cricopharyngeus muscle is also crucial for opening of the upper esophageal sphincter. Relaxation of the smooth muscle and thus opening of the lower esophageal sphincter (option a) is not affected by hyolaryngeal excursion. The tensor and levator palati muscles lift the velum (option c) up and backwards, closing off the entrance to the nasal cavities above by coming into contact with the pharyngeal wall and are not directly influenced by hyolaryngeal excursion, although they move simultaneously during swallowing. Vocal fold adduction, not abduction (option d), occurs during the swallow to protect the airway. Finally, hyolaryngeal excursion does not affect the labial closure (option e) during swallowing.

28. d. Reduced lingual range and mobility can make moving more viscous material, such as semisolids and solids, a challenge. Transit of less viscous materials such as liquids (option a) is more easily facilitated by gravity and thus less likely to pose a problem. The labial seal (option b) is unlikely to be affected after a glossectomy, because the anterior facial muscles should be intact. Aspiration (option c) resulting from a weakened lingual pump is a potential problem, either before the pharyngeal response (as a result of incoordination of the bolus within the oral cavity) or after the pharyngeal response (as a result of increased postswallow residue); however, it is unlikely to occur because the hyolaryngeal mechanism should be well able to protect the airway during the pharyngeal response. In general, most patients are able to retain near-normal swallowing after glossectomy.

29. c. Auditory stimulation has not been shown to be an effective treatment tool to facilitate swallowing function. Increased texture (option a), cold temperature (option b), and tart taste (option d) of food have been shown in some populations to improve bolus awareness, thus improving the timing of swallowing

biomechanics and airway protection. Touch pressure cues to the faucial pillars and/or pharyngeal walls are also used to improve the timing of the swallow.

30. b. Occlusion of the posterior inferior cerebellar artery or one of its branches or of the vertebral artery, in which the lateral part of the medulla oblongata infarcts, results in LMS, characterized by incomplete opening of the upper esophageal sphincter. Oropharyngeal swallowing symptoms such as oral stasis (option a) nasal regurgitation (option c) and labial spillage of food (option e) are generally not associated with LMS. Sensory function of the larynx is intact in LMS, and thus silent aspiration (option d) is rare.

31. d. Although protection of the airway is a critical aspect of safe swallowing, clinicians and clinical researchers do not identify any phase of the swallow as laryngeal. For clinical and research purposes, the continuous swallow is divided into four consecutive phases: the preparatory phase, in which the bolus is masticated and formed into a bolus; (option e) the oral phase (option a), in which the bolus is moved into the pharynx through intrinsic lingual muscle contractions; the pharyngeal phase (option b), in which peristaltic contractions propel the bolus through the upper esophageal sphincter; and the esophageal phase (option c), which is characterized by sequential contractions of the esophagus and relaxation of the lower esophageal sphincter as the bolus is moved into the stomach.

32. b. Slower initiation of the pharyngeal response has been reported in normal, healthy older adults. This slowed response has been described as an "uncoupling" of the more volitional oral phases of the swallow with the more automatic pharyngeal phase. Nasal regurgitation (option a) is not associated with healthy aging but could be observed in patients with age-related neurological diseases. Increased stasis is not generally observed in healthy adults in the vallecula (option c) or in the upper esophageal sphincter (option d); however, elderly persons are more likely to be taking medications that dry the mucosa, which could predispose them to pharyngeal stasis. The upper esophageal sphincter also stiffens with age.

33. a. Sarcopenia is associated with age-related reductions in muscle mass and cross-sectional area, a reduction in the number or size of muscle fibers, and a transformation or selective loss of specific muscle fiber types. Sarcopenia is inherently associated with diminished strength. Healthy older persons demonstrate significantly reduced isometric (i.e., static) tongue pressures in comparison with younger counterparts.

In contrast, maximal tongue pressures generated during swallowing (i.e., dynamic) remain normal in magnitude because swallowing is a submaximal pressure-demanding activity. However, functional reserve is something from which elderly people can draw upon during physiologically stressful situations; thus, if this reserve is diminished, elderly people are at greater risk for dysphagia. There is no evidence of increased lingual rigidity (option b) with aging. Although lingual hemiparesis (option c) could cause changes in lingual pressure generation, it is not observed in healthy aging.

34. d. Eating is a psychosocial activity that is often associated with celebrations and often closely linked with interaction with other people. Patients on altered diets may become embarrassed to eat with others, or the poor palatability of modified foods may decrease their quality of life. Other interventions, including active rehabilitation and postural changes, should be explored before a diet is modified (option c). Diet modification can be useful, however, particularly in combination with active rehabilitation to maintain a healthy pulmonary system and with the cognitively challenged patient who may not be able to participate with other interventions. Diet modification is employed in all health care settings and homes (option a) and encompasses modifying not only the texture of liquids and solids (option b) but also their flavors and temperatures. Diet modification, if appropriate, is used across the lifespan.

35. c. Having (or not having) teeth is not a risk factor for pneumonia. However, poor oral hygiene (option b) allows bacteria to flourish in the oral cavity and, with aspiration (option a), predisposes a person to develop pneumonia. It has also been shown that dependence for feeding (option d) is likely to increase the risk of pneumonia if patients are fed by poorly or inappropriately trained staff. The care providers may deliver food or liquid too rapidly or in large amounts, putting the patient at risk for aspiration. Dependence for feeding is also associated with an extremely dependent state, and overall functional status is an important predictor of pneumonia. Persons with motor speech disorders (option e) also have concomitant feeding problems and are at risk for pneumonia.

36. b. All options for treatment (or nontreatment) should be explained to patients, along with relevant risks and benefits to each choice. Ultimately, a patient with intact cognition has the final decision in the treatment plan, and the SLP providing information for an informed decision. Although nonoral intake (option a) may be a viable option, it should be selected only after full consideration of other

options. Adequate nutrition is crucial for patients with ALS, and thus option (option c) could be potentially harmful. Gastrostomy tubes (option d) have not been shown to prevent pneumonia.

37. c. Although the tongue plays an important role in propelling the bolus through the upper esophageal sphincter, lingual protrusion is not a movement crucial for swallowing. The Mendelsohn maneuver (option a) is designed to increase the extent and duration of laryngeal elevation and therefore increase the duration and width of the opening of the upper esophageal sphincter. Shaker exercises (option b) aim to improve function of the anterior neck muscles and have been shown to improve the opening of the upper esophageal sphincter. Chemical myotomy of the cricopharyngeus muscle using botulinum neurotoxin type A (option d) has been shown to be effective in reducing dysphagia-associated hypertonicity of the upper esophageal sphincter.

38. d. An oncologist specializes in the diagnosis, prevention, and treatment of tumors (benign and malignant) and would typically be the specialist coordinating the multidisciplinary care of a patient with cancer. An oncologist would typically not play a role in the care of a patient after neurological insult (i.e., stroke). The SLP (option a) is the consultant with the greatest knowledge about swallowing and who performs the diagnostic evaluations and dysphagia therapeutic interventions. The dietitian (option b) must coordinate nutritional intake with regard to the recommendations provided by the SLP and the physician. The neurologist (option c) is typically the specialist coordinating total care in the acute poststroke period. Nursing staff (option e) provide and carry out interventions prescribed by the other professionals.

39. c. In general, suckling and swallowing can sustain nutritional needs at approximately 34 weeks of gestational age. Additional development of at least 4 weeks is necessary to institute exclusive oral feeding.

40. b. The period for transitioning to solid foods is generally ages 4 to 6 months. A normally developing baby is initially fed formula or breast milk. During the period of 4 to 6 months of age, solids are first introduced.

41. a. All four of these statements are true with regard to infant anatomy and physiology. However, the flexibility of the thyroid cartilage does not improve airway protection. The close approximation of the velum to the epiglottis (valleculae; option b) helps separate the oral route for bolus transit and the nasal route for breathing. The higher position of the larynx in the neck (option c) helps protect the airway. Infants do not swallow and breathe at the same time, and so the larynx remains elevated and adducted during sequential swallowing (option d).

42. d. Tongue protrusion with solids is common during the transitional period for eating solid foods but should be suppressed by approximately 7 months of age. Thus, 12 months (option e) is incorrect. Persistence of this behavior is called *tongue thrust* and is also seen in acquired neurological impairment. The strategies of changing texture (option a) and training the parent in exercises to reduce tongue thrust (option c) are appropriate intervention strategies only if this behavior persists. Placing the food on the hard palate (option b) is not effective in treating this behavior or in feeding in general.

43. c. Botulinum toxin injections constitute the preferred and common medical intervention for sialorrhea. Increasing swallowing frequency (option a) and strengthening exercises (option b) are behavioral, not medical, interventions. Surgical removal of the salivary glands (option d) is not common. Biofeedback (option e) has been used experimentally on a limited basis with variable results.

44. e. Although the typical trigger for a pharyngeal swallow occurs as the bolus passes the anterior faucial pillar (option a), there are normal variations (options b and c) that are based on bolus size and consistency, as well as on age.

45. a. The trigeminal nerve mediates pain and temperature sensation and touch and proprioception in the face, mouth, and anterior two thirds of the tongue, as well as efferent nerves to the tensor veli palatini, mylohyoid, anterior belly of the digastric and tensor tympani muscles, and the muscles of mastication. The facial nerve (option b) mediates taste for the anterior two thirds of the tongue, as well as efferent nerves to the muscles of facial expression, the stapedius muscle, and the sublingual and submandibular salivary glands (autonomic function). The glossopharyngeal nerve (option c) mediates taste to the posterior third of the tongue, as well as general sensation to the tonsils and soft palate, and efferent nerves to the stylopharyngeus muscle and the parotid gland (autonomic function). The hypoglossal nerve (option d) is a motor nerve to the intrinsic and extrinsic tongue muscles.

46. d. Percutaneous gastrostomy (PEG) is the most commonly recommended alternative to oral nutrition and hydration. Feedings through Dobhoff (option a)

and nasogastric (option b) tubes are considered short-term or temporary alternatives to oral nutrition and hydration and should remain in place no longer than 4 weeks. Total parenteral nutrition (option c) is used only in rare cases of severe digestive disruption.

47. a. The lesion is on the left side (ipsilateral to the lesion), impairing the left-sided musculature of the velum (levator veli palatini). Upon elevation, the intact side (right side) does function, causing the velum to deviate to the strong side. This is mediated by cranial nerve X. The hypoglossal nerve, (CNXII) mediates the intrinsic and extrinsic tongue musculature. The facial nerve (CNVII) has both sensory and motor fibers that are active during the swallowing process.

48. c. Videofluoroscopy is considered the most sensitive and specific tool for detecting aspiration. A clinical or bedside swallowing evaluation (option a) may reveal signs or symptoms of aspiration, but 40% to 60% of aspiration is "silent" or undetected and thus may be missed. FEES (option b) may detect aspiration, but there is a period of "whiteout" during the pharyngeal swallow when this may be missed. Ultrasonography (option d) is typically used to visualize tongue movement (oral stage), and imaging of the pharynx and larynx is not appropriate for detecting aspiration. Scintigraphy (option e) provides a two-dimensional picture of a body radiation source through the use of radioisotopes.

49. a. After a total laryngectomy, the alimentary and respiratory pathways are separated (the patient is breathing directly through the tracheostoma), and aspiration is not a concern. Stricture (a narrowing) of the upper esophageal sphincter (option b) and fistula abnormal tissue pockets in the pharynx (option c) are common postoperative sequelae in total laryngectomy that can interfere with swallowing.

50. d. Although taste (option a) and temperature (option b) have been shown to modulate and facilitate the pharyngeal swallow, mechanoreceptors (responsible for touch sensation) have the greatest density in the sensory fields and therefore are the most likely to trigger and modulate a swallow. Pain (option c) is not an effective stimulus for triggering a swallow nor is smell (option e).

51. b. The boy is severely delayed in his feeding development. Spoon feeding normally starts by approximately 6 months of age, and frequent gagging on new textures is normally seen in healthy infants 5 to 6 months of age. Furthermore, at this age, feeding periods should not be longer than 40 minutes. Longer feeding periods

(even at an earlier age) indicate difficulties during feeding and that feeding could be an unpleasant experience for the infant or child and the caregiver. Thus, these behaviors are not typical of this child's age (option a). Also, delaying a complete evaluation would further compromise his development and nutrition (options c and d). A home treatment plan would not be appropriate until a comprehensive evaluation has been completed. The child should be referred for a complete swallowing and feeding evaluation.

52. a. The coordination of sucking-swallowing and breathing is not completely developed for successful oral feeding until approximately 34 weeks of gestational age. Thus, in premature infants, the sucking-swallowing-breathing sequence is frequently not well coordinated. Respiratory rates of higher than 80 to 85 breaths per minute during oral feeding put the infant at higher risk for penetration and aspiration. If the infant's respiratory rate is that high during oral feeding, then the infant has less time to complete the sucking-swallowing-breathing sequence. Faster breathing interferes with this sequence. Thus, the SLP should not continue oral feeding with interspersed breaks (option b) or continue feeding after the respiratory rate returns to normal (option c). The SLP may recommend nonnutritive sucking stimulation but without continuing oral feedings (option d). The SLP should stop oral feedings immediately and consult with the neonatologist on whether orogastric or nasogastric feedings are appropriate for this infant at this time.

53. a. The major factors to consider when deciding what is the best instrumental technique in the diagnosis of a patient are (1) which technique will provide the most information necessary to establish a diagnosis and (2) which technique puts the patient at lower risk for further complications. In the case of a child with spastic cerebral palsy, an attempt to insert a flexible endoscope through the nasal cavity (option b) could potentially injure the child, if a spastic movement or a spasm occurs during the examination. Ultrasonography (option c) would provide information regarding the oral components of swallowing but no information on the pharyngeal stage of the swallow. Auscultation (option d) provides information regarding the sound of the swallow. Any other sounds that could potentially be heard during auscultation cannot be easily interpreted in terms of what they represent. Scintigraphy (option e) is an imaging procedure that uses radioisotopes but would not be the best choice for this child. Videofluoroscopy furnishes the most information on the physiology of both the oral and pharyngeal stages of the swallow. In addition, if radiation safety guidelines are followed, exposure to this limited

amount of radiation should not put the child at greater risk for further complications.

54. b. Jenny's symptoms—including poor bolus formation and control, long feeding periods, frequent coughing with liquids, and inability to gain weight—indicate that she has severe swallowing difficulties. The SLP should refer Jenny for a videofluoroscopic examination of her swallowing function to determine whether it is safe for her to receive oral feedings. Although her parents insist on oral feedings, the SLP must first determine whether oral feeding is safe for Jenny before suggesting any treatment recommendations (options a and c). Inserting a fiberoptic endoscope (to perform FEES) in the nasal cavity of a child with athetoid cerebral palsy (option d) could potentially lead to injuries of the nasopharynx if an athetoid movement occurs during the examination.

55. b. Frequent gagging on new textures, ejecting food involuntary with the tongue after removal of the spoon from the mouth, and use of sucking pattern during spoon feeding are not typical for a 9-month-old; they are typical of the developmental feeding age of 5 months (option a). Drooling with teething is a typical behavior at 7 to 9 months of age (option d) as is hand to mouth eating foods such as crackers (option e). Thus, most of his symptoms indicate that the infant is mildly delayed in his feeding development (option c).

56. d. Infants can express stress through numerous reactions. Some of the most common signals include irregular or faster breathing (option a) and becoming lethargic during feedings (option b). Frequent pushing of the nipple away after taking only a small amount of liquid can also be considered a stress sign, but not when it is an uncommon behavior that occurs after several minutes after feeding initiation (option c).

57. b. Orofacial hyposensitivity and hypotonia are common characteristics of children born with Down syndrome. To reduce the orofacial hyposensitivity, several methods can be utilized. Applying firm but gentle stroking around the mouth and on the tongue is often a technique used to heighten sensory awareness of the orofacial structures. Applying deep and sustained pressure in and around the mouth (option a) is often used to treat orofacial hypersensitivity, not hyposensitivity. Mouth play with toys (option c) may reduce jaw thrusting (i.e., sudden, forceful jaw opening and exaggerated up-and-down jaw movements), which is usually associated with cases of hypertonia, not hypotonia. Drinking through large-diameter straws (option d) can increase lip

and cheek motor activity but not sensory awareness. Stimulation of the tongue (option e) may help the patient but is not the area to direct stimulation at this time.

58. c. Transition from suckling to spoon feedings (typically at 4 to 6 months of age) is an important milestone in the feeding development. It is also crucial that this transition is made with the right type of feeding technique and utensils. Ideally, the feeder should use a flat spoon and place it at midtongue. A flat spoon (in contrast to a long, round spoon) helps place all food inside the mouth and precludes inappropriate scraping of any remaining food off the palate or upper gums of the infant. The placement of the spoon at midtongue is also important because this is the location that encourages formation of the bolus and appropriate timing and coordination of the swallows. A slight downward pressure also ensures lip closure around the spoon, which should eliminate the need for scraping the food off the palate.

59. c. The tonic bite reflex is characterized by clenching of the jaw when a nipple or an object is inserted in the oral cavity and contacts the gums or the teeth of the infant. It is a normal reflex that typically disappears by 9 to 12 months of age and should not be present at 16 months (option a). Release of the bite reflex can be difficult, and pulling against the bite reflex (option b) usually has the opposite effect (i.e., it increases the force of the bite). One way to reduce the frequency of the occurrence of the reflex is to provide an inhibitory sensory environment, such as dimming the lights and using quiet voices during feedings. Sensory stimulation to the faucial pillars is not appropriate in this case.

60. c. Pierre Robin sequence is characterized by three major features: micrognathia, posterior cleft palate, and glossoptosis. The presence of a posterior cleft creates inability to develop sufficient negative intraoral pressure, which is necessary for effective sucking to occur. Thus, it is very possible that this infant exhibits weak and ineffective sucking (option a). In addition, this can further result in excessive air intake that is frequently followed by frequent gagging and choking (option d). Glossoptosis (the pathological retraction of the tongue) can also frequently cause airway obstruction, resulting in frequent choking and aspiration of liquids. A cleft palate also results in inability to seal off the nasal cavity, which leads to nasal regurgitation during feeding (option b). Anterior loss of liquid could be seen in infants with Pierre Robin sequence if additional structural or neurological problems are present; however, it is not commonly expected.

PART V

Audiology and Hearing

CHAPTER 13

Hearing Science

John A. Ferraro

PRINCIPLES OF HEARING

1. The notation "dB HL," or "HTL" (hearing threshold level), refers to:
   a. The average thresholds at different frequencies of a group of young persons with normal hearing
   b. The lowest sound pressure level detectable by a person at different frequencies
   c. The amount of decibels above a person's threshold
   d. The highest sound level at which a person can discriminate different frequencies
   e. The decibel range between threshold and when sounds are uncomfortably loud

2. Dynamic range is:
   a. The range of frequencies humans can hear
   b. The decibel range between threshold and the level at which sounds become "felt"/uncomfortably loud
   c. The decibel range between threshold and the level at which sounds become painful to hear
   d. The decibel range beyond which humans can hear
   e. The decibel range below which sounds are inaudible

3. The range of frequencies that humans with normal hearing can detect is:
   a. 20 to 20,000 Hz
   b. 125 to 8000 Hz
   c. 500 to 5000 Hz
   d. 100 to 10,000 Hz
   e. 250 to 4000 Hz

4. The frequency range in which most speech sounds occur is:
   a. 20 to 20,000 Hz
   b. 125 to 8000 Hz
   c. 500 to 5000 Hz
   d. 100 to 10,000 Hz
   e. 250 to 4000 Hz

5. In general, crossover does not occur when:
   a. The sound entering one ear is loud enough to be heard in the other ear through bone conduction
   b. Sounds delivered to the ear through air conduction are louder than 40 to 45 dB HL
   c. Sounds delivered to the ear through air conduction are softer than 40 to 45 dB HL
   d. Sound is delivered to the ear through a bone vibrator
   e. A loudspeaker is used to deliver the stimulus

ANATOMY AND PHYSIOLOGY OF THE HEARING AND VESTIBULAR MECHANISMS

6. The primary type of energy transferred through the outer ear is:
   a. Acoustical
   b. Mechanical
   c. Hydraulic
   d. Electrical
   e. Electroacoustical

7. Which of the following tissue types is *not* found in the tympanic membrane?
   a. Skin
   b. Muscle
   c. Cartilage
   d. Mucous membrane
   e. All the above

8. The middle ear functions to match the impedance of _____ and _____ in transmitting mechanical vibrations to the cochlea.
   a. The ear canal; middle ear space
   b. The tympanic membrane; auditory ossicles
   c. The auditory ossicles; middle ear muscles
   d. Air; cochlear fluid
   e. The tympanic membrane; middle ear muscles

9. At rest under normal conditions, the nasopharyngeal ostium of the eustachian tube is:
   a. Open
   b. Closed
   c. Surrounded by bone
   d. Occluded by the adenoids
   e. Partially opened and partially closed

10. The eustachian tube of a child is _____ and _____ than that of an adult.
    a. Longer; wider
    b. Longer; more elevated
    c. Shorter; more elevated
    d. Shorter; more horizontal
    e. Shorter; more open

11. Contraction of the middle ear muscles in response to sound:
    a. Protects the inner ear from loud sounds
    b. Amplifies the mechanical vibrations of the tympanic membrane
    c. Occurs only when the sound is very soft
    d. Is measured via tympanometry
    e. Does not occur with other stimuli

12. Of the following structures, which is *not* a part of the organ of Corti?
    a. Modiolus
    b. Inner hair cells
    c. Outer pillar cells
    d. Phalangeal cells of Deiter
    e. Tectorial membrane

13. Of the following features of the basilar membrane, which is *not* essential to the maintenance of the traveling wave?
    a. Its mass
    b. Its elasticity
    c. Its width
    d. Its fluid environment
    e. None of the above

14. High tones are coded in the _____ turns of the cochlea.
    a. Basal
    b. Middle
    c. Middle and apical
    d. Apical
    e. All of the above

15. At the level of the organ of Corti:
    a. Acoustical energy is transduced into mechanical energy
    b. Mechanical energy is transduced into hydromechanical energy
    c. Hydromechanical energy is transduced into bioelectrical energy
    d. Mechanical energy is transduced into neural energy
    e. Acoustical energy is transduced into hydromechanical energy

16. Of the following statements, which is false?
    a. The ear only receives and transmits sounds to the brain
    b. The ear receives, transmits, and produces sounds
    c. The inner ear sends and receives information to and from the brain
    d. The brain transmits neural messages to both the middle and inner ears
    e. All of the above

17. Of the following nerves, which does *not* course through the internal auditory meatus?
    a. Facial
    b. Auditory
    c. Trigeminal
    d. Vestibular
    e. Nervus intermedius of the facial nerve

18. The central auditory pathways consist of a complex, sequential series of _____ and _____ that extend from the brainstem to the cerebral cortex and back down again.
    a. Ganglia; nerves
    b. Ganglia; nuclei
    c. Nuclei; nerves
    d. Nuclei; fiber tracts
    e. Sulci; gyri

19. Of the following structures, which is *not* a part of the vestibular apparatus?
    a. Saccule
    b. Utricle
    c. Semicircular canals
    d. Ductus reuniens
    e. Crista ampullaris

20. Of the following senses, which does *not* contribute to maintenance of balance?
    a. Proprioception
    b. Vision
    c. Hearing
    d. Vestibular function
    e. All of these senses contribute to balance

ANATOMICAL AND PHYSIOLOGICAL BASES FOR HEARING LOSS

21. Which of the following causes of hearing loss is not associated with the outer ear?
    a. Microtia
    b. Impacted cerumen
    c. Otosclerosis
    d. Cholesteatoma
    e. Swimmer's ear

22. Of the following treatments, which is common for middle ear infection in children?
    a. Cerumen removal
    b. Hearing aid
    c. Pressure-equalization tube
    d. Cochlear implant
    e. Ear plugs

23. Hearing loss caused by disorders of the inner ear or auditory nerve, or of both, are classified as:
    a. Conductive
    b. Sensorineural
    c. Mixed
    d. Central
    e. Sensory only

24. In a child with a diagnosis of auditory processing disorder, the suspected site of lesion or dysfunction is:
    a. The middle ear
    b. The inner hair cells of the cochlea
    c. The outer hair cells of the cochlea
    d. The central auditory pathways
    e. The inner ear and auditory nerve

25. Congenital abnormalities of the ear are often accompanied by congenital abnormalities of the _____, inasmuch as both these organs develop embryologically at about the same time.
    a. Heart
    b. Lung
    c. Kidney
    d. Pancreas
    e. Skin

Answers

1. a. The notation "dB HL" represents the decibel notation used for calibration of audiometers. The lowest sound pressure level detectable at different frequencies (option b) is an individual value, and the decibel notation for the amount of decibels above a person's threshold (option c) is "SL" (sensation level). No decibel value corresponds to the highest sound level at which different frequencies can be discriminated (option d), and the level between threshold and when sounds are uncomfortably loud (option e) is the "dynamic range" of hearing. Because speech-language pathologists (SLPs) review audiograms and the results of other audiometric tests, it is important for them to be familiar with "dB" notation.

2. b. The dynamic range is the range between threshold and when sounds are uncomfortably loud. This is an important concept in the fitting and adjusting of hearing aids, design of classroom acoustics, and setting of cochlear implants, all of which may come under the purview or be assisted by SLPs. The term *dynamic range* has nothing to do with frequency perception (option a), and the range between threshold and pain (option c) is the range below the dynamic range. The range beyond which humans can hear (option d) is infinite. Inaudible sounds (option e) are at levels that not high enough to be heard.

3. a. The human ear is ideally designed to be most sensitive to speech sounds (option c), but it can hear at frequencies of 20 to 20,000 Hz. The range of 125 to 8000 Hz (option b) is the audiometric test frequency range. The other ranges listed (options d and e) are just general ranges of frequencies to which humans are sensitive.

4. c. Speech sounds usually occur at frequencies of 500 to 5000 Hz. The range 125 to 8000 (option b) is the audiometric test frequency range. The other ranges listed (options a, d, and e) are just general ranges of frequencies to which humans are sensitive.

5. c. Sounds less than 40 to 45 are too soft to initiate crossover. Hearing in the opposite ear through bone conduction (option a) defines crossover. Crossover occurs when the sounds delivered to one ear are louder than 40 to 45 dB HL (option b) and also when sound is delivered to the ear directly through a bone vibrator (option d). If sounds from a loudspeaker (option e) are loud enough, crossover can occur. To interpret an audiogram correctly, the examiner must understand the conditions under which crossover does or does not occur.

6. a. The ear transduces sound (i.e., acoustical) energy into a bioelectrical impulse. This transduction begins at the tympanic membrane, where acoustical energy in the ear canal is transduced into mechanical vibrations (option b), which is the mode of energy processed by the middle ear. Hydraulic energy (option c) is initiated at the oval window and gives rise to the mechanical displacement of inner ear structures, which eventually leads to the electrical excitation of cochlear hair cells (option d). Electroacoustical transduction (option e) occurs when an electrical signal (e.g., from a microphone) is delivered to a speaker phone or earphone.

7. c. The tympanic membrane comprises skin (option a), muscle (option b), and mucous membrane (option d), but no cartilage or bone. SLPs often perform otoscopic examinations, especially in children, to check for middle ear infection. It is important to have good knowledge of the anatomy of this structure to know how a normal or abnormal tympanic membrane should look.

8. d. The middle ear functions to match the impedance of air and cochlear fluid. This is an important concept that relates to the nature and understanding of conductive hearing loss. This type of loss is caused when the impedance match between air (the medium of both the outer and middle ears) and cochlear fluid is altered by, for example, middle ear infection. In such conditions, energy is reflected back at the tympanic membrane instead of being transmitted to the inner ear.

9. b. The nasopharyngeal ostium of the eustachian tube is normally closed. Eustachian tube dysfunction is a primary cause of middle ear infection in children, which can lead to hearing loss and speech and language delay. A chronically open (option a) or partially open eustachian tube (option e) is a pathological condition. The nasopharyngeal ostium is surrounded by muscle, not bone (option c), which allows it to open and close in response to atmospheric pressure changes. Adenoid-occluded eustachian tubes (option d) represent another pathological condition that can lead to middle ear infection.

10. d. The shortness and relatively horizontal flat plane of the eustachian tube makes it easy for upper respiratory and other oropharyngeal and nasopharyngeal infections to spread to the middle ear. This is the major reason why small children are more

susceptible to middle ear infection. As children grow, the eustachian tube becomes longer and more elevated (option b). This explains why they tend to "outgrow" this condition.

11. a. One of the functions of the middle ear muscles is to protect the inner ear from loud sounds. The muscles do not amplify the vibrations of the tympanic membrane (option b), and they generally contract when sound levels exceed 80 dB, not when sounds are soft (option c). Several types of stimuli, including swallowing, blinking, and blowing on the ear, can cause contraction of the muscles (option e). Tympanometry (option d) measures the compliance of the tympanic membrane, not the contraction of the middle ear muscles. Knowledge of specific tests of middle ear function is important for SLPs, especially those working with children with hearing loss.

12. a. The modiolus (option a) is the only structure listed that is not considered to be part of the organ of Corti. A general knowledge of the anatomy of the organ of Corti is important for SLPs because it is the primary "organ" of hearing.

13. c. The traveling wave, which gives rise to the excitation of cochlear hair cells leading to hearing, is dependent on the mass (option a) and elasticity (option b) of the basilar membrane and on the fluid forces that surround it (option d). The width of the basilar membrane really does not contribute to the traveling wave.

14. a. Pitch perception is dependent on the site of stimulation on the basilar membrane and the organ of Corti. High-pitched tones are coded in the basal regions of the cochlea, whereas middle-pitched tones are coded in the middle regions (option b) and low-pitched tones in the apex (option d). Knowledge of the tonotopicity of the basilar membrane is important for such tasks as interpretation of the audiogram and identification of possible sites of lesion, fitting hearing aids, and programming cochlear implants.

15. c. The essential transduction from hydromechanical to bioelectrical energy is accomplished at the level of the organ of Corti. Transductions of acoustical energy into mechanical energy (option a) and of mechanical energy into hydromechanical energy (option b) take place at the tympanic membrane and oval window, respectively. The transduction of mechanical energy alone into a neural impulse (option d) does not take place in the ear, nor does a direct transduction of acoustic to hydromechanical energy (option e).

16. a. The ear not only receives and transmits sounds to the brain but also produces them, in the form of otoacoustic emissions (option b). Measurement of otoacoustic emissions has become an important clinical test for the identification of, for example, hearing loss in newborns. The function of inner hair cells is to send impulses to the brain, but the outer hair cells act more like a motor system that receives messages from the brain (option c). The brain sends neural messages to both the outer and inner hair cells and also to the middle ear muscles (option d).

17. c. Cranial nerve V, the trigeminal nerve, is the only nerve listed that does not course through the internal auditory meatus.

18. d. *Ganglia* and *nerves* (options a, b, and c) are terms used almost exclusively to refer to the peripheral nervous system. Sulci and gyri (option e) are the grooves and folds of tissue, respectively, on the cerebral cortex. The auditory pathways consist of nuclei (collections of neuronal cell bodies in the central nervous system) and fiber tracks (dendrites and axons in the central nervous system).

19. d. The ductus reuniens connects the cochlear duct to the vestibular apparatus, but it is not considered to be exclusive to the apparatus, as the saccule (option a), utricle (option b), semicircular canals (option c), and crista ampullaris (option d) are. A general knowledge of the structure and function of the vestibular apparatus, because it is part of the inner ear, is important for SLPs. In addition, speech and language disorders resulting from stroke, for example, are often accompanied by balance disorders, for which the site of the lesion may or may not be in the vestibular system.

20. c. The only sense listed that is not essential for the maintenance of balance is, interestingly enough, hearing. Balance is maintained by a complex system of neurological interactions that involve vision (option b), proprioception (option a), and vestibular function (option d).

21. c. Otosclerosis is a disorder of the middle ear. All of the other conditions listed are associated with the outer ear and should be recognizable by SLPs.

22. c. The placement of pressure-equalization tubes is a common treatment for middle ear infection in children. SLPs working with children should be aware of the implications of this treatment for the relationship between middle ear disorders and speech-language delays. Cerumen removal (option a) is confined to the outer ear; hearing aids (option b),

cochlear implants (option d), and ear plugs (option e) are never used to treat middle ear infections.

23. b. Disorders of the inner ear and auditory nerve cause sensorineural hearing loss. Knowledge of the different types of hearing loss and of the general sites of lesion or dysfunction is essential to anyone providing speech-language-hearing services to children and adults. Conductive losses (option a) are generally associated with the outer and middle ears, and central losses (option d) signify dysfunction or lesion in the central nervous system. For a purely sensory loss (option e), the lesion would be confined to the inner ear.

24. d. Identification of and therapy for auditory processing disorder are often under the purview of SLPs. Both the diagnosis and treatment of auditory processing disorder remain controversial issues, but the suspected sites of lesion or dysfunction for this disorder are the central auditory pathways.

25. c. It is not unusual for children with congenital hearing loss to also have kidney disorders. SLPs working with children who have congenital hearing loss need to be aware of the possibility of other, related disorders, as well as the effects of medications used for treating these conditions.

CHAPTER 14

Audiological Assessment

Ashleigh A. Payne

1. Your patient is a 5-year-old boy who received a diagnosis of hearing loss at birth. He has no history of ear pain, ear surgery, or otitis media. His mother reports a normal birth history, no complications during pregnancy, and no serious illnesses. One of his brothers also has a substantial hearing loss. The patient reached normal developmental milestones for sitting, walking, and other physical activities; however, his mother is concerned about his speech and language development. She reports that he is "withdrawn and shy." His current audiometric results are as shown in Figures 14-1 and 14-2 and Table 14-1 on p. 199. Which of the following best describes the audiogram (Fig. 14-1)?
   a. Mild to moderate sensorineural hearing loss
   b. Moderately severe sloping to profound sensorineural hearing loss
   c. Profound rising to moderately severe sensorineural hearing loss
   d. Moderately severe sloping to profound conductive hearing loss
   e. Profound rising to moderately severe conductive hearing loss

2. For the patient described in question 1, his tympanograms (Fig. 14-2) are of what type?
   a. Type A
   b. Type As
   c. Type Ad
   d. Type C
   e. Type B

3. For the patient described in question 1, on the basis of the case history and audiometric results, what is the most likely cause of his hearing loss?
   a. Chronic otitis media
   b. Congenital atresia
   c. Congenital heredity (Connexin 26)
   d. Noise-induced hearing loss
   e. Ototoxicity

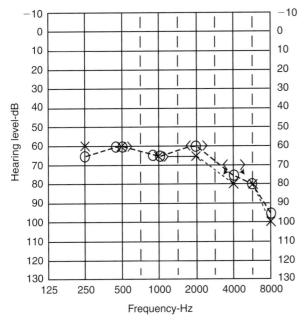

Figure 14-1 Audiogram of the patient showing air and bone conduction thresholds.

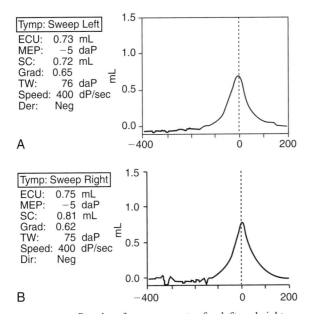

Figure 14-2 Results of tympanometry for left and right ears.

TABLE 14-1			
Ear	Speech Reception Threshold (SRT)	Sensation Level (SL)	Word Recognition Score
Right	65 dB HL	30 dB	76%
Left	65 dB HL	30 dB	72%

4. For the patient described in question 1, all of the following are appropriate recommendations for this patient *except:*
   a. Bilateral hearing aids
   b. FM system for the classroom
   c. Preferential seating
   d. Unilateral cochlear implant
   e. Aural rehabilitation

5. Which of the following statements best describes the purpose of the speech reception threshold (SRT) behavioral audiometric test?
   a. SRT provides a reference for the sensation level at which suprathreshold speech testing is presented
   b. SRT is a measure of the lowest level that spondaic words can be repeated 100% of the time
   c. SRT scores determine candidacy for hearing aids
   d. SRT scores are obtained with phonetically balanced monosyllabic words
   e. SRT scores can be used as a diagnostic tool to determine whether a hearing loss is conductive or sensorineural

6. If an infant does not pass an initial hearing screening of otoacoustic emissions (OAE) in the hospital shortly after birth, what is the most appropriate action?
   a. Referral to a pediatric audiologist for a cochlear implant evaluation
   b. Referral to an audiologist for a hearing aid fitting
   c. Referral to an audiologist for a follow-up evaluation to confirm the hearing loss
   d. Referral to a specialist for genetic counseling
   e. Referral to an otolaryngologist for an assessment of the outer and middle ear

7. When performing audiometric screening for preschool children aged 3 to 5 years, which of the following would constitute as a passing response?
   a. One conditioned play audiometry (CPA) response at each test frequency obtained with good reliability to 20-dB HL tones presented at 1000, 2000, and 4000 Hz
   b. Two consecutive CPA responses to each 20-dB HL tone presented at 1000, 2000, and 4000 Hz
   c. Two consecutive conventional audiometric (i.e., hand raise) responses to each 30-dB HL tone presented at 1000, 2000, and 4000 Hz
   d. Two consecutive CPA responses to speech presented at 20 dB HL
   e. Two consecutive conventional audiometric (i.e., hand raise) responses to broadband noise presented at 20 dB HL

8. If an 8-month-old produces a normal tympanogram, displays a normal auditory brainstem response (ABR),

and has no otoacoustic emissions (OAE), what is the most likely cause of the child's hearing loss?
a. Otitis media
b. Otosclerosis
c. Presbycusis
d. Congenital hereditary
e. Auditory neuropathy

9. All of the following are associated with a conductive hearing loss except:
a. Type B tympanograms
b. Type C tympanograms
c. Impaired air conduction and normal bone conduction
d. An air-bone gap of 20 dB HL
e. Impaired bone conduction and impaired air conduction

10. Patients with which type of hearing loss would typically display the poorest word recognition scores when test items are presented at 40dB SL?
a. Retrocochlear
b. Mild conductive
c. Moderate conductive
d. Mild sensorineural
e. Moderate sensorineural

11. In a normally developing 24-month-old, the behavioral audiological test most appropriate for determining frequency-specific hearing sensitivity is:
a. CPA
b. Behavioral observation audiometry
c. Visual reinforcement audiometry
d. ABR testing
e. SRT testing

12. Type B (flat) tympanograms are abnormal audiometric findings that can be attributed to all of the following except:
a. Tympanic membrane perforation
b. Impacted cerumen
c. Interrupted ossicular chain
d. Probe against the canal wall
e. Pressure equalization tube

13. A 56-year-old man has recently received a diagnosis of an acoustic neuroma in his left ear. Of the following findings, which best describes the acoustic reflex results?
a. Absence of ipsilateral acoustic reflexes on the left side
b. Absence of ipsilateral acoustic reflexes on the right side
c. Absence of ipsilateral acoustic reflexes bilaterally
d. Absence of contralateral acoustic reflexes bilaterally
e. Normal acoustic reflexes ipsilaterally on the left side

14. Your patient, a 36-year-old woman, presents with spontaneous episodes of intense vertigo lasting minutes to hours; a sense of aural fullness; unilateral, fluctuating, low-frequency sensorineural hearing loss in the right ear; and low pitched tinnitus that seems to intensify during attacks of dizziness. Head movements do not increase dizziness, and she reports no imbalance or dizziness between episodes. What is the most likely cause of her symptoms?
a. Vestibular schwannoma
b. Disequilibrium of aging
c. A central nervous system disorder
d. Benign paroxysmal positional vertigo (BPPV)
e. Ménière disease

15. A total communication rehabilitative method would be most appropriate for children with which of the following types of hearing loss?
a. Mild conductive hearing loss
b. Mild sensorineural hearing loss
c. Fluctuating conductive hearing loss
d. Moderate sensorineural hearing loss
e. Profound sensorineural hearing loss

16. When a 1000-Hz tone is presented through air conduction by supra-aural earphones, what pathway is followed?
a. Auditory nerve, inner ear, middle ear, outer ear
b. Outer ear and middle ear
c. Outer ear, middle ear, inner ear, auditory nerve
d. Outer ear, inner ear, auditory nerve
e. Inner ear, auditory nerve

17. Which of the following is a likely cause of feedback in hearing aids?
a. A blockage of cerumen in the ear canal
b. A low battery
c. A T-coil that is turned on
d. Clogging of the ear mold tubing with moisture
e. Complete occlusion of the receiver of the hearing aid by cerumen

18. Of the following situations, which is *not* a reason for prompt medical referral?
a. Tinnitus as a primary symptom
b. Pain or discomfort in the ear
c. History of sudden hearing loss within the previous 90 days
d. Noise exposure
e. Active drainage in the ear

19. Children with specific risk factors for hearing loss need to be monitored every 6 months until age 3 years for progressive and delayed-onset hearing loss. Which of the following conditions is *not* a specific risk factor for permanent childhood hearing loss?

a. Hyperbilirubinemia necessitating exchange transfusion
b. Neurodegenerative disorders
c. Head trauma
d. In utero infections
e. Autism

20. Of the following patients, which should be referred for an electrophysiological evaluation with neurodiagnostic ABR testing?
a. Patient with asymmetrical sensorineural hearing loss
b. Patient with asymmetrical conductive hearing loss
c. Patient with symmetrical sensorineural hearing loss
d. Patient with symmetrical conductive hearing loss
e. Patient with auditory processing disorder

21. Which of the following is *not* a common cause of tinnitus?
a. Excessive noise exposure
b. Auditory processing disorder
c. Ototoxicity
d. Menière disease
e. Acoustic neuromas

22. An 88-year-old woman exhibits a mild sloping to moderate sensorineural hearing loss. She lacks the finances, dexterity, and motivation for pursuing amplification at this time; however, she would like to be able to hear her granddaughter better over the telephone. She also lives in a nursing home and does not have a strong family support network in the area. You have discussed hearing aid options with her, but she does not want a hearing aid. What would be the best rehabilitative option for this patient?
a. Telephone amplifier
b. An audio loop system

c. An FM system
d. Speech reading training
e. Personal voice amplification system

23. A school-aged child with a mild hearing loss may exhibit all of the common psychological aspects and communication difficulties related to hearing loss except:
a. Negative impact on self-esteem
b. Loss of ability to hear selectively
c. Difficulty suppressing background noise
d. Increased fatigue as a result of expending more effort to listen
e. Increased identity with Deaf culture

24. Of the following disorders, which is a medical emergency in which immediate referral is necessary?
a. Tinnitus
b. Otosclerosis
c. Sudden hearing loss
d. Pseudohypacusis
e. Presbycusis

25. Of the five following possibilities in communication situations, which is the most detrimental to effective communication for people with significant hearing loss?
a. Listeners know they have understood what has been said
b. Listeners understand what is said but do not confirm this to the speaker
c. Listeners know they did not understand what has been said
d. Listeners are not sure they understood what was said
e. Listeners think they understood but did not understand correctly

1. b. This audiogram is most accurately described as moderately severe sloping to profound sensorineural hearing loss, on the basis of the conventional categories of hearing loss: Thresholds in the range of 56 to 70 dB HL are considered moderately severe, and thresholds exceeding 90 dB HL are considered profound. Sensorineural hearing loss is determined by equal air and bone conduction thresholds or no air-bone gap. Sloping hearing losses have better thresholds in the lower frequencies, worsening in the higher frequencies. The hearing loss is not mild (option a) because the thresholds on the audiogram exceed the moderate range of hearing loss (41 to 55dB HL). In profound rising to moderately severe loss (option c), thresholds are poorer in the lower frequencies and better in the higher frequencies. Conductive hearing losses (options d and e) imply normal bone conduction thresholds and reduced air conduction thresholds.

2. a. The measure of static acoustic admittance and peak pressure are within the normal range; therefore, this result is a type A tympanogram. Type As (option b) and type Ad (option c) tympanograms would also have normal peak pressure; however, the static acoustic admittance would be low for type As or high for type Ad. A type C (option d) tympanogram would exhibit negative peak pressure, and a type B (option e) tympanogram would display no peak pressure.

3. c. This is a sensorineural hearing loss, not a conductive disorder such as chronic otitis media (option a) and congenital atresia (option b). Although noise-induced (option d) hearing loss is a sensorineural type of hearing loss, this child's condition was identified at birth, and noise damage is therefore an unlikely cause. Ototoxicity (option e) also causes a sensorineural type of hearing loss; however, the child did not exhibit a serious illness in which ototoxic drugs would have been needed. Connexin 26 is one of the more common causes of congenital hereditary hearing loss and would be the most likely cause of this child's hearing loss.

4. d. The patient's degree of hearing loss does not meet the current criteria for cochlear implantation in children (ages 3 to 18 years): bilateral hearing loss that is severe (>70 dB HL) in the low frequencies to profound (>90 dB HL) in the middle and high frequencies, along with a best aided word score of 30% or less. Bilateral hearing aids (option a), a classroom

FM system (option b), preferential seating (option c), and aural rehabilitation (option e) would all be recommended for a 5-year-old child with a moderately severe sloping to profound sensorineural hearing loss.

5. a. The SRT is measured with spondaic words, not phonetically balanced monosyllabic words (option d); however, the threshold is determined by the level at which the patient can repeat the words 50% of the time, but not 100% (option b). Although the SRT is an important audiometric tool, candidacy for hearing aids (option c) is based on the entire audiological test battery and case history. Determination of conductive or sensorineural hearing losses is based on the comparison of air and bone conduction results, not SRT score (option e). The word recognition test is a suprathreshold test in which the sensation level used for presentation of the word list is based on the SRT score.

6. c. Although a hearing aid (option b) or a cochlear implant (option a) may be options for this infant, the first step of audiological management would be to confirm the hearing loss. Once a sensorineural hearing loss is confirmed by diagnostic OAE testing and auditory brainstem response (ABR) testing, genetic counseling (option d) may be warranted. Assessment by an otolaryngologist (option e) for outer and middle ear evaluation would be needed if additional testing suggested a conductive component.

7. b. According to screening guidelines for preschool-aged children, frequency-specific responses are required; therefore, speech (option d) and broadband noise (option e) would not be acceptable stimuli. In addition, the screening protocols developed by the American Speech-Language-Hearing Association (ASHA) recommend 20 dB HL, not 30 dB HL (option c), as the acceptable intensity for hearing screenings. In order to obtain a dependable measure for this population, two responses, not one (option a), to the same frequency need to be obtained.

8. d. Congenital hereditary hearing losses are often sensorineural in nature. In OAE testing, function of outer hair cells is examined, and absence of responses is suggestive of a problem with the inner ear. Otitis media (option a) is a conductive problem; therefore, tympanometry would be abnormal. Otosclerosis (option b) is also a conductive disorder, and onset typically occurs in young adulthood. Presbycusis

(option c) is a sensorineural problem; however, it occurs in geriatric, not pediatric, patients. Auditory neuropathy (option e) is a sensorineural disorder that affects infants; however, it is a retrocochlear problem, and the ABR would be abnormal.

9. e. Impaired air and bone conduction thresholds indicate a sensorineural hearing loss. Type B (option a) and type C (option b) tympanograms are abnormal findings that are suggestive of conductive disorders, such as middle ear effusion or otitis media. "Impaired air conduction with normal bone conduction" (option c) and "air-bone gap of 20 dB HL" (option d) are essentially the same way of describing conductive hearing loss because in both cases, the bone conduction hearing is normal.

10. a. Word recognition scores are typically less affected by conductive hearing losses than by sensorineural hearing losses. Patients with retrocochlear types of hearing loss display disproportionately low word recognition in comparison with pure tones. Although patients with sensorineural hearing losses generally have poorer word recognition than those with conductive hearing losses, the patients with mild (option d) and moderate (option e) sensorineural hearing losses would display better scores than someone with a retrocochlear disorder. Patients with mild (option b) or moderate (option c) conductive hearing losses should have excellent (88% or above) word recognition scores when the presentation level is 40 dB SL.

11. c. Visual reinforcement audiometry is a behavioral method of testing based on operant conditioning that is commonly used to determine frequency-specific hearing in toddlers. Behavioral observation audiometry (option b), based on reflexive and orienting responses to sounds, yields information that does not have absolute sensitivity or is not frequency specific. CPA testing(option a) is indicated only for older children; a 24-month-old would not be able to perform the task. ABR testing(option d) can be used to determine frequency-specific hearing; however, it is a physiological, not a behavioral, test. SRT testing(option e) would not be indicated because the speech and language of a 24-month-old are too limited. In addition, the SRT is not a frequency-specific measure of hearing.

12. c. Patients with an interrupted ossicular chain typically produce type Ad tympanograms. Patients with the other conditions may produce type B tympanograms; however, the ear canal volumes, along with otoscopic results, would be methods of aiding in differentiating between the conditions. Tympanic

membrane perforations (option a) and pressure equalization tubes (option e) would create an abnormally large ear canal volume, whereas impacted cerumen (option b) and a probe against the canal wall (option d) would lead to extremely small ear canal volumes.

13. a. Acoustic neuromas are abnormal growths on cranial nerve VIII. The acoustic reflex pathway travels through this nerve on the ipsilateral side; therefore, the ipsilateral pathway would be interrupted on the left side in this patient. The ipsilateral reflexes on the right side (options b and c) would not be affected. The left contralateral reflex (option d) would be absent.

14. e. All of the stated symptoms are common in patients with Menière disease. Patients with vestibular schwannomas (option a), disequilibrium of aging (option b), and central nervous system disorders (option c) commonly complain of more slowly progressing constant disequilibrium and imbalance, not episodic true vertigo. Benign paroxysmal positional vertigo (option d) is a common cause of episodic vertigo; however, the symptoms are typically precipitated by head movements and have a duration of approximately 1 minute.

15. e. To gain the most access to information, children with profound hearing loss often need sign language, fingerspelling, lipreading, writing, gesture, and visual imagery along with amplification or cochlear implants. Mild (options a and b), fluctuating (option c), and moderate (option d) degrees of hearing loss would not be significant enough to implement a total communication approach unless additional disabling conditions were present. In addition, conductive hearing losses (options a and c) can often be corrected with medical intervention.

16. c. When presented through the air, the sound wave must travel through the outer ear (i.e., the ear canal), the middle ear (i.e., the ossicles), and the inner ear (i.e., the cochlea) to the auditory nerve. The path of auditory nerve, inner ear, middle ear, and outer ear (option a) is the pathway in the reverse order. The other options do not include all of the sections of the ear.

17. a. Excessive cerumen in the ear canal is a common cause of feedback, or "whistling," in hearing aids. A low battery (option b) would cause a hearing aid to sound weak or to cease working. The hearing aid would also appear dead with the T-coil (option c) in place because this setting is for use on the telephone and with loop systems. When ear mold tubing has

excessive moisture (option d) or when the receiver is clogged with cerumen (option e), the hearing aid may also stop working. If the hearing aid is weak or not working, it would not be possible to produce feedback.

18. d. Noise exposure definitely warrants investigation for hearing loss, counseling on aspects of noise exposure and prevention of future damage to the ear, continued audiological monitoring, and potential rehabilitative measures such as amplification. However, a patient with noise exposure and no additional complaints or abnormalities does not need an immediate medical referral. Patients with any of the other conditions listed should be advised to seek prompt medical attention from a physician.

19. e. Research into hearing loss and autism is limited; however, autism is not recognized by the ASHA as a pediatric risk factor for hearing loss. In addition, autism is often not diagnosed until the age of 3 years. All the other conditions listed increase the risk of progressive and delayed hearing loss in children and should be monitored.

20. a. For patients who have asymmetrical sensorineural hearing losses, ABR tests are often used to determine abnormalities that may suggest retrocochlear problems, such as acoustic neuromas. Patients with acoustic neuromas often exhibit unilateral hearing loss, tinnitus, dizziness, and dysequilibrium. An ABR test could be performed for the other types of hearing loss listed; however, the main purpose of a neurodiagnostic ABR test is to look for signs of retrocochlear disorders.

21. b. Although the exact mechanism of tinnitus ("ringing in the ears") is unknown, it is thought to be associated with damage to the hair cells in the cochlea. No strong relationship has been established between tinnitus and auditory processing disorders After excessive noise exposure (option a) and otoxicity (option c), which damage cochlear hair cells, most people exhibit some form of tinnitus. Many patients with common disorders such as Menière disease (option d) and acoustic neuromas (option e) also complain of tinnitus.

22. a. Telephone amplifiers are relatively inexpensive and can sufficiently improve hearing over the telephone for people with mild to moderate hearing losses. Audio loop (option b) and FM systems (option c) must be used in conjunction with a hearing aid. Speech reading training (option d) and a personal voice amplification system (option e) may aid this patient in face-to-face communication but not over the telephone.

23. e. Children with mild hearing loss would not display enough hearing loss to identify with Deaf culture. Typically, only persons with greater degrees of hearing loss (severe to profound) identify with Deaf culture and use sign language to communicate. All other aspects listed more accurately describe a child with mild hearing loss.

24. c. With sudden hearing loss, patients need medical attention immediately because certain types of medical intervention are most effective the earlier they are given. If the patient waits for an extended time period, hearing may not recover as well. Although a medical referral is warranted for patients with tinnitus (option a) as a primary complaint and those with otosclerosis (option b), the need for medical attention is not urgent. Patients displaying pseudohypacusis (option d) or nonorganic hearing loss have no physical reason for hearing loss; therefore, a medical referral would not be necessary. Presbycusis (option e) is hearing loss resulting from primarily the aging process; without any additional concerns or findings, patients with presbycusis would not need medical clearance before proceeding with audiological management.

25. e. Many of the communication breakdowns experienced by patients with hearing loss occur when the listener thinks that he or she understood the message but actually did not understand correctly. When patients know they have understood the message (options a and b), communication is most effective. On the other hand, when patients know that they do not understand what is said (option c) or are not sure what is said (option d), they can ask for repetitions or rephrasing of the message.

CHAPTER 15

Auditory Habilitation and Rehabilitation

Nancy Tye-Murray

1. Of the following newborns, which would not be at particularly high risk for hearing loss?
   a. Babies who weigh more than 9 lbs (4 kg) at birth
   b. Babies whose mothers had cytomegalovirus during pregnancy
   c. Babies with craniofacial anomalies
   d. Babies with high Apgar scores
   e. All the above

2. In most classic auditory training programs, the aim of training is for the patient to progress from one skill level to the next. The hierarchy of skills is typically composed of the following:
   a. Formal and then informal
   b. Sound awareness, sound discrimination, identification, comprehension
   c. Words, phrases, sentences
   d. Auditory perception only, visual perception only, and then audiovisual speech perception
   e. Formal, sound awareness, words, visual perception only

3. An audiologist finds that a 75-year-old patient has a sloping sensorineural hearing loss. The patient performs more poorly on a test of speech recognition than would be predicted by her pure-tone average. This patient most likely has:
   a. Otosclerosis
   b. Dementia
   c. Cholesteatoma
   d. Presbycusis
   e. Conductive hearing loss

4. Of the following statements about cued speech, which is true?
   a. Cued speech is a system of manually coded English
   b. Cued speech involves the use of phonemically based hand gestures to supplement speechreading
   c. Cued speech is another name for a communication mode that is characteristic of a "multisensory approach"
   d. Cued speech replaces speechreading as a child's communication mode
   e. None of the above

5. Charles is a 10-year-old who has a mild to moderate hearing loss. He has worn a hearing aid since the age of 18 months. He was recently referred to a speech-language pathologist for speech therapy. Which statement probably characterizes his articulation difficulties?
   a. He neutralizes his vowels and tends to produce voiced-voiceless confusions and errors in consonant clusters
   b. He often produces vowels in the form of diphthongs and produces such consonantal errors as substitutions, omissions, and distortions
   c. Whereas vowel production is appropriate, he has difficulty in producing affricates, fricatives, glides, and laterals
   d. He pronounces most sounds with good accuracy, but he often mispronounces the fricatives /s/ and /sh/
   e. The fricative and affricate manners of articulation are problematic for the child to produce

6. For some relief from the sensation of tinnitus, various options are available. Of the following methods, which is not typically considered an option?
   a. Sound maskers
   b. Cognitive therapy and counseling
   c. Medication
   d. Tinnitus retraining therapy
   e. Relaxation training

7. A member of the Deaf culture seeks services from a speech and hearing professional. The individual is most likely inquiring about:
   a. A hearing test
   b. Sign interpreting
   c. Speech therapy
   d. Cochlear implants
   e. Use of amplification

8. A man has a significant hearing loss. His wife asks the speech and hearing professional about how she might facilitate conversation with her husband. The professional suggests that she learn to speak using a technique known as "clear speech." The wife should learn to speak:
   a. With a somewhat slowed speaking rate and with good but not exaggerated enunciation
   b. With simple syntax, such as speaking predominantly subject-verb-object sentences
   c. With semantically straightforward utterances, avoiding unclear references and unspecified pronouns
   d. With animated facial expressions and exaggerated lip and jaw movements so that speechreading is easier for the husband
   e. With a slightly increased rate of speech and exaggerated oral movements

9. Of the following statements, which best characterizes the difficulty of the lipreading task?
   a. Most people recognize fewer than 20% of the words they see when they cannot simultaneously hear the speech signal
   b. About 60% of the sounds of the English language are visible on the mouth and about 40% cannot be readily seen
   c. Viseme groups, such as /p/, /b/, /f/, and /v/, magnify the difficulty of the lipreading task
   d. Most words are homophonous, meaning that other words that sound very similar exist in the language; the existence of homophones is one reason that many people experience difficulty in lipreading
   e. All the above

10. According the American Academy of Audiology, the recommended components of a routine auditory assessment include which of the following?
    a. Documentation of a case history, audiography, otoscopic inspection, speech audiometry, determination of the need for physician referral, counseling, assessment of candidacy for and motivation to use amplification, and determination of medical clearance as determined by the U.S. Food and Drug Administration (FDA)
    b. A hearing screening, speech discrimination testing, patient counseling, and documentation of a case history
    c. Audiography, otoscopic inspection, fitting for a hearing aid if indicated, and determination of medical clearance as determined by the FDA
    d. A hearing screening, immittance testing, speech audiometry, determination of medical clearance as determined by the FDA, and patient counseling
    e. None of the above

11. Many aural rehabilitation specialists encourage their patients to avoid using nonspecific repair strategies. Of the following statements, which is *not* true of nonspecific repair strategies?
    a. This is the kind of repair strategy most commonly used by adults who have hearing loss
    b. An example of a nonspecific repair strategy is "Would you please repeat that?"
    c. When a listener uses a nonspecific repair strategy, the communication partner typically repeats what he or she just said verbatim

d. When an individual with hearing loss uses nonspecific repair strategies, conversational partners sometimes perceive the individual in an unfavorable light

e. Nonspecific repair strategies typically do not interfere significantly with the course of an existing conversation

12. What is the definition of an acoustic lexical neighborhood?

a. A set of words that contain the speech sounds with the same frequency in which they occur in everyday conversations

b. A set of words that have similar meanings and similar frequency of occurrence, such as *house, home,* and *apartment*

c. The result of a statistical analysis that indicates the transmission of speech features; test stimuli are grouped on the basis of the presence or absence of those features, and confusions between these stimuli are scored

d. A set of words that are acoustically similar and have approximately the same frequency of occurrence

e. All the above

13. Of the following statements, which best summarizes the primary goal of communication strategies training for adults who have hearing loss?

a. To enhance a patient's ability to recognize the audiovisual speech signal

b. To enhance a patient's conversational fluency

c. To eradicate a patient's passive communication behaviors

d. To increase the use of repair strategies by patients who have hearing loss

e. To introduce a passive conversational style

14. Continuous discourse tracking is:

a. Often used as an assessment procedure to determine how well patients can understand connected discourse

b. A procedure used by teachers to track the language development of children who have significant hearing loss

c. A training activity in which the receiver (listener) attempts to repeat text that is presented by a sender (speaker) verbatim

d. An instructional strategy used to teach children how to read

e. An instructional strategy used to facilitate fine motor development

15. The so-called McGurk effect is important because:

a. It helps explain why learning effects occur with repeated exposure to the items on a speech recognition test

b. It helps explain why patients who have hearing loss prefer to receive communication strategies training and personal adjustment counseling in small groups rather than in one-on-one sessions with an audiologist

c. It explains why many patients who have hearing loss believed that they have benefited from receiving auditory training even if pretraining and posttraining speech test results do not show a change

d. It is an unequivocal demonstration of audiovisual integration

e. All the above

16. Of the following statements about classroom acoustics, which is *not* true?

a. Noise may average about 50 to 60 dBA sound comparison with human ear pressure level (SPL) in the typical American classroom

b. Angling mobile whiteboards is one way to help optimize classroom acoustics

c. SoundField FM systems are not an option for a child who is in a regular classroom placement because the amplified signal may be distracting to the children who do not have hearing loss

d. Reverberation magnifies the effects of classroom noise

e. Installing draperies on windows can reduce reverberation

17. Children who have hearing loss have a good chance of developing spoken language skills:

a. That are similar to those of their peers who have normal hearing if they are identified as having hearing loss before the age of 6 months and if they receive early intervention services

b. That are similar to those of their peers who have normal hearing if they receive a cochlear implant before the age of 5 years

c. That are similar to those of their peers who have normal hearing if they began to use American Sign Language (ASL) in preschool

d. That are delayed by 12 months or more in comparison with those of their peers who have normal hearing, regardless of the communication mode that their parents select for them

e. All the above

18. Asking a child to discriminate nasal versus nonnasal unvoiced consonants that differ in place of production (e.g., "mean" from "teen") is an example of:

a. A synthetic auditory training activity

b. An informal auditory training activity

c. A very advanced auditory training exercise

d. An analytic auditory training activity

e. A comprehension activity

19. Ms. Jones, who has a profound hearing loss, is taking a lipreading test. Which word is she most likely to identify incorrectly?
    a. *Cracker*
    b. *Telephone*
    c. *Baseball*
    d. *Thumb*
    e. All the above

20. Mr. Thompson has a hearing loss. He tends to blame others for misunderstandings, and does not shy away from pointing fingers at his conversation partners. Mr. Thompson may be said to have:
    a. A passive-aggressive conversational style
    b. A passive conversational style
    c. An assertive conversational style
    d. An aggressive conversational style
    e. A noninteractive behavior mode

21. One disadvantage of using a questionnaire to characterize a patient's hearing-related disability is that:
    a. Most questionnaires were designed to assess hearing sensitivity and not disability
    b. Scoring can be subjective
    c. It is possible that a patient's hearing-related disabilities will not be identified because the questionnaire does not query about them
    d. The information is not relevant to the use of a hearing aid
    e. Questionnaires provide subjective information

22. Tim is an 8-year-old who has pure-tone averages of 10 dB hearing level (HL) in both ears. His teacher reports that he does not seem to understand verbal instructions as well as his classmates and believes that he is not paying much attention during class. An audiologist reported that he has a hard time counting the number of pips that occur in a short series. Tim most likely has:

    a. Auditory neuropathy
    b. Central auditory processing disorder (CAPD)
    c. Persistent tinnitus
    d. Alport syndrome
    e. Cleft palate

23. Theresa is 5 years old. She was born with a bilateral profound sensorineural hearing loss, which was diagnosed at the age of 2 months. Three months ago, she received a cochlear implant. She is able to articulate the following sounds accurately:
    a. Central vowels
    b. Back vowels
    c. Front vowels
    d. Voiceless stops
    e. Voiced stops

24. An audiologist has just tested Ms. Kerley. The test results indicate that she has a moderate hearing loss. Until today, Mrs. Kerley had never had a hearing test. At this point, the audiologist is most likely to provide:
    a. Personal adjustment counseling
    b. Communication strategies counseling
    c. Desensitization
    d. Informational counseling
    e. All the above

25. In interacting with a patient who has hearing loss, a speech and hearing professional behaves in a genuine manner, avoids assuming a façade of professionalism, and avoids using professional jargon. The professional is said to have:
    a. Unconditional positive regard
    b. Empathetic understanding
    c. Congruence with self
    d. Rational emotive behavior
    e. Cognitive counseling orientation

1. a. Hearing loss sometimes co-occurs with low birth weight but not high birth weight. Infants born to women who are infected with cytomegalovirus (option b) for the first time during pregnancy are at risk for hearing loss and other complications, such as microcephaly, circulation problems, mental retardation, and visual impairment. Co-occurring craniofacial abnormalities (option c) and hearing loss are characteristic of many syndromes, such as Edward syndrome (trisomy 18) and Crouzon syndrome. Children with low Apgar scores—which refer to appearance, pulse, grimace, activity, and respiration—have been shown to be at higher risk for hearing loss than have babies who have high Apgar scores (option d).

2. b. Norman Erber was one of the first practitioners to suggest that auditory training be organized in such a way that the student progresses from stages of sound awareness, sound discrimination, identification, and comprehension. This suggestion has served as the starting point for many subsequent auditory training programs. "Formal and then informal" (option a) refers to the types of training activities that might be included in an auditory training lesson. Sometimes a lesson may include one type or the other and, often, includes both types. "Words, phrases, sentences" (option c) refers to the types of stimuli that may be used during an auditory training lesson. "Auditory only, visual only, and then audiovisual speech perception" (option d) refer to possible modalities that students may rely on when receiving speech perception training. On occasion, a student may first be asked to perform training tasks in an audiovisual condition and then, when performance is very good, be asked to perform training tasks in an auditory-only condition. "Formal, sound awareness, words, visual only" (option e) is a combination of items across training activities, levels of training, stimuli, and modality.

3. d. *Presbycusis* is a global term used to refer to hearing loss associated with the aging process. It is characterized by a sensorineural hearing loss in the higher frequencies and decreased word recognition. Otosclerosis (option a) is abnormal growth of bone in the middle ear, and results in conductive rather than sensorineural hearing loss. Dementia (option b), also a common physical problem among older persons, is an irreversible decline in cognitive functioning. Persons with dementia may or may not also have presbycusis. Cholesteatoma (option c) is a tumor-like mass of squamous epithelium in the middle ear cavity that may also invade the mastoid; it is often associated with chronic otitis media or tympanic membrane perforation. Conductive hearing loss (option e) is the result of outer or middle ear involvement and would be an unlikely cause of hearing loss in this case scenario.

4. b. Cued speech is a communication system in which phonemically based hand configurations and placements are used to supplement speechreading. Eight hand shapes are used to distinguish consonants, and six locations on the face and neck are used to distinguish vowels. Manually coded English (option a) is composed of manual signs corresponding to the words of English and can convey messages with or without concomitant speaking. A multisensory approach (option c), a variant of aural-oral language, refers to instances when children use both vision and hearing to recognize the spoken word. Cued speech is used to clarify ambiguity in the visual speech signal; it cannot stand alone, apart from the spoken word, and therefore cannot replace speechreading (option d).

5. d. Children who have mild to moderate hearing loss, especially children who receive appropriate amplification early on, tend to develop nearly normal speech articulation, but they may mispronounce fricatives such as /s/ and /sh/. The errors described in the alternative options are characteristic of children who have significant hearing loss and wear hearing aids. Receipt of a cochlear implant at an early age often enables children with severe and profound hearing loss to develop speech that is more like that of children who have mild to moderate hearing loss.

6. c. There is no known cure for tinnitus and no prescribed medication affords relief. Sound maskers (option a) deliver sound to the ear that masks the tinnitus. Cognitive therapy and counseling (option b) help patients learn to control where they direct their attention and to change the content of their thoughts about tinnitus. Tinnitus retraining therapy (option d) entails a combination of counseling and sound therapy. Relaxation training (option e) involves a direct focus on decreasing muscle tension through the use of different exercises.

7. b. Adult members of the Deaf culture typically lost their hearing early in life and rely on sign language for face-to-face communication. They consider

themselves to be culturally and linguistically distinct from hearing society and may request sign interpreting services. Many do not communicate with spoken language, and so they would not seek speech therapy (option c). They do not use hearing aids, and so they are not interested in amplification (option e) and thus do not routinely seek audiography (option a), and they are opposed to cochlear implants (option d).

8. a. Clear speech involves a somewhat slowed speaking rate and good but not exaggerated enunciation. It has been shown to be more intelligible than conversational speech for persons who have hearing loss. Speaking with simple syntax (option b) and semantically straightforward utterances (option c) may also be helpful to the person who has hearing loss, but those techniques are not encompassed under the rubric of "clear speech." Exaggerated lip and jaw movements (option d) rarely enhance the speech-reading task and often make a spoken message even more difficult to speechread, as would increasing rate of speech (option e).

9. a. Lipreading is difficult, and most people can recognize fewer than 20% of the words when a speech sample is presented in a vision-only condition. Fewer than 40% of the sounds of English are visible on the face (option b), and this is a reason that lipreading is difficult. Viseme groups (option c) contain sounds that look alike on the face; however, the production of /p/ and /b/ entails a bilabial lip closure, whereas that of /f/ and /v/ entails a labiodental closure. Homophenes (option d) are words that look the same on the mouth, even though they may sound different; for instance, the words "grade" and "yes" sound different, but they look similar on the face.

10. a. The American Academy of Audiology. www.audiology.org Clinical Practice of Algorithms and Statements (Journal Audiology Today Special Issue 2000) suggested that the auditory assessment include documentation of a comprehensive case history, pure-tone audiography and measurement of loudness discomfort levels, otoscopic inspection, determination of the need for physician referral, counseling, assessment of candidacy for and motivation to use amplification, and determination of medical clearance as determined by the FDA. A hearing screening (options b and d) is not a comprehensive audiogram. Fitting for a hearing aid (option c) does not occur during an initial or routine auditory assessment; instead, it occurs after the hearing status of a patient has been determined and amplification options have been considered.

11. b. In a nonspecific repair strategy, the communication partner is not told what to do to repair a communication breakdown; this strategy includes such utterances as "Huh?" and "What?"

12. d. Word lists used in speech assessments have been based on the principles of acoustic lexical neighborhoods. Words that have a similar frequency of occurrence (i.e., how often the words occur during everyday language use) and that have similar acoustic-phonetic characteristics belong to the same neighborhood. For example, the words *cat, kit,* and *kiss* are members of the same neighborhood. "A set of words that contain the speech sounds with the same frequency in which they occur in everyday conversations" (option a) is the definition of a phonetically balanced word list. "A set of words that have similar meanings and similar frequency of occurrence" (option b) is the definition of a semantic neighborhood. The statistical procedure (option c) is known as information transmission analysis, which is sometimes used to analyze the results of a test of phonemes and nonsense syllables.

13. b. The primary goal of communication strategies training is to enhance conversational fluency. Conversational fluency is described in terms of time spent in repairing communication breakdowns, exchange of information and ideas, sharing of speaking time among conversational partners, and time spent in silence. The goal of speech perception training is to enhance recognition of the speech signal (option a). One goal of assertiveness training is to encourage patients to use assertive behaviors in lieu of passive communication behaviors (option c). Using repair strategies (option d), particularly specific repair strategies, more often and more effectively is one way to enhance conversational fluency. A passive conversational style (option e) is one wherein the person limits communicative interactions, as opposed to engaging in conversational repair.

14. c. In continuous discourse tracking, the sender reads aloud a selection from a printed passage, phrase by phrase. After each phrase, a receiver attempts to repeat it. If the receiver cannot do so, then he or she may use repair strategies to elicit additional information from the sender. The procedure provides both speech perception practice and communication strategies training. Performance on a continuous discourse tracking task is affected by the skill of the sender in speaking the materials and in providing repair, and by the level of the difficulty of the passage, among other extraneous variables. As such, it is not very reliable as a means to document a patient's speech recognition abilities (option a). Continuous discourse tracking is not used for

tracking language development (option b), for reading instruction (option d), or for fine motor development (option e).

15. d. In the McGurk paradigm, patients see a talker speak one syllable as they simultaneously hear the talker speak a different syllable. For instance, they may see "ba" and hear "ga." For some discrepant syllable combinations, the patients will perceive a third syllable that differs from the two syllables. In this example, a common percept is "da." The fact that patients combine the signals suggests that when people recognize speech, they integrate auditory and visual speech information in the process of decoding the signal and that this integration is obligatory (i.e., they cannot help but do it).

16. c. SoundField FM systems are listening system in which sound from the teacher's microphone is transmitted to the students by loudspeakers that are positioned throughout the classroom. The system is advantageous for children who have either normal or impaired hearing because it offers a better signal-to-noise ratio for hearing the teacher's speech. Most classrooms are noisy (option a), and thus are not optimal environments for children who have hearing loss to hear the teacher. Angling mobile whiteboards reduces the amount of reverberation (option b). Reverberation is the persistence of a sound caused by reflection of the signal from the wall, ceiling, and floor surfaces. Reverberation prolongs a noise and may cause a speech signal, such as the teacher's speech, to merge with other signals and to lose clarity (option d). The installation of draperies or other such window treatments (option e) is recommended in order to reduce reverberation.

17. a. Research has demonstrated that if hearing loss is identified, and intervention starts, before a baby reaches the age of 6 months, the child will achieve language scores that are comparable with those of to children who have normal hearing by the time the child reaches 3 years of age. Research has shown that the earlier a child receives a cochlear implant, the more favorable will be the language outcome (option b); however, common practice has increasingly been to provide a cochlear implant to a child before the age of 2 years. By the age of 4 or 5 years, the child will have missed out on some if not much of the critical period for acquiring spoken language. ASL (option c) and spoken language typically do not develop in unison. ASL is a system of communication used by members of the Deaf Culture in the United States. Its syntax is different from that of spoken English and cannot be used simultaneously with speaking. Sometimes children who have hearing

loss learn ASL as their first language and then learn English later in school (this is known as a *bilingual/ bicultural model*). Although many children who have significant hearing loss experience language delay, the use of appropriate listening devices, early identification and intervention, and parental involvement can mitigate against delay (option d).

18. d. Analytic training emphasizes the recognition of individual speech sounds or syllables, and this activity would focus the child's attention on distinguishing / m/ from /t/. This is an example of a formal auditory training, not informal (option b), because it implies a highly structured activity that may involve drill. In a synthetic auditory training activity (option a), individuals are taught to comprehend the meaning of spoken utterance even if they do not identify every sound or word. Discrimination activities (option c) tend to occur fairly early on in a hierarchy of auditory training exercises, and discriminating a nasal consonant from a nonnasal consonant is relatively easy for persons with hearing loss; in comparison, discriminating between two voiceless stop consonants is more difficult. Comprehension activity (option e) refers to the understanding of spoken messages.

19. a. The word *cracker* is composed of sounds that are not very visible on the face, such as /k/, and so this word would be difficult to recognize in a vision-only condition (the term *lipreading* typically refers to using only the visual signal to recognize speech). Very few words look like *telephone* (option b) on the mouth, and it contains a "visible" sound, /f/. The spondee *baseball* (option c) also entails visible movements, and few words resemble it when spoken in a vision-only condition. Both the initial and final consonant of *thumb* (option d) are quite visible when spoken.

20. d. A person with an aggressive conversational style may display characteristics such as hostility, and belligerence. A person with a passive-aggressive conversational style (option a) is likely to express aggression in an indirect way. A person with a passive conversation style (option b) would withdraw from conversation rather than confront others or attempt to repair communication breakdowns. An assertive conversational style (option c) suggests that the patient takes responsibility for managing communication difficulties in a manner that is considerate of others. A noninteractive behavior mode (option e) is a conversational strategy that is typically associated with a passive conversational style.

21. c. Hearing-related disability is a loss of function imposed by hearing loss, and the term denotes a multidimensional phenomenon. One drawback in

administering a questionnaire is that it is possible to miss information about a patient's specific communication difficulties because those difficulties are not covered by the questionnaire. Moreover, some questions may be irrelevant. For instance, a true-false statement such as "I ask a coworker to take notes during presentations" may be irrelevant to a patient who spends the day gardening in a yard. Many questionnaires are available, and some are designed to assess disability (option a). Many questionnaires contain closed-ended questions; when they pose open-ended questions, the questions typically elicit qualitative information that does not entail "scoring" per se (option b). The information that may be collected with a questionnaire is often relevant to hearing aid use (option d); a well-designed questionnaire can elicit information about whether a patient's hearing-related disability has declined as a result of hearing aid use. Questionnaires are used to assess in a subjective manner (option e) a person's conversational fluency and communication handicap, which is helpful for both the person and conversation partners.

22. b. CAPD, an inability to differentiate, recognize, and understand sounds, is not caused by either hearing loss or cognitive impairment. Although tinnitus (option c) can distract a listener's attention, it is probably not the cause of Tim's seeming inattention. In auditory neuropathy (option a), pure-tone thresholds may or may not be in the normal range, but acoustic reflexes may be absent, auditory brainstem response may be abnormal, and word discrimination may be impaired. Alport syndrome (option d) is characterized by sensorineural hearing loss and nephritis. Children born with cleft palate (option e) are at risk for conductive hearing loss.

23. a. Children with profound hearing loss tend to neutralize their vowels, including back vowels (option b) and front vowels (option c). Upon receipt of a cochlear implant, vowel production improves. Children with profound hearing loss often have voiced-voiceless confusions (options d and e). After extended experience with a cochlear implant, some children begin to articulate these stops correctly, especially if they receive their cochlear implants at a very early age.

24. d. The audiologist would first provide Ms. Kerley with information about the hearing loss and about the benefits and limitations of amplification. Later on, if necessary, she might receive personal adjustment counseling (option a), communication strategies training (option b), or desensitization (option c). These latter interventions might alleviate her communication difficulties and help her adjust to the presence of hearing loss.

25. c. Congruence with self is a first tenet of person-centered counseling in which clinicians act as themselves in interactions with patients and do not assume an imposing professionalism. They speak to patients honestly and sincerely. Unconditional positive regard (option a), another tenet of person-centered counseling, is related to the assumption that patients know best and that they have the inner resources to overcome their conversation difficulties. Empathetic understanding (option b) is another tenet of person-centered counseling, in which a counselor listens to the patient's concerns and feelings about a hearing problem, reflects those communications back to the patient, and helps the patient identify solutions. The goal of rational emotive behavior therapy (option d), a solution-oriented counseling or therapy approach, is to resolve specific problems by using cognitive, behavioral, and affective elements; a key to this approach is the idea that emotions result from beliefs rather than from events or circumstances. In cognitive counseling (option e), the aim is to modify the client's underlying thought processes, such as incorrect assumptions or inappropriate emotional reactions.

Bibliography

American Academy of Audiology. www.audiology.org Clinical Practice Algorithms and Statements (Journal Audiology Today Special Issue 2000).

PART VI

Clinical
Management

CHAPTER 16

Alternative and Augmentative Communication

Kathleen Franklin

1. Of the following items, which represents an unaided communication symbol?
   a. Line drawing symbol
   b. Vocalization
   c. Photographic symbol
   d. Speech-generating device
   e. Blissymbol

2. In the hierarchy of symbolization, which of the following is the most iconic?
   a. Braille
   b. Written words
   c. Line drawings
   d. Photographs
   e. Sign language

3. In order to use advanced audio coding (AAC), a person needs to have:
   a. Intact receptive language skills
   b. Intact expressive language skills
   c. Sensorimotor cognitive skills of object permanence and of means and end
   d. The physical motor skills to point to communication symbols
   e. An inability to communicate effectively to support daily needs and wants

4. An aided communication symbol is represented by which of the following?
   a. Low-tech communication board with photograph symbols
   b. American Sign Language
   c. An informal gestural system

d. Vocalizations or intelligible words, or both

e. Facial expression

5. Of the following techniques for enhancing communication rate, which is the most difficult to learn?
   a. Color encoding
   b. Iconic encoding
   c. Numerical encoding
   d. Alphanumerical encoding
   e. Alphabetical encoding

6. The most successful AAC intervention consists of:
   a. Creating communication systems in which multiple communication strategies are used
   b. Ensuring that a speech-generating device is available
   c. Using low-tech options exclusively
   d. Using gesture system approaches
   e. Using formal sign language systems

7. Alternative access to a communication device in which a switch is used for scanning requires matching a scanning technique best suited to an individual's motor capabilities. For an individual who has difficulty maintaining contact with a switch to keep scanning in operation but can access a switch effectively for short period of time, _____ is the best choice.
   a. Step scanning
   b. Direct scanning
   c. Automatic scanning
   d. Circular scanning
   e. Linear scanning

8. AAC vocabulary for nonliterate individuals generally consists of:
   a. Letters to teach spelling in order to develop literacy skills
   b. One symbol to represent each semantic category
   c. One symbol to represent a whole message
   d. Coverage vocabulary based on the age of the individual using AAC
   e. One symbol to represent each grammatical category

9. One concern in AAC use is the slow rate of message formulation. Techniques have been developed to increase rate. One technique, encoding, involves:
   a. Using letter, number, and word codes to represent messages
   b. Using direct selection access in AAC rather than scanning
   c. Spelling messages
   d. Using graphic symbols
   e. Using word abbreviations

10. One AAC device allows a person to access an electronic screen that, when activated, automatically changes pages on the screen. This device is referred to as:
    a. Fixed display
    b. Rigid display
    c. Hybrid display
    d. Visual scene display
    e. Dynamic display

11. The ability to activate or access AAC devices (low-tech and high-tech) by using pointing or touching is referred to as:
    a. Direct selection
    b. Speech recognition
    c. Scanning
    d. Encoding
    e. Decoding

12. A patient evaluated for AAC access methods was able to point with eyes to letters on a Plexiglas board. This access strategy is an example of:
    a. Timed activation
    b. Inverse scanning
    c. Directed scanning
    d. Release activation
    e. Direct selection

13. Individuals with limited motor control who cannot use direct selection need to use electronic or partner-assisted scanning. A scanning pattern that involves identifying a group of items and then eliminating options gradually until a final selection is made is called:
    a. Low-tech scanning
    b. Circular scanning
    c. Linear scanning
    d. Group-item scanning
    e. Step scanning

14. The model of assessment in AAC that promotes ongoing analysis of communication needs for both now and the future is the:
    a. Communication needs model
    b. Participation model
    c. Candidacy model
    d. Traditional language model
    e. Needs assessment model

15. Many individuals referred for AAC evaluation and intervention services have some natural speech abilities remaining. In a multimodal approach to communication use, a speech-language pathologist (SLP) should:
    a. Focus directly on AAC strategies in which aided techniques are used
    b. Incorporate natural speech skills as part of overall AAC system
    c. Concentrate on maximizing natural speech abilities
    d. Focus directly on AAC strategies in which unaided techniques are used
    e. Focus directly on AAC strategies in which sign language is used

16. Parents of young children with AAC needs often question the effects of these interventions on the development of natural speech skills. Current research indicates that:
   a. Natural speech will be replaced by AAC
   b. Natural speech may be enhanced by use of AAC
   c. Children become confused by too many communication strategies
   d. AAC strategies slow the development of natural speech skills
   e. AAC strategies do not change the development of natural speech skills

17. For individuals with complex motor impairments, the evaluation of motor skills should be completed by:
   a. An occupational therapist who specializes in AAC assessments
   b. An SLP who specializes in AAC assessments
   c. A physical therapist who specializes in AAC assessments
   d. A vision specialist who specializes in AAC assessments
   e. A team of professionals who specialize in AAC assessments

18. Formal and informal language assessment as part of an AAC evaluation is completed to provide insight into:
   a. Test scores
   b. Developmental level
   c. Functional profile of current capabilities
   d. Ability to match device to language skills
   e. Criterion-referenced performance

19. In an AAC assessment, identifying an individual's level of recognition of print and phoneme, phonological processing, reading comprehension, and spelling skills is useful for determining:
   a. The extent to which words and letters can be used as part of the AAC system
   b. Whether the student will be able to speak
   c. The extent to which photographic symbols can be used as part of the AAC system
   d. The extent to which line drawing symbols can be used as part of the AAC system
   e. Low-tech versus high-tech device acquisition

20. Funding for AAC devices through an insurance vendor (e.g., Medicaid, Medicare, private insurance) requires documentation that the device will be used:
   a. To meet spelling goals
   b. To meet language goals
   c. To meet math goals
   d. To teach reading and writing skills
   e. To meet daily and health care need

21. A patient with newly diagnosed amyotrophic lateral sclerosis (ALS) is referred to an SLP for consultation. According to current practice, the SLP should:
   a. Direct the patient to return when speech is unintelligible
   b. Direct the patient to return when writing skills are impaired
   c. Direct the patient to return when reading skills are impaired
   d. Provide patient education on AAC options and inform the patient to return when AAC is needed
   e. Provide patient education on AAC options and allow the patient to develop skills in AAC use

22. AAC services in an acute care medical setting are necessary to provide access to communication for individuals who may temporarily be unable to speak. In this environment, AAC services are best delivered by:
   a. An AAC consultant
   b. Transporting the patient to an outpatient center
   c. An on-site staff SLP
   d. Deferring intervention; wait until natural speech returns
   e. AAC vendors who can demonstrate equipment to the patient

23. An individual with an acute medical condition was evaluated by an SLP. Results indicated orientation ×3, good receptive language skills, and sufficient oral-motor control for speech, but inadequate voicing to produce words. AAC strategies are recommended and initially should be:
   a. Trials with a speech-generating device
   b. Trials with a low-tech communication board
   c. Trials with an eye gaze board
   d. Trials with an electrolarynx
   e. Trials with unaided strategies such as signing

24. AAC can be an effective strategy for an individual with a traumatic brain injury (TBI). The goal of AAC within this population is to:
   a. Defer intervention until patient stabilizes so that a long-term AAC solution can be determined
   b. Provide AAC that may change over time early in the treatment process, focusing on a strategy for the patient to communicate needs
   c. Provide long-term AAC applications so that there is time for training
   d. Defer intervention completely because of possible cognitive or linguistic impairments
   e. Defer intervention completely because of possible motor impairments

25. Individuals who are in the recovery stage after a TBI generally benefit from:
   a. Electronic speech-generating devices
   b. Letter boards

c. Context-specific communication displays

d. Written word boards

e. Line drawing boards

26. After a cerebral vascular accident, a 60-year-old man displayed severe upper limb motor impairment and severe speech dysarthria. Initially, the SLP created a communication board, using words to assist the patient in meeting communication needs at home. His wife was instructed to sit next to him with the board and point from row to row until the correct row was identified and then point item by item in a row until the desired item was touched. This procedure is referred to as:

a. Linear scanning

b. Direct selection

c. Partner-assisted scanning

d. Circular scanning

e. Step scanning

27. Individuals classified as beginning communicators rely on nonsymbolic strategies for communication. Of the following scenarios, which illustrates the use of non-symbolic strategies?

a. A student uses an AAC device to answer questions during science class

b. An adult with intellectual disabilities orders fast food, using a low-tech communication board

c. A preschooler uses a voice-output device to describe weather during circle time

d. A high school student communicates frustration by screaming during activity and environment transitions

e. An adult recovering from TBI uses head shaking and nodding to indicate "yes" and "no"

28. In early intervention, AAC use with a child supports

a. The incorporation of goals to develop natural speech

b. Delay in developing literacy skills until the child enters school

c. The assumption that not all children will enter kindergarten

d. The use of norm-referenced measures to assess a young child's abilities

e. A focus on impairments rather than on strategies

29. Communication symbols, presented either on an electronic device or on low-tech communication board, must be organized to promote effective and efficient communication for the individual using them. The organization of displays with regard to themes or routines is referred to as:

a. Taxonomic display

b. Semantic-syntactic display

c. Visual scene display

d. Activity-based display

e. Letter-based display

30. Several approaches are available to teach language skills to individuals who use AAC. Strategies that focus on teaching symbol use and language in a contextually rich natural environment are reflected in:

a. An aided language stimulation model

b. A discrete trials-teaching model

c. A conversational coaching model

d. An adapted strategic instruction model

e. A naturalistic teaching model

31. Individuals with severe speech and physical disabilities who use AAC generally have limited literacy skills. More than 50% and as many as 90% cannot read or write or have skills well below age-level expectations. These findings can be attributed mainly to:

a. The severity of the language impairment

b. The severity of the motor impairment

c. The severity of visual and auditory perceptual difficulties

d. The severity of cognitive impairment

e. The limited opportunities to engage in reading and writing tasks

32. A student who is integrated into a regular education classroom is provided with enlarged copies of class notes and visual access to concepts presented on a SMART Board mounted in the front of the class. The teacher allows other children access to notes if they want them so that they do not have to write out everything the teachers says. These classroom strategies are examples of:

a. Selected inclusion for learning

b. Universal design for learning

c. Full integration for learning

d. Competitive educational participation

e. Active educational participation

33. Communication boards for people with late-stage dementia should:

a. Combine words with pictures (line drawings and photographs)

b. Provide letters for spelling messages

c. Display written words

d. Display written phrases

e. Communicate "yes" and "no"

34. The use of communication boards with words to clarify messages for individuals with dysarthria to supplement unintelligible natural speech is an example of:

a. Alphabet supplementation

b. Topic supplementation

c. Voice amplification supplementation

d. Natural speech supplementation

e. Strategic supplementation

35. Which statement best reflects the role of the person being assessed for AAC and family members in the decision-making process?
    a. Decision making about AAC devices and strategies should be based on the expertise of the AAC professionals
    b. Decision making about AAC devices and strategies requires input from AAC vendors
    c. Decision making about AAC devices and strategies should include input from all constituents involved in the evaluation process
    d. Decision making about AAC devices and strategies should be based on available funding
    e. Decision making about AAC devices and strategies should be based on the wishes of the individual being evaluated or of the family members, or of both

36. Abandonment of the AAC device is commonly the result of:
    a. Lack of appropriate training of the AAC facilitator
    b. Complexity of the AAC device
    c. Inability of the person using the AAC device to program the device
    d. Frequent malfunction of the AAC device
    e. Obsolescence of the AAC device

37. Individuals with significant fine motor disorder may be unable to use a standard mouse to use a computer for writing. Of the following devices, which represents an alternative to a standard mouse?
    a. Voice recognition software
    b. Pencil and paper
    c. Trackball
    d. Adapted switch
    e. Scanning

38. Joe is a student in a public school who recently received a high-tech communication device that was funded by the school district. At the end of his first week of using the device within the school setting, he was getting ready to leave school for the weekend and was putting the device in his backpack so that he had it available for communication over the weekend. The school's principal stopped in the classroom at dismissal and told Joe's teacher that the device had to remain at school and could not be transported back and forth between home and school. This is an example of:
    a. Policy barrier
    b. Practice barrier
    c. Knowledge barrier
    d. Skill barrier
    e. Attitude barrier

39. In choosing vocabulary for individuals who use AAC, selecting words that are common and frequently used by a group of individuals is referred to as:
    a. Fringe vocabulary
    b. Informant vocabulary
    c. Individual vocabulary
    d. Core vocabulary
    e. AAC vocabulary

40. A rate enhancement technique that allows for words to be "predicted" on the basis of beginning letters typed into a computer or AAC device is referred to as:
    a. Message prediction
    b. Icon prediction
    c. Encoding prediction
    d. Color prediction
    e. Alphabet prediction

1. b. Symbols can be categorized as aided and unaided. Aided symbols require an external element for production, such as a communication board or a device. Unaided symbols do not require an external element; vocalizations, speech, gestures, and sign language are examples of unaided symbols.

2. d. *Symbol iconicity* refers to how closely a symbol resembles its referent or the item or concept that it represents. Highly iconic symbols closely resemble its referent; abstract symbols have little to no relationship to the thing it represents. For example, a photograph of an apple is a good representation of the item, whereas the sign for apple has no relationship and is considered abstract.

3. e. No prerequisite skills are necessary for an individual to be considered for AAC options, although this was not always the case. Early in the history of the AAC field, clients were thought to need specific cognitive skills before AAC was considered for them. Today, if the need for communication supports with AAC is identified, it should be provided, regardless of a person's disability or its severity.

4. a. Aided communication symbols require some type of physical device to be displayed. In this case, the communication board is the physical device. American Sign Language (option b), informal gestures (option c), vocalizations (option d), and facial expression (option e) represent unaided symbols; they do not require a device for representation.

5. b. Encoding is a strategy that allows an individual to combine specific codes (e.g., number, letters, icons, colors) to express a longer message. For example, the alphanumerical code G4 might represent a greeting message such as "Hey, how is everything going?" According to research into the ease of learning different types of encoding systems, combining different icons together to create messages requires the most practice in order to memorize the codes than do the other strategies available.

6. a. Successful AAC interventions allow an individual access to multiple methods of communication. Multimodal communication provides access to different communication strategies, depending on communication partners, environments, and other variables. For example, at home an individual may use gestures and vocalization to communicate because this may be the most efficient way of interacting with family members. Within the community, a communication device or communication boards may be necessary to ensure that unfamiliar communication partners understand the messages being communicated.

7. c. Automatic scanning allows for a cursor to move directly from location to location until the scanning is interrupted by activation of a switch. For direct scanning (option b), the movement of a cursor is advanced by the person's holding down on a switch; the person releases it when the desired location is reached. Step scanning (option a) requires that a switch be activated for each movement of the cursor. Options d and e are scanning patterns not access techniques as per a, b, and c.

8. c. AAC strategies should be matched to an individual's language and cognitive skills. Individuals who do not have literacy skills may need to use a strategy in which one symbol represents an entire message. In AAC applications, strategies are designed to provide immediate access to communication; therefore, they are matched to a person's skills. AAC strategies can also be used to teach new skills as part of an overall educational plan, but this should not be the primary focus.

9. a. Encoding strategies allow for combinations of a few symbols (letter codes, number codes, picture codes) to represent full messages. This allows individuals to save time in that they do not have to either spell out entire messages or use separate symbols for each word in an utterance string.

10. e. Dynamic displays are computer-based and allow the user to "navigate" between screens by touching symbols to move from one location to another. Fixed displays (option a) represent communication displays that are "fixed" in a set location; they are also called *static displays.* Low-tech communication boards and simple-tech speech-generating devices are examples of fixed displays. Option b rigid refers to a display that is static or does not change. Hybrid displays (option c) have both fixed and dynamic capabilities. Visual scene displays (option d) use pictures or virtual environments that contain conversational elements. Additional cells can be added to the display can provide content related to the picture or environment.

11. a. Direct selection techniques are strategies for access of AAC devices and strategies through the use of fingers, hands, and adapted pointing devices. Eye gaze to

specific symbols can also be considered a direct selection technique. Computers and communication devices that allow for eye tracking (a camera that reads eye movement) enable individuals with severe motor impairment to operate an electronic device screen's cursor as an alternative to standard mouse control.

12. e. Eye pointing is an example of a direct selection technique. Timed activation and release activation are scanning-related cursor control strategies.

13. d. Group-item scanning involves moving through groups of items, selecting the group that contains the desired item, and then scanning item by item until the cursor reaches the desired item. Group-item scanning functions as a rate enhancement strategy. Low tech scanning (option a) refers to an introductory scanning technique that is frequently used to teach scanning. A circular scanning pattern (option b) scans items presented in a circle. Linear scanning (option c) requires the movement of a cursor across each item in a row before moving to the next row. Step scanning (option e) is a method of activation that changes the cursor one step at a time.

14. b. The participation model is the assessment or intervention model supported by practitioners in the AAC field. In this model, decisions about AAC use are based on the participation needs of the individual who may need AAC in relation to the functional participation patterns of peers of similar age. This model also promotes the development of AAC interventions that are useful today with planning for next steps needed in the future.

15. b. As communicators, people use a variety of methods in addition to speech: gesture, facial expressions, body language, and written communication. SLPs should encourage the use of multimodal strategies, including natural speech skills, for individuals who use AAC. In this way, they have a variety of strategies to use that can be combined in different ways to maximize communication within the various environments and activities accessed throughout the day.

16. b. Current research supports the use of AAC with young children. It has been documented that the use of AAC does not slow down or replace natural speech skills. Rather, AAC strategies have been found to promote the development and use of natural speech in some children.

17. e. A team approach should be used in AAC assessment for individuals with complex needs. Staff from different disciplines can raise important considerations that might otherwise be overlooked. For example, an SLP is interested in physical access of a communication device, whereas an occupational therapist and a physical therapist need to think about the person's positioning needs and device mounting, if needed.

18. c. In AAC assessment, the goal is to identify what an individual can do from a communication perspective. The goal is to further develop appropriate communication skills through the use of AAC strategies to maximize an individual's participation in the activities and environments accessed throughout the day. Formal test scores and developmental levels can provide information on how to organize communication devices and strategies.

19. a. Literacy assessment is important for determining the overall reading, writing, and spelling skills of the individual who needs AAC. Often, literacy is overlooked in formal teaching of individuals with severe expressive communication disorders. Scatter skills among the components of literacy may be evidenced. SLPs need to understand the extent to which literacy can be incorporated into the AAC strategy and how literacy may assist in determining interventions goals focused on further developing the scatter skills.

20. e. Insurance carriers consider AAC devices to be speech-generating devices classified under durable medical equipment. In this instance, AAC can be reported only as a strategy to provide a way for an individual to meet daily living needs and communicate about health care. Educational goals such as spelling, language, math, reading, and writing cannot be stated; insurance carriers would argue that educational goals are the domain of the education system and that the education system should therefore provide access to an AAC device.

21. e. Patients with ALS inevitably require the use of AAC. Providing opportunities to develop low-tech boards and teaching electronic device use before the patient needs these strategies will ensure that there is continuity in access to communication as the disease progresses.

22. c. In view of the dynamic nature of the acute care medical setting, on-site staff should be available to provide AAC services. This will ensure that AAC strategies are put into place quickly.

23. d. In the acute care setting, providing AAC strategies that are quick and efficient are encouraged so that a patient can communicate about health care needs. In this case, because the patient has good oral motor control for speech, trials with an electrolarynx is warranted.

24. b. Research supports the use of AAC strategies early with patients who have TBI. The visual nature of AAC strategies can provide appropriate scaffolding for patients with cognitive and linguistic deficits. Because of the ongoing improvements seen in these patients during first weeks and months, it is important to know that AAC strategies and techniques will need to change in response to the patient's developing skills.

25. c. Individuals with TBI can develop a range of cognitive, linguistic, or motor deficits, or a combination of these. Providing AAC communication displays that relate to specific topics (e.g., family, health care, physical comfort) can assist in focusing the patient on relevant topics related to immediate needs. These strategies may or may not need a voice output component. The use of letter boards and written word formats can be used only if the patient has maintained literacy skills.

26. c. Partner-assisted scanning is a strategy in which communication symbols are physically scanned by another person. This technique is often used in an acute care setting in which quick access to communication is needed. It is also a technique used as a preliminary technique for individuals with significant motor impairments who need to have access to a variety of techniques for communication.

27. d. Beginning communicators may use behaviors such as screaming, tantrums, hitting, and other physical acting out to communicate a message. For example, a person might scream, and the consequence is that someone pays attention to the person. Over time, the person might identify screaming as the communication used to gain another person's attention. Use of an AAC device (option a), a low-tech communication board (option b), a voice-output device (option c), and head movements (option e) are symbolic strategies.

28. a. Early intervention philosophy focuses on identifying strengths, building on them, and adhering to the "least dangerous assumption" principle, in which the expectation is that all children will build skills and perform at the same level as peers. Consequently, the goal would be the development of natural speech if possible.

29. d. Activity-based displays organize displays according to schemes, routines, and activities. In taxonomic displays (option a), symbols are grouped on the basis of categories. Semantic-syntactic displays (option b) organize displays according to the parts of speech. Visual scene displays (option c) use contextually rich photographs or other symbols to communicate about

topics. In letter-based displays (option e), the alphabet is used for letter-by-letter spelling.

30. a. Aided language stimulation involves the organization of physical environments and activities in such a way that communication symbols are available and used at all times. They are available for students to use to relay messages to others, but teachers, therapists, and family members are encouraged to use the symbols as well; this provides an additional way for learners to receive information from others verbally. Information is supplied both verbally and visually.

31. e. Regardless of an individual's disability or degree of disability, literacy experiences should be provided. Research findings indicate that people with disabilities have limited opportunities to participate in reading and writing tasks. Assistive technology and AAC are available to provide support in introducing and adapting materials to promote reading and writing activities for all patients.

32. b. The concept of universal design for learning is becoming widely used in the educational arena. The principles of universal design are to make available to all learners a variety of strategies to enhance the overall educational experience. In this way, students can pick methods and strategies for learning that meet their needs. These strategies are available not only for learners with disabilities but also for other members of the class.

33. a. For patients with advanced dementia, the key to the usefulness of communication boards is creating the fewest memory demands. The goal is to create communication strategies that reduce distraction and allow for information to be chunked, such as combining words with pictures. Communication boards that use words and phrases may be too cognitively demanding for individuals with advanced dementia.

34. b. In topic supplementation, specific words are used to help set communication topics so that communication partners have words cues to identify what a person is discussing. In alphabet supplementation (option a), letters are used to spell out unintelligible words until a communication partner can figure out the word an individual is trying to say. Voice amplification (option c) is method for increasing the intensity of a speaker's voice, and is not effective in improving intelligibility. Option d refers to any type of AAC strategy such as gesture to communicate. Strategic supplementation refers to strategies such as rate enhancement.

35. c. Decision making should include input from all relevant individuals involved. The opinions and concerns of the individual being evaluated and the family members are very important in the decision-making process. Their preferences and attitudes about equipment suggested and overall recommendations must be considered in order for implementation to be successful.

36. a. An AAC facilitator can be a family member, professional, or communication partner who takes on the responsibility for programming the device and keeping it current. Without appropriate commitment and training of a facilitator, patients are highly likely to abandon the device.

37. c. There are a number of standard mouse alternatives for people who need access to a computer for writing. A number of different types of trackball mice exist. A joystick can also be used to operate as a mouse. The most current technology allows mouse functions to be controlled by eye movement that is read by cameras that allow for mouse use.

38. b. The barrier described is not a regulatory or legislative policy (option a); it is a school district's independent belief about device use and ownership. This is an example of a practice barrier, in which are procedures and practices that have become common are not actual policies. Knowledge barriers (option c) deal with lack of information that can limit an individual's access to AAC. Skill barriers (option d) involve a lack of appropriate skills in the area of AAC that may limit an individual's access or success in using AAC. Attitude barriers (option e) refer to the thoughts and beliefs that can limit an individual's access or participation.

39. d. Core vocabulary consists of the words and messages that are common and frequently used by a group of people. Informant vocabulary (option b) is obtained through interviewing the AAC user and caregivers and tends to be specific to that individual user. Individual vocabulary (option c)—that is, fringe vocabulary (option a)—can be collected by talking with people most familiar to that person; they can serve as a vocabulary informant. AAC vocabulary refers to preprogrammed vocabulary that is provided by AAC device manufacturer's.

40. a. Message prediction is a message retrieval strategy that enables predication of letter, word, and phrase or sentence.

CHAPTER 17

Counseling

Audrey L. Holland

1. According to the American Speech-Language-Hearing Association (ASHA) Scope of Practice statements, counseling:
   a. Is outside the profession's responsibilities, and patients who are believed to be in need of counseling should be referred to other related disciplines, such as psychiatry or clinical psychology
   b. Is within the scope of practice for speech-language pathologists (SLPs) but, when practiced, must pertain specifically to disorders of communication
   c. Must be limited to patients who have communication disorders, not their family members
   d. Can be engaged in by only professionals whose training has included specific coursework in counseling
   e. Can be practiced by anyone who is a sensitive and good listener

2. Counseling clients with communication disorders (and their families) is *not* intended to:
   a. Convince the client of the specific cause of his or her disorder
   b. Help the client make sensible adjustments to the disorder
   c. Help the client understand as fully as possible what has happened
   d. Substitute for traditional intervention
   e. a and c

3. Depression is a frequent accompaniment to many communication disorders. Thus, SLPs need to do which of the following in relation to depression?
   a. Be grounded and educated in the clinical techniques that are effective in the management of depression and, once they have such training, be willing and able to intervene
   b. Develop a professional relationship with a psychologist or psychiatrist who can manage

depression and refer clients to that professional when depression is suspected

c. Attempt to manage clients' depression themselves, because (particularly with adult clients with language disorders) some clinicians have trouble understanding the depression of the clients with communication disorders who are referred to them

d. Understand the *DSM* (American Psychiatric Association, 2000) criteria for depression, and when appropriate, refer to the primary care physician and provide information concerning a range of appropriate referrals

e. Find a physician for the depressed client who will prescribe antidepressants

4. Competent counseling in communication disorders requires knowledge about which of the following?
   a. Relevant community resources
   b. Disorder-specific support groups
   c. Access to public transportation for people with disabilities
   d. Internet resources and responsible Web sites
   e. All of the above

5. A competent counselor should possess all of the following counseling skills. Of them, which is the most important?
   a. The ability to translate professional jargon into lay terms
   b. The ability to listen to what the client is communicating, at both a surface and deep level
   c. Sensitivity to cultural differences
   d. Flexibility
   e. An understanding of the limitations of counseling

6. In many ways, counseling addresses more than the particular problem that a client or family might be manifesting. Why, therefore, is it important for a competent counselor to keep up with clinical research and professional developments?
   a. To be able to inform clients that much of the information they may find on the Internet or the popular press is untrustworthy
   b. To communicate the clinician's role as the authority convincingly
   c. To link the clinician's role as a competent counselor with best practices in the field
   d. To gain rapport
   e. To avoid having to say "I don't know" when a client asks for clarification concerning something he or she has been told or read.

7. "We are going to have to be careful about the consistency viscosity of Mrs. S's oral intake, to avoid her aspirating." Translate this statement into a sentence that nonmedical professionals, such as, perhaps,

Mr. S, can understand and that provides a rationale for action.

a. "Mrs. S could get liquid in her lungs, and if this happens, she could develop pneumonia. One way to help avoid this is by being careful about the thickness and the textures of the food she eats. We need to avoid thin liquids, like water, particularly. Thin liquids are most likely to travel into her lungs."

b. "I am putting your wife on a diet of pureed foods. This will keep her from aspirating, which is very important if we want her to get better. Do you want to talk to a dietitian? Do you have any questions?"

c. "Here is some thickening substance. Make sure you use it in all the liquids she takes. She needs to swallow only thick liquids at this stage."

d. "We are going to have be careful about what Mrs. S swallows. There is a risk that she can develop pneumonia if we don't. And this would be very bad for her, given her overall condition."

e. "We must work together to prevent Mrs. S from choking. Choking is not only unpleasant, it can be life-threatening."

8. "Clarifying" is a counseling strategy in which the counselor:
   a. Uses examples from his or her own life to illustrate a concept
   b. Provides the client with previously unknown information
   c. Helps a client to give more precise descriptions of his or her own ideas and feelings
   d. Restates the client's message
   e. Builds on the statement with one relating to the counselor's own personal experience

9. "Reflecting back" to the client the underlying message of his or her utterance:
   a. Is a psychoanalytic technique and therefore off-limits for SLPs
   b. Is a counseling technique of Carl Rogers' client-centered therapy that can be used by SLPs
   c. Is traditionally used by SLPs to make sure that they understand what a client means
   d. Is used to challenge accuracy in a polite way
   e. Involves the use of mirror work designed, for counseling purposes, to help the client more fully understand some principles of face reading as outlined by Paul Ekman

10. The reason why clinicians are warned to be careful in their use of the technique of personal disclosure is that:
    a. It tends to distract the client from the important issues
    b. Personal disclosure can change the nature of clinical relationship into one of friendship instead of counseling, thus complicating the counseling function

c. Telling a client about oneself is unethical and always unwarranted

d. The proper counseling role in SLP is always one of distance and impersonality

e. Research has shown that disclosure is a poor way to demonstrate empathy, even when it is skillfully done

11. What is the rationale for pausing to think through a question or comment and consider how to respond to it before answering?
    a. It gives the counselor time to think of something to say on the topic
    b. It enables the counselor to think through various alternative responses that might capitalize on other skills, as well as to communicate the counselor's attentiveness to the question
    c. It conveys the seriousness of the situation
    d. It gives the client the impression that the clinician is taking his or her comment or question seriously, and even if such is not the case, it builds clinical trust and respect
    e. Pausing such as this differentiates counseling encounters from a more natural conversational flow, and this distinction is important to successful counseling

12. According to Webster (1977), which of the following is *not* a feature of counseling in communication disorders?
    a. To receive information that the individual and his or her family wish to share with the clinician
    b. To give information
    c. To provide solutions to problems
    d. To help individuals clarify their ideas, attitudes, emotions, and beliefs
    e. To provide options for changing behaviors

13. Which of the following is within the scope of practice for counseling Mrs. A and her family with regard to the consequences of a stroke last week that led to Mr. A's moderate to severe aphasia?
    a. Discussing in detail the outcome and course of recovery for Mr. A's aphasia
    b. Discussing in detail what is known about the outcomes of aphasia, and the general outline of its course, but clarifying that only broad generalizations can be made
    c. Discussing with Mrs. A what the medical course of Mr. A's recovery will be and what steps will be taken next, including issues such as the likelihood of subsequent seizures, the likelihood that Mr. A will have an additional stroke, and the importance of general health status in his recovery

d. Initiating a discussion with Mrs. A about family finances and perhaps the need to rethink plans for retirement and related issues

e. Sharing with Mrs. A something confidential that Mr. A has shared with you

14. Of the following issues (in addition to speech and language development), which is *not* likely to be a major concern for the parents of a 7-year-old son with Down syndrome as they worry about his potential limitations in development?
    a. His ability to live independently
    b. His safety
    c. His happiness
    d. His ability to have friends
    e. None of the above

15. The counselor asks Mrs. J, the mother of Billy, a 10-year-old with severe cognitive problems, to envision what she would like him to be doing 10 years from now. Mrs. J says that she would like him to be ready to attend junior college. Which of the following is an appropriate reply?
    a. "Then let's help him to take a step in that direction. Let's begin right away to get serious about toilet training. Shall we get some help in this from the behavioral specialist?"
    b. "Mrs. J, it is important that you develop more realistic goals for Billy."
    c. "I am worried that you don't seem to recognize Billy's limitations."
    d. "We have been over this before. College is not going to happen for Billy in 10 years, or even in 15 years."
    e. "*That* is going to require a miracle."

16. A frequent complaint of persons with aphasia and their families is that no one told them about the consequences of stroke, or the implications of aphasia, in the early post-onset period. What is the likeliest explanation for this?
    a. Physicians and other caregivers in acute care settings (and in early rehabilitation) are too busy getting the recovery process started to explain such things to families
    b. Hospital personnel assume that families have knowledge of stroke and other conditions that bring about aphasia and do not see the need to explain
    c. Persons who have sustained stroke, and their families, are in the middle of a crisis, and information provided at that time is probably not going to be understood and digested
    d. Most hospitals and speech pathology staffs hand out very complete information, but people do not tend to read such material and are not encouraged to ask about it
    e. Not enough is known to make this an ethical topic for discussion

17. Which of the following is likely to be a counseling issue for school-aged children who stutter?
    a. Controlling their anger
    b. Being bullied or teased
    c. Being ridiculed by teachers
    d. Parental insensitivity to stuttering as a problem
    e. All of the above

18. Of the following counseling issues, which is outside the scope of practice of SLPs who work with aging adults?
    a. Financial concerns
    b. Playing a role in a decision concerning whether to place a feeding tube
    c. Providing guidelines for the selection of extended-care facilities with communication enrichment
    d. Providing advice on how to communicate with one's physician more effectively
    e. Helping families in the use of communication aids for family members with dementia

19. Suzie is a cheerleader at her high school, where she is a senior. She is experiencing the effects of vocal abuse, and her parents are concerned that the cheerleading is contributing to her voice problems. Of the following issues, which constitutes counseling concerns?
    a. Getting Suzie to quit the cheerleading team
    b. Helping Suzie see the relationship between cheerleading and her voice problem
    c. Helping Suzie's parents to calm down about her problem, because it is likely to be transitory inasmuch as Suzie will be off the cheerleading squad in a few months
    d. Persuading Suzie to increase her hydration
    e. All of the above

20. A client with amyotrophic lateral sclerosis (ALS) whose symptoms involve primarily the extremities has entered counseling so that he can have a head start on communication once he begins to have speech symptoms. He starts a session by noting, "I feel I may have brushed my own teeth for the last time this morning." What is your clinical responsibility at this moment?
    a. To sympathize briefly but then to point out that your purpose here is to work on communication and that there is work to be done
    b. To ignore this comment because it is outside the scope of your skills
    c. To put your lesson plan aside until you have listened to him and permitted him to grieve about his worsening condition
    d. To tell him that you think he is exaggerating and it is probably not very likely to be true
    e. To politely excuse yourself and tell him you are going to find a staff member who is qualified to help him with this problem

21. According to David M. Luterman, which of the following are essential components of the counseling process?
    a. Deep listening and silent witnessing
    b. Empathic responding and careful analysis
    c. Advising and guiding
    d. In-depth interviewing and information seeking
    e. Empowering and advocating

22. Which of the following concepts best describes an acceptable counseling attitude?
    a. Pity
    b. Empathy
    c. Sympathy
    d. Transference
    e. Benevolence

23. Building and maintaining rapport with a client or family is thought to be an important clinical skill for both direct service delivery and counseling. Which of the following is most likely to increase rapport in clinical encounters?
    a. The clinician's ability to share his or her experiences with the client
    b. The clinician' similarity to the client in terms of age, ethnic and cultural background, and education
    c. The clinician's ability to convey a genuine sense of concern and understanding
    d. The clinician's knowledge and grasp of clinical techniques that are appropriate in treating a particular client
    e. All of the above

24. Cross-cultural understanding is important for all clinical endeavors, but it is perhaps most pertinent for activities that are related to the counseling function in speech and language pathology. Why?
    a. Without sensitivity to the beliefs, attitudes, and values of the client, it is extremely difficult to build the trust and understanding on which counseling relationships depend
    b. Because counseling requires verbal interchange, it necessarily means that the counselor must work cross-linguistically when counseling someone from another culture
    c. In the case of most speech and language disorders, different cultures place differing values on the importance of intervention; thus, it is important in direct practice to counsel clients of differing cultures to accept the importance of language and speech therapy
    d. It helps a clinician identify individuals whose culture might make it unpleasant for the clinician to accept and therefore to help.
    e. All of the above

25. Some clinicians prefer to provide group counseling for families and spouses of persons with communication disorders. Of the following reasons, which might explain a preference for groups?
    a. Groups enable the clinician to use time more effectively and efficiently
    b. Groups provide a clinical situation that resembles everyday life
    c. Groups present an opportunity for individuals to learn from other group members
    d. Groups enable members to see that they are not alone and that others have similar problems
    e. All of the above

Answers

1. b. As in most helping professions (e.g., marital counseling, intimacy counseling), the professional counseling responsibilities of SLPs are constrained: They must be relevant to the disorders for which such professionals have been trained to provide more direct services.

2. e. Clinicians who counsel their clients should be as free as possible of biases concerning specific causes of disorders, particularly those whose cause is controversial. In addition, counseling is also not a substitute for more disorder-focused treatment.

3. d. Understanding *DSM* criteria for depression and referring clients as appropriate is the most appropriate solution to the problem of dealing with depression. It is important for SLPs to be educated and grounded in the basics of depression (option a), of course. It is also laudable to work out a relationship with a particular professional who might be of help to clients with communication disorders (option b), but not all clients relate to the same therapist. Because SLPs lack relevant training, they should not attempt to manage this problem on their own (option c). It is inappropriate to consider prescribing antidepressants (option e) because medication may not be needed or could be harmful to clients.

4. e. Relevant community resources (options a) and support groups (option b), access to public transportation (option c), and Internet resources (option d) all can facilitate counseling by increasing access to other sources that can help individuals manage and adjust to their communication disorders.

5. b. Good listening skills are the bedrock of counseling. The ability to elucidate professional jargon (option a), sensitivity to cultural differences (option c), flexibility (option d), and understanding the limits of counseling (option e) are important skills in the counseling process, but good listening skills are paramount.

6. c. Effective counseling is grounded in comprehensive clinical knowledge. The counselor must be aware of new trends in clinical research and incorporate such information in practice.

7. a. Options b and c contain somewhat less jargon but provide only sketchy rationales. Options d and e provide some information but may alarm Mr. S unnecessarily at the same time.

8. c. "Clarifying" is a counseling technique that assists the client is better expressing feelings. The other responses are other types of different strategies that are used by counselors.

9. b. "Reflecting back," described by Carl Rogers, is a technique in which the counselor paraphrases what the client has said, in order to ensure that the counselor understands the client's message.

10. b. There is nothing unethical about disclosure when it is used properly and when it is judiciously applied (e.g., "When my mother was sick, I felt helpless, too"). However, disclosure has the potential for changing the clinical role when the nature of the relationship becomes "buddy-buddy" instead of an empathic "client-clinician."

11. b. The counselor needs to consider the client and select the most appropriate response for the context. Fast responding often results in failure to adequately assess the comment or question and thus to provide less help than a more studied response might offer. It also tends to give the client the impression that the clinician is serious about her or his response; however, if the time is not well spent by the clinician, it is an insincere response.

12. c. Clinicians (and counselors) are never in a position to provide solutions to problems; they can merely provide options and suggestions for implementing them. One person can never solve another's problems successfully.

13. b. Clinicians (of any kind) are not in a position to make explicit statements about outcome and course of recovery (options a and c). They can discuss these things only in general, because each patient has an individual course. Discussing medical steps to take (option c) is in the scope of medical practice; a discussion of family finances (option d) is a problem for social work involvement. Sharing a confidence (option e) breaks trust, even though the information might be important to the welfare of both Mr. and Mrs. A. (A better solution might be to help Mr. A to understand why he should share the information if it is important and then to follow up with him.)

14. e. All are issues for potential concern and may require for parental or client counseling as well.

15. a. If Billy is not toilet trained, the first approach invites the parent to participate in achieving the goal.

The other options are, in various degrees, confrontational. The likeliest outcome of confrontation is that the confronted person will become defensive, which makes rapport difficult and undermines the clinical process.

16. c. Early stages of crisis make it difficult for affected persons to absorb information. In the case of aphasia, of course, this is complicated by the language disorder of the persons with aphasia.

17. b. The issue of bullying and teasing is significant for many children who stutter and is the subject of a number of papers and publications concerning the clinician's role in its management. It is not necessarily the case that stuttering children are angry (option a), few teachers ridicule stuttering kids (option c), and parents are typically quite aware of the problem (option d).

18. a. SLPs would not be involved in counseling a client with regard to financial concerns. All of the other options involve expertise that relates to communication and swallowing issues.

19. b. In order for Suzie to understand and improve her vocal hygiene, it is necessary that she make the connection between her behavior and its consequences. Whether Suzie remains on the team (option a) or increases hydration (option d) are not major counseling concerns. There is no information about whether the problem is actually transitory (option c).

20. c. The client has a progressive condition that is terminal, and he should be given the opportunity to discuss his feelings. The SLP is concerned with the client's communication skills but should also be aware of and understanding of the patient's needs to discuss any perceived or potential problems. The other responses are not appropriate in the described scenario.

21. a. Luterman has developed a counseling process that includes deep listening and silent witnessing. According to this perspective on counseling, the client talks about particular issues, and the clinician listens. Clinicians are trained to understand that they must listen carefully to what the client has to say; that is, they need to withstand the inclination to furnish instant feedback and advice and must listen to the messages, which underlie the words of their clients. The other choices are also techniques that may be used when counseling clients.

22. b. It is important for the SLP to empathize with a client and the family during the therapy process. The SLP needs to identify with and understand the client and family's feelings and problems. Pity (option a), sympathy (option c), and benevolence (option e) are feelings that would not be appropriate to project in a counseling context. Transference (option d) is a process in psychotherapy in which a person redirects feelings or emotions to a new entity, such as the therapist.

23. c. Rapport might be influenced by all the factors listed, but the most foundational is having and communicating, both verbally and nonverbally, the counselor's concern and understanding of the client as a person.

24. a. The SLP needs to be sensitive and understanding in regard to the beliefs, attitudes, and values of the client, if the SLP is to build trust and understanding. The other options all contain flaws of logic or inappropriate inferences concerning cultural biases.

25. e. All of the options are advantages of providing group counseling for families and spouses of persons with communication disorders.

Bibliography

American Psychiatric Association. (2000). *Diagnostic and Statistical Manual of Mental Disorders, Fourth Edition, Text Revision.* Washington, DC: Author.

Webster, E. J. (1977). *Counseling with parents of handicapped children: Studies for ongoing communication.* Grune & Stratton: Newyork.

CHAPTER 18

Documentation and Monitoring of Patient Progress

Leslie C. Graebe

Karen B. Haines

1. A patient appears depressed and is frequently talking about suicide. For a speech-language pathologist (SLP), what would be the most appropriate course of action?
   a. Most patients are depressed, so nothing should be done; the mood most likely will pass
   b. This is not within an SLP's realm of training
   c. Notify the patient's primary care physician
   d. Recommend a friend who has a background in psychology
   e. None of the above

2. Your 85-year-old nonverbal patient shows severe bruising on his legs. He frequently points to them and cries. In addition, he appears fearful when a particular nursing assistant is around. What would be your course of action to remediate this problem?
   a. Ignore it
   b. Notify the charge nurse
   c. Report it immediately to the Department of Human Services
   d. Explain to the patient that he has a history of falls and the bruises are most likely a result of those falls
   e. All of the above

3. You are writing a SOAP note for your adult patient with traumatic brain injury (TBI) in an acute care facility. He frequently uses profanity and talks about how stupid and worthless his therapy is. In what section of the note would you include these statements?
   a. S
   b. O

c. A

d. P

e. Do not include these statements in the note.

4. For persons who are 65 years of age or older, primary health care costs are generally covered by which of the following?
   a. Medicaid
   b. Private pay
   c. Third-party payers
   d. Medicare
   e. None of the above

5. The SLP working with an elderly patient receiving home health care notices that the caregiver, who is the patient's spouse, is tired and seems to be in poor health. Suggestions that the SLP might provide to help the spouse better manage the difficult caregiving situation might include:
   a. Get adequate rest
   b. Take vitamins
   c. Investigate community resources that might help in the home or provide financial assistance
   d. All of the above
   e. a and c only

6. When treating an elderly patient in a long-term care setting who has recently suffered a cardiovascular accident (CVA), the SLP should first be considering discharge issues:
   a. During the initial evaluation
   b. About midway through the treatment program
   c. One day before discharge
   d. At the clinical team's discharge planning conference
   e. It is not part of the SLP's role to be concerned about discharge planning

7. To ensure adequate reimbursement for speech-language pathology services, your appropriate documentation should include:
   a. Measurable goals
   b. Your signature on all documentation
   c. A summary of your findings
   d. All of the above
   e. a and c

8. Person-first language is used when individuals with disabilities are described. Of the following terms, which is an example of person-first language?
   a. "The aphasic"
   b. "Stutterers"
   c. "The hearing impaired"
   d. "Persons who stutter"
   e. None of the above

9. You are an SLP in a skilled nursing facility. Your patient is having difficulty self-feeding because of positioning issues. The best course of action would be:
   a. Provide adaptive equipment to the patient
   b. Position the patient yourself so that he or she is able to feed himself or herself better
   c. Refer the patient to an occupational therapist
   d. Refer the patient to a physical therapist
   e. a and b only

10. Documentation of speech-language therapy in geriatric rehabilitation should:
    a. Follow Medicare guidelines
    b. Emphasize functional outcomes
    c. Not include the occupational therapist's and physical therapist's assessments
    d. Include long- and short-term goals
    e. All of the above

11. You are covering for another SLP in a rehabilitation setting, and you disagree with that SLP's treatment plan. You would:
    a. Follow the treatment plan anyway; the other SLP knows the patient best
    b. Refuse to see the patient
    c. Change the plan of care during the period that you are seeing the patient
    d. Address other goals in the plan of care that you believe are appropriate
    e. None of the above

12. Bryan is a 65-year-old man with impulsive behavior, poor table manners, and very few teeth. His speech is unintelligible, and he very rarely makes eye contact. He eats with his fingers and has been observed stuffing an entire sandwich into his mouth, which results in coughing episodes. The SLP observes that when his sandwich is cut into bite-size pieces and he is given no more than two pieces at a time, he slows his eating pace to a normal level. Of the following, which is the most appropriate short-term goal for Bryan?
    a. Bryan will demonstrate good table manners
    b. Bryan will demonstrate decreased impulsivity
    c. Bryan will make eye contact with three individuals during Bingo
    d. Bryan will chew and swallow each piece of his sandwich before placing the next in his mouth four of five times at meals in the dining room, with no coughing observed
    e. All of the above are appropriate short-term goals

13. An SLP providing consulting services to a long-term care facility should do all of the following *except*:

a. Provide input on selection of forms and the documentation process

b. Advise on enhancement of group dynamics and resident involvement to improve communication skills

c. Suggest ways staff can do introduce physical therapy activities to cover the lack of physical therapists

d. Train nursing assistants on effective strategies to communicate with hearing-impaired patients

e. Interact with the dietary staff on appropriate food textures and consistency of thickened liquids

14. During a home visit in which the SLP is conducting a family training session, the daughter (caregiver) of the an elderly woman with Parkinson disease states that she is having difficulty controlling her feelings of frustration and anger toward her communicatively impaired mother. An appropriate response by the SLP would be:

a. "I am here to treat your mother; your issues are of no concern to me."

b. "Ask your physician for a referral so that we can establish an arrangement for billing my services."

c. "Getting away is important. Why not go to the mall this afternoon?"

d. "Anger is not a good thing to have when taking care of someone because you cannot focus on what your mother needs."

e. "Expressing your anger is important. Is there a person you know, such as a minister or counselor, with whom you could discuss your feelings?"

15. When giving elderly hearing-impaired patients directions, keep information short and to the point, and:

a. Use technical words as well as common language

b. Ask the patient to repeat the information back to you

c. Yell at the patient; the louder you talk, the more the patient will understand

d. Provide written directions once you know that the patient is capable of reading

e. b and d

16. You are writing a SOAP note for an elderly woman whom you are seeing in her home. You are writing goals for next week. In what section of the note would you include goals?

a. S

b. O

c. A

d. P

e. You would not include goals for next week in the SOAP note

17. You are treating a patient with TBI in a rehabilitation facility who has severe cognitive deficits. Visitors are asking you questions about your treatment plan and the patient's progress. Your best response should be:

a. Show them the patient's treatment plan and, using layman's terms, explain his progress

b. Refer them to the physical therapist

c. Encourage them to ask the patient himself

d. First ask them if they have the power of attorney (POA); if they do not, explain that you cannot release any information to anyone other than the person who has POA

e. None of the above

18. You are conducting an interview with a parent of a child during a diagnostic evaluation. Which of the following should *not* occur?

a. Allow the family member adequate time to respond to your questions

b. Use "parent-friendly" language

c. Ask only "yes"/"no" questions

d. Ask open-ended questions

e. All are correct

19. You are treating an elderly gentleman who recently sustained a CVA. He has excellent potential for improvement; however, his depression is interfering with progress. His wife has promised to take him home after his course of therapy. He cries during your sessions and says he wants to die. What should you do as an SLP?

a. Tell him that if he does not cooperate, Medicare will not pay the bill and he will be responsible

b. Provide encouragement about the potential that he does have and the progress he has shown

c. Speak with his primary care physician regarding a psychological evaluation because of the depression

d. Discharge him from therapy; he obviously does not want to get better

e. b and c

20. You are treating a 2-year-old patient with language delay, using "play therapy." To facilitate play therapy, you would do which of the following?

a. Eliminate all distractions in the room

b. Follow the child's lead

c. Make the session enjoyable on the basis of the child's chronological age

d. Maintain an accurate record of the child's responses

e. All of the above are correct

21. A 62-year-old man presents with mild ataxic gait and dysarthria. He reports that he saw his primary care physician, who referred him to a neurologist. The neurologist was reportedly unable to determine the cause of these symptoms and did not suggest any medical follow-up. The neurologist referred him to you for management of his dysarthria. Your first course of action for this patient would be to:

a. Begin treatment of dysarthria

b. Refer him to another neurologist for a second opinion

c. Refer him to an otolaryngologist

d. Explain that you cannot treat dysarthria but you can provide him with strategies to improve his speech intelligibility

e. Refer him to his primary care physician

22. You are a public school SLP, and you are treating a 5-year-old kindergartener for speech sound, and language therapy disorders. The child's teacher has asked you to add a goal for handwriting skills because the child does not hold a pencil correctly and is unable to write any letters. The most appropriate response to the teacher would be to:

a. Refer the child to the occupational therapist for an evaluation

b. Suggest that the teacher develop a home program for the child to practice handwriting every day with parents

c. Develop handwriting goals in conjunction with the speech sound and language goals and implement handwriting practice in therapy

d. Refer the child to the physical therapist for an evaluation

e. Tell the teacher that you do not deal with handwriting

23. You are evaluating a 21-year-old woman who has cerebral palsy, cognitive impairment, and severe speech and language impairment and who is nonambulatory. According to the case history form, the patient is 5 feet, 4 inches tall and weighs 53 pounds. She is fed orally and does not have a gastrostomy tube. During the evaluation, you note that the patient is lethargic and generally nonresponsive. She has a baclofen pump but no history of seizures or other medications. Formal testing produces limited information. The family states that she produces a few vocalizations but seems to follow general conversation. Your first course of action is to:

a. Begin therapy to minimize the gap between her receptive and expressive language

b. Initiate feeding and swallowing therapy

c. Refer to the physical therapist because she in nonambulatory

d. Refer to the neurologist for evaluation of the baclofen pump

e. Perform, or refer for a feeding and swallowing evaluation

24. You are working in a private facility, and a parent brings you his 6-year-old child who has a diagnosis of childhood apraxia of speech. The child's history includes Birth to Three services from ages 18 months to 3 years of age and speech sound therapy through the local schools from age 3 to the present. When asked about previous therapy, the parents tell you that they know the child was working on sounds but they are uncertain about which ones. Your evaluation reveals that the child's speech is generally unintelligible to the unfamiliar listener, with numerous sound omissions and substitutions. It would be most important for you to:

a. Initiate supplemental therapy immediately

b. Suggest the parent consider an augmentative communication system

c. Obtain a signed release of information form so you can contact the child's prior therapists to determine previous therapy goals and treatment techniques used

d. Refer the child to the school SLP for continued therapy

e. Recommend increased therapy

25. You are working with a 6-year-old who exhibits the phonological process of stridency deletion for the phonemes /s/, /z/, /ʃ/, /tʃ/, /ʒ/, /θ/, and /ð/. For the past 6 months, you have worked on the production of /s/, /ʃ/, ts, /θ/ in all words and positions. The child is currently correctly producing these sounds in her connected speech. The most appropriate next step in this child's treatment would be to:

a. Initiate therapy for /z/, /ʒ/, and /ð/

b. Readminister a formal articulation test

c. Probe the child's production of /z/, /ʒ/, and /ð/

d. Dismiss this child from therapy

e. Continue treatment for /s/, /ʃ/, /tʃ/, and /θ/

26. You are working in a private practice and a parent has requested that you discuss her child's speech and language issues with his classroom teacher. Your next course of action would be to:

a. Contact the teacher

b. Ask the parent to relay your information

c. Explain that it is not your responsibility to talk to the teacher

d. Ask the parent to have the teacher contact you

e. Have the parent sign a release of information form allowing you to discuss her child with his teacher

27. You have just completed a language assessment for a 4-year-old. The child received a standard score of 105 on the Peabody Picture Vocabulary Test, a standard score of 112 on the Auditory Comprehension subtest of the Preschool Language Scale (PLS), and a standard score of 89 on the Verbal Ability Subtest of the PLS. The mean standard score for the tests is 100, and the standard deviation is 15. The most appropriate course of action would be to:

a. Initiate therapy for expressive language

b. Initiate therapy for receptive and expressive language

c. Schedule additional language assessment

d. Determine that the child's language skills are within normal limits

e. Recommend a reevaluation in 1 year

28. Your patient has received response accuracy scores of 95% and 98% during the past two therapy sessions. The goal is to respond correctly to "who" questions in a structured drill activity. Your next treatment step will be to:
a. Move to introduce other "wh" questions
b. Continue structured drill activities with "who" questions
c. Work on "who" questions in a variety of functional less structured activities, gradually moving to conversation
d. Discontinue work on "who" questions
e. Assess the patient's responses to other "wh" questions

29. Your 6-year-old patient has successfully mastered all of his speech sound goals. You note, however, that he continues to distort /r/ or substitute /w/ for /r/. He is not stimulable for /r/ or any of the /r/ diphthongs. You recommend that the child:
a. Remain in therapy until he masters /r/ and the /r/ diphthongs
b. Be discharged from therapy because he is likely to develop /r/ and the /r/ diphthongs when he is older
c. Be discharged from therapy but his production of /r/ and /r/ diphthongs be reevaluated when he turns 10
d. Be discharged from therapy but that his production of /r/ and /r/ diphthongs be reevaluated when he turns 8
e. Receive formal assessment of /r/ and /r/ diphthongs

30. Molly is 15 years old and has a severe cognitive disability. Her receptive language skills are at approximately the 24-month level, and her expressive output consists of 15 words that are intelligible only to familiar listeners. She lives with her parents, and the majority of her day is spent in a self-contained special education classroom. Molly has attended traditional pull-out therapy since she was 3 years old. She has made no measurable progress on her goals in the past 2 years and has begun to refuse to leave the classroom for therapy. However, her parents expect you to continue individual pull-out therapy as long as Molly is enrolled in public school. The best course of action would be to:
a. Continue pull-out therapy as long as Molly is enrolled in the public schools
b. Discharge Molly from therapy as her receptive language skills are commensurate with her expressive language skills
c. Educate Molly's family about other service delivery models, such as consultation, that would allow her goals to be addressed functionally and across environments

d. Develop new treatment goals

e. Initiate a positive reinforcement schedule to encourage Molly to attend therapy

31. To determine whether a patient's skills are generalizing to other contexts, it is most appropriate to perform periodically which of the following during a treatment program?
a. Measure base rate skills
b. Perform formal tests
c. Graph data
d. Probe the skills
e. Review data from the most recent session

32. When a patient works on a communication skill, a response accuracy rate of 65% for a specific treatment goal indicates that:
a. The patient is learning the skill
b. The task is too difficult and the goal should be dropped
c. The task is too difficult and a branching step is needed
d. The task is too easy
e. None of the above

33. To evaluate a patient's progress on a communication skill over a period of time across treatment sessions, it is most appropriate to:
a. Measure the base rate of the skill before treatment
b. Probe the skill during treatment
c. Graph the patient's daily performance data
d. Assess the skill with a formal assessment tool
e. Review the data from the most recent session

34. To measure generalization performance on a specific communication skill from the beginning of a treatment program to the end, it is most appropriate to use:
a. Probes with standardized tests
b. Graphs
c. Periodic formal assessment
d. Using single-subject A × B design to measure performance
e. Patient's response data from the most recent session

35. A patient's pediatricians informs the patient's parents that therapy is no longer needed, even though the patient's SLP has not dismissed the patient from therapy. The most appropriate course of action for you is to:
a. Explain to the parents why you feel that continued therapy is needed
b. Discontinue therapy
c. Tell the parents that the pediatrician does not know what he is talking about
d. Do nothing and continue therapy
e. Reassess the patient to determine whether he continues to need therapy

36. You are evaluating a 28-month-old. According to the parents, you are the first professional to evaluate the child. The pediatrician has reportedly told the parents that development appears normal. Language assessment reveals a receptive language age of 15 months and an expressive language age of 21 months. The patient is observed to produce primarily single words and some two-word combinations that are composed of mainly vowels and only an occasional consonant. Your first course of action would be to:
    a. Refer this child for a complete audiological evaluation
    b. Immediately initiate language therapy
    c. Refer the child to his pediatrician for additional assessment
    d. Reevaluate the child in 6 months
    e. Immediately initiate speech sound therapy

37. You are evaluating a 28-month-old. According to the parents, you are the first professional to evaluate the child. The pediatrician has reportedly told the parents that development appears normal. Language assessment reveals a receptive language age of 15 months and an expressive language age of 21 months. The patient is observed to produce primarily single words and some two-word combinations that are composed of mainly vowels and only an occasional consonant. On the basis of the results of a complete audiological assessment to rule out hearing loss, which of the following interpretations is most appropriate?
    a. Severe impairment in receptive and expressive language
    b. Significant delay in receptive and expressive language and speech sound skills
    c. Mild delay in receptive language and moderate delay in expressive language
    d. Mild delay in speech sound skills
    e. Moderate to severe delay in receptive language skills, mild delay in expressive language skills, and severe delay in speech sound skills

38. You are working in a rehabilitation hospital with an 8-year-old patient who suffered a TBI in an automobile accident. The patient is due to be released soon, and the public school SLP from this patient's county school system contacts you to discuss continued treatment through the public schools. Your initial response should be to:
    a. Share the appropriate information because the family told you to relay the information
    b. Obtain a signed release of information form allowing you to share information with this SLP
    c. Instruct the SLP to contact the child's parents
    d. Instruct the patient's case manager to contact the SLP
    e. Send a copy of your most recent report

39. You have administered a formal assessment tool to a patient who has a disorder with presenting characteristics that were not represented in the normative population with that disorder. When reporting the results, you should:
    a. Not include the test score
    b. Explain that the test score may be invalid and why
    c. Report the test score in the same manner you do for patients who were represented in the normed population
    d. Report only the standard scores
    e. Report only the raw scores

40. Your patient has a diagnosis of amyotrophic lateral sclerosis. The patient's connected speech is generally unintelligible to the unfamiliar listener. Your first course of action would be to:
    a. Initiate language therapy
    b. Perform an augmentative and alternative communication evaluation
    c. Initiate speech sound therapy
    d. Teach the patient compensatory behaviors
    e. Refer the patient to an audiologist

Answers

1. c. It is the primary care physician's responsibility to make the appropriate referral for psychological intervention. An SLP should alert the physician to the presence of suicidal tendencies in the patient. Doing nothing (option a) would not be correct because depression may not pass and it is the SLP's responsibility to alert the physician. An SLP is not a psychologist, but it is within the SLP's realm of training to make the appropriate referral (option b). Recommending a friend with a psychology background (option d) would be a violation of Health Insurance Portability and Accountability Act (HIPAA).

2. b. It is your responsibility to contact the most appropriate professional to address this situation. You would want the charge nurse to be aware of the problem and to determine the next course of action. You would not ignore the situation (option a), because abuse may be occurring, and the charge nurse will determine whom to involve next. However, no abuse may be occurring; thus, you need not immediately notify the Department of Human Services, because this department would conduct an investigation, which may not be needed. No information is given as to whether the patient has a history of falls; furthermore, the patient might not understand an explanation (option d).

3. a. This is the subjective (S) portion of the note, and statements from the patient should be included in this section. The objective (O) part of the note (option b) includes facts that support statements mentioned in the S section. The assessment (A) section (option c) is an interpretation of the subjective observation and objective data; in that section, the problem would be summarized and can even include a discussion of the patient's strengths and weaknesses. In the plan (P) section (option d), recommendations for future therapy are documented.

4. d. Medicare is the primary health care insurance for people 65 years of age and older. They may have a supplemental insurance in addition to Medicare, but Medicare is the most common insurance for elderly people. Medicaid (option a) is not the primary health care coverage for seniors. Some patients do have the funds to pay privately (option b), and some use third-party payers (option c), but this is not true of the majority of older patients.

5. e. You want the spouse to be in adequate health in order to care for the patient. Adequate rest and the help of community resources may alleviate some of the stress in this caregiving situation. Advising the spouse only to get adequate rest (option a) is insufficient because it is difficult to obtain adequate rest when a person is acting as a caregiver. Taking vitamins (option b) may not be the only course of action to alleviate the stress; you may want to leave that recommendation up to the physician. The availability of community resources alone (option c) is not enough to help the spouse without adequate rest.

6. a. Discharge planning should be addressed as soon as the patient is evaluated, and it should be planned throughout the course of the patient's stay at the facility. About midway through treatment (option b) is too far into the treatment program to make appropriate recommendations, as is one day before discharge (option c). Because there are many factors to consider regarding discharge and adequate time is needed to complete discharge planning for a patient, the discharge planning conference is too late. It is indeed part of the SLP's role to be concerned and involved in discharge (option e) and to consider options such as developing a home health care program or making a referral to a home health care SLP.

7. d. Documentation should include a summary of the evaluation findings (option c) along with appropriate goals (option a). In addition, all paperwork generated by the clinician should be signed (option b). The SLP is required to sign all documentation and correspondence and to report assessment and treatment findings in writing to alert the physician of the results and to ensure adequate reimbursement.

8. d. The emphasis should be on the person, not the disability; therefore, "persons who stutter" is the most appropriate answer. "The aphasic" (option a), "stutterers" (option b), and "the hearing impaired" (option c) emphasize the disability, not the person.

9. c. The occupational therapist addresses positioning issues, as well as self-feeding issues. SLPs would not address these issues independently because they are not trained properly in those areas. An SLP would not provide adaptive equipment to the patient (option a). It is not within the scope of practice for SLPs to position a patient (option b); SLPs could injure themselves as well as the patient. Physical therapists (option d) would not be trained in positioning and feeding, as opposed to occupational therapists.

10. e. Adequate documentation in geriatric rehabilitation should follow Medicare guidelines (option a), which include emphasizing functional outcomes (option b), documenting long- and short-term goals in the communication domain (option d), and excluding the physical therapist's and occupational therapist's assessments (option c).

11. d. The patient does need to be treated, and you have agreed to be the treating SLP; therefore, address goals in the plan that you do feel comfortable handling. You should not do anything with a patient that you do not feel professionally comfortable doing (option a); you may end up hurting, not helping, the patient. You would not, however, change another SLP's treatment plan (option c).

12. d. A well-written goal includes a performance component, a condition component, and a criterion component. Chewing and swallowing each piece of sandwich at a time with no coughing includes all of these components. Demonstrating good tables manners (option a) does not include a condition or criterion component. Demonstrating decreased impulsivity (option b) also does not include any information on criterion. Making eye contact (option c) does not focus on the patient's primary deficits; it is important to establish eye contact with other residents, but this scenario is focusing on feeding and swallowing and on safety at meals, as opposed to recreation and eye contact. Answer (e) is not correct as (a,b,c) are incorrect. The correct answer is (d) as it is measureable, contains a condition component, as well as a criterion component.

13. c. Even if the facility lacks physical therapy service, it is not within the SLP's scope of practice to provide any examples of physical exercises to any staff member. SLPs do provide input on forms and the documentation process (option a) and advise recreational and activities directors on how to improve communication and interaction during group activities (option b). SLPs also train nursing assistants on how to more effectively communicate with hearing-impaired individuals. In addition, SLPs do interact with dietary staff and dietary managers on appropriate food textures and consistency of thickened liquids (option e).

14. e. A caregiver must know that feelings are important and that caring for a loved one can be a frustrating situation. However, caregivers need to talk with the most appropriate professional regarding these feelings so that they are able to care for their loved one. Dismissing the caregiver's feelings (option a) would be inappropriate. Payment services (option b)

are not discussed with family members during a treatment session; that is done with the home health agency before treatment. Although getting away (option c) would be a good idea, it does not address arrangements needed for someone to stay with the patient while the caregiver is away, and the person staying should not be the SLP. Merely telling the caregiver that anger is "not a good thing to have" (option d) is not helpful.

15. e. Technical words (option a) may not be understood by patients. Common words, however, are useful. Repeating the information back to you (option b) and written directions (option d) will help patients comprehend the directions. Yelling (option c) only frustrates the patient and worsens the situation further.

16. d. The P (planning) section of the SOAP note includes future action and goals. The S (subjective) section addresses statements from the patient (the patient's problems and situation) and any observations by the clinician. The O (objective) section addresses current goals and accuracy rates, not what will be addressed in the future. The A (assessment) section is used to interpret the subjective observations and objective data and possibly to make a statement regarding the severity of the deficits.

17. d. You first should determine whether visitors have the POA. If they do not, you then indicate that no information can be released without written consent regarding the patient, and therefore you cannot discuss anything about the patient. Showing the treatment plan and providing further information (option a) to visitors who do not have POA would be incorrect. Referring visitors to the physical therapist (option b) would be incorrect because the physical therapist is under the same HIPAA guidelines as the SLP. Questioning the patient directly (option c) would be inappropriate because the patient has severe cognitive deficits and probably could not answer the questions.

18. c. "Yes"/"no" questions do not elicit important information. The parent or caregiver should be provided adequate time (option a) to respond to your questions. Terminology that a parent or caregiver understands (option b) is appropriate; "technical" or "jargon-like" terminology should be avoided. Open-ended questions allow caregivers to provide the information that they believe is pertinent to the interview and to the questions you are asking.

19. e. Emotional lability and depression frequently accompany a CVA; therefore, you should provide

encouragement and motivation (option b) and make a referral to a psychologist through the primary care physician (option c) to possibly eliminate the depression or find ways to cope with his deficits. It is not your place to tell him that Medicare will not pay the bill (option a). The patient needs encouragement, not admonishment, which may further alienate him from the therapy process. If he does have potential, he deserves the opportunity to achieve functional gains with therapy and should not be discharged (option d).

20. e. All of the actions are appropriate. You should eliminate all distractions in the room (option a) to encourage the child to pay attention to one item. You would want to follow the child's lead (option b) in order to engage them in the "play therapy." The child should have an enjoyable experience, geared to her/his age which would promote attention, interaction, and development of language. You must maintain a record of all responses (option d) in order to build from those responses during future sessions.

21. b. Because the patient's symptoms are suggestive of a neurological problem that may be in the initial stages, it is very important that the patient seek a second opinion and appropriate medical care. Although treatment of dysarthria (option a) may be appropriate and explaining strategies to improve speech intelligibility (option d) is important in the treatment, the first course of action must be the referral. The primary care physician is unlikely to be able to assist with this difficult diagnosis (option e), and referral to an otolaryngologist (option c) is not appropriate.

22. a. Because the teacher's concern involves fine motor skills, it is most appropriate to refer this child to an occupational therapist for an evaluation. The evaluation must be performed by the occupational therapist to determine the course of action; the teacher cannot independently develop an appropriate home program (option b), and an SLP cannot independently develop handwriting goals. A physical therapist (option d) evaluates gross motor skills, not fine motor skills. Telling the teacher that you do not deal with handwriting (option e) does not provide the student with the needed assessment.

23. e. This patient is dangerously underweight. Lack of nutrition could account for her lethargy. It is imperative that she receive an immediate feeding and swallowing evaluation. Although she may benefit from therapy (option a), she will not receive the full benefit until she has adequate nutrition. Initiating

feeding and swallowing therapy (option b) without assessment is not appropriate. Referring her to a physical therapist (option c) is not appropriate because her being nonambulatory is not an urgent issue. Referral to a neurologist (option d) is not appropriate because you have no indication that the pump is not working effectively.

24. c. In order to determine appropriate recommendations, you must have thorough background information regarding previous treatment goals and approaches used with this child. Only when you fully understand what has and has not been effective will you be able to determine the appropriate approach for this child; therefore, immediate supplemental therapy (option a) cannot take place without this vital background. You have too little information to discuss an augmentative communication system (option b) or to suggest increased therapy (option e). Referring the child for continued therapy (option d) without a full understanding of past history is not appropriate.

25. c. The most appropriate next step would be to probe the child's productions of the phonemes /z/, /ʒ/, and /ð/ to determine whether these sounds have acquired through the acquisition of their cognate pair; therefore therapy (option a) is not appropriate, because the child may have already acquired these phonemes. Dismissing this child from therapy (option d) is not appropriate, because the child may *not* have acquired these phonemes. Formal assessment tools (option b) should not be readministered within an academic year. Continuing treatment for the other phonemes (option e) is not appropriate, because the child is correctly producing these sounds in conversation.

26. e. Before you can discuss a patient's situation with another professional, you must have a signed form for release of information. Therefore, you must not contact the teacher (option a) or have the teacher contact you (option d) until you obtain this signed form. It is not appropriate to ask the parent to relay the information (option b), inasmuch as the parent has already asked you to speak to the teacher. Once you have a signed release form, it is your responsibility to relay appropriate information (option c).

27. d. These scores are within one standard deviation of the mean; therefore, the child's language skills are within normal limits. It would not be appropriate to initiate intervention (options a and b), and these scores do not indicate the need for additional language assessment (option c). In addition, there is no indication that a reevaluation (option e) is necessary.

28. c. To encourage generalization, a concept must be practiced in a variety of functional activities to simulate more naturalistic settings with many materials. It is not appropriate to continue structured drill activities with "who" questions (option b), because the patient has mastered this level. It is also not appropriate to discontinue work on "who" questions (option d), to assess other "wh" questions (option e), or switch to other "wh" questions (option a), because you have no indication that responding correctly to "who" questions has generalized to conversation.

29. d. Some children do not develop competency with correct production of /r/ until age 8. Therefore, it is not good practice to work on /r/ at age 6 (option a) or to wait until he is 10 to reevaluate (option c). It is also not good practice to discharge a patient with an existing error (option b) without a follow-up plan. Because you already know that he is not stimulable for /r/ and /r/ diphthongs, formal assessment (option e) is not likely to yield new information.

30. c. Therapy can be provided in a variety of models, including consultation. A consultation model would allow Molly's goals to be addressed functionally and across environments. Addressing her goals in functional environments may increase Molly's motivation to improve her communication. Also, working across environments may increase generalization of her skills to a variety of environments. However, because her parents have requested traditional pull-out therapy, it is necessary to educate them about other delivery models that might be more appropriate in view of her reluctance to attend therapy and her lack of progress. Therefore, continuing pull-out therapy (option a) or initiating a positive reinforcement schedule (option e) will not address her lack of progress. Molly's receptive language skills (24 months) are more advanced than her expressive language skills (15 months), not commensurate with them (option b). Initiating new treatment goals (option d) will not necessarily improve her motivation to attend therapy.

31. d. Periodic probes will reveal whether the skills being taught are generalizing to other contexts. Base rates are measured (option a) to provide a pretreatment baseline for the skills being taught. Formal tests are performed (option b) before treatment begins, and graphing data (option c) provides a visual representation of progress on the therapy tasks but does not provide information about generalization. Reviewing data from the most recent session (option e) furnishes information regarding the patient's response to treatment activities but does not provide information about generalization.

32. c. A branching step is needed to help the patient achieve the goal. At 65% accuracy, the patient is obviously producing many error responses; therefore, the patient might be learning (option a), but with obvious difficulty. The task is not too easy (option d). Dropping the goal (option b) will not help the patient attain the desired skills. An accuracy rate of 50%, not 65%, is at the level of chance (option e).

33. b. The most appropriate way to view a patient's performance on a therapy task over a period of time is by probing the skill during the treatment sequence. Graphing the data (option c), measuring base rate (option a), reviewing data from the most recent session (option e), and formal assessment (option d) will reveal information about a skill but not generalization performance over the therapy time period.

34. d. Single-subject A × B design is used to measure generalization of a treatment goal. A pretreatment baseline is established to determine the patient's level of performance before treatment, and periodic probes are conducted during treatment to measure generalization. Standardized test probes (option a), graphing (option b), periodic formal assessment (option c), and data from the most recent session (option e) will provide information about a skill but not generalization information.

35. a. It is most appropriate for you to explain why you believe that continued therapy is needed. It would also be appropriate to provide the patient's performance data, which shows that the patient has not generalized the communication skills that are being treated. It is unprofessional for you to tell the parent that the pediatrician does not know what he is talking about (option c) or to do nothing and continue therapy (option d). There is no reason for you to discontinue therapy (option b), because you obviously believe it is still needed; otherwise, you would have discharged the patient. Reassessment (option e) should not be needed, because you should always know how the treatment process is progressing and whether continued therapy is necessary.

36. a. This child should be referred for a complete audiological evaluation because it is most important to rule out a hearing loss. Although initiating language therapy (option b) and initiating speech sound therapy (option e) are important, you will be unable to develop a treatment plan until you know the hearing status of this child. There is no reason to refer this child to his pediatrician (option c), inasmuch as the

pediatrician has already stated that development appears normal. It would be inappropriate to wait 6 months to reevaluate the child (option d) because this child needs follow-up now.

37. e. According to these test results, the most appropriate interpretation is that the child has moderate to severe delay in receptive language skills, mild delay in expressive language skills, and severe delay in speech sound skills. The patient does not have a severe impairment in expressive language skills (option a). The child's delay is not consistent across all areas (option b). Receptive language skills are more impaired than expressive language skills (option c). A child of this age should have a more extensive consonant inventory (option d).

38. b. You must have a signed release of information to share information regarding a patient. Even when the patient or family has verbally given you permission to share the information (option a), you must not share the information without the signed release. In addition, you must have a signed release of information form before you may send a copy of your report (option e). You are the most appropriate professional to relay this type of information;

therefore, it does not make sense to have the speech-language pathologist contact the parents (option c) or have the case manager contact the SLP (option d).

39. b. It is not always possible to use a test that has normative data for the population you are assessing. Therefore, you must always explain in your report that the test score may be invalid and the reason why. It would be inappropriate to report the test score as if the patient were represented in the normative group (option c). There is no reason not to include the score (option a), to report only the standard score (option d), or to report only the raw scores (option e).

40. b. Because amyotrophic lateral sclerosis is a progressive neurological disorder in which the ability to produce speech is gradually lost, augmentative communication techniques are generally needed. Most affected patients do not require language therapy (option a), benefit from speech sound therapy (option c), or develop a hearing loss (option e). Although they may benefit from therapy for compensatory behaviors to produce verbal communication (option d), it is important to first perform the augmentative assessment.

CHAPTER 19

Efficacy

Mary Pannbacker

1. _____ is the extent to which an intervention or service produces a desired outcome under ideal conditions.
   a. Efficacy
   b. Effectiveness
   c. Clinical outcome
   d. Intervention
   e. None of the above

2. _____ is the extent to which an intervention or service produces a desired outcome under usual clinical conditions.
   a. Efficacy
   b. Effectiveness
   c. Clinical outcome
   d. Patient satisfaction
   e. None of the above

3. A 6-year-old boy is dismissed from therapy on the basis of results on a standardized test of speech-sound production. His parents and teachers are concerned because his speech is very difficult to understand. What should be recommended?
   a. An analysis of a conversational speech sample
   b. Proceed with termination of therapy
   c. Monitor speech-sound development
   d. Re-administer the standardized test of speech-sound production
   e. None of the above

4. Which of the following is the best preoperation criteria for speech outcome after pharyngeal flap surgery?
   a. Lateral pharyngeal wall movement
   b. Palatal elevation
   c. Palate tension
   d. Posterior pharyngeal wall movement
   e. None of the above

5. The most important outcome of cleft palate surgery is
   _____.
   a. Feeding
   b. Hearing
   c. Speech
   d. Facial appearance
   e. None of the above

6. As a supervisor of a speech-language pathology department, you are responsible for developing a program for outcomes management. The program will require
   _____.
   a. Administrative support
   b. Staff support
   c. Technology
   d. Sufficient time to collect and analyze outcome data
   e. All the above

7. Program standards for master's degree programs in speech-language pathology are related to all the following *except:*
   a. Administration
   b. Faculty
   c. Location
   d. Students
   e. Curriculum

8. The primary purpose of the examination of oral structure and function is _____.
   a. To evaluate dental hygiene
   b. To assess the relationship between oral findings and speech
   c. To determine whether to refer the patient for orthodontic evaluation
   d. To determine whether to refer the patient for dental follow-up
   e. To determine oral resting posture

9. Ms. Smith is a 35-year-old school teacher who has made excellent progress in voice treatment for hoarseness secondary to vocal nodules. Her voice quality is now normal, as is her score on the Voice Handicap Index (VHI). What other outcome measures are warranted?
   a. Audiological evaluation
   b. Cognitive assessment
   c. Laryngoscopic examination
   d. Resonance evaluation
   e. None of the above

10. Failure of a speech-language pathologist to develop a functional outcomes management program may be related to lack of measurement and monitoring of outcomes. Of the following problems, which would be a barrier to outcome measurement?
    a. Lack of administration support
    b. Preoccupation with other clinical programs

c. Significant problems with technology
d. Insufficient time to manage outcome data
e. All the above

11. A speech-language pathologist wants to examine the outcome of cleft palate surgery. Of the following assessment measures, which would be most appropriate as a direct assessment of velopharyngeal function?
    a. Examination of oral structure and function
    b. Low-technology assessment of resonance
    c. Nasometry
    d. Assessment of speech-sound production
    e. Nasoendoscopy

12. For describing an outcomes management plan, which of the following should be given greatest consideration?
    a. The agent responsible for data analysis and interpretation
    b. The mode of data collection
    c. The source of data collection
    d. The source of information
    e. None of the above

13. Coston and associates (1992) reported a specificity of 99.6% for the Quick Screening for Congenital Malformations, which is a screening examination for the identification of different craniofacial anomalies. The specificity is _____.
    a. A high percentage of negative cases that were correctly identified
    b. A high percentage of positive cases that were correctly identified
    c. The percentage of cases that were correctly identified
    d. The percentage of cases that were incorrectly identified
    e. None of the above

14. The speech-language pathologist's careful assessment of specific treatment outcomes includes:
    a. Baseline performance
    b. Change over time
    c. Conducting retrospective studies
    d. Conducting prospective studies
    e. All the above

15. A false-negative identification of a client on some assessment or test means that:
    a. The client failed the test and does have the problem
    b. The client passed the test and does not have the problem
    c. The client failed the test but does not have the problem
    d. The client passed the test but does have the problem
    e. None of the above

16. The input-process-output model for outcomes management focuses on which of the following factors?
    a. Financial risk
    b. Generic or population focus
    c. Staffing
    d. Value of health care quality
    e. All the above

17. The primary purpose of efficacy research is _____.
    a. To study the benefit of certain clinical practice conditions occurring in the real world
    b. To study outcomes under typical clinical conditions
    c. To study outcomes under controlled experimental conditions
    d. To measure the effect of some intervention
    e. None of the above

18. Which is the most common barrier to outcomes measurement in a clinical setting?
    a. Problems with data collection
    b. Staff and administration resistance
    c. Limitations of time and resources
    d. All the above
    e. None of the above

19. An outcome of primary interest to payers of speech-language pathology services is related to _____.
    a. Clinically devised outcomes
    b. Financial outcomes
    c. Functional outcomes
    d. Social outcomes
    e. All the above

20. According to the American Speech-Language-Hearing Association's (ASHA's) Code of Ethics, a speech-language pathologist must do which of the following when providing services to a client?
    a. Evaluate the outcome of services
    b. Guarantee the outcome of service
    c. Obtain informed consent
    d. All the above
    e. None of the above

21. Which of the following is primarily a measurable administrative outcome?
    a. Employability
    b. Functional outcome
    c. Quality of life
    d. Rate of missed appointments
    e. All the above

22. Phase I research of the five-phase model of clinical research involves:

a. Examining the intervention with an alternative intervention or with a control group
b. Establishing the internal validity of the intervention
c. Examining the clinical viability of the intervention
d. Identifying an intervention to be examined
e. Identifying the clients whose condition improves with the treatment

23. Phase II research of the five-phase model of clinical research involves:
    a. Examining the intervention with an alternative intervention or with a control group
    b. Establishing the internal validity of the intervention
    c. Examining the clinical viability of the intervention
    d. Identifying an intervention to be examined
    e. Identifying the clients whose condition improves with the treatment

24. Phase III research of the five-phase model of clinical research involves:
    a. Examining the intervention with an alternative intervention or with a control group
    b. Establishing the internal validity of the intervention
    c. Examining the clinical viability of the intervention
    d. Identifying an intervention to be examined
    e. Identifying the clients whose condition improves with the treatment

25. Phase IV research of the five-phase model of clinical research involves:
    a. Examining the intervention with an alternative intervention or with a control group
    b. Establishing the internal validity of the intervention
    c. Examining the clinical viability of the intervention
    d. Identifying an intervention to be examined
    e. Identifying the clients whose condition improves with the treatment

26. Phase V research of the five-phase model of clinical research involves:
    a. Examining the intervention with an alternative intervention or with a control group
    b. Establishing the internal validity of the intervention
    c. Examining the clinical viability of the intervention
    d. Identifying an intervention to be examined
    e. Identifying the population of clients whose condition improves with the treatment

27. The term *cost utility* refers to which of the following?
    a. Cost versus benefit
    b. Cost to improvement
    c. Quality of life
    d. All the above
    e. None of the above

28. Practitioners need to provide clinical services within the context of evidence-based practice, and they have a responsibility to be knowledgeable of the current research evidence for a particular assessment or intervention instrument. The level of evidence for a particular instrument can be classified according to credibility. The highest level or most credible evidence is:
    a. Level I
    b. Level II
    c. Level III
    d. Level IV
    e. All the above

29. Practitioners need to provide clinical services within the context of evidence-based practice, and they have a responsibility to be knowledgeable of the current research evidence for a particular assessment or intervention instrument. The level of evidence for a particular instrument can be classified according to credibility. The lowest level or least credible evidence is:
    a. Level I
    b. Level II
    c. Level III
    d. Level IV
    e. None of the above

30. Which of the following levels of evidence apply to clinical practice guidelines?
    a. Class I
    b. Class II
    c. Class III
    d. Class I and class II
    e. Class II and class III

1. a. Efficacy is the study of outcomes under ideal conditions. Effectiveness (option b) is the real effect reported in research experiments that are examining a treatment under typical clinical conditions. Clinical outcomes (option c) pertain to the findings of investigations of different treatments and their application in the clinical treatment of patients. An intervention (option d) is a treatment plan with measurable goals that is employed to modify various communicative or feeding disorders.

2. b. Effectiveness concerns the extent of a desired outcome of treatment under usual clinical conditions. Efficacy (option a) is the study of outcomes under ideal conditions. Clinical outcomes (option c) pertain to the findings of investigations of different treatments and their application in the clinical treatment of patients. Patient satisfaction is a type of outcome measure that pertains to the patient's satisfaction with a particular clinical treatment.

3. a. Differences between speech sound production in single words and conversational speech are well known. It is likely that the client can produce the targeted sounds at the single word level but experiences difficulty at the contextual speech level and requires additional treatment. Monitoring speech-sound development (option c) and re-administering the speech-sound production test (option d) are unlikely to influence his intelligibility or ability to be understood by others. Decisions about dismissal from treatment of a speech-sound disorder (option b) should include data from a conversational speech sample.

4. a. Velopharyngeal closure (VPC) is typically sphincteric, that is dynamic and involves movement of the lateral and posterior pharyngeal wall and velar elevation. Movement of the lateral pharyngeal walls during preoperative assessment is a positive indicator of potential for surgical intervention. Placement of a flap requires movement of the lateral pharyngeal walls to occlude the portals on either side of the pharyngeal flap during speech production.

5. c. Speech outcome is the primary consideration in cleft palate surgery. In general, about 75% of children who undergo cleft palate surgery before the age of 18 months develop normal speech. Feeding (option a), hearing (option b), and facial appearance (option d) are also important outcomes, but speech is the principal one.

6. e. Administrative support (option a), staff support (option b), technology (option c), and sufficient time for data collection and analysis (option d) are all necessary for outcomes management. The supervisor develops the outcome management program, but each of the aspects just mentioned is important for the success of the program.

7. c. Geographic location of a graduate program is not a program standard. Administration (option a), faculty (option b), students (option d), and curriculum (option e) are compared against standards in program evaluation for accreditation of speech-language pathology programs.

8. b. The main purpose of the oral examination is to determine the existence of any problems with oral structure or function that adversely affect speech production. It is possible that some patients may exhibit obligatory errors; that is, the observed errors are a function of some structural variable such as a malocclusion.

9. c. Laryngoscopic examination is a prerequisite for dismissal from voice treatment. Laryngeal status, voice quality, and the client's perception of his or her voice problem are the primary outcome measures for voice treatment. It should be noted that the VHI is a measure of the patient's perception of his or her voice problem. Audiological evaluation (option a), cognitive assessment (option b), and resonance evaluation (option d) are part of patient assessments for different communication disorders.

10. e. Administration support (option a), focus specifically on outcomes measurement (option b), technology (option c), and sufficient time to manage outcome data (option d) are necessary for outcomes management. Problems in these areas create significant barriers to outcomes management.

11. e. Nasoendoscopy provides direct visual observation of velopharyngeal function during speech. Examination of oral structure and function (option a), low-technology assessment of resonance (option b), nasometry (option c), and assessment of speech-sound production (option d) are also important components of an outcome assessment but are considered indirect measures of velopharyngeal function.

12. c. The source of data collection is the primary consideration in developing a plan for outcomes

management. The other activities are also important but should be considered later and in the following sequence: source of information (option d), mode of data collection (option b), and the agent responsible for data analysis and interpretation (option a).

13. a. Researchers examine different questions, and one is validity: Does a particular assessment or measure actually measure what it purports to measure? The validity of an assessment or measure can be studied in terms of specificity and sensitivity. Specificity, or true negative findings, is the percentage of persons that were correctly identified as not having the disease or disorder. According to the statistic reported, the screening has high specificity; that is, it is a valid tool for identifying patients without craniofacial anomalies. Sensitivity, or true positive findings, is the percentage of persons who are at risk for a particular problem or disorder. An appropriate assessment or measure would have satisfactory specificity and sensitivity.

14. e. Efficacious treatment is appropriate and effective treatment that results in improved patient communication skills. Treatment outcomes describe the results of treatment without specific research controls but under typical treatment conditions. To validate effective treatment outcome, the speech-language pathologist needs to collect data in a number of different ways. Monitoring of short-term and long-term treatment outcomes should include base line performance (option a), changes over time (option b), and periodic retrospective (option c) or prospective studies (option d) to evaluate outcomes.

15. d. The questions deals with the specificity and sensitivity of a specific test or assessment measure. "False-negative" means that the client passed the test but does have the problem. This means that the client may not receive needed treatment, and there is a potential risk of liability. A false-positive judgment indicates that the client did not pass the test but does not have the problem (option c). A true-positive judgment means that the client failed the test and does have the problem (option a). A true-negative judgment indicates that the client passed the test and does not have the problem (option b). The validity of an assessment or measure can be studied in terms of specificity and sensitivity. Specificity, or true-negative results, is the percentage of clients who were correctly identified as not having the disease or disorder. Sensitivity, or true-positive results, is the percentage of clients who are at risk for a particular problem or disorder. An appropriate assessment or measure would have satisfactory specificity and sensitivity.

16. b. The input-process-output model focuses on the generic or specific population with regard to the outcomes. The Doerger model focuses on monitoring and managing financial and clinical risk (option a). The effort of staffing (option c) is the major focus of Cho's model. The value of care model concentrates on the importance of value (option d) in the assessment of health care quality.

17. c. Efficacy research is the study of outcomes under various degrees of controlled clinical conditions. The purpose is to study different treatments and determine their clinical effectiveness. Efficacious treatment results in a desired effect. The other options refer to outcomes research. *Treatment outcome* refers to the results of treatment without the use of stringent experimental control. One variation is efficiency research, which is the study of outcomes under usual clinical conditions (option b).

18. d. Problems with data collection (option a), staff and administration resistance (option b), and time and resource limitations (option c) are common barriers to developing, implementing, and maintaining an outcomes measurement program.

19. b. Financial or cost measures are of primary interest to payers. Among these cost measures are cost-benefit ratios, cost effectiveness, and cost utility. Clinically devised outcomes (option a), functional outcomes (option c), and social outcomes (option d) are of more importance to clients, families, and clinicians.

20. a. The outcome of service must be evaluated. According to the ASHA's Code of Ethics, "Individuals shall evaluate the effectiveness of services rendered and of products dispensed and shall provide services or dispense products only when benefit can reasonably be expected." The speech-language pathologist cannot guarantee the outcome of services to a client (option b). Informed consent (option c) is obtained in when clients participate in research or in teaching presentations, which does not always occur in the provision of services.

21. d. Rate of missed appointments, clinical referral patterns, and productivity levels in direct client care are administrative outcomes that provide important data for the practitioner. Employability (option a), functional outcome (option b), and quality of life (option c) are outcomes related to other areas: Employability is a social outcome, the ability to communicate is a functional outcome, and quality of life is a client-defined outcome.

22. d. Like other rehabilitation disciplines, the discipline of communication sciences and disorders is increasingly

guided by intervention research within an organized framework. A number of professionals have proposed specific frameworks, such as the five-phase model of intervention research. In this particular model, interventions are examined systematically, so that there is a gradual progression from identifying an intervention to examining the intervention in different research paradigms. Phase I research involves the identification of an intervention that will be studied in later phases of research.

23. c. During phase II of the five-phase model of intervention research, preliminary research studies such as case studies and small group cohort studies are carried out to scrutinize the clinical viability of the intervention.

24. b. Small group experimental and quasi-experimental studies are undertaken in phase III of the five-phase model of intervention research, with the primary goal of establishing the internal validity of the intervention: that is, determining whether research data support a causal relationship.

25. a. Phase IV of the five-phase model of intervention research consists of further experimental studies, which investigate the intervention against an alternative intervention or with a no-treatment control condition. Research data may be used to make clinical choices, but the data are not at the highest level of evidence for supporting specific clinical decisions.

26. e. In the five-phase model of intervention research, Phase V consists of research studies designed to examine generalization of the intervention to the specific population under normal and variable clinical environments (e). Are the clinical effects similar to the findings of phase IV research.

27. c. Speech and language therapy are interventions that generally do not affect survival but do improve quality of life. To examine the value of an intervention for improved quality of life, a cost-utility analysis is useful. In such an analysis, the researcher considers the treatment's effect on quality of life. Cost-versus-benefit analysis (option a) is used to evaluate the efficiency of an intervention to determine whether the benefits outweigh the cost. Cost to improvement (option b) is a process for establishing a goal-oriented cost analysis that will facilitate future cost reductions in services, such as the delivery of an intervention.

28. a. The primary objective of evidence-based practice is to incorporate clinical practice, state-of-the-art evidence, and client values in order to supply high-quality services that are consistent with the patient's interests, values, wants, and preferences. *Level of evidence* refers to a hierarchy of experimental designs that are used to minimize research bias. No single hierarchy is generally used; however, randomized controlled trials are judged to be the least subject to bias. Different experimental hierarchies encompass observational studies and nonexperimental designs. Level I evidence is the most credible and is produced by one or more well-designed, randomized, controlled trials.

29. d. The primary objective of evidence-based practice is to incorporate clinical practice, state-of-the-art evidence, and client values in order to supply high-quality services that are consistent with the patient's interests, values, wants, and preferences. *Level of evidence* refers to a hierarchy of experimental designs that are used to minimize research bias. No single hierarchy is generally used; however, randomized controlled trials are judged to be the least subject to bias. Different experimental hierarchies encompass observational studies and nonexperimental designs. Level IV is the least credible evidence and is based on the clinical opinion of "authorities" in the discipline.

30. e. The primary objective of evidence-based practice is to incorporate clinical practice, state-of-the-art evidence, and client values in order to supply high-quality services that are consistent with the patient's interests, values, wants, and preferences. *Level of evidence* refers to a hierarchy of experimental designs that are used to minimize research bias. No single hierarchy is generally used; however, randomized controlled trials are judged to be the least subject to bias. Different experimental hierarchies encompass observational studies and nonexperimental designs. Clinical practice guidelines reflect a moderate degree of certainty and are usually based on class II evidence or on a strong consensus from class III evidence. Within these classes, research on the topic of interest ranges from controlled studies without randomization (class II) to nonexperimental studies such as correlational or case study designs (class III).

Bibliography

American Speech-Language-Hearing Association. (2003) *Code of ethics.* Available at www.asha.org/policy (accessed July 7, 2009).

Coston, G. N., & Sayetta, R. B. (1992). Craniofacial screening profile: Quick Friedman, H. I. et al. Screening for congenital malformations. *Cleft Palate Craniofacial Journal, 29,* 87–91.

CHAPTER 20

Instrumentation

J. Anthony Seikel

1. Work with dialect reduction involves modification of into-nation. This information may be found in displays of:
   a. The vocal fundamental frequency plotted over time
   b. The formant frequency plotted over time
   c. The waterfall appearance of formant structure over time
   d. The spectral slice of the individual vowel
   e. All the above

2. Individuals who are being treated to reduce the effect of nonnative dialect often have stop consonant voicing errors according to the perception of an English lis-tener. To examine their speech to determine the nature of the error, a useful instrumental means is:
   a. A display of fundamental frequency, as in Visi-Pitch
   b. A display of amplitude of fundamental frequency, as in Visi-Pitch
   c. A display of frequency changes over time, as in spectrography
   d. A display of vocal fold open and closed phases, as in electroglottography
   e. Palatometry

3. An adult client has a hoarse voice and can sustain a vowel for only 4 seconds before taking a breath. The otolaryngologist must determine the presence or absence of vocal nodules. Which procedure is used?
   a. Palatometry
   b. Spectroscopy
   c. Electroglottography
   d. Endoscopy
   e. Nasometry

4. A client has a history of repaired cleft palate, and the speech-language pathologist (SLP) is seeking a means of instrumental assessment of his speech in relation to the repaired defect. Of the following methods, which will provide the best evidence of the effect of the repair on speech production?

a. Nasometry
b. Palatometry
c. Electroglottography
d. Spectrography
e. All the above

5. A deaf child is receiving treatment for vowel production. Of the following instruments, which will provide the most appropriate feedback of accuracy?
   a. Visi-Pitch
   b. Nasometer
   c. Speech Viewer
   d. Electroglottograph
   e. Aerodynamic measurement

6. The SLP's perception is that a patient with Parkinson disease has a reduced fundamental frequency range. What measure will provide the most effective evaluation of this?
   a. Spectrographic display
   b. Waterfall display of formants
   c. Pitch contour
   d. Nasalance
   e. All the above

7. The SLP questions whether a patient aspirates while consuming thin liquids. To determine the presence of aspiration, the SLP will:
   a. Provide thin liquids in small quantities and listen for voice change
   b. Provide progressively thinner liquids, listening for coughing by the patient
   c. Observe the transit of thin liquids by using radiography (modified barium swallow study [MBSS])
   d. Observe the patient during mealtime for signs of aspiration
   e. Do none of the above

8. The SLP is concerned that a patient may have pharyngeal residue secondary to reduced contraction of the pharyngeal constrictor muscles. Which method will provide the most effective evidence of the presence and degree of residue?
   a. Fiberoptic endoscopic examination of swallowing (FEES)
   b. MBSS
   c. Clinical evaluation, with the five-finger evaluation method
   d. Clinical evaluation, with focus on vocal quality after swallowing
   e. Bedside feeding assessment

9. The SLP wants to examine the bolus during the oral preparation stage. The best means of performing this examination is:

a. FEES
b. Clinical examination
c. MBSS
d. Esophagography
e. None of the above

10. The SLP needs to assess the timing of the pharyngeal swallow. The best way to do this is by:
    a. Clinical examination
    b. Two-channel electromyography (EMG), with electrodes reading the genioglossus and hyoid elevators
    c. FEES
    d. MBSS
    e. Presenting food of different viscosities to the patient

11. The SLP mixes dye in water and presents it to a patient during a swallowing evaluation, although the patient does not have a tracheostomy tube. What procedure is being using?
    a. MBSS
    b. Clinical examination
    c. EMG
    d. FEES
    e. All the above

12. A patient has demonstrated nasal regurgitation during swallowing, and the SLP wishes to assess velar function. The most appropriate means for doing this entails the use of:
    a. Nasoendoscopy
    b. MBSS
    c. Clinical swallowing examination
    d. Nasometry
    e. Pressure/flow measurement

13. A patient with amyotrophic lateral sclerosis has severe dysarthria secondary to muscular weakness that limits range of movement and force in the superior direction. The SLP is considering use of a prosthesis to assist in articulation. What device might assist the assessment of tongue and palate function?
    a. Palatometer
    b. Spectrograph
    c. Visi-Pitch
    d. Nasometer
    e. Photodetection device

14. On the basis of an oral mechanism examination, the SLP suspects palatal-pharyngeal-laryngeal myoclonus. Which instrumental procedure provides the best evidence of this condition?
    a. Spectrography of speech signal, with the use of sustained vowel productions
    b. Visi-Pitch or Speech Viewer, with pitch as the monitoring function

c. Nasoendoscopy, with patient at rest
d. MBSS
e. None of the above

15. The SLP questions whether a patient has adequate esophageal stage function during swallowing. The procedure to determine this is:
a. MBSS
b. FEES
c. Clinical swallowing examination
d. Clinical swallowing examination plus the monitoring of vocal quality between swallows
e. All the above

16. The SLP suspects esophageal reflux after a patient swallows. What procedure provides the best evidence of this?
a. MBSS
b. Case history and questioning of patient (if communication function is adequate)
c. FEES
d. Clinical swallowing examination
e. Instrumental assessment by a gastroenterologist

17. A client is perceived as hoarse, which may be an indication of variability in periodicity of vocal fold vibration. Which measure will allow the SLP to determine the degree of variability of vocal fold vibration?
a. Vocal intensity, in decibels
b. Fundamental frequency, in hertz
c. Closed quotient, as measured by electroglottography
d. Perturbation or vocal jitter
e. None of the above

18. An 8-year-old has been referred to an SLP with the notation that his "speech is muffled." Which instrumental procedure will help the SLP assess whether this is an issue of hypernasality or articulatory precision?
a. Sound spectrography
b. Electroglottography
c. Nasometry
d. Palatometry
e. Pressure/flow measurement

19. A patient with a history of right hemisphere stroke has pneumonia and may be at risk for aspiration. Which procedure would best determine the nature of swallowing deficit, if it is present?
a. Clinical examination, with the use of five-finger evaluation to determine trigger timing and degree of laryngeal elevation
b. Case history, in which the patient is asked about difficulties that she is experiencing with mastication and deglutition
c. FEES, focusing on oral and pharyngeal stages
d. MBSS, focusing on oral and pharyngeal stages
e. Ultrasonography

20. Of the following instruments, which provides evidence of sufficient intraoral pressure for speech?
a. Manometer
b. Spirometer
c. Spectrometer
d. Hygrometer
e. None of the above

21. A patient has symptoms of spastic dysarthria after a cerebrovascular accident. The perception is of hard glottal attacks, and the SLP wants to verify the presence of phonatory attack for this patient. Which instrument is most effective for this evaluation?
a. EMG
b. Electroglottography
c. Spectrography
d. Endoscopy
e. All the above

22. A 6-year-old produces voicing of voiceless phonemes, but the SLP suspects that the child is in a transitional stage in the development of the contrast. How can the SLP determine whether the client has achieved the phonemic voicing distinction, although it is not yet perceptible?
a. Examine fundamental frequency traces for variations in pitch fluctuation that would signal phonemic knowledge of the voicing distinction
b. Examine electroglottographic evidence, specifically for timing differences between voiced and voiceless cognates
c. Examine voice onset time by using spectrography, and compare with norms for age
d. Use EMG to measure timing differences between larynx and lingual muscles
e. All the above

23. A patient with a history of chronic obstructive pulmonary disease, hypertension, and cerebrovascular accident exhibits low vocal intensity. The SLP needs to differentiate the effects of resonance and respiration on speech production. What combination of instruments would assist in this differentiation?
a. Nasometer and sound spectrograph
b. Nasometer and spirometer
c. Electroglottograph and sound spectrograph
d. Manometer and spirometer
e. Spirometer and sound spectrograph

24. A patient with a history of cerebrovascular accident has spastic dysarthria, resulting in reduced duration of phonation. Which instrument enables the SLP to determine vital capacity?
a. Manometer
b. Spirometer

c. Hygrometer
d. Palatometer
e. None of the above

25. The SLP knows that a client needs to be able to generate between 5 and 7 cm H_2O of subglottal pressure for sustained speech at conversational levels. Of the following devices, which enables the SLP to determine a patient's pressure reserves?
    a. Spirometer
    b. Oral manometer
    c. Sound spectrograph
    d. Nasometer
    e. All the above

26. A child has tongue thrust, and the SLP is working with him on increasing superior lingual force during the oral phase of swallow. The SLP can objectively measure superior force by using:
    a. The Iowa Oral Pressure Instrument (IOPI)
    b. The Speech Viewer (articulation module)
    c. MBSS
    d. FEES
    e. Oral mechanism examination

27. A child has a suspected oromyofunctional disorder. By palpating the masseter muscles during the oral mechanism examination, the SLP detects possible asymmetrical contraction. How can the SLP objectively evaluate this perception?
    a. FEES, with tip aimed toward the oral cavity
    b. MBSS, with focus on oral structures
    c. EMG, with both masseter muscles monitored simultaneously
    d. Palatography, with monitoring for asymmetry of articulatory precision
    e. Ultrasonography, with observation of tongue function during dry swallows

28. The SLP wants to examine the vibratory pattern of a patient's vocal folds. Which instrumental procedure provides that information?
    a. Nasoendoscopy and stroboscopy
    b. Electroglottography and nasometry
    c. Sound spectroscopy and electroglottography
    d. Oscilloscopic trace and manometry
    e. All the above

29. Which analysis provides information about the transfer function of the vocal tract?
    a. Fast Fourier transform
    b. Cepstral analysis
    c. Linear predictive coding

d. Sound spectrography
e. All the above

30. Of the following instruments, which would provide a display of the speech waveform?
    a. Oscilloscope
    b. Endoscope
    c. Sound spectrograph
    d. Laryngoscope
    e. Palatometer

31. What display will allow the SLP to provide acoustical evidence of laryngeal tremor?
    a. Display of fundamental frequency over time
    b. Display of formant structure over time
    c. Display of glottal closure quotient
    d. Display of speech waveform
    e. Display of oral air pressure during the production of pressure sounds

32. What instrument allows the SLP to measure point of articulation?
    a. Sound spectrograph
    b. Spirometer
    c. Manometer
    d. Palatometer
    e. All the above

33. An SLP needs to determine whether oral motor exercises are helping to strengthen the dorsum of the tongue in a patient with dysphagia. Force data can be derived from:
    a. MBSS
    b. Perception of the force applied by the tongue to a tongue depressor
    c. A labial goniometer
    d. The IOPI
    e. Ultrasonography

34. Of the following methods, which measures an impedance drop across the vocal folds?
    a. Electroglottography
    b. Sound spectrography
    c. EMG
    d. Nasometry
    e. Pressure/flow measurement

35. Of the following measures, which allows the SLP to determine the duration of the second formant (F_2) transition in speech?
    a. Display of fundamental frequency over time
    b. Indirect laryngoscopy
    c. Oscilloscopy
    d. Sound spectrography
    e. All the above

1. a. The fundamental frequency represents the basic vibration of the vocal folds and dominates the perception of vocal pitch. Intonation is the change in vocal pitch over time, and thus a temporal display is essential. Formant structure (option b) represents the filter function of the vocal tract, and intonation is a function of the vocal source. The other choices waterfall display (option c) and the spectral slice (option d) also provide acoustical information but not about fundamental frequency over time.

2. c. The voicing distinction is carried primarily in the voice onset time of the prevocalic stop and in vowel duration in the postvocalic stop. A spectrographic display allows the clinician to examine both voice onset time and vowel duration. Displays of the fundamental frequency (option a) and amplitude of the fundamental frequency (option b) do not provide information about voice onset time, and electroglottography (option d) shows only data about vocal fold opening and closure. The palatometer (option e) provides a visual record of tongue-palate contact during speech.

3. d. Endoscopy is a procedure that allows introduction of a flexible or rigid tube into the oral or nasal cavity as a means of observing activity and structures within the nasal and pharyngeal spaces. None of the other measures provides evidence of physical processes of the larynx. Palatometry (option a) is an instrumental procedure that provides a visual record of tongue-palate contacts during speech production. Spectroscopy (option b) and nasometry (option e) are acoustic study methods, and electroglottography involves the measurement of impedance between the vocal folds to estimate the degree of vocal fold contact.

4. a. Nasometry (option a) provides the most effective means of determining the degree of nasal resonance present in nonnasal speech. The nasometer measures oral and nasal acoustic sound energy and computes a ratio known as nasalance. Spectrography (option d) would provide qualitative evidence of hypernasality, but nasometry can provide quantitative evidence. Palatometry (option b) and electroglottography (option c) are also important instrumental methods but would not provide the information that the SLP is seeking.

5. c. The Speech Viewer has speech-recognition software that allows the clinician to identify the correct productions by a client and to use those as targets. The software provides visual feedback for speech accuracy. The Visi-Pitch (option a) measures acoustic parameters (e.g., fundamental frequency, amplitude, and spectral characteristics) during speech and voice production and displays the desired measurement parameters in real time. The nasometer (option b) measures oral and nasal acoustic sound energy and computes a ratio known as nasalance. The elecroglottograph (option d) measures impedance between the vocal folds to estimate the degree of vocal fold contact. In aerodynamic measurement (option e), air pressure and air flow in the vocal tract are assessed.

6. c. Pitch contour provided by instruments such as Dr. Speech, Visi-Pitch, or Speech Viewer enable the SLP to examine the degree of frequency excursion in running speech. This information can be extracted from spectrography (option a) but with difficulty, and much time is needed. The waterfall display of formants (option b) and nasalance (option d) do not provide the information that the SLP is seeking.

7. c. Although all the choices could be used, only radiography provides a direct record of the patient's pharyngeal phase of swallowing. The MBSS allows the SLP to view the bolus enter the laryngeal aditus. The clinical study methods (options a, b, and d) may furnish evidence of penetration, but confirmation of penetration or aspiration requires visualization.

8. a. Both FEES and MBSS (option b) provide the ability to visualize residue, but FEES provides better ability to characterize the amount of residue, inasmuch as the SLP is in direct view and not using a radiographic procedure. The clinical evaluations (options c and d) and bedside feeding assessment (option e) would not provide the information needed by the SLP.

9. c. Although mastication function can be estimated through the clinical examination (option b), the MBSS enables the SLP to visualize bolus movement in real time. The FEES (option a) does not image the oral cavity, and esophagography (option d) is used to study the physiology of the esophagus.

10. d. The MBSS allows determination of the timing of the pharyngeal swallow. Neither clinical examination (option a) nor EMG (option b) provides the timing information that is needed. The FEES (option c) image "whites out" during the trigger of swallow. The presentation of food (option e) is a variable that is manipulated during both bedside and instrumental measurement of swallowing.

11. d. The use of dye in FEES helps the SLP visualize the liquid. It is not needed in MBSS (option a), because barium is added for visualization. Clinical examination (option b) and EMG (option c) do not involve the use of dye for contrast purposes.

12. b. MBSS enables the SLP to visualize the velum in a coordinated manner during the act of swallowing. Nasoendoscopy (option a) is useful for determining velar elevation and function, but it cannot show activity of the velum during swallowing. The clinical swallowing examination (option c), nasometry (option d), and pressure/flow measurement (option e) also do not provide visualization of the velum during the act of swallowing.

13. a. The palatometer provides a measure of the degree of lingual contact on the palate during speech, which could be used in fabrication of a prosthesis. The spectrograph (option b), Visi-Pitch (option c), nasometer (option d), and photodetection device (option e) provide acoustic or physiological data but would not be appropriate for fabricating a prosthesis.

14. c. A physiologically based instrumental procedure is required, and nasoendoscopy is suitable for this scenario. Although MBSS (option d) would provide evidence, it would expose the patient to unnecessary radiation. Spectrography (option a) and Visi-Pitch or Speech Viewer (option b) are instrumental procedures that provide acoustic data, but they are not physiologically based instruments.

15. a. The MBSS enables direct visualization of esophageal motility during swallowing. The other visualization procedure, FEES (option b), does not provide evidence of esophageal motility. A clinical or beside examination (options c and d) would not provide such diagnostic information.

16. e. A gastroenterologist is the professional who deals with problems such as esophageal motility and would conduct an instrumental assessment. The MBSS (option a) provides evidence of reflux if it occurs during the swallowing study, but patient safety requires limiting exposure to radiation. FEES (option c) allows the clinician to observe the period after swallowing without exposure to radiation, but it may not provide the necessary information. The clinical swallowing examination (option d) would not provide the evidence needed. Case history and questioning (option b) are important information sources; they do not provide direct evidence, but they would provide information that may lead to appropriate referral for an assessment by a gastroenterologist.

17. d. Vocal quality is a function of the vibration of the vocal folds. Hoarse voice quality is typically caused by abnormality of the vocal folds, as in the cases of laryngitis or vocal abuse. Measurements of perturbation and vocal jitter reflect the degree of vocal fold variability, expressed as a percentage, and would provide an index of vocal fold variability. Measures of vocal intensity (option a), fundamental frequency (option b), and closed quotient (option c) are not appropriate for determining variability.

18. c. An acoustic index of hypernasality is the comparison between oral and nasal acoustic energy, reflected by nasometric measurement. Palatometry (option d) would provide evidence of articulatory precision or imprecision but would not help differentiate between hypernasality and articulatory precision. Spectrography (option a) can provide evidence of hypernasality and articulatory function, but the spectral evidence for hypernasality is weaker than that of nasalance. Electroglottography (option b) entails measurement of the impedance between the vocal folds to estimate degree of vocal fold contact. Pressure/flow measurement (option e) entails examination of oral air pressure, nasal airflow, and nasal air pressure during speech production.

19. d. The MBSS furnishes direct visual information about the oral and pharyngeal stages of swallowing. FEES (option c) provides information about pharyngeal function before and after the trigger of the swallow but not about the oral stage. Ultrasonography (option e) allows visualization only of lingual function. Case history (option b) and clinical examination (option a) are only indirect means of determining difficulty.

20. a. The manometer is an instrument used to measure the pressure of liquids and gases and has been used by SLPs. The spirometer (option b) is used to measure air volume or flow. The spectrometer (option c) is used to assess the properties of light over a specific portion of the electromagnetic spectrum. The hygrometer (option d) is used to measure relative humidity.

21. d. Endoscopy allows direct visualization of the larynx in order to directly assess the degree of force being exerted at onset. Electroglottography (option b), spectrography (option c), and EMG (option a) can provide different types of physiological or acoustic evidence through magnitude of the trace, but direct visualization allows the examiner to confirm the force being exerted at onset.

22. c. Phonemic awareness of the voicing contrast has been identified through spectroscopy, even though

the contrast was not perceptible to adult listeners. Fundamental frequency traces (option a), electroglottographic evidence (option b), and EMG (option d) would not provide evidence of the voicing contrast.

23. b. The nasometer provides evidence of velar activity or lack thereof, and the spirometer can provide evidence of respiratory volume insufficiency. The sound spectrograph (options a, c, and e), electroglottograph (option c), and manometer (option d) would not provide the information needed to evaluate the resonance and respiratory systems.

24. b. Vital capacity is the total volume of air that can be expelled from the lungs after a maximum inspiration. The spirometer enables estimation of respiratory volumes for speech and is appropriate for this patient. The manometer (option a) is used to measure the pressure of liquids and gases. The palatometer (option d) is used to examine the tongue-palate contacts. The hygrometer (option c) is used to measure relative humidity.

25. b. The oral manometer allows indirect measurement of subglottal pressure. Since it is used to measure the pressure of liquids and gases. The spirometer (option a) allows measurement of air volumes inhaled and exhaled from the lungs. The sound spectrograph (option c) and the nasometer (option d) allow acoustic measurement, not the physiological information needed to answer this question.

26. a. The IOPI allows direct measurement of force generated by articulators. Speech Viewer (option b) allows the SLP to examine perceptual elements. The MBSS (option c) allows the SLP to observe the movement of the structures, not the force generated. FEES (option d) does not address oral-stage dysphagia or the measurement of muscle force. In the oral mechanism examination (option e), structure and function of the oral mechanism are assessed, but an objective index of tongue force is not provided.

27. c. The paired masseter muscles are used in mastication. The superficial part of these muscles inserts from the zygomatic process of the maxilla and from the anterior two thirds of the border of the zygomatic arch. The muscle fibers course downward and backward with insertion to the lateral surface of the ramus of the mandible. The two-channel EMG provides evidence of timing of the masseter contraction that cannot be obtained by FEES (option a), MBSS (option b), palatography (option d), or ultrasonography (option e).

28. a. A stroboscopic light source that is synchronized with the fundamental frequency of vocal fold vibration allows re-creation of vocal fold vibration in slow motion, so that the SLP can see, through the endoscope, the mode of vibration of the vocal folds. Electroglottography (options a and c), nasometry (option a), sound spectroscopy (option c), and oscilloscopic trace and manometry (option d) provide important instrumental information but are not appropriate for this assessment of vocal fold function.

29. c. Transfer function is the involvement of vocal tract resonance with the source function and resulting speech sound. Although the fast Fourier transform (option a) provides information about the filter function, linear predictive coding is more appropriately suited for the speech signal and for estimation of the vocal tract transfer function. Cepstral analysis (option b) consists of a variety of signal processing applications that are based on the concept of the complex cepstrum. The complex cepstrum of a signal is defined in terms of its Z transform. Sound spectrography (option d) is an acoustic measurement technique that yields information about the frequency, intensity, and duration of a sound.

30. a. The oscilloscope provides a plot of amplitude of a waveform displayed over time. The endoscope (option b) and laryngoscope (option d) allow direct visualization of the vocal tract. The sound spectrograph (option c) provides acoustic information about frequency, intensity, and duration of a sound. The palatometer (option e) is used to measure points of contact between the tongue and palate.

31. a. Because tremor is typically in the range of 4 to 10 Hz, it would be visible in a fast trace of the fundamental frequency. The displays of formant structure over time (option b), glottal closure quotient (option c), speech waveform (option d), and oral air pressure during the production of pressure sounds (option e) provide different acoustic and physiological information that is used by SLPs for assessment, treatment, and research purposes.

32. d. The palatometer provides direct evidence of lingual contact with the hard palate, which is the point of articulation. The sound spectrograph (option a) provides indirect evidence through the acoustic signal. The spirometer (option b) and manometer (option c) do not provide information about the point of articulation. The spirometer is used to measure air volumes inhaled and exhaled from the lungs; a manometer is used to measure the pressure of liquids and gases.

33. d. The IOPI measures lingual force from the dorsum of the tongue. Although the MBSS (option a) and

ultrasonography (option e) allow the SLP to observe and record function, they do not give information about force. Perception of tongue depressor force (option b) is subjective, not objective, data. A labial goniometer measures lip symmetry (option c).

34. a. Electroglottography is used to measure impedance between the vocal folds in order to estimate degree of vocal fold contact. Sound spectrography (option b) furnishes acoustic information in terms of frequency, intensity, and duration of a sound. EMG is a physiological technique that measures the electrical activity of neuronal muscle stimulation.

Nasometry (option d) is used to assess acoustic sound energy from the oral and nasal cavities and computes a ratio between the two. Pressure/flow measurement is used to examine oral air pressure, nasal airflow, and nasal air pressure during speech production.

35. d. Sound spectrography allows the SLP to visualize formants displayed over time. Fundamental frequency display (option a) and waveform display, or oscilloscopy (option c), do not reveal this information, and indirect laryngoscopy (option b) reveals physiological, not acoustical, information.

CHAPTER 21

Speech-Language Assessment

Karen B. Haines

Leslie C. Graebe

1. A 5-year-old is referred for a speech evaluation with the complaint of "air passing through the nose during speech production." The child has never been enrolled in a speech treatment program, and parents report that cognitive, motor, and social development are normal. As part of a comprehensive assessment, the speech-language pathologist (SLP) evaluates the speech-sound skills of the child and identifies nasal emission during the production of the /s/ and /z/ phonemes. Other pressure sounds are produced with satisfactory oral placement and without nasal emission. The oral mechanism examination is unremarkable. On the basis of the assessment data, the appropriate recommendation for the youngster is:
   a. Referral to a cleft palate–craniofacial team
   b. Referral for an aerodynamic study
   c. The initiation of oral motor exercises for the nasal emission
   d. Speech-sound treatment for the nasal emission
   e. No treatment and a reevaluation in 6 months because of developmental concerns

2. An SLP is evaluating an 8-year-old child for a speech-sound disorder and identifies dentalization of all alveolar sounds. Manner of articulation and voicing are correct, but placement is anterior to the alveolar place. An oral mechanism examination reveals a class III malocclusion. The child's placement errors would be classified as:
   a. Developmental errors
   b. Obligatory errors
   c. Compensatory errors
   d. Fronting errors
   e. Backing errors

3. During a kindergarten screening, an SLP identifies a 4-year-old child with lateral emission of /s/ and /z/. Other speech and language skills are judged to be within normal limits. The SLP should inform the parents that the child is:
   a. Exhibiting nondevelopmental errors that necessitate treatment
   b. Exhibiting developmental errors that may necessitate treatment when the child is older
   c. Producing speech-sound substitutions
   d. Producing speech-sound omissions
   e. In need of a hearing screening

4. An 18-year-old man with Down syndrome is referred by his employer to an SLP for a diagnostic evaluation. The client currently works under supervision in a local thrift shop. His responsibilities include interacting with customers, making change, and carrying out other work-related duties such as cleaning and dusting the store. He is a very pleasant individual and is well-liked by his supervisors and peers. The diagnostic evaluation should focus on:
   a. Establishing his current level of communication
   b. Generating recommendations for communication in the workplace
   c. Assessing his narrative skills
   d. a and b
   e. a and c

5. Ellen is undergoing an evaluation at the request of her parents because their older daughter has a speech and language disorder and is receiving treatment. If Ellen has a problem, they wish to seek remediation as soon as possible. Ellen is 1 year, 8 months of age and appears to have reached all appropriate developmental milestones, according to parental report. She can be understood by most people and appears to enjoy talking. Unlike her older sister, she will participate in a conversation. She has no reported major medical problems, but she has had approximately five middle ear infections since birth. These have been managed through drug therapy and pressure-equalization tubes. Current results of hearing tests indicate normal hearing bilaterally. Standard English is spoken in the home. Speech and language testing indicate age-appropriate communication skills. An appropriate management plan for Ellen is:
   a. Referral to Birth to Three services
   b. Parent counseling
   c. Language treatment
   d. Referral to an otolaryngologist
   e. All the above

6. A 5-year-old was referred to a school-based SLP for a feeding consultation because of her refusal to eat certain foods at school lunch. She will drink thin liquids and eat puree-consistency and solid foods, but she refuses mixed textures such as vegetables in soups. Her mother also indicated that the youngster was a selective eater and would refuse foods at home. She informed the clinician that the child had severe gastroesophageal reflux disease during the first 2 years of life but had outgrown the problem. The mother had never sought services for the child, because she believed that the child would begin to eat mixed textures. A feeding assessment showed no signs of any oral or pharyngeal motility disorders such as residue in the mouth, food loss, choking, or gagging. Oral hypersensitivity was noted. The SLP should recommend the following:
   a. Referral for a modified barium swallow study
   b. Referral to a gastroenterologist
   c. Parent counseling
   d. Treatment for dysphagia
   e. Treatment for dysphagia and parent counseling or training

7. A 60-year-old man was diagnosed with a T4 squamous cell cancer of the tongue base. He was treated with a combination of radiation and chemotherapy. After treatment, the patient developed mucositis, which occurs frequently in many patients who have undergone chemoradiation. This delayed his dysphagia assessment and treatment for 1 month. At the initial assessment, he exhibited a number of problems frequently found in these patients that may include which of the following?
   a. A delay in triggering the pharyngeal swallow
   b. Reduced laryngeal elevation
   c. Reduced tongue base retraction
   d. All the above
   e. None of the above

8. A 4-year-old underwent a sound system assessment and was found to have a very limited consonant inventory: /m/, /w/, /p/, /t/, and /f/. Oral structure and function are within normal limits, and hearing acuity was normal. No cognitive, motor, or social development issues were identified. Expressive and receptive language testing indicated a delay of approximately 12 months for both communication processes. The most appropriate treatment recommendation for the sound system disorder is:
   a. Phonetic placement training
   b. A phonemic approach
   c. A phonetics approach
   d. An imitative modeling teaching sequence
   e. A stimulability assessment

9. A 6-year-old with spastic dysarthria and normal cognitive skills has received approximately 4 years of speech treatment. Documentation indicates limited progress in speech production skills. A recent reevaluation indicates that intelligibility remains a problem for both familiar and unfamiliar listeners. The client is also

beginning to exhibit frustration during communication interactions because of the intelligibility problem. An appropriate recommendation for this client is:
a. More intensive speech-based treatment
b. Intensive parent practice sessions at home
c. An augmentative/alternative assessment
d. Nonspeech oral motor treatment
e. Minimal pairs treatment

10. A 5-year-old boy was referred by his family doctor because of poor speech. The parents explained that the boy has been difficult to understand since he first began to talk. His pediatrician told the family that he would outgrow the speech problem, but the boy has not, to date. His kindergarten teacher expressed concern to the parents, and they contacted the pediatrician. The pediatrician then initiated a referral for the evaluation. One of the child's speech-sound production problems is that stops, fricatives, and affricates are deleted in the postvocalic position. The process error is as follows: + stop, + fricative, + affricate→ φ ____#. What is the general error?
a. Assimilation
b. Gliding
c. Stopping
d. Initial consonant deletion
e. Final consonant deletion

11. A 5-year-old client with a repaired cleft palate has just transferred to your school. According to parent report, pharyngeal flap surgery has been scheduled for this child in approximately 6 months. Your assessment indicates that the client is hypernasal and uses glottal stops in place of /t/, /d/, /k/, and /g/. Your recommendation for this child is:
a. Enroll the child in treatment and teach correct oral placement of speech sounds currently substituted by glottal stops
b. Postpone therapy until after surgery
c. Treat the hypernasality using oral motor exercises
d. Initiate tongue-strengthening exercises
e. None of the above

12. A 7-year-old is undergoing a diagnostic assessment. The following exchange occurs between the SLP and client, while speech-sound discrimination is being assessed:
SLP: This is picture of a rope. Say rope.
Client: Wope.
SLP: Did you say wope?
Client: No, I said wope.

The exchange provides evidence that the client has:
a. A problem with the external discrimination of /r/
b. Correct external discrimination of /r/
c. A problem with the internal discrimination of /r/
d. Correct internal discrimination of /r/.
e. All the above

13. An 11-year-old with an /r/ distortion error is referred for an assessment. Case history information indicates that the client has undergone treatment for 3 years but has been unable to achieve correct production of /r/. The child is not stimulable for /r/. The clinician may recommend:
a. A phoneme-based treatment approach
b. Placing the child on a recheck list and postponing treatment
c. Biofeedback treatment
d. The use of exclusive parent practice with the client
e. Imagery

14. SLPs conduct assessments of adults with neurogenic communication disorders for a variety of purposes, which may include:
a. Diagnosing the patient's communication disorder
b. Formulating a prognosis for the patient
c. Developing recommendations for treatment
d. Assessing the effectiveness of treatment
e. All the above

15. Some adults with right-hemisphere damage may exhibit a variety of communication impairments that include suprasegmental and expressive or receptive deficits. During an assessment, the SLP may identify suprasegmental variations such as:
a. Reduced pitch variability
b. Lack of narrative cohesion
c. Confabulatory connected speech
d. Impaired discourse comprehension
e. Impaired nonliteral meaning comprehension

16. John is a 70-year-old patient living in a nursing home who suffered a cerebrovascular accident. The SLP is administering the Boston Diagnostic Aphasia Examination. The patient has a severe hearing loss but uses speechreading. Nevertheless, he still misses some of the intended message. What is one way to modify the assessment in order to obtain information about his communication skills and still use formalized testing?
a. Do not use this test to evaluate patients with severe hearing loss
b. Incorporate written instructions in conjunction with verbal instructions
c. Speak loudly when presenting the questions
d. Refer to the patient for an audiological assessment, and postpone testing until the results of the hearing test are completed
e. None of the above

17. The SLP is evaluating a 69-year-old woman with dementia. The SLP notes during testing that the patient is uninterested and labile and presents with a flat affect. This could indicate:

a. Dysarthria
b. Apraxia
c. Depression
d. Aphasia
e. None of the above

18. Where in a SOAP note is measurable information, including testing results documented by the SLP?
a. S section
b. O section
c. A section
d. P section
e. S and P sections

19. An SLP is evaluating a 50-year-old woman in her home after discharge from a rehabilitation hospital, where she was recovering from a cerebrovascular accident. She is alert but complains of word-finding problems and difficulty with reading comprehension. Of the following formalized testing instruments, which might be appropriate to test her deficit areas?
a. The Traumatic Brain Response Inventory
b. Peabody Picture Vocabulary Test
c. Boston Diagnostic Aphasia Examination
d. Goldman Fristoe Test of Articulation
e. a and c

20. Greg is a 30-year-old who sustained a traumatic brain injury and is being evaluated in a rehabilitation hospital. He is easily distracted and makes inappropriate comments but wants to return home after therapy to resume his job as a mechanic. The optimum place to assess Greg's communication skills is in what area of the hospital?
a. The dining room
b. The therapy gym
c. A quiet therapy room
d. A group therapy room with other patients present
e. c and d

21. During an evaluation of a 62-year-old woman with Parkinson disease, she relates that she does not have difficulty swallowing her medications, because she crushes her pills and mixes them with applesauce. Of the following concerns regarding this practice, which necessitates that the patient must be counseled?
a. Putting pills in applesauce will cause the patient to dislike applesauce
b. This is not a concern because crushing pills is a standard practice
c. Some medications prescribed for Parkinson's patients are time released and should not be crushed
d. Liquid medications can be substituted for pills
e. All the above

22. An SLP evaluated a 4½-year-old boy and obtained the following results on the Preschool Language Scale—Fourth Edition: for auditory comprehension, an age equivalent of 4 years, 2 months, and for verbal ability, an age equivalent of 2 years, 2 months. Results of a speech-sound inventory indicate that the child is producing the consonants /m/, /w/, and /n/, but all other consonant speech sounds are omitted. Vowel distortions are present. The child also exhibits frequent syllable simplification. Prosody and intonation are intact. Intelligibility is significantly reduced because of the numerous omitted consonants and syllable restrictions. Resonance appears normal, as does voice quality. A language sample reveals that the child is producing primarily one- and two-word utterances, although they are unintelligible. On the basis of these results, you recommend the following:
a. Oral-motor therapy
b. Intensive phonological treatment and an augmentative communication evaluation
c. Intensive phonetics-based treatment
d. Speech and language treatment
e. Oral-motor therapy with phonetics-based treatment

23. The SLP is evaluating a 15-year-old boy who is struggling academically. According to the case history, testing with the Wechsler Intelligence Scale for Children—Revised (WISC-R) yielded a full-scale IQ score of 98. There is a significant difference between his verbal and performance subtest scores; his verbal score is in the below-average range. Complaints include the observation that he rarely speaks in class, has difficulty with written tasks, is a poor reader, and has few friends. The SLP assessed the boy's receptive vocabulary with the Peabody Picture Vocabulary Test, and the boy received a standard score of 101. What other components of communication should the evaluation cover?
a. Determine that the boy's language skills were not responsible for his academic difficulties
b. Refer the boy for assessment of learning disabilities
c. Perform additional assessment of spoken language
d. Perform assessment of speech sound skills
e. Reevaluate in 1 year

24. The SLP is evaluating a patient for an augmentative communication system; the patient has received a diagnosis of amyotrophic lateral sclerosis (ALS). It is very important that:
a. The assessment be performed in a timely manner
b. The patient has an active role in selecting the system
c. The representative from the company that manufactures the voice output device be present during the evaluation
d. a and b
e. a, b, and c

25. An SLP is conducting an augmentative communication evaluation of a 4-year-old girl with Rett syndrome. It is most important that the SLP consider which of the following in identifying the most optimum augmentative system?
   a. Assessing the child by using sign language
   b. Assessing the child by using eye gaze
   c. Assessing the child by using pictures
   d. Assessing the child in cooperation with an autism specialist
   e. All the above

1. d. The child is exhibiting phoneme-specific nasal emission. The problem is one of mislearning, not velopharyngeal dysfunction. Because the nasal emission is not present during the production of other pressure sounds, it is not related to a structural defect and is readily amenable to speech-sound treatment. Referral to a cleft palate–craniofacial team (option a) is not necessary because the child's velopharyngeal mechanism is normal. An aerodynamic study (option b) is an instrumental measurement technique that provides physiological information on air pressure and airflow in the vocal tract. It would be an appropriate procedure for a child with a suspect velopharyngeal closure mechanism but is not necessary in this case. There is no evidence to support the use of oral motor exercises (option c) for phoneme-specific nasal emission. Postponing treatment (option e) is not appropriate, because the speech-sound error is nondevelopmental and should be treated at the time of diagnosis.

2. b. In a class III malocclusion, the mandible (lower jaw) is ahead of the maxilla (upper jaw). With this jaw occlusion, tongue resting posture and movement are generally anterior to the alveolar ridge. The dentalized alveolar speech-sound errors are the result of the structural deficit and therefore classified as obligatory errors. Obligatory errors are usually distortions and cannot be corrected with speech-sound treatment. Oral structure must be modified through surgical, orthodontic, or dental treatment. After medical intervention, obligatory errors generally correct spontaneously. Developmental errors (option a) are normal variations in sound development. Compensatory errors (option c) are sound substitutions that are learned responses. For example, some children with velopharyngeal closure deficits produce a glottal stop in place of oral stops; this substitution is a compensatory error. Fronting errors (option d) are sound substitutions that are anterior to the expected point of articulation and reflective of developmental variation, not obligatory caused by a structural deficit. Backing errors (option e) are speech sounds made posterior to the expected point of articulation and are nondevelopmental phonological processes.

3. a. Lateral emission is a nondevelopmental speech-sound error, and it is highly unlikely that the child will outgrow the error. Treatment is indicated now, despite the child's age (option b). The error type is classified as a distortion, not a sound substitution (option c) or a sound omission (option d). A hearing screening (option e) is an important component of an assessment and should be conducted, but it is not the priority for this scenario.

4. d. It is important first to establish the client's current level of communication (option a) and to develop meaningful recommendations that will assist the client is his daily work duties (option b). He has a number of assigned tasks, and satisfactory communication skills are important for his success in the workplace. Assessing narrative skills (option c) might be a part of the diagnostic process but would not be a primary focus of treatment.

5. b. Ellen has normal language skills, but several issues need to be emphasized by the SLP when counseling the parents. First, there is a history of language disorder in the family, and the parents were wise in seeking an evaluation. They should be instructed and given materials regarding communication development, but Ellen is not a candidate for treatment at this time (options a and c). Second, Ellen has a history of middle ear infection, which could affect speech and language development. Referral to an otolaryngologist (option d) is appropriate, but Ellen has no infection at this time. However, long-term attention to Ellen's audiological needs in terms of hearing testing and medical follow-up should be stressed to the parents.

6. e. Treatment for dysphagia and parent counseling and training are recommended. This case is an example of a behavioral feeding problem that was probably caused by an early medical problem (gastroesophageal reflux disease). The medical problem resolved, but the child refuses certain food textures. Treatment would focus on reducing oral hypersensitivity and the gradual introduction of mixed textures. The mother would be counseled in regard to the problem and how to deal with the problem at home. Treatment activities would also be introduced for the home after parent training. Because no signs of a pharynx-based dysphagia were observed, an imaging study (option a) or referral to a medical doctor (option b) would not be necessary at this time.

7. d. Frequent problems of patients who have undergone chemoradiation treatment for cancer of the tongue base include delay in triggering the pharyngeal swallow (option a), reduced laryngeal elevation (option b), and reduced tongue base retraction

(option c). These patients are also at risk for the development of a stricture in the area of the cervical esophagus.

8. b. Because the client has a very limited consonant inventory, treatment must be structured in a way that facilitates the development of phonological rules; therefore, a phonemic approach is appropriate. In addition, the SLP needs to treat the language disorder that was also identified in the assessment. A sound-by-sound phonetics-based approach (option c) would not be appropriate for this client because of the severe sound system disorder. Phonetic placement training (option a) and an imitative modeling teaching sequence (option d) are treatment techniques that are used with clients; they are not theoretical treatment approaches. A stimulability assessment (option e) is used to establish a child's phonetic production skills and it also is not a treatment approach.

9. c. Limited progress over the 4-year period indicates that the communication needs of the client are not being met, and an augmentative/alternative assessment is necessary to identify more effective communication options. It is unlikely that exclusive speech treatment with the clinician (option a) or parents (option b) will have a significant effect on intelligibility. There is no evidence that nonspeech oral motor treatment (option d) has an effect on speech production skills. Minimal pairs (option e) is a phonological treatment and would not be appropriate, because the history of limited improvement and poor intelligibility.

10. e. The error is final consonant deletion. The client is deleting the sound classes listed in the postvocalic position of words. Assimilation, gliding, stopping, and initial consonant deletion are other phonological processes that correspond to different error patterns. Assimilation (option a) is context-sensitive variation wherein one sound influences another. Gliding (option b) is the substitution of a glide (/w/, /j/) is place of one or more sounds. Stopping (option c) is the substitution of one or more stops in place of sounds from other sound classes. Initial consonant deletion (option d) is deletion of consonant speech sounds in prevocalic position of words.

11. a. The child should receive treatment to teach correct placement of sounds being substituted by glottal stops. Compensatory articulation errors such as glottal stops should be corrected as soon as possible because they become ingrained sound substitutions. For that reason, therapy should not be postponed (option b). Hypernasality is a resonance disorder,

which should improve after surgery. Oral motor exercises (option c) have not proved effective in the treatment of velopharyngeal closure deficits. The general population of children with cleft palate do not present with muscle weakness; consequently, tongue-strengthening exercises (option d) are not necessary.

12. b. The exchange is an example of an external discrimination task, since the client is being asked to discriminate the target sound from the error sound when produced by the SLP. The client does identify the error as produced incorrectly by the clinician (option a). The problem does not pertain to internal discrimination (options c and d). Internal discrimination is the ability of the child to discriminate the error sound and the correct sound in her or his own speech.

13. c. Research indicates that children with residual errors may benefit from biofeedback treatment, when traditional phonetics- or phoneme-based treatments have not been effective. A phoneme-based treatment approach (option a) is therefore not appropriate now. Exclusive parent practice with the client (option d) is not optimal because the client needs to produce the target sound correctly is some context before enlisting the aid of caregivers. Postponing treatment (option b) is also inappropriate, because it is unlikely that the client will acquire correct target sound production without treatment. Imagery (option e) is a phoneme-based treatment procedure. The SLP attempts to make a distinction between an error feature and target feature by trying to establish an internal image for the client.

14. e. An assessment is conducted for a number of different reasons, according to which data are needed. In initial diagnostic testing, the SLP administers tests and conducts a chart review to diagnose the communication disorder (option a). The data help the SLP to make a prognosis or prediction in regard to the patient's outcome (option b). Test data are also used to make recommendations concerning general and specific treatment goals (option c). Assessment is also conducted periodically to assess the effectiveness of a particular treatment (option d).

15. a. Suprasegmental features are the prosodic aspects of speech that are superimposed on phonemes and words and are produced through variations in pitch, intensity, and rate. For example, reduced pitch variability could affect intonation shifts that signal information, such as rising pitch at the end of an utterance to signal a question or a downward pitch shift at the end to denote a statement. Lack of

narrative cohesion (option b), confabulatory connected speech (option c), impaired discourse comprehension (option d), and impaired nonliteral meaning comprehension (option e) are deficits in expressive and receptive language that are seen in patients with right-hemisphere damage.

16. b. You can incorporate written instructions with verbal instructions to obtain assessment information. You can use the Boston Diagnostic Examination with hearing-impaired patients (option a) if you modify the testing. Yelling (option c) would only frustrate the patient and the clinician. You should not wait to test this patient, because he is in a nursing home and scheduling an audiological assessment (option d) may take several weeks, inasmuch as nursing homes generally do not employ full-time audiologists. Instead, the resident would need to be transported to another facility for a hearing test.

17. c. Depression is frequently present in patients with early-stage dementia. The description does not include any characteristics of dysarthria (option a), apraxia (option b), or aphasia (option d).

18. b. Measurable information, including the results of testing, is contained in the "O" (objective documentation) section. The "S" section (option a) contains only subjective information regarding the patient. Information in the "A" section (option c) summarizes the SLP's colleted data and interprets subjective assessments. The "P" section includes the SLP's plan for the next treatment session.

19. c. The Boston Diagnostic Aphasia Examination would provide information about her difficulties with naming and reading comprehension. The Traumatic Brain Response Inventory (option a) is not a diagnostic test. The Peabody Picture Vocabulary Test (option b) would furnish an only estimation of receptive vocabulary skills. The Goldman Fristoe Test of Articulation (option d) would provide information about speech sound production skills.

20. c. Because Greg is distractible, initial testing should not take place in crowded areas or places with other people, who may serve as distracters (options a, b, and d). Later in his recovery, testing may take place in a room that simulates his vocational interest, to assess the effects of different distractions.

21. c. Some medications are time released and should not be crushed, because they may lose their effectiveness. Putting pills in applesauce may result in the patient developing a dislike for applesauce (option a), but this is not a primary concern. Even though crushing pills is a standard practice (option b), all patients should check with their physician to see whether crushing is acceptable for a particular medication. Some medications are not available in liquid form (option d).

22. b. This profile indicates a significant impairment in speech-sound production and a concurrent language disorder. Current evidence suggests that the child requires intensive phoneme-based therapy to improve his speech-sound production and an augmentative communication system to improve his ability to communicate expressively and repair communication breakdowns and to provide him with an output method to acquire language structure and function. There is no evidence that a child with this profile will benefit from oral-motor treatment (option a) or oral-motor treatment with phonetics-based treatment (option e). Although intensive phonetics-based treatment (option c) is possibly beneficial, a phonetics approach, or sound-by-sound treatment, is not appropriate for this child. The use of speech and language treatment (option d) without an alternative output mode is likely to be of limited benefit because his speech-sound impairment will reduce his ability to produce language.

23. c. The Peabody Picture Vocabulary Test is only a measure of receptive vocabulary, and the WISC-R profile is suggestive of specific language impairment. A more in-depth assessment of spoken language is needed to determine whether a language impairment is present. The Peabody Picture Vocabulary Test cannot establish whether the boy's language skills were responsible for his academic difficulties (option a). Similarly, there is no communication assessment data to indicate that the boy should be referred for learning disabilities assessment (option b). Such a decision would be based on the collective results of all specialists evaluating the client. Neither assessment of speech sound skills, (option d) nor reevaluation in 1 year (option e) would be an appropriate recommendation.

24. d. Because ALS is a progressive neurological disorder, it is very important that the assessment be performed as soon as possible (option a), because it will take some time to obtain the necessary augmentative equipment. It is also very important that the patient be an active participant in selecting the system that he or she will ultimately use (option b). It is not necessary for a representative from the company that manufactures the device to be present during the evaluation (option c).

25. b. Children with Rett syndrome typically have no functional use of their hands; therefore, it is imperative that you use eye gaze as the response mode. Sign language (option a) is thus not an appropriate response mode. Some girls with Rett syndrome use eye gaze for pictures and others use it for objects; therefore, using pictures alone (option c) is not appropriate. Although Rett syndrome is on the autism spectrum, it is not necessary for an autism specialist to be present during the assessment (option d).

CHAPTER 22

Speech-Language Intervention

Betsy Partin Vinson

1. Olson, a 19-year-old man, has Down syndrome. He exhibits receptive language skills loosely equivalent to those of a 5-year-old child. He knows the letters of the alphabet but cannot decode to read. He recognizes the orthographic representations of his name and those of his family members, and he can recognize a few sight words. His expressive abilities are primarily single words and two- to three-word phrases. Currently, he experiences much frustration, including intense temper tantrums, when he is misunderstood in his communication attempts. These attempts are characterized by mis-articulations (primarily omission of final consonants) and the use of single words from which, without additional context, the listener has to infer Olson's intent. He participated in individual private speech therapy off and on from birth to 5 years of age. Between the ages of 4 and 18 years, he received speech and language therapy and occupational therapy as part of his educational program. In the final two years of school, Olson's education focused on developing basic vocational skills. Since graduating from school, Olson has worked in a hospital laundry. For the past year, Olson has been receiving one-on-one speech and language therapy for two 50-minute sessions per week from a speech-language pathologist (SLP) in private practice. This therapy was initiated at the request of Olson's family because of his increasing levels of frustration associated with his communication efforts. In view of Olson's history, at this time the most prudent course of action would be to focus on which of the following?
   a. Increasing intelligibility through intense focus on improving articulation, because speech is more accepted in society than the use of augmentative communication devices
   b. Pursuing the use of augmentative and alternative communication (AAC)

c. Working intensely on improving oral-motor skills in hopes of improving intelligibility through strengthening and refining oral motor movements

d. Focusing on increasing his semantic skills so that he uses repair strategies, such as being able to use alternative words to iterate his messages

e. Refer Olson to a psychologist or behavioral specialist for anger management strategies

2. With regard to Olson, the 19 year-old man with Down syndrome referred to in question 1, which of the following treatment goals, does *not* conform to the concept of functional outcomes?

a. Olson will successfully travel from home to work (and, after work, back home) by using the public bus system

b. Olson will appropriately ask for assistance or clarification when he does not understand a task

c. Olson will increase his expressive language skills in order to enhance his conversational abilities

d. Olson will independently go to the bank and deposit his paycheck

e. Olson will use repair strategies (e.g., pointing) in order to request information and to clarify requests that are misunderstood by his conversation partner

3. Beth, who is 64 years old, sustained an ischemic stroke that resulted in right-sided paralysis and a paucity of speech. She does not respond to simple commands. Beth is considered to have aphasia with intermittent auditory imperceptions. At 72 hours after onset of the stroke, the SLP, Sue, conducts a bedside evaluation, using the Aphasia Language Performance Scales (ALPS) (Keenan & Brassell, 1975). Before the stroke, Beth, who is considered to be clinically obese, was in poor health, having dealt with diabetes for most of her adult life. Beth is not considered to be "medically stable" by her physician. On the basis of Sue's observations, her review of Beth's medical records, her discussion with Beth's family, and Beth's performance on the tasks of the ALPS, Sue needs to develop a treatment plan. At this stage of Beth's recovery, which of the following actions best describes the most reasonable approach to developing the intervention plan for Beth?

a. Wait for 2 weeks to see whether Beth's apparent global aphasia evolves into another type of aphasia

b. Reevaluate in 48 hours by using a more comprehensive assessment tool

c. Educate the family about aphasia and treatment approaches, and obtain information about Beth's education, interests, and work before the stroke

d. Begin diagnostic therapy to further analyze Beth's abilities with regard to speech, language, and cognition

e. Develop a communication board that Beth can use to express basic needs

4. With regard to Beth, the 64-year-old who sustained ischemic stroke that resulted in right-sided and a paucity of speech, Which of the following approaches to treatment of individuals who have aphasia would be the most logical, if Beth's neurological status remains consistent or slightly better throughout the immediate recovery period and when she is medically stable?

a. Life participation approach to aphasia (LPAA)

b. Language treatment in a controlled setting

c. Structured therapy groups

d. Cognitive stimulation

e. Development of compensation strategies

5. Of the following intervention models for child language therapy, which is *not* characteristic of a functional model of treatment?

a. Conversational techniques designed to emphasize exchange of a message

b. Use of spontaneous conversations and social interactions

c. Stressing of imitation, practice, and drill to develop skills

d. Provision of therapy in contextually meaningful settings

e. Treating language as a set of rules that vary according to setting and communication partners

6. The first step in a mand-model of language intervention is to:

a. Establish joint attention

b. Model the desired behavior

c. Request a previously learned communication behavior

d. Elicit questions from the child

e. Provide indirect linguistic cues to facilitate the desired response from the child

7. The use of judgment tasks in therapy requires the development of metalinguistic skills. Therefore, these types of therapy activities are not appropriate for children who are not functioning cognitively and linguistically at age _____ or more.

a. 1 year

b. 2 to 3 years

c. 4 to 5 years

d. 6 to 7 years

e. 8 to 9 years

8. Of the following activities, which is not a component of therapy designed to improve metapragmatic skills in children with language deficits?

a. Discussing the differences between effective and ineffective conversations

b. Teaching interpretation of nonverbal communication behaviors

c. Teaching interpretation of idioms

d. Role-play of interactive or communication scenarios

e. Developing coherent narratives that are based on events in the child's life

9. A child who is performing at the level of _____ should be able to analyze information, synthesize facts, organize information by category and sequence, and make inferences.
   a. Kindergarten through grade 2
   b. Grades 3 and 4
   c. Grades 5 and 6
   d. Grades 7 and 8
   e. Grades 9 to 12

10. Of the following statements, which is *not* characteristic of a strategy-based language intervention model as a basis of therapy with adolescents who have language or learning deficits?
    a. Language impairment is based on inadequately developed interactions between the child, the child's primary communication partners, and the child's teachers
    b. Therapeutic focus is based on learning strategies needed to solve problems
    c. Therapy includes teaching methods of organizing and retrieving information
    d. Strategy-based language intervention should be paired with a systems model to facilitate learning in the classroom
    e. Strategy-based intervention is a tool that can facilitate curriculum-based intervention

11. Postural techniques are frequently recommended by SLPs as a method to reduce aspiration during the swallowing process. The aspiration is often caused by reduced laryngeal closure or unilateral laryngeal dysfunction. Two of these techniques are to have the patient tuck the chin and rotate the head toward the damaged side. Of the following results, which is *not* a rationale for employing these maneuvers?
    a. The maneuvers result in narrowing of the laryngeal entrance
    b. The maneuvers cause increased vocal fold adduction
    c. The maneuvers put the epiglottis in a more protective position
    d. The maneuvers direct the bolus to the stronger side of the oral cavity, thereby minimizing aspiration
    e. The maneuvers widen the vallecula

12. Of the following results, which is an expected outcome of neuromuscular stimulation—achieved through surface electromyography (sEMG)—as a treatment for swallowing disorders?
    a. Muscle facilitation
    b. Prevention of muscle atrophy
    c. Muscle reeducation
    d. Muscle strengthening
    e. All the above

13. Increasing sensory awareness is a treatment approach to swallowing in all but which of the following disorders?
    a. Swallow apraxia
    b. Hyperactive gag reflex
    c. Food aversion
    d. Delayed laryngeal elevation
    e. Delayed onset of the oral phase of the swallow

14. Focusing on the elimination of errors affecting classes of sounds is a primary purpose of phonological therapy at what age range?
    a. 12 to 18 months
    b. 18 to 24 months
    c. 2 to 5 years
    d. 5 to 8 years
    e. after 8 years of age

15. In a cycles approach to phonological therapy, the clinician analyzes the results of phonological assessments and develops a hierarchy of the phonological processes on which the child is stimulable in a minimum of _____ of the contexts.
    a. 20%
    b. 40%
    c. 60%
    d. 80%
    e. 90%

16. The reversal of the position of two sounds in a word (e.g., "aminal" for "animal") is:
    a. Metathesis
    b. Epenthesis
    c. Migration
    d. Assimilation
    e. Reduplication

17. Of the following achievements, which is a standard component of Hodson and Paden's (1983) cycles approach to treatment of phonological disorders?
    a. Production of emerging sounds
    b. Learning a few sounds containing the targeted distinctive features
    c. Phonetic placement
    d. Shaping
    e. Development of a hierarchy of phonological processes on which the child is stimulable and auditory bombardment

18. A 38-year-old woman whose speech is characterized by strained vocal quality and vocal fatigue is a seen by an SLP. While giving the clinician her history, she indicated

that she has had difficulty for more than a year. Onset followed a bout with an upper respiratory illness. She pursued speech therapy on the advice of her general practitioner but experienced little change as a result and quit after 6 weeks. A month ago, an otolaryngologist diagnosed adductor spasmodic dysphonia. Of the following treatments, which is the most reasonable and most evidence-based approach to treatment of this woman's condition?

a. Surgical transection of the recurrent laryngeal nerve
b. Botulinum toxin type A (Botox) injection into the thyroarytenoid muscle in conjunction with speech therapy
c. Botox injection into the posterior cricoarytenoid muscle, followed by speech therapy
d. Implantation of laryngeal nerve stimulators
e. Additional speech therapy with no other interventions

19. A 38-year-old woman whose speech is characterized by strained vocal quality and vocal fatigue is a seen by an SLP. While giving the clinician her history, she indicated that she has had difficulty for more than a year. Onset followed a bout with an upper respiratory illness. She pursued speech therapy on the advice of her general practitioner but experienced little change as a result and quit after 6 weeks. A month ago, an otolaryngologist diagnosed adductor spasmodic dysphonia. Of the following therapeutic procedures, which would *not* be appropriate to suggest during a course of speech therapy in the early stages of spasmodic dysphonia?

a. Reduction of laryngeal tightness
b. Increasing expiratory breath flow rate
c. Speaking on inhalation
d. Raising the patient's pitch
e. Vocal fold thinning with a laser, followed by polytetrafluoroethylene (Teflon) injection

20. Patients who opt for unilateral botulinum toxin type A (Botox) injections can expect which of the following?

a. Diminished intrinsic laryngeal muscle hyperfunction, as indicated by reduced vocal fold rigidity and a more normal glottic closure
b. Diminished extrinsic laryngeal muscle hyperfunction, as indicated by reduced vocal fold rigidity and a more normal glottic closure
c. Normal volume in conversational speech
d. Permanently increased risk of aspiration
e. Permanent resolution of the spasmodic dysphonia

21. Six-year-old Amy has cerebral palsy associated with upper motor neuron damage. She demonstrates limited phonation, a hyperactive gag reflex, increased muscle tone, and difficulty with eating. Nonverbal cognition is relatively intact (at the lower range of normal), although she has approximately an 8-month delay in

expressive language skills. Of the following protocols, which would *not* be an initial focus of speech-language therapy?

a. Oral-motor therapy focused on normalization of oral-motor reflexes
b. Therapy focused on increasing vocalizations and, eventually, verbalizations
c. Intervention focused on task specific oral-motor functions necessary for feeding
d. Enhancement of academic potential by focusing on facilitation of receptive language abilities
e. Development of an AAC system

22. Adam, 28 years old, sustained a head injury while serving in Iraq. Although he has some mild short-term memory deficits and demonstrates moderate word retrieval difficulties, his primary problem is moderate apraxia of speech. Of the following therapies, which represents the best initial approach for Adam?

a. Developing an AAC system to facilitate word finding through the use of visual cues, and to minimize possible frustration when his speech is not understood by others
b. Diagnostic therapy over several sessions to determine in what contexts, particularly sentence completion, Adam is able or unable to produce specific speech sounds
c. Therapeutic intervention focusing on oral musculature–strengthening exercises
d. Developing goals designed to address articulation skills on the basis of observation and standardized assessment results
e. Engaging in spaced-retrieval training

23. Of the following treatment approaches designed to remediate apraxia of speech, which is most supported by evidence from analyses of clinical practice and dedicated research studies?

a. Sensory stimulation
b. Repeated practice of oral musculature exercises
c. Contrastive practice
d. Articulatory-kinematic and integral stimulation
e. Improving diadokokinetic rate

24. Of the following skills, which would *not* be emphasized in therapy for dysarthria?

a. Resonance
b. Inspiratory muscle training
c. Facilitation of motor programming
d. Decreasing sound distortion
e. Relaxation of respiratory muscles

25. Of the following schedules of reinforcement, which is most likely to result in generalization of a newly acquired skill that has been mastered in the clinical setting?

a. Fixed-ratio schedule
b. Fixed-interval schedule
c. Variable-ratio schedule
d. Variable-interval schedule
e. Continuous-reinforcement schedule

26. Of the following statements about evidence-based practice (EBP), which is most accurate?
    a. EBP provides guidelines for the interpretation of test scores and the use of that interpretation to formulate appropriate, functional therapy goals
    b. EBP is the definitive component of clinical decision-making process when a treatment plan is designed for a patient
    c. EBP removes subjective and assumptive analysis of clinical intervention from the clinical decision-making process
    d. EBP provides an intervention framework through which the clinician can integrate best practice measures, critical review of the science governing intervention, and clinical observation to determine therapy goals
    e. A clinician should use only techniques that are documented in the literature as being effective

27. In 2001, the World Health Organization offered a revised framework for evaluating the implementation and effectiveness of treatment on the basis of the concept of the patient's levels of functioning. With regard to communication delays and disorders, which of the following statements about this revision is most accurate?
    a. The previously used term *impairment* has been redefined as the degree to which a person's communication disorder affects his or her daily activities
    b. The previously used term *handicap* is now defined in terms of "participation" and interpreted as the effect of the communication deficit on the individual's ability to participate in various social activities
    c. The previously used term *impairment* is now defined in terms of "participation" and interpreted as the effect of the communication deficit on the individual's ability to participate in various social activities and in personal interactions and relationships
    d. The previously used term *disability* now refers to the anatomical and physiological effects of any medically based condition that affects a patient's communication abilities
    e. The new terminology does not reflect functional goals and outcomes any more than did the old terminology

28. Of the following statements regarding a child's therapy outcome, which would be considered a "functional outcome statement"?

a. Edward successfully communicates his needs and wants by using his AAC device
b. Edward has increased his expressive vocabulary by 68%
c. Edward has improved his ability to make refined movements of his tongue and lips
d. Edward has learned 15 American Sign Language signs
e. Edward can successfully complete two-step commands in sequence

29. Through research and clinical application, the pharmacological industry worked to develop medications that may result in redevelopment of linguistic skills in individuals with aphasia caused by stroke, as well as linguistic deficits resulting from right-hemisphere damage, traumatic brain injury, or dementia. Mr. Smithson, aged 48 years, suffered a traumatic brain injury in a head-on automobile accident. As a result of the head injury, Mr. Smithson demonstrates a variety of linguistic impairments and impairments of executive functioning. Two months after the accident, he comes to you, the SLP, for treatment. While in your office, his wife asks whether there is any medication he can take to help restore his linguistic abilities. Of the following statements, which would be the most appropriate response to her question?
    a. "There are some drugs currently on the market that could restore linguistic functions in individuals with aphasia"
    b. "Although there are some medications that restore linguistic functioning, they should be paired with behavioral therapy, including speech-language therapy, for the patient to see maximum benefit"
    c. "Such an idea is not backed in the research; there are no drugs that can potentially enhance linguistic functioning"
    d. "There are medications that have been used in various studies and clinical trials but, as of now, the findings are inconsistent"
    e. "I suggest that you ask your local pharmacist for an answer to this question"

30. Through research and clinical application, the pharmacological industry worked to develop medications that may result in redevelopment of linguistic skills in individuals with aphasia caused by stroke, as well as linguistic deficits resulting from right-hemisphere damage, traumatic brain injury, or dementia. Mr. Smithson, aged 48 years, suffered a traumatic brain injury in a head-on automobile accident. As a result of the head injury, Mr. Smithson demonstrates a variety of linguistic impairments and impairments of executive functioning. Two months after the accident, he comes to you, the SLP, for treatment. While in your office, his wife asks whether there is any medication he can take to

help restore his linguistic abilities. What is the role of the SLP in evaluating the effectiveness of medications prescribed for patients with neurogenic language disorders?

a. Advise her as to which medication would have the most potential effect on her husband's recovery

b. Suggest that she ask her husband's physician to prescribe a neurostimulant to facilitate her husband's recovery of communication

c. Evaluate Mr. Smithson's language and cognition skills and develop a baseline against which to measure change if Mr. Smithson begins taking medication

d. Observe Mr. Smithson and report to the prescribing physician the changes (positive and negative) that you observe

e. It is beyond the scope of practice for SLPs (according to the American Speech-Language-Hearing Association) to address issues related to pharmaceutical effectiveness

31. Of the following statements regarding therapy approaches for aphasia, which is most accurate?

a. Therapies that simultaneously integrate all aspects of sentence production processing are most supported by the research

b. It is important to break down sentence production into components (i.e., syntax, lexicon, and function), then intensively train each aspect

c. Therapy approaches based on typical development and use of a variety of sentence structures are helpful in pediatric language therapy, but they are not effective in treatment of adults with aphasia

d. Training sentence production in hopes that it will lead to increasing overall sentence comprehension has proved to be efficacious in the treatment of aphasia

e. Facilitating language recovery is dependent on neural regeneration; therefore, treatment should not begin until spontaneous recovery is complete and the clinician has a more realistic picture of the patient's deficits

32. Eloise Jackson, a 77-year-old widow with moderately severe dementia (as measured on the Mini-Mental State Examination), resides in a long-term care facility. The family discussed their growing concerns regarding her ability to function independently after several instances over the previous 2 weeks. For example, on arrival for her daily visit, Mrs. Jackson's daughter smelled something burning and discovered that her mother had left a pot of soup on a hot burner. Furthermore, the daughter found that her mother had not taken her medications that morning. The following week, Ms. Jackson had wandered away from her home late one night. She had been picked up by a local law enforcement

agent, who took her to the hospital when she could not tell the agent where she lived. After a review of Mrs. Jackson's recent history and a frank discussion with the daughter, the physician recommended that Mrs. Jackson be admitted to a long-term care facility. Of the following activities, which is *not* a reasonable area of focus in Ms. Jackson's speech-language therapy?

a. Engaging in clinical activities designed to improve Ms. Jackson's measured levels of cognitive functioning

b. Developing skills to facilitate performance of daily living skills and routines

c. Reducing demands on her episodic and working memories

d. Educating family members and the staff of the care facility about communication strategies

e. Creating a "memory book" with pictures of family members, vacations, friends, and so forth, to facilitate engaging Mrs. Jackson in conversation

33. Of the following therapeutic approaches, which addresses the learning of new information and recall of previously learned information in persons with dementia?

a. Stimulation of procedural memory

b. Interaction with children that is modeled on the Montessori approach

c. Spaced-retrieval training

d. Sensory stimulation

e. Stimulation of episodic memory

34. With regard to fluency therapy with an adolescent or adult, which of the following statements is most accurate?

a. If a client expresses anxiety about speaking in a specific situation, the SLP should reassure the client that the anxiety will disappear when the client masters the fluency control strategies

b. If a client expresses anxiety and feelings of stress about speaking in a specific situation, the SLP should target that anxiety, focusing on stress management techniques, before beginning fluency control measures

c. If a client expresses anxiety about speaking in a specific situation, the SLP should explain that muscle tension results from anxiety and should target muscle relaxation and fluency control strategies in treatment

d. If a client expresses moderate anxiety about speaking in a specific situation, the SLP should refer the client to a psychologist to address the fear component; when that is accomplished, speech therapy to learn control strategies can begin

e. If a client expresses anxiety about speaking in a specific situation, the SLP should work on muscle relaxation, expecting that the relaxation will minimize the dysfluencies

35. Of the following statements, which best reflects current theory with regard to fluency-enhancing strategies that should be used in treatment?
    a. Rhythmic stimulation is the most effective treatment because it reduces the variability of stress between stressed syllables
    b. Delayed auditory feedback is the most effective treatment because it results in a decreased rate in the speech of the person with dysfluency
    c. Use of melodic intonations is the most effective treatment because it is well documented that people who stutter do not stutter when singing
    d. All of the above are effective means to enhance fluency, and they all should be incorporated into treatment
    e. There is much variation in clients' responses to fluency treatment; thus, none of the above is an acceptable response to this question

1. b. Olson has received intensive speech-language therapy for most of his life. In addition, he is demonstrating escalating frustration when he is not understood or his intent is misinterpreted. Therefore, it is not reasonable to expect that additional phonological therapy is going to be efficacious. Pursuing the use of AAC is the most reasonable approach because, cognitively, Olson can learn the techniques, whether he uses a "homemade" communication notebook or a sophisticated electronic device. Use of AAC would enable Olson to communicate effectively and, as a result, should decrease his frustration in his communication attempts. Focusing on oral motor skills is not likely to make a significant difference in his speech. Increasing his semantic skills in order to use repair strategies (option d) could be a part of therapy, but it would not result in the improvement of his communication with others nearly as much as AAC would. Referral to a psychologist (option e) is not a bad idea, but most of Olson's temper tantrums and aggressiveness are associated with communication attempts. Until Olson has a chance to use AAC and the family and clinician can see if it resolves Olson's frustrations, it is not recommended. Parents of children with communication deficits have enough expenses and therapies to monitor. One more should not be added until other possibilities have been ruled out.

2. c. According to the "Communication First" theory, functional outcomes are the result of functional goals that are designed to facilitate communication in a client's natural environments. Using public transportation (option a), increasing expressive language skills (option b), depositing a paycheck (option d), and using repair strategies (option e) are all goals that will facilitate Olson's ability to function in a supervised vocational setting. There is no reason to think that a child functioning at Olson's language age will easily generalize generic "expressive language skills" to activities of daily living.

3. c. Family members can provide Sue with information she can use to make preliminary plans for further testing and treatment. Also, family members may have questions about what has happened to Beth and what to expect in the future. Waiting 2 weeks for further developments (option a) allows time for some spontaneous recovery, which some clinicians would see as reasonable and give her time to be more medically stable, but it does not contribute to forming an intervention plan. It is doubtful that

Beth will have the stamina to participate in a more comprehensive assessment in 48 hours (option b). For the same reasons, diagnostic therapy (option d) and use of a communication board (option e) are possibilities for the future but are not feasible at present.

4. a. LPAA is designed to help the patient with aphasia to participate in life activities, thereby increasing quality of life. LPAA is a form of group therapy that focuses on the effect of personal factors and environmental influences on daily functioning. Language treatment in a controlled setting (option b) has historically been a frequent approach. The attainment of skills in a controlled setting, however, does not guarantee the generalization of those skills to the patient's daily living environments. Structured group therapy (option c) is thought to be effective with patients with aphasia, but the term *structured* implies that it is based more on question-answer, stimulus-response formats that do not necessarily carry over into daily life. Cognitive stimulation (option d) is often the focus of therapy for dementia of the Alzheimer's type, but aphasia is defined more as a language loss, not a cognitive loss. Development of compensation strategies, combined with a program such as LPAA, would be beneficial, but it would not be as effective alone.

5. c. Stressing imitation, practice, and drill are typically addressed in regulated settings such as a therapy room in a clinic. Sometimes circumstances dictate that therapy be provided in controlled settings, but it is not the optimal method. In these cases, parents and siblings should be encouraged to participate in the therapy in order to facilitate skills such as conversational techniques (option a), use of spontaneous social interactions (option b), contextually meaningful settings (option d), and treating language as a set of flexible rules (option e). The clinician could also develop schemes and role-plays to encourage the development of communication skills that can be generalized to the child's natural settings.

6. a. Mand-model intervention is a type of milieu treatment. When a child demonstrates interest in an activity or toy, the clinician offers communication starters and traditional approaches such as prompting, cuing, and modeling or imitation to facilitate participation in communication. The best foundation of these skills is the establishment of joint attention. Before the clinician models the behavior (option b),

requests a previously learned behavior (option c), elicits questions (option d), or provides cues (option e), the child must actively attend to the cycle of the adult capitalizing on the child's interest in an activity or object and then to engage in an interaction with the adult, focusing on that stimulus. Those four activities are valid approaches but can succeed only if the child is attentive to the clinician.

7. c. Developmentally, the skills encompassed in the umbrella of metalinguistics emerge around 4 to 5 years of age. Metalinguistics is the ability to think and comment about language. This includes understanding and use of synonyms and antonyms, multiple meanings, grammatical structures and rules, phonological awareness, and different morphological structures, and parts of speech. Children who do not develop metalinguistic skills experience social and academic challenges. Living in a home where children are encouraged to understand words and how they are used facilitates the development of metalinguistics.

8. c. Metapragmatics is the analyzing and understanding of appropriate use of language in a variety of contexts. Interpretation of idioms is more of a metalinguistic skill than a metapragmatic skill, and it does not require social use of language. Discussing the differences between effective and ineffective conversations (option a), teaching interpretation of nonverbal communication behaviors (option b), role-playing interactive or communication scenarios (option d), and developing coherent narratives (option e) all focus on the use of language.

9. b. The curriculum for grades 3 and 4 builds on the earlier skills while increasing the application of linguistic and symbolic knowledge and skills needed for the cognitive-linguistic demands of school. By grades 5 and 6, children should have these skills firmly integrated in order to handle the increasing complexity of the academic curriculum. The curriculum for kindergarten through grade 2 (option a) focuses on the development of perceptual-cognitive abilities. Children at this level should be able to talk about some abstract concepts but, in general, are not cognitively and linguistically sophisticated enough analyze, synthesize, and organize information in academic and social situations.

10. a. In the statement about "language impairment," the term is defined, but no intervention model or strategy for learning language is described. The statement about therapeutic focus (option b) describes teaching the child how to solve problems and is a strategy-based intervention plan, encompassing conversational repair strategies and other

pragmatics-based intervention. The statement about what therapy includes (option c) also reflects a specific focus that involves teaching the student one or more methods that the student can use to facilitate academic progress and improve conversational fluency. The two statements about strategy-based intervention (options d and e) reflect the current trend toward collaborative programs in the schools. This model is usually curriculum based, which facilitates the integration of therapy skills with the child's academic focus. A systems model is one in which learning occurs as the student engages in interactions. A combination of the systems model with the strategy-based intervention program would best assist the student in the development of strategies that will improve social and academic prowess.

11. d. Directing the bolus to the stronger side is not a rationale for using swallowing maneuvers, because it reflects the oral preparatory stage of swallowing. Chin tuck combined with rotation of the head narrows laryngeal closure (option a) by facilitation of vocal fold adduction (option b) and therefore reflects an effective technique to minimize aspiration. The chin tuck pushes the epiglottis posteriorly (option c), thereby minimizing the risk of aspiration. By tucking the chin, the base of tongue is pushed backward toward the pharyngeal wall, which widens the vallecula and thereby minimizes aspiration and vallecular residue.

12. e. Neuromuscular stimulation through sEMG can serve as a biofeedback technique to enhance muscle facilitation (option a), prevent muscle atrophy (option b), achieve muscle reeducation (option c), and strengthen muscles (option d), all of which are addressed in improving the swallowing process.

13. d. Laryngeal elevation does not have a sensory component. Sensory awareness is a proven technique for improving the oral phase of a swallow. Swallow apraxia (option a), hyperactive gag reflex (option b), and delayed onset of the oral phase of swallowing (option e) are all involved with the oral phase. Sensory awareness can also be used to assist those with food (option c) or food texture aversions. Improvement of sensory awareness helps to "send a signal" to the central nervous system that initiation of swallowing (i.e., stimulation of the pharyngeal swallow) is about to occur.

14. c. Phonological development is most pronounced at ages 2 to 5 years, and therapy for children in this age range focuses on sound processes (e.g., fronting, backing, stopping, gliding) or feature errors. Stimulating sound acquisition in single words and

acquiring syllable production in specified words is a focus at 12 to 24 months of age (options a and b). Therapy for children aged 5 years and older (options d and e) typically focuses on elimination of errors in increasingly complex syllabic structures.

15. b. The cycles approach, developed by Hodson and Paden (1983),reflects the classes and organization of speech sounds. It focuses on a combination of sound production and auditory stimulation and is designed to use with a child who has numerous misarticulations and whose speech is highly unintelligible. The authors set the criteria of 40% after extensively evaluating and treating children with speech disorders. After assessing a child, the clinician should develop a hierarchy of the phonological processes that is based on the processes in which the child is stimulable in at least 40% of the production contexts. The processes with the highest degree of stimulability should be the initial focus of therapy. Treatment of speech-sound errors usually focuses on encouraging production of emerging sounds, correction of errors in key words needed by the child, phonetic placement and shaping, and stimulability. Emerging sounds are those that a child produces correctly in 19% to 49% of the time in one or more phonetic environments.

16. a. The reversal of the position of two sounds in a word is metathesis. Epenthesis (option b) is the insertion of an additional sound into a word; migration (option c) as the moving of a sound from a correct position in an utterance to an incorrect position; assimilation (option d) as the alteration of a phoneme so that it takes on characteristics of another sound; and reduplication (option e) is the repetition of all or part of a syllable.

17. e. The cycles approach is based on a hierarchy of processes that a child exhibits in phonological assessment. Those processes, on which the child is stimulable in a minimum of 40% of the contexts, then forms the basis of the child's therapy program. Auditory bombardment focusing on words and sentences containing the target sounds and words is the first activity in therapy. The "emerging sounds" approach (option a) focuses on increasing the number of correct productions of a sound in a variety of contexts. The distinctive features approaches (option b) involve the teaching of a few sounds at a time that contain the targeted distinctive feature in hopes that the features will generalize to other sounds. Phonetic placement (option c) and shaping (option d) are sound elicitation techniques used to develop correct placement of speech-sound errors, if the child is not stimulable.

18. b. Injection of Botox into the thyroarytenoid muscle temporarily paralyzes one vocal fold, thereby reducing laryngeal spasms and improving breath flow through the glottis, which results in improved phonation. Surgical transection of the recurrent laryngeal nerve (option a) was developed in 1976 to reduce larygeal tightness and increase air flow through the glottis by paralyzing one vocal fold. However, the improvements did not hold up over time, and support for this procedure has waned. Botox injection into the posterior cricoarytenoid muscle (option c) is a treatment for abductor (not adductor) spasmodic dysphonia. The implantation of laryngeal nerve stimulators (option d) needs further study; at this time, evidence of its results is insufficient for it to be considered a first-line treatment. Speech therapy (option e) is sometimes helpful in the early stages through the implementing of techniques designed to reduce laryngeal tightness and to increase air flow and breath support. Other adaptations include whispering, speaking at a higher pitch, easy voice onset, and speaking on inhalation. However, evidence shows that patients rarely implement these techniques beyond the confines of the therapy room, and they are not effective beyond the early stages unless combined with more aggressive medical intervention.

19. e. Vocal fold thinning by laser and Teflon injection would not be recommended as an "early" treatment. Even for treatment in later stages of the patient's course, it is rarely implemented because studies have demonstrated that Teflon is unstable; it breaks down and migrates to other parts of the body. Reduction of laryngeal tightness (option a), increasing expiratory breath flow rate (option b), speaking on inhalation (option c), and raising the patient's pitch (option d) are techniques that represent a reasonable approach to treating spasmodic dysphonia in the early stages.

20. a. Patients who have unilateral Botox injections typically experience decreased shimmer and jitter. Shimmer is a measure of cycle-to-cycle variation in amplitude; jitter is a measure of cycle-to-cycle variation in frequency. Clinical research studies have clearly demonstrated that extrinsic laryngeal muscles do not change (option b) after Botox injections. The majority of patients with adductor spasmodic dysphonia who have Botox injections actually experience reduced speech volume (option c). It is possible for patients who have Botox injections to experience aspiration, but it is usually temporary (option d), and it is worse in patients who have bilateral injections than in patients who have unilateral injections. Patients have to undergo reinjection

periodically; most Botox injections are effective for an average of 3 to 8 months (option e), at which time the patient seeks reinjection.

21. b. Therapy focused on increasing vocalizations and, eventually, verbalizations is not reflective of a functional outcome. Also, because of Amy's age, clinicians need to focus on skills that would enhance her immediate abilities to achieve academic and social success. Oral-motor therapy (option a) has been shown to be effective in normalizing aberrant oral-motor reflexes in children with cerebral palsy. Intervention focused on task specific oral-motor functions necessary for feeding (option c) would possibly lead to improved nutrition and, thus, general health enhancement. Focusing on facilitation of receptive language abilities (option d) would enable Amy to be more successful in the classroom. The development of an AAC system (option e) is certainly warranted, to enable her to interact with her teachers and classmates.

22. b. Individuals who have apraxia of speech typically make inconsistent errors, have difficulty initiating speech, and attempt to self-correct their speech errors. Oftentimes, apraxia of speech is comorbid with nonfluent aphasia. Because Adam's speech is considered moderately disordered, it is reasonable to further evaluate his verbal productions to determine the effects of context on his intelligibility. A trial of diagnostic therapy would provide evidence that could be used to support or refute the other options. Adam may, at some point, benefit from an AAC system (option a), oral muscular–strengthening exercises if muscle weakness is present (option c), and addressing articulation skills (option d). Spaced-retrieval training (option e) is a technique shown to facilitate short-term memory recall in individuals with dementia and would not be particularly appropriate for Adam.

23. d. Articulatory-kinematic techniques designed to foster improvement in symptoms of apraxia of speech and aphasia have been supported in clinical research since the 1930s. Articulatory-kinematic techniques focus on having the patient repeat movements and vocalizations that are modeled by the clinician. In the 1970s, integral stimulation combined awareness of how oral-motor movements look and sound with simultaneous practice. Sensory stimulation (option a), practicing oral musculature exercises (option b), contrastive practice (option c), and diadokokinetic practice (option e) focus on either sensory or motor approaches, not both. The combination of the sensory and motor approaches found in the articulatory-kinematic and integral stimulation approaches has proved to be most efficacious.

24. c. Facilitation of motor programming would be a reasonable approach for individuals with apraxia of speech, not dysarthria. Resonance (option a), inspiratory muscle training (option b), decreasing sound distortion (option d), and relaxation of inspiratory muscles (option e) all address the core dimension of dysarthria, which is muscle weakness, not motor programming. Movements of the muscles that are involved with articulation, phonation, resonance, and respiration are impaired differentially in individuals who have dysarthria.

25. d. In a variable-interval schedule, the reinforcer is presented on the basis of a behavioral response mean or average. The individual whose behavior is being modified is not aware of when reinforcement will occur; thus the response rate will be higher because there is no postreinforcement pause. A variable-interval schedule more closely approximates the "real world" than does a fixed-ratio (option a), fixed-interval (option b), or variable-ratio schedule (option c). Continuous reinforcement (option e) is the presentation of a reinforcer immediately after each occurrence of the target behavior or after each time period during which the target behavior is exhibited.

26. d. EBP includes the role of literature review, clinical observation, and clinical experience, knowledge, and skills in determining the best treatment plan for a specified patient. EBP does not provide guidelines for interpreting test scores (option a), although interpretation of test scores is *one* component of formulating therapy goals. EBP is a component, but not the definitive component (option b), of decision making; the strengths and weaknesses of the patient must be the primary area of concern for making clinical decisions. It is recognized in EBP that subjectivity cannot always be excluded from clinical decision-making (option c); if only scientifically proven techniques were used (option e), the field of speech-language therapy would never improve. Clinicians should systematically evaluate the evidence from tests of a clinical hypothesis, eventually documenting its efficacy or refuting it as a reasonable approach.

27. b. The term *handicap* is now interpreted as the effect of the communication deficit on the individual's ability to participate in various social activities; this statement reflects the current terminology. The term *impairment* (option a) is no longer in use; when it was used, it was defined as the disruption or abnormality in mental or physical functioning, or both, not in terms of the effect on daily functioning. Furthermore, *handicap*, not *impairment*, is now

defined in terms of "participation" (option c). The term *disability* referred to impairment in functioning as the result of a condition, not the anatomical or physiological effects of a condition (option d). The primary purpose of the adoption of new terminology was to more appropriately reflect functional goals and outcomes (option e).

28. a. Successfully communicating needs and wants by using an AAC device is an outcome that has a functional impact on Edward's communication ability in his natural environments. Increasing expressive vocabulary by 68% (option b) and learning 15 signs (option d) certainly could have an impact on his communication effectiveness, but the wordings do not indicate that those skills have generalized beyond the therapy setting. Refined movements of the tongue and lips may lead to improved communication; however, pretherapy and posttherapy assessments are needed to determine whether (1) Edward's speech has been positively affected by the oral-motor improvement (not always a sequelae to oral-motor treatment) and (2) Edward has generalized his improved speech from a controlled setting to his everyday environments. Successfully completing two-step commands (option e) may indicate an improvement in auditory memory, but does not reflect a change in Edward's daily communication.

29. d. Answering this question requires the clinician to be familiar with the literature that addresses medical treatment for expressive and receptive language skills. There have been numerous clinical trials (option c), but the medications have shown no consistent ability to improve communication deficits caused by brain injury or insult (option a). Pairing other therapies with such medications would be efficacious, but these medications do not exist (option b). Pharmacists certainly are knowledgeable about approved medications and those in clinical trials (option e), but they do not have access to the patient's medical records, which they would need to study before making a reasonable response to such a question.

30. d. Medications can have side effects that could inhibit a response to speech and language therapy. Some of these side effects might include drowsiness, lethargy, decreased hearing, and other undesirable conditions. Because these types of changes need to be reported to the patient's physician, the SLP should monitor Mr. Smithson and report changes to his prescribing physician; it may not be possible to establish a baseline (option c). It is not within the scope of practice to discuss or recommend the effectiveness of medications (option a); No studies have shown conclusively that medications can facilitate recovery

of communication skills lost through brain injury; therefore, the SLP should not suggest prescribing a neurostimulant (option b). SLPs may address evidence that pharmaceuticals have an impact on skills associated with communication (option e), but they cannot prescribe medications.

31. a. Current evidence shows that working on comprehension and production simultaneously results in the most functional gains in treating patients with aphasia. Historically, breaking down sentence production and intensively training in each aspect (option b) was an accepted approach to therapy, but it is not as efficacious as working on comprehension and production simultaneously. Focusing on form of language, as opposed to use of language, has not been shown to generalize to use in social situations (option d); therefore, it does not truly fit the concept of being a functional outcome. Following typical developmental norms for children is an accepted practice in treatment but not typically used for the treatment of adults. Current theory leans toward the need to begin intervention, or even diagnostic therapy, as soon as the patient is medically stable, not until spontaneous recovery (option e).

32. a. Dementia is a progressive disease that negatively affects cognitive and communication abilities. Activities to improve Ms. Jackson's levels of cognitive function are not efficacious; moreover, they are not functional in terms of Mrs. Jackson's immediate needs. Developing skills to facilitate performance of daily living skills and routines (option b), educating family members and the staff of the care facility about communication strategies (option d), and creating a "memory book" (option e) all have an impact on Ms. Jackson's immediate ability to function within her environment and, hence, meet the profession's emphasis on functional goals with functional outcomes. Reducing demands on her episodic and working memories (option c) is also a reasonable therapy strategy because it is based on research that shows episodic and working memories are more affected by dementia than are procedural and declarative memory.

33. c. Spaced-retrieval training is designed to help the patient practice recalling information over progressively longer intervals of time by tapping into implicit, automatic memory functions (which are less impaired than other memory systems, such as episodic and working memory) without taxing the cognitive system. Because procedural memory (option a) is one of the less affected memory systems in patients with dementia, therapy should not focus on its stimulation at the expense of time

needed for focusing on other memory systems. Montessori-type interaction with children (option b) and sensory stimulation (option d) are approaches used to facilitate socialization, but they do not address directly improving memory. Because episodic memory (option e) is negatively affected by dementia, particularly dementia of the Alzheimer's type, treatment protocols should focus on reducing the demands on episodic memory, not on stimulating episodic memory.

34. c. The SLP should focus on strategies for reducing muscle tension while simultaneously exploring fluency control measures that the client can implement in conversations. Fluency therapy has sometimes been based on the assumption that the anxiety will disappear once fluency control is mastered (option a), but there is little or no evidence that supports this approach. The reverse, that anxiety reduction should minimize the dysfluencies (option e), implies that control strategies do not need to be incorporated into treatment. Using stress management techniques alone does not specifically address the problem of muscle tension provoked by anxiety. Psychotherapy (option d) would be a somewhat reasonable approach if the client has significant anxiety, but the speech therapy should not be postponed until the psychotherapy is over.

35. e. Scientific and anecdotal reports clearly illustrate the fact that no single treatment strategy works for everyone. Furthermore, a client may incorporate a variety of strategies, depending on the situation. Rhythmic stimulation (option a), delayed auditory feedback (option b), and use of melodic intonations (option c) all represent techniques of fluency enhancement that have support in speech pathology. Introducing a variety of management strategies to see which is or are most effective (option d) would be more a period of diagnostic therapy than actual treatment.

Bibliography

Hodson, B., & Paden, E. (1983). Targeting intelligible speech: A phonological approach to remediation. San Diego: College Hill Press.

Keenan, J., & Brassell, E. (1975). Aphasia Language Performance Scale (ALPS) Murpheesboro, TN: Pinnacle Press.

CHAPTER 23

Syndromes and Genetics

Linda D. Vallino

GENETICS

1. Saethre-Chotzen syndrome has a population frequency of approximately 1 per 50,000. If the most likely mode of inheritance is that shown in Figure 23-1, what is the probability that the daughter of the proband (*arrow*) is affected?
   a. 1 per 4
   b. 1 per 2
   c. 1 per 100
   d. 0
   e. 1 per 50,000

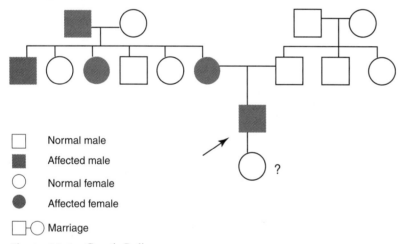

□	Normal male
■	Affected male
○	Normal female
●	Affected female
□─○	Marriage

Figure 23-1   Genetic Pedigree

2. Lola is 9 months old and has popliteal pterygium syndrome. She had bilateral cleft lip and palate, oral synechiae, multiple lower lip pits, and marked popliteal webbing over the elbows and knees. Upon meeting the parents, you observe that the father has the same syndrome as his daughter but appears to be less affected. He has bilateral cleft palate and also reports that he has toe syndactyly. The best explanation for this occurrence is:
   a. High recurrent mutation rate
   b. Autosomal recessive inheritance with incomplete penetrance

c. Autosomal recessive inheritance with variable expressivity

d. Autosomal dominant inheritance with variable expressivity

e. Autosomal dominant disorder with late onset

3. A child has a cleft palate, microcephaly, polydactyly, and severe developmental disabilities for which a diagnosis could not be established. There is no family history of the disorder. Genetic testing revealed that neither parent has a genetic defect. While pregnant, the mother did not smoke, use drugs, or drink alcohol. The geneticist reported to the family that this disorder is most likely sporadic. Of the following statements, which is most accurate about the recurrence of this birth defect?

a. There is no increased risk beyond the general population risk for subsequent children of these parents because the condition is the result of a new mutation

b. There is a 5% risk to pass the gene on to a subsequent child because the condition is a new mutation

c. There is no recurrence risk because the condition is a single-gene defect

d. There is a 5% risk to pass the gene on to a subsequent child because the condition is an autosomal dominant disorder with reduced penetrance

e. There is no recurrence risk because the condition is the result of teratogens

4. A 7-year-old boy is referred to you for an assessment. He has significant developmental delay; dysmorphic facial features, including a long and narrow face, large ears, prominent jaw, and prominent forehead; attention difficulties; and autistic-like behavior that affects communication and social interaction. The genetic pedigree showed that the grandfather was affected and passed the mutation to none of his sons but to all of his daughters, who are considered carriers. The sons of these carrier women have a 50% chance of inheriting this disorder. Some of the female carriers may show no symptoms of the disease and others may show only mild symptoms. The pedigree best describes the clinical characteristics of which type of disorder?

a. Fetal alcohol syndrome

b. Trisomy 21

c. 22q11.2 deletion syndrome

d. Syndrome of coloboma, heart disease, atresia choanae, retarded growth and development, genital hypoplasia, and ear anomalies (CHARGE syndrome)

e. Fragile X syndrome

5. A 9-month-old with cleft palate has been referred to you for assessment before surgery to repair the palate. According to the genetic history, this child's anomaly can best be explained as a single problem in morphogenesis that led to a cascade of subsequent defects. What would be the best diagnosis for this child?

a. Fetal alcohol syndrome

b. CHARGE syndrome

c. Pierre Robin sequence

d. 22q11.2 deletion

e. Apert syndrome

6. In determining whether a child has Apert syndrome, what distinct feature would have to be present in order to distinguish this condition from other types of craniosynostosis?

a. Elbow anomalies

b. Midface retrusion

c. Ocular proptosis

d. Symmetrical syndactyly of the hands and feet

e. Narrow palate

7. Tina is a 16-year-old high school student who is concerned about her speech. Although she said she is not teased, she reported that her voice does not sound like those of other girls her age. She has never been enrolled in speech therapy, and this is her first speech assessment. She has hypernasality in the absence of a cleft palate, difficulty with reading and math, and a childhood history of chronic middle ear effusion. Her mother mentions that some time ago, Tina had a blood test for an immunodeficiency disorder, but she is unable to provide any other information about it. On the basis of the targeted history information, you recommend referral to a geneticist, and the mother agrees. In making the referral, all of the following documentation is important to convey *except:*

a. Features noted in the patient

b. Cause for concern

c. Communication assessment results

d. Information about the blood test obtained from the other health care provider

e. Suspected diagnosis

8. Tina is a 16-year-old high school student who is concerned about her speech. Although she said she is not teased, she reported that her voice does not sound like those of other girls her age. She has never been enrolled in speech therapy, and this is her first speech assessment. She has hypernasality in the absence of a cleft palate, difficulty with reading and math, and a childhood history of chronic middle ear effusion. Her mother mentions that some time ago, Tina had a blood test for an immunodeficiency disorder, but she is unable to provide any other information about it. On the basis of the targeted history information, you recommend referral to a geneticist, and the mother agrees. Of the following syndromes, which is most frequently associated with this phenotype?

a. Stickler syndrome

b. Treacher Collins syndrome

c. 22q11.2 deletion syndrome

d. Usher syndrome

e. VATERR association

SPEECH, LANGUAGE, AND HEARING

9. Petra is a 16-year-old patient with Crouzon syndrome. During the assessment, she expresses concern about difficulty producing /s/, /z/, /tʃ/ ("ch"), /ʃ/ ("sh"), /dʒ/ ("j"), and /ʒ/ ("zh" as in "treasure"), saying that they sound "slushy." She also reported that she sounds as if "I talk through my nose." She enjoys school and her friends and is interested in improving her speech. During the examination, you observe that Petra maintains an open-mouth posture at rest and breathes audibly. Oral inspection reveals a high, narrow palatal vault; maxillary hypoplasia; and class III open-bite malocclusion. Perceptually, you agree with her that her sibilant and affricate productions are distorted and that her resonance is abnormal. On mirror testing, nasal emission was judged to be reduced on words containing /m/, /n/, and /ŋ/. Pressure-flow studies revealed reduced nasal airflow on /m/ in the word "hamper," and the mean nasalance score on nasal sentences was 36% (norm: 61.06; standard deviation: 6.94). On the basis of findings of Petra's oral examination and instrumental assessment, her resonance can be most accurately described as:
   a. Hyponasal
   b. Hypernasal
   c. Denasal
   d. Cul-de-sac
   e. Mixed hyper-hyponasal

10. Petra is a 16-year-old patient with Crouzon syndrome. During the assessment, she expresses concern about difficulty producing /s/, /z/, /tʃ/ ("ch"), /ʃ/ ("sh"), /dʒ/ ("j"), and /ʒ/ ("zh" as in "treasure"), saying that they sound "slushy." She also reported that she sounds as if she "I talk through my nose." She enjoys school and her friends and is interested in improving her speech. During the examination, you observe that Petra maintains an open-mouth posture at rest and breathes audibly. Oral inspection reveals a high, narrow palatal vault; maxillary hypoplasia; and class III open-bite malocclusion. Perceptually, you agree with her that her sibilant and affricate productions are distorted and that her resonance is abnormal. On mirror testing, nasal emission was judged to be reduced on words containing /m/, /n/, and /ŋ/. Pressure-flow studies revealed reduced nasal airflow on /m/ in the word "hamper," and the mean nasalance score on nasal sentences was 36% (norm: 61.06; standard deviation: 6.94). Petra's articulation errors are most typical of which of the following causes?
   a. Phoneme-specific nasal emission
   b. Mild conductive hearing loss
   c. Velopharyngeal inadequacy
   d. Dental malocclusion
   e. Specific phonological disorder

11. Petra is a 16-year-old patient with Crouzon syndrome. During the assessment, she expresses concern about difficulty producing /s/, /z/, /tʃ/ ("ch"), /ʃ/ ("sh"), /dʒ/ ("j"), and /ʒ/ ("zh" as in "treasure"), saying that they sound "slushy." She also reported that she sounds as if "I talk through my nose." She enjoys school and her friends and is interested in improving her speech. During the examination, you observe that Petra maintains an open-mouth posture at rest and breathes audibly. Oral inspection reveals a high, narrow palatal vault; maxillary hypoplasia; and class III open-bite malocclusion. Perceptually, you agree with her that her sibilant and affricate productions are distorted and that her resonance is abnormal. On mirror testing, nasal emission was judged to be reduced on words containing /m/, /n/, and /ŋ/. Pressure-flow studies revealed reduced nasal airflow on /m/ in the word "hamper," and the mean nasalance score on nasal sentences was 36% (norm: 61.06; standard deviation: 6.94). Of the following, which strategy would be most effective in improving Petra's speech?
   a. Orthodontic treatment
   b. Nonsurgical maxillary protraction device
   c. Septoplasty
   d. Mandibular advancement
   e. Maxillary advancement

12. George is a 13-year-old patient with Stickler syndrome. He has mandibular hypoplasia, a repaired submucous cleft palate, and a pharyngeal flap. He also has a history of snoring and sleep apnea; 2 years earlier, he underwent mandibular distraction to lengthen the jaw, which improved the condition. His mother reported that George has recently resumed snoring loudly at night. Listening to the tape recording his mother brought to the session, you hear the snoring and also perceive short cessations of breathing. The patient exhibits moderate hypernasal speech and weak pressure consonants that reduce overall intelligibility. What would be the most important assessment recommendation in establishing a treatment for this person?
   a. Cephalometric radiography
   b. Polysomnography
   c. Nasoendoscopy
   d. Orthodontic evaluation
   e. Multiview videofluoroscopy

13. During your assessment of a 20-month-old patient with Beckwith-Wiedemann syndrome, you notice that at rest, her tongue protrudes beyond the central incisors. During her babbling, you also observe that she produces /p/ and /b/ labiodentally and interdentalizes /t/ and /d/. The velar stop consonants /k/ and /g/ are produced accurately. The best reason for her error in sounds is that she exhibits:
   a. Macroglossia
   b. Generalized development delay
   c. Oromotor impairment

d. Retrognathia

e. Childhood apraxia of speech

14. Nellie is a 12-month-old patient with Nager syndrome. In addition to the other anomalies associated with this disorder, she has cleft palate, esophageal reflux, upper limb anomalies, tracheotomy, and hypoplastic left heart syndrome, which causes a bluish appearance. Nellie remained in hospital for the first 5 months of life and has had recurrent intermittent short-stay readmissions since discharge. The parents express great concern about Nellie's communication development, stating that she produces only /a/ during vocal play. Repair of the cleft palate has been postponed until her medical condition is stable. What is the best course of intervention?

a. Waiting until the palate is repaired

b. Enrolling Nellie in a formal speech therapy program at a local agency

c. Instructing the parents in a home speech-language stimulation program with ongoing monitoring

d. Recommending monitoring of communication development every 3 months

e. Teaching sign language

15. Jon is 10 years old and has 22q11.2 deletion syndrome and submucous cleft palate. He has a history of fluctuating middle ear effusion with concomitant hearing loss. Jon is a pleasant child who enjoys communicating with his teachers and friends. He produces utterances of up to five words, but these utterances are unintelligible. Articulation errors are characterized by omissions of consonants at the initial and final positions of words and by hard glottal attacks. Jon is unable to elevate his tongue for the tip-alveolar consonants /t/ and /d/ and elevates his mandible so that the tongue can touch the palatal region in an attempt to produce /n/. Modeling and cueing during stimulability testing for bilabial stops and tip alveolar stops have been unsuccessful. Nasality is variable, ranging from normal to mildly hypernasal. Jon shows speech behaviors that are typical of children in whom which of the following is diagnosed?

a. Hyperkinetic dysarthria

b. Velopharyngeal inadequacy

c. Apraxia of speech

d. Phonetic speech disorder

e. Conductive hearing loss

16. Jon is 10 years old and has 22q11.2 deletion syndrome and submucous cleft palate. He has a history of fluctuating middle ear effusion with concomitant hearing loss. Jon is a pleasant child who enjoys communicating with his teachers and friends. He produces utterances of up to five words, but these utterances are unintelligible. Articulation errors are characterized by omissions of consonants at the initial and final positions of words and by hard glottal attacks. Jon is unable to elevate his

tongue for the tip-alveolar consonants /t/ and /d/ and elevates his mandible so that the tongue can touch the palatal region in an attempt to produce /n/. Modeling and cueing during stimulability testing for bilabial stops and tip alveolar stops have been unsuccessful. Nasality is variable, ranging from normal to mildly hypernasal. As part of the ongoing assessment, the speech-language pathologist's most appropriate action is:

a. To obtain additional information about the velopharyngeal function and articulation by using multiview videofluoroscopy

b. To obtain additional information about velopharyngeal function and articulation by using nasopharyngoscopy

c. To obtain spectrographic measures of perceived hypernasality and articulation

d. To obtain information about nasalance by using the Nasometer

e. To obtain information on articulatory patterns of tongue and palatal contacts by using electropalatography

17. Mitchell is 14 years old and has Moebius syndrome. He has been referred to you because of poor speech intelligibility and concerns about facial expression. The neurological report states that he has cranial nerve VII involvement. He is doing well in school and has several close friends. What would you predict to be the most difficult sound class for Mitchell to produce?

a. Lingual dental fricatives

b. Glottal fricatives

c. Velar stops

d. Lingual alveolar stops

e. Labials

18. Mitchell is 14 years old and has Moebius syndrome. He has been referred to you because of poor speech intelligibility and concerns about facial expression. The neurological report states that he has cranial nerve VII involvement. He is doing well in school and has several close friends. In view of Mitchell's age and concerns, what would most likely be the most effective strategy for speech and language intervention?

a. Oromotor exercises to improve neuromuscular control

b. Compensatory articulation strategies to maximize intelligibility

c. Postponement of speech therapy until Michael has undergone facial reanimation surgery

d. Strategies to supplement spoken output in order to establish the context of the message

e. An assistive communication device

19. Which of the following hearing disorders best typifies a case of craniosynostosis?

a. Delayed auditory maturation

b. Sensorineural hearing loss

c. Conductive hearing loss

d. Mixed hearing loss

e. Central hearing loss

20. A 9-year-old with fetal alcohol syndrome has a repaired cleft palate and a history of middle ear effusion. The most recent peripheral audiological assessment revealed normal hearing sensitivity. Articulation is characterized by gliding of liquids. Resonance is slightly hypernasal but inconsistently. His performance on the receptive and expressive subtests of the Clinical Evaluation of Language – (3rd Edition) was in the low average range. Also, he recently received a diagnosis of attention deficit disorder. On the basis of these findings and what is supported by the current literature on fetal alcohol syndrome, the most critical assessment that now needs to be done in order to provide the most effective intervention is:

a. Central auditory testing

b. Neuropsychological testing

c. Nasopharyngoscopic examination of velopharyngeal function

d. Neurological testing

e. Psychiatric assessment

21. To assist the adolescent with Prader-Willi syndrome in developing better behavioral interactions, which of the following would be considered to be appropriate treatment goal?

a. Improving narrative skills

b. Improving intelligibility

c. Improving articulation

d. Improving receptive language

e. Facilitating self-monitoring skills

22. The literature on CHARGE syndrome suggests that although physical disorders, vision loss, and hearing loss may adversely affect communication ability, these factors do not preclude the development of symbolic language. There is evidence that a major factor in the successful acquisition of symbolic language in children with CHARGE syndrome is highly correlated with:

a. Cognitive ability

b. Early consistent audiological intervention

c. Prelinguistic communication skills

d. Degree of visual impairment

e. Enrollment in early intervention programs

23. Maura is an 8-year-old with Treacher Collins syndrome. She has moderate hypernasality and a muffled voice quality. Her articulation is marked by pharyngeal fricatives and affricates. What is the most critical factor in making a decision about physical management to correct hypernasality in a patient with Treacher Collins syndrome?

a. Glossoptosis

b. Anomalous shape of the nasopharynx

c. Severity of mandibular hypoplasia

d. Airway

e. Restricted mouth opening

24. A girl was born with lip pits and a complete unilateral cleft lip and palate. The case history revealed that other family members—including an aunt, an uncle, and a male cousin—had orofacial clefts of varying degrees, lip pits, and speech problems. In view of this family pedigree and description of the disorder, which of the following best typifies this condition?

a. Van der Woude syndrome

b. Pierre Robin sequence

c. Orofacial digital syndrome

d. Otopalatodigital syndrome, type I

e. Stickler syndrome

25. Carol is a 9-year-old with right-sided hemifacial microsomia. On the affected side, she has a mild auricular deformity and a moderate-severe hearing loss; on the unaffected side, she has normal hearing. Her parents recently received reports from the school indicating that Carol has difficulty understanding speech in the classroom, especially when it is noisy, and that she has difficulty responding correctly to questions. Her language skills fall within the broad range of normal and are routinely monitored. Carol's hearing loss can best be attributed to:

a. Auditory neuropathy

b. Ossicular discontinuity

c. Atresia of the external ear

d. Middle ear effusion

e. Underdevelopment of the cochlea

26. Carol is a 9-year-old with right-sided hemifacial microsomia. On the affected side, she has a mild auricular deformity and a moderate-severe hearing loss; on the unaffected side, she has normal hearing. Her parents recently received reports from the school indicating that Carol has difficulty understanding speech in the classroom, especially when it is noisy, and that she has difficulty responding correctly to questions. Her language skills fall within the broad range of normal and are routinely monitored. You consult with the educational audiologist. Which of the following amplification strategies would be most effective in maximizing educational potential?

a. Preferential seating in the classroom

b. Contralateral routing of signals (CROS) aid

c. FM system

d. Conventional hearing aid

e. Bone-anchored hearing aid

27. Consideration of mandibular lengthening by distraction osteogenesis in an infant who has a Pierre Robin sequence would most appropriately improve:

a. Airway
b. Speech
c. Feeding
d. Cosmesis
e. Dental occlusion

28. May is an 8-year-old with Treacher Collins syndrome. She has a class II open bite malocclusion. She also has a moderate-severe conductive hearing loss and wears a bone-anchored hearing aid. In her classroom, she uses an FM system. At rest, May maintains an anterior tongue posture. Resonance is within normal limits. Articulation is marked by interdentalization of sibilants and inconsistent f/θ and n/m substitutions. Language skills are judged to be age appropriate. What is considered to be the best recommendation for treatment for this child?
a. Insertion of a tongue crib to correct tongue thrust
b. Orthodontic intervention to correct the anterior open bite
c. No treatment at this time
d. Enrollment in articulation therapy
e. Surgery to advance the mandible

29. Jackie is an 8-year-old with 22q11.2 deletion syndrome. Her speech is characterized by moderate hypernasality, audible nasal emission, and weak pressure consonants. Nasoendoscopic examination of the velopharyngeal mechanism has been recommended to assist in treatment planning. In addition to assessing the pattern and degree of closure, what information are you seeking before making a definitive surgical decision?
a. Medial displacement of the carotid artery
b. Unilateral vocal paralysis
c. Swallowing disorder
d. Tongue function during articulation
e. Contribution of Passavant's ridge to closure

30. In an infant with Goldenhar syndrome, what feature would probably be responsible for difficulty with feeding?
a. Pharyngeal stenosis
b. Glossoptosis
c. Maxillary hypoplasia
d. Unilateral facial weakness
e. High narrow palate

31. A 19-month-old with Beckwith-Wiedemann syndrome and cleft palate has been referred to you for a communication assessment. Her medical records show that she underwent tongue reduction at 12 months and palate repair at 15 months. This is her first visit since the palate was repaired. During the session, this child vocalized "mama," "dada," and "gaga." Resonance was judged to be normal. Hearing was tested in sound field and was normal in the better ear. The parents reported

that their daughter appears to understand what is said to her but are concerned about her expressive abilities. Language testing show age-level receptive skills and expressive skills that are poorer than expected for a child 16 months of age. What would be an optimal goal for treatment?
a. Increase lingual strength
b. Develop oromotor function for speech
c. Expand consonant inventory
d. Develop basic sign language vocabulary
e. Increase tongue mobility

32. According to the literature, with regard to the language abilities of typically developing school-aged children, those with Williams syndrome have specific difficulty with:
a. Concrete vocabulary size
b. Conceptual and relational vocabulary
c. Short-term memory
d. Grammar
e. Expressive vocabulary

33. Lou is an 11-year-old with Down syndrome and repaired cleft palate. He has a fistula at the junction of the hard and soft palates. He exhibits nasal turbulence on /sk/ blends and several phonological errors that interfere with intelligibility. With regard to what is known about the speech of children with Down syndrome, of the following phonological problems, which would you most expect to occur in this child?
a. Deletion of nasal consonants
b. Deletion of final consonant
c. Posterior nasal emission
d. Lateralization of sibilants
e. Liquid simplification

34. A 6-year-old boy presents with large ears and long face. His speech is rapid and is difficult to understand. His pragmatic skills have been described as "peculiar." Furthermore, his teachers report that he has difficulty in maintaining the topic during conversation and in answering direct questions. These speech behaviors are typical of children in whom which of the following is diagnosed?
a. Treacher Collins syndrome
b. Down syndrome
c. Sotos syndrome
d. Fragile X syndrome
e. Pierre Robin sequence

35. Anna is an 8-month-old with Apert syndrome. This is her first visit to the speech-language pathologist. The mother, who stated that Anna is not babbling like other children her age, is interested in learning more about the features of this syndrome that might imperil Anna's communication progress. Anna is a pleasant infant who

focuses on the clinician's face when she is spoken to and exhibits responsive smiling. Among the many factors that contribute to communication impairment in this syndrome, it is most important during this visit to focus on:

a. The effect of dental malocclusion on speech
b. The effect of the crowded nasopharynx on resonance
c. The reduced phonetic inventory present during babbling and early word attempts
d. The specific learning difficulties that impede language learning
e. The effect of the earlier cranial vault surgery on brain development

1. b. Saethre-Chotzen syndrome is a condition involving premature craniofacial synostosis. It is an autosomal dominant disorder; therefore, the chance that an affected parent, male or female, will pass the mutant gene on to offspring is 50%, or 1 per 2. For an autosomal recessive disorder in which both parents are carriers, the probability of having an affected child is 25%, or 1 per 4 (option a). Frequencies of 1 per 100 (option c) and 0 (option d) are incorrect because they reflect the probability of a chance occurrence. A rate of 1 per 50,000 (option e) represents the prevalence of the disorder, not the rate of recurrence in offspring.

2. d. Popliteal pterygium syndrome is an autosomal dominant disorder. The gene can be passed equally to both sons and daughters; in this case, it was passed from father to daughter. One of the characteristics of an autosomal disorder is variable expressivity: that is, the extent of severity in an affected person does not affect the severity of expression in the next generation. In this case, the offspring of a mildly affected father is severely affected. In the case of a disorder involving a high recurrent mutation rate (option a), both parents would be normal. Incomplete penetrance and variable expressivity occur only in autosomal dominant disorders and never in autosomal recessive disorders (options b and c). Popliteal pterygium syndrome is not a disorder of later onset (option e), an example of which is Huntington chorea.

3. a. Because the characteristics are not part of a syndrome, and because family history and genetic test results for the parents are negative, this condition represents a new mutation; therefore, the risk of recurrence is no greater than that of the general population. No gene or chromosome anomalies were identified (options b and d); the 5% recurrence risk is associated with cleft lip and palate alone and not that associated with other defects. Tobacco, drugs, and alcohol (option e) are known teratogens implicated in causing a birth defect, but this mother did not ingest those substances.

4. e. Fragile X syndrome is an X-linked inherited condition involving several physical and cognitive disabilities. It is caused by a genetic mutation on the X chromosome. Men with the fragile X syndrome cannot transmit it to any of their sons (because men contribute a Y chromosome, not an X, to their male offspring) but do transmit it to all their daughters, because men

contribute their X chromosomes to daughters. Fetal alcohol syndrome (option a) is the result of alcohol consumed during pregnancy, and this was not suggested in the case presented. Trisomy 21 (option b), 22q11.2 deletion syndrome (option c), and the CHARGE syndrome (option d) are autosomal chromosome defects involving an extra chromosome, a partial deletion of a chromosome, and a chromosomal mutation, respectively.

5. c. The Pierre Robin sequence is a disorder in which an anomaly leads to a cascade of events. It is generally characterized by cleft palate, micrognathia, and glossoptosis. The initiating event for this sequence is the interference in the normal development of the mandible during early gestation. Because the mandible is small, the tongue is forced to remain high in the oral cavity, thereby interfering with palatal fusion. Fetal alcohol syndrome (option a) is a constellation of birth defects that is caused by maternal ingestion of alcohol, which interferes with normal embryological processes. The 22q11.2 deletion (option d) is a single-gene defect, and Apert syndrome (option e) is caused by an abnormal gene. CHARGE syndrome (option b) is the nonrandom occurrence of a pattern of multiple anomalies and is a diagnosis of exclusion.

6. d. Syndactyly, or fusion of the fingers and of the toes, is the characteristic that most differentiates Apert syndrome from the other craniofacial dysostosis syndromes. Although other forms of craniosynostosis, such as Pfeiffer syndrome, may include partial soft tissue syndactyly of the hands, it is not an obligatory finding. Elbow anomalies (option a) are associated with Pfeiffer syndrome. Midface retrusion (option b), ocular proptosis (option c), and narrow palate (option e) are features that are common to other types of craniosynostosis, including Apert syndrome, but are not defining features.

7. d. Information or test results provided by another provider cannot be shared without consent of the family. When a target history is documented, information is collected with regard to a specific suspected condition or group of conditions, whereas a comprehensive history and pedigree are best completed by the geneticist. A speech-language pathologist is in a position to document a history that would help determine the need for referral, as in this case. The referral should document the features noted in the patient (option a); cite the causes for concern (option b), including communication assessment results; and even provide

a suspected diagnosis (option e). Providing a suspected diagnosis based on valid evidence often serves as a starting point for the genetics professional.

8. c. All the characteristics described in this case are associated with 22q11.2 deletion syndrome. An immunodeficiency disorder often associated with a different manifestation of 22q11.2 deletion syndrome is referred to as DiGeorge syndrome. The other conditions listed are not associated with immunodeficiency. Stickler syndrome (option a) is characterized by micrognathia, cleft palate, myopia, and joint problems. Treacher Collins syndrome (option b) is characterized by retrognathia, downward-slanting palpebral fissures, and microtia. Usher syndrome (option d) is a condition that affects both hearing and vision, and most affected patients do not exhibit craniofacial anomalies. The VATERR association (option e) is characterized by vertebral defects, anal atresia, tracheoesophageal fistula, and radial and renal dysplasia.

9. a. Petra exhibits posterior midface retrusion, which results in a class III malocclusion, and probable airway obstruction, which results in snoring during sleep and audible breathing at rest. Airflow on the nasal consonant /m/ is reduced, and the nasalance scores are significantly lower than the normative data provided for nasal sentences. These findings together are consistent with the diagnosis of hyponasality. If the airway were completely occluded (option c), nasal emission airflow would be absent on the nasal consonants /m/, /n/, and /ŋ/ and their production would approach /b/, /d/, and /g/, respectively. Hypernasality (option b) is a result of acoustic sound energy diverting into the nasal passage as a result of incomplete velopharyngeal closure. Cul-de-sac resonance (option d) is a variation of hyponasality in which the place of obstruction is anterior; in Petra's case, however, the obstruction is posterior. Mixed hyper-hyponasality (option e) may co-occur if the patient exhibits velopharyngeal inadequacy and also experiences airflow resistance as the result of a nasal deformity. This did not occur in Petra's case.

10. d. According to the literature, the sounds most frequently affected by skeletal and dental malocclusions are the sibilant and affricate phonemes. Petra's class III open-bite malocclusion, a common finding in persons with Crouzon syndrome, is extreme enough to preclude a narrow anterior air stream necessary for adequate sibilant production; as a result, sound is distorted. Phoneme-specific nasal emission (option a) is the result of faulty articulation mislearning and not an anatomical cause. Conductive hearing loss (option b) has been reported

in persons with Crouzon syndrome; however, speech sound distortions or omissions would be most likely attributed to the hearing loss if the loss were moderate to severe loss, not mild. Petra does not have velopharyngeal inadequacy (option c), a condition that would result in hypernasality. Petra has developed sibilants and affricates (option e) that are used at her age; the problem is that they are distorted.

11. e. Published data demonstrate that hyponasality is eliminated and articulation is improved by maxillary advancement in patients with Crouzon syndrome. Orthodontic treatment (option a) is undertaken to align the teeth on the dental arches only in preparation of orthognathic surgery; it does not alter the maxillary-mandibular relationship. A maxillary protraction device (option b) is used to correct mild maxillary retrusion. A septoplasty (option c) is a surgical procedure used to straighten the nasal septum, not to correct maxillary retrusion. Advancing the mandible forward (option d) would worsen the relationship between the maxilla and mandible.

12. b. Although the patient's speech is of great concern, the snoring and episodes of breathing cessation during sleep suggest that he is experiencing airway difficulties that necessitate immediate attention. Polysomnography, which is conducted during sleep, identifies the presence or absence of sleep apnea and, if apnea is present, the type of apnea. Nasoendoscopy (option c), orthodontic evaluation (option d), and multiview videofluoroscopy (option e) are valuable imaging procedures used to understand how the pharyngeal flap contributes to airway obstruction. However, these tools would be recommended after the findings of polysomnography. Cephalometric radiography (option a) is helpful in determining the severity of the retrognathia often noted in a patient with Stickler syndrome, but it would not be helpful in determining the cause of the sleep apnea.

13. a. Macroglossia is a characteristic feature of Beckwith-Wiedemann syndrome. The tongue is too large to stay within the confines of the oral cavity and therefore protrudes past the maxillary and mandibular incisors, resulting in placement errors. The child is attempting to produce age-appropriate consonants, which contradicts the notion of developmental delay (option b). The errors are obligatory, relating to the structural abnormality, and not a result of oromotor impairment (option c) or childhood apraxia of speech (option e). Children with Beckwith-Wiedemann syndrome have a tendency toward mandibular protrusion, not retrognathia (option d).

14. c. In Nellie's case it is important to consider her condition, the desires of her parents for Nellie to communicate, the impact of her recurrent hospitalizations, and the fact that her speech and language are delayed. Having the parents serve as the intervention agents is the best course of intervention at this time. Her medically compromised condition precludes palate repair (option a); even in cases in which the patient's health is good and palate repair could be considered, patients with Nager syndrome have mandibular hypoplasia and limited jaw opening, both of which could be hazardous to the airway. Nellie's frail condition makes travel to receive speech therapy (option b) difficult. Although monitoring communication development (option d) is important, Nellie's communication delays warrant more immediate intervention than ongoing observation. Because Nellie has upper limb anomalies in association with Nager syndrome, she cannot use sign language (option e).

15. c. Although Jon has 22q11.2 deletion syndrome, in which hypernasality is often a prominent feature, he is showing symptoms consistent with verbal childhood apraxia of speech. According to a growing amount of literature, this speech disorder is more prevalent than previously known. Hyperkinetic dysarthria (option a) results from lesions of the basal ganglia and is a speech characteristic often associated with Huntington chorea. Although Jon might have symptoms of velopharyngeal inadequacy (option b), the errors made are not considered to be compensatory errors associated with this condition. Jon does not have a phonemically based speech disorder (option d) that affects the phonetic level. Hearing loss (option e) in children with 22q11.2 deletion can occur as a result of the middle ear effusion. However, the errors Jon exhibits are not consistent with a conductive hearing loss. If this were the case, consonants would more than likely be distorted or omitted.

16. a. From the lateral view on multiview videofluoroscopy, the clinician is able to view the length and contour of the velum. In addition, tongue movement during articulation can be observed. Lingual coordination patterns and tongue movement (particularly if used to assist in elevating the velum or used during compensatory movements during speech) can also be observed. All this information is useful in understanding the speech disorder and facilitates intervention planning. Although nasopharyngoscopy (option b) is widely used to obtain valuable information about the function of the soft palate and surrounding structures, it provides only a limited view of the relationship between the tongue and other articulators in speech errors related to oromotor dysfunction. Neither spectrographic measures of perceived hypernasality and articulation nor the Nasometer provide images of velar or lingual movement. Electropalatography (option e) is a useful technique for recording the tongue's contact with the hard palate during speech and has been used successfully to diagnose and treat disordered speech. However, because of the fabrication of a customized artificial plate embedded with electrodes, it is difficult to use as a routine diagnostic tool.

17. e. The cranial nerves involved in Moebius syndrome include the abducens (VI), facial (VII), and, on occasion, trigeminal (V), glossopharyngeus (IX), and hypoglossus (XII). Cranial nerve VII is responsible for facial expression. Bilateral involvement of the buccal or mandibular branches of this nerve, or both, reduces lip rounding on vowels. As a result, all consonants requiring labial movement articulation (/p/, /b/, /m/, /f/, and /v/) would be involved. These sounds are often replaced by compensatory sounds produced by the tongue behind, against, or between the frontal teeth. Some affected patients also have difficulty with tongue mobility. Lingual dental fricatives (option a), glottal fricatives (option b), and lingual alveolar stops (option d) are incorrect because damage to cranial nerve V would probably affect sibilant and affricate productions adversely. Although velar stops (option c) can be produced pharyngeally, they are not affected by cranial nerve VII involvement.

18. d. In view of Mitchell's age, speech difficulties, and concern about the lack of facial expression, the most effective goal of treatment at this time would be to help Mitchell develop strategies to supplement spoken output in order to establish the context of the message. Oromotor stimulation (option a) might be used to improve neuromuscular control in a younger child, but it is less effective in older children. Compensatory strategies to maximize intelligibility (option b) alone might not provide optimal results. Facial reanimation surgery (option c) has been shown to have some promising results and facial exercises after surgery to strengthen the transplanted muscle are often recommended. However, because of Mitchell's current communication needs, postponing a treatment program aimed toward optimizing communication would not be considered the best treatment option at this time. Assistive technology (option e) might be used better to augment oral language than to supplant it.

19. c. The type of hearing loss that occurs most frequently in patients with craniosynostosis is a conductive

hearing loss. It is caused by a variety of otological conditions that affect the middle ear, including middle ear effusion, external canal anomalies, and ossicular fixation. The auditory pathway is not immature (option a) in these cases. The remaining options are incorrect because although sensorineural (option b), mixed (option d), and central hearing losses (option e) can occur in craniosynostosis, they occur less frequently than does conductive impairment.

20. b. Children with fetal alcohol syndrome often exhibit mild to moderate cognitive deficits in the areas of recall, concepts and directions, and social communication. Neuropsychological testing reveals a profile of strengths and weaknesses in a variety of cognitive areas relating to language such as memory and executive function, as well as behavior; this information is crucial for selecting appropriate goals and intervention strategies. Although central auditory processing is often impaired in children with fetal alcohol syndrome, testing (option a) for this would be better deferred pending results of the neuropsychological test. Inconsistent hypernasality suggests that the child is displaying marginal velopharyngeal closure. Articulation is marked only by developmental errors, and there is no suggestion that this child exhibits errors related to velopharyngeal function (option c); however, routine monitoring of resonance is supported. The major problem in these children is brain development and the neurological impairments caused by the alcohol exposure; the prime consideration for care in this case is educational, not neurological (option d). A psychiatric evaluation (option e) may be warranted if the child is taking medication for the attention deficit disorder or if there are other behavioral conditions that necessitate the skills of a psychiatrist.

21. a. Although adolescents with Prader-Willi syndrome have persistent deficits in articulation and in receptive and expressive language, the narrative difficulties and poor conversational skills are notable. Improving intelligibility (option b), improving articulation (option c), improving receptive language (option d), and facilitating self-monitoring skills (option e) are reasonable goals in younger children with Prader-Willi syndrome; however, developing more appropriate skills that facilitate peer and adult interactions would be more reasonable for the adolescent.

22. b. Severe to profound hearing loss is prevalent among patients with CHARGE syndrome. Although selecting and fitting amplification is often difficult, consistent audiological intervention is of paramount importance when communication intervention is implemented for symbolic language development. Because of the communicative challenges and visual and auditory handicaps, it is difficult to ascertain an accurate picture of cognitive ability (option a) and ultimately its relationship to symbolic language. Affected children who do not acquire symbolic language may learn to use prelinguistic communication (option c) such as use of gestures and vocalizations. Although a visual impairment (option d) may adversely affect communication development, there is evidence of better success with amplification. Enrollment in early intervention (option e) for children with CHARGE syndrome is crucial for their communication development, social interaction, and learning, but the progress made is enhanced with optimal audiological intervention.

23. d. Upper airway obstruction is a common, serious problem and can be life-threatening in some patients with Treacher Collins syndrome. Glossoptosis (option a) may be problematic in infancy but is generally not a problem in an 8-year-old; instead, the child exhibits an anterior tongue posture. The anomalous shape of the nasopharynx (option b) can complicate prosthetic fitting. The severity of mandibular hypoplasia (option c) and restricted mouth opening (option e) may complicate access for surgery. Physical management, whether prosthetic or surgical, may serve to further restrict an already restricted airway.

24. a. Although occurring in various forms, lip pits and various forms of orofacial clefting are characteristic features of Van der Woude syndrome. Both the Pierre Robin sequence (option b) and Stickler syndrome (option e) are associated with micrognathia and cleft palate; lower lip pits are not a feature of these disorders. Multiple frenuli, not lower lip pits, are notable features of orofacial digital syndrome (option c), whereas cleft of the soft palate is a feature of otopalatodigital syndrome, type I (option d).

25. c. A frequent finding in patients with hemifacial microsomia is absence of the external ear and auditory canal, which precludes hearing in that ear. The absence of an external ear does not cause an auditory neuropathy (option a). Patients with hemifacial microsomia usually have ossicular fixation and not ossicular discontinuity (option b). Depending on the extent of the middle ear anomaly, an affected patient may experience middle ear effusion (option d), but this is rare in hemifacial microsomia. Underdevelopment of the cochlea (option e), resulting in a sensorineural hearing loss, is a rare occurrence in this disorder.

26. c. An FM system minimizes background noise, reduces the effect of distance between the teacher and Carol, and overrides poor classroom acoustics. Preferential seating (option a) alone would not be considered an optimal recommendation; Carol has a unilateral moderate-severe hearing loss and needs optimal speech-to-noise ratio because the classroom acoustics and speech of the teacher are not constant. A CROS aid (option b) is more useful in a quiet listening situation and is not recommended in situations in which noise could enter on the impaired side and be sent to the "normal" side. This could make it more difficult for the child to understand what is being said. A conventional air-conduction hearing aid (option d) may be appropriate for some children with a unilateral hearing aid; it is recommended if the impaired ear has some usable hearing, but Carol has an atretic ear canal and cannot wear it. Little is known about the effects of a bone-anchored hearing aid (option e) in children with a unilateral hearing loss.

27. a. Infants with Pierre Robin sequence often exhibit retrognathia and glossoptosis severe enough to cause airway obstruction, which is life-threatening. Mandibular lengthening provides for an increase in the anteroposterior dimensions of the airway, making it easier to breathe. Mandibular lengthening may provide for better access to the oral cavity in order to repair the cleft palate, which would aid in speech (option b); however, it would generally not be performed for only this purpose. Although severe retrognathia may adversely affect feeding (option c), nutrition can be supplemented by other means until the airway is issue is resolved. Mandibular lengthening is undertaken in an infant to facilitate breathing and not for cosmetic reasons (option d). The mandible grows during the first year of life and improves facial esthetics. Mandibular lengthening would not be performed to improve dental occlusion (option e), which has no effect on airway.

28. c. No treatment is recommended at this time. May's sibilant errors are related to the dental malocclusion, for which speech therapy (option d) would be ineffective, and the other errors are related to development. According to evidence, orthodontic management (option b) alone cannot correct the skeletal deformity in these patients. May is too young for orthognathic surgery (option e). The tongue crib (option a) is an appliance used to control visceral swallowing and tongue thrusting in infants and to encourage somatic tongue posture and function; May has an obligatory anterior tongue posture in relation to the restricted size of the oral cavity.

29. a. Medial displacement of the carotid artery is commonly seen in patients with 22q11.2 deletion syndrome, the pulsations of which can be viewed on the pharyngeal wall during nasoendoscopy. Knowledge of this is important before the incision site is established for creating the pharyngeal flap used to correct velopharyngeal dysfunction for speech. Most cases of unilateral vocal fold paralysis (option b) may be idiopathic or be the result of injury; it is not a congenital condition associated with 22q11.2 deletion syndrome. Swallowing is generally not impaired (option c) in this syndrome; an infant with 22q11.2 deletion is more likely to experience difficulty drinking because of an unrepaired palatal cleft or other noncleft velopharyngeal dysfunction. Tongue function during articulation (option d) and Passavant's ridge (option e) pose no threat to surgical intervention.

30. d. The unilateral weakness can affect the lips and tongue, which, in turn, compromises an adequate lip seal around a bottle and the adequate formation of a bolus, respectively. Pharyngeal stenosis (option a) is rare in Goldenhar syndrome; however, it is a condition that certainly should not ruled out if feeding continues to be difficult. Glossoptosis (option b) is a typical finding in infants with the Pierre Robin sequence and Stickler syndromes and not in those with Goldenhar syndrome. The mandible, not the maxilla, is hypoplastic (option c) in Goldenhar syndrome. Children with Goldenhar syndrome typically do not have a high narrow palate (option e) but may have a cleft palate or symmetrical palatal elevation.

31. c. Although this child is producing oral consonants after palate surgery, her repertoire is limited. An optimal goal at this time is to expand her consonant inventory. Weak lingual function (option a), poor oromotor control (option b), and decreased tongue mobility (option e) are associated characteristics of Beckwith-Wiedemann syndrome, but improving them would not increase speech and language skills. Learning sign language (option d) is not necessary because the child is adding oral stops to her inventory, which is to be expected after palate repair.

32. b. Conceptual and relational vocabulary is weakest in children with Williams syndrome. Concrete vocabulary (option a), short-term memory (option c), grammar (option d), and expressive vocabulary (option e) are relative strengths in children with Williams syndrome.

33. b. In the older child with Down syndrome, deletion of final consonants is a frequent phonological speech sound error. Deletion of nasal consonants (option a), posterior nasal emission (option c), and

liquid simplification (option e) generally occur with less frequency, particularly at this age. Most errors in sibilants (option d) in a child with Down syndrome are marked by interdentalization and less often by palatalizations.

34. d. Difficulty with pragmatics is a characteristic associated with the fragile X syndrome. The majority of children with Treacher Collins syndrome (option a) and the Pierre Robin sequence (option e) have age-appropriate pragmatic skills. The evidence suggests that children with Down syndrome (option b) have a normal range of pragmatic skills and communicative intentions for their specific developmental level. Children with Sotos syndrome (option c) have average social-behavioral pragmatic characteristics skills.

35. c. The important point is that the child is 8 months old and produces limited babbling. The discussion should focus on what is known about phonological development in infants with Apert syndrome: that they have a reduced phonetic inventory during babbling and early word attempts in comparison with their typically developing peers. The effect of the malocclusion on speech (option a) becomes more obvious as the child gets older. The crowded nasopharynx (option b) results in hyponasality, a resonance disorder, and does not have a direct impact on phonological development. Specific learning difficulties (option d), if present, are generally identified when the child reaches school age. The purpose of the cranial surgery (option e) is to increase intracranial volume to allow for brain growth, and this is discussed with the neurosurgeon.

PART VII

Professional Issues, Psychometrics, and Research

CHAPTER 24

Ethical Practices

David L. Irwin

DISCLAIMER

All case scenarios presented as follows are fictitious and do not depict any specific individual or situation. Any resemblance to an actual situation or person is purely coincidental. Nothing in these questions should be construed as legal advice.

The term *individuals* is used in the following items and can refer to someone who is (1) a member of the American Speech-Language-Hearing Association (ASHA), whether certified or not; (2) a nonmember holding the Certificate of Clinical Competence (CCC) from the ASHA; (3) an applicant for membership or certification; (4) a clinical fellow seeking to fulfill standards for ASHA certification, or (5) a professional licensed by a state with applicable standards and rules for speech-language pathologists (SLPs).

1. Allison is an ASHA-certified SLP in private practice. A patient tells her during a treatment session about his plan to commit suicide. Allison's most important step would be which of the following?
   a. Tell the patient that his life is not that bad and continue speech-language services
   b. Confide in the patient that she at one time considered suicide and that it is important not to act upon those feelings
   c. Refer the patient to the appropriate mental health professional to address the issue of suicide
   d. Have the patient put his plan in writing so she can document the conversation
   e. Ignore the statement since it is a mental health issue and not a speech-language pathology issue

2. An SLP with the CCC from ASHA and licensed by the state works for a public school system. A first-grader is referred to the SLP because of some concerns regarding speech sound errors. During the screening, the SLP also notes that the child has considerable hoarseness and low pitch. The most significant issue for this child is:

a. Refer the child to an otorhinolaryngologist because of the hoarseness and low pitch

b. Determine whether the child fails or passes the screening examination

c. Talk with the classroom teacher about referring all children with hoarseness

d. Administer a test to determine a pattern to the speech sound errors

e. Delay screening until a journal article is located to support proper procedures

3. An SLP has a close friend with a child suspected of having attention deficit disorder (ADD). The close friend asks the SLP to talk with the child and determine whether the child does have ADD. The SLP should do which of the following?

a. Explain to the mother that children with ADD usually require some type of medication

b. Make a direct referral to a psychiatrist

c. Ask the mother to consult with the child's primary care physician and determine the appropriate referral

d. Talk with the child to determine whether there is the presence of a speech-language delay

e. Encourage the mother to do a Web-based search regarding ADD

4. John, CCC-SLP, has full-time employment with a public school and holds a license from the state. Seth, a child at the school, sees John for treatment two times per week for 30 minutes in a small group at the school. Seth's mother thinks more progress would be made if he were served after school for individual treatment for an additional hour per week. She asks John to provide treatment in their home. She assures John that he will be compensated for his time while treating Seth at home. What is the solution for John?

a. John should explain that he has a strict policy not to see patient in their homes or his home

b. John should explain to Seth's mother that group treatment usually ensures interaction with peers during conversation

c. John should provide to Seth's mother a list of other SLPs with CCC-SLP who can also treat Seth after school hours

d. John should ask Seth's mother to give him a call so that they can discuss it outside of school hours

e. John should investigate whether insurance will pay for treatment

5. An SLP earned a master's degree and the CCC about 15 years ago. An adult with a swallowing disorder is referred to her. During the master's degree program, this SLP did not receive any instruction about swallowing disorders. The best solution for this SLP is which of the following?

a. Refer the patient to an SLP who holds the CCC and has proper training and education in the area of swallowing disorders

b. Seek the advice of a recent graduate of a master's degree program about evaluation and treatment strategies

c. Ask her employer to schedule her attendance at a continuing education activity pertaining to swallowing disorders

d. Conduct a screening for the patient referred and then determine whether the swallowing disorder is significant for referral to another source

e. Screen the patient for all speech-language concerns except swallowing

6. Kristin, CCC-SLP, holds a master's degree. She has been oriented and trained regarding securing proper records for her patients. One day at work, an administrator from the State Department of Education comes to Kristin and states that she is there to review Individualized Education Plans (IEPs) for several students. What should be Kristin's first step?

a. Asking the administrator whether she can pull the records or whether the administrator can randomly select them

b. Asking the administrator to properly identify herself as an employee for the State Department of Education and has the authority to request records for review

c. Directing the administrator to the locked filing cabinet where student records are maintained

d. Asking the administrator to wait a few minutes so that Kristin can rearrange her schedule to be present for any questions coming from the review

e. Seek parental consent so the administrator can view records

7. A CCC-SLP who is living in a remote rural area of the United States with a large caseload has a part-time employee as support personnel with a degree in speech communication. This is permitted by the state licensure board, but the SLP wants to have the employee perform speech-language screenings for a local school system. What is the solution for the SLP?

a. Have the employee enroll online at a university and take a course in normal speech and language development before beginning screenings

b. Provide adequate training and supervision to the employee for conducting speech-language screenings

c. Ask the support person to establish a procedure to be used for screenings and check with the SLP before implementing it

d. Limit the support person's activities to only making materials for treatment

e. Conduct a background check regarding the possibility of any prior convictions

8. An ASHA-certified SLP provides treatment for a man with a fluency disorder. After about eight treatment sessions, the patient asks the clinician to go on a trip for the weekend with no other adults present. What should the clinician say to the patient?
   a. Ask the patient to wait and check with the immediate supervisor
   b. Politely decline because the clinician is not interested in dating the patient
   c. Let the patient know that he will be treated by another clinician starting with the next visit
   d. Tell the patient that it is unethical for a professional to have personal relationship for which he or she exercises professional authority
   e. Encourage the patient to communicate by using Facebook or MySpace

9. Sarah, CCC-SLP and a member of ASHA, has recently hired a part-time SLP for the private practice. After about a month, Sarah learns that the person she recently hired is homosexual. Sarah believes that she may have been misled about the employee's qualifications and that the part-time SLP should have disclosed sexual orientation during the interview. What ethical principle of the ASHA (2003) Code of Ethics should guide her decision?
   a. Principle I, which basically states that the welfare of persons served is paramount
   b. Principle II, which primarily states that a professional should achieve and maintain the highest level of professional competence
   c. Principle III, which basically states that professionals should promote the profession to the public
   d. Principle IV, which primarily states that relationships with colleagues, students, and members of allied health professions shall uphold dignity and harmonious relationships
   e. None of the above

10. Kelley, CCC-SLP, is getting on the elevator and sees a physician who referred a patient for a voice evaluation. There are other people on the elevator, with Kelley and the physician in a corner. Kelley tells the physician that the patient, John M., is probably experiencing a period of depression. Kelley tells the physician about her intent to refer John M. to a psychologist. The referring physician nods and agrees. Which of the following ethical rules from ASHA did Kelley primarily violate?
    a. Individuals should not guarantee the results of any treatment or procedure
    b. Individuals shall not reveal, without authorization, any professional or personal information about identified persons served professionally
    c. Individuals shall use every resource to ensure that high-quality service is provided

d. Individuals shall not engage in dishonesty, fraud, deceit, misrepresentation, sexual harassment, or any other form of conduct that adversely reflects on the professions or on the individual's fitness to serve persons professionally
e. Individuals shall treat a patient solely by correspondence

11. A child with very poor speech intelligibility is being served by an SLP who holds the CCC from ASHA. The SLP is meeting with the child's mother and is making a recommendation for an augmentative communication system. The electronic speech-generating device being considered would be used both at home and school. The SLP also holds a contract with a vendor that dispenses augmentative communication devices as a part-time consultant. The SLP should be guided primarily by which of the following rules of ethics?
    a. Individuals shall not charge for services not rendered, and they shall not misrepresent services rendered, products dispensed, or research and scholarly activities conducted
    b. Individuals shall continue their professional development throughout their careers
    c. Individuals' statements to the public shall adhere to prevailing professional standards and shall not contain misrepresentation
    d. Individuals shall not participate in professional interactions that constitute a conflict of interest
    e. Individuals shall use every resource possible when treating patients

12. A certified SLP has established a Web page that provides general information about speech and language disorders. The Web page has information about developmental milestones and indicators of potential delays. An e-mail address is provided for people to contact the SLP with questions. Under which of the following conditions may this situation be an ethical violation?
    a. If the SLP requires a fee to answer any questions
    b. If the SLP provides an additional link to the ASHA Web site
    c. If the SLP asks the person who sends and is asked (sender) to provide general information about a child without identifying data or protected health information
    d. If the SLP provides more information about general speech and language behaviors
    e. If the SLP provides a checklist of developmental milestones

13. A speech and hearing clinic at a university charges for treatment services on a semester basis. The patient pays one fee ($200) at the beginning of the semester for 15 treatment sessions. A certain patient misses 6 sessions during the semester. The director of the clinic,

who holds ASHA CCC, could be violating which of the following rules of ethics?

a. Individuals shall engage in the provision of clinical services only when they hold the appropriate CCC or when they are in the certification process and are supervised by an individual who holds the appropriate CCC

b. Individuals shall not provide clinical services solely by correspondence

c. Individuals shall not charge for services not rendered and shall not misrepresent services rendered, products dispensed, or research and scholarly activities conducted

d. Individuals shall prohibit anyone under their supervision from engaging in any practice that violates the ASHA (2003) Code of Ethics

e. Individuals shall use persons in research or as subjects of teaching demonstrations only with their informed consent

14. An SLP is the owner of a local rehabilitation company. Several years ago, the SLP let her CCC lapse. The SLP has employed two clinical fellow–SLP clinicians and did not disclose that her certification is not current with ASHA. At the end of the clinical fellowship, the clinicians are told by ASHA that their supervisor is not currently certified. What is their first step?

a. The persons employed during the clinical fellow year with the non-CCC SLP should be allowed to count a portion of their time, because they were misled

b. The non-CCC SLP should be reported to the appropriate agencies, including third-party payers, state licensure board, and so forth, about her conduct

c. The non-CCC SLP should contact ASHA immediately to inquire about getting the CCC-SLP reinstated and made retroactive

d. Because the non-CCC SLP does not hold ASHA certification, there is little that can be done in terms of a reprimand or correcting the behavior

e. The persons employed during the clinical fellow year with the non-CCC SLP cannot count their time.

15. Treating patients with a tracheotomy is required as part of a job in a local hospital. This information was made known during an interview. An SLP who worked with children for several years decides to accept the job. After 2 weeks of employment, the supervisor at the local hospital requires a patient with a tracheotomy to be seen in the intensive care unit. What should the new employee's first action be?

a. The evening before the evaluation of the patient, the new employee should read all materials and books about treating patients with a tracheotomy that were taught during graduate school

b. Explain to the patient that in a few days someone will be able to provide services regarding the tracheotomy

c. Immediately resign the position

d. Refer the patient immediately to an SLP who has the competence, training, and experience with patients who have a tracheotomy

e. Consult the ASHA Board of Ethics regarding the violation with an anonymous letter

16. An SLP with the CCC who works in a community-based center provides hearing screenings. Because of budgetary problems, however, the portable audiometer has not been calibrated in 2 years. The supervisor of the SLP is not an SLP and does not support having the audiometer calibrated because of continuing budget problems. Who is primarily at greater risk for an ethical violation?

a. The SLP conducting the hearing screenings

b. The supervisor of the SLP who does not have the CCC and is a special educator

c. The supervisor and the SLP because of not implementing appropriate safeguards for patients

d. The director of the community-based agency who oversees funding from grants and other organizations

e. Another SLP who knows that the audiometer has not been calibrated

17. An SLP is director of a speech and hearing department in a large hospital. The SLP's list of credentials includes the CCC in SLP and audiology (CCC-A). The SLP holds the CCC-SLP; however, the SLP holds only a license as a hearing aid dispenser in another state and does not hold the CCC in audiology. What is the best solution for the SLP?

a. List the credentials as holding the CCC-SLP and the appropriate listing as an audiology assistant

b. Resign the position as director because credentials to the public have been misrepresented

c. List the credentials as holding the CCC-SLP and the license to dispense hearing aids by state, and not list the CCC in audiology

d. Talk with the administration at the hospital about including hearing aid dispensing as part of the services

e. Clearly post all certificates on the wall of an office

18. An adult with aphasia has been referred to a local outpatient clinic. The outpatient clinic offers an array of therapy services, including physical therapy, occupational therapy, and speech-language treatment. The patient is informed that several other clinics are available in the same town for services, but many do not have an SLP with extensive experience with adults. The SLP at the outpatient clinic talks with the family and provides a list of workshops attended in the past

5 years about dealing with aphasia. For the SLP, this may be an ethical dilemma for which of the following reasons?
a. The SLP has not continued professional development throughout the career
b. The SLP has provided a statement to the public that may not adhere to prevailing professional standards and may contain misrepresentations
c. The SLP may have engaged in fraud or deceit
d. The SLP is providing misleading information and possibly violating patient rights
e. The SLP may be practicing by telecommunication when it is not allowed by law

19. In the advertising section of the phone book, the advertisement for a licensed SLP with the CCC includes the description "state-certified swallowing therapist"; however, the licensure board does not provide specific endorsement or specialty recognition. What is the best option for the SLP?
a. Determine from the licensure board whether specialty recognition will be available for swallowing therapy by the next time the phone book is published
b. Display the certification as a "state-certified swallowing therapist" on the wall of the patient waiting room
c. Ask the licensure board if an exception can be made and provide the board with extensive documentation about trainings
d. Seek specialty recognition from ASHA as a swallowing therapist
e. Remove the designation from the advertisement at the next opportunity and place a sign at the front desk that the state does not designate a specialty as a swallowing therapist

20. In a hospital, an SLP who holds the CCC is supervising graduate students from a local university. During the internship, a graduate student is asked by the supervisor to perform a diagnostic evaluation without having previously consulted about the case; no supervision is provided during the evaluation. What is most important about this situation?
a. The welfare of the patient is paramount, and it is important that the student consult with the supervisor before evaluating a patient
b. The supervisor has signed an evaluation report without supervising the student
c. The student should be allowed to show independent judgment during the internship
d. The student should be referred to the Academic Misconduct Committee at the university
e. The supervisor is extremely busy and the student provides some help with managing the workload

21. A professor who holds the CCC-SLP has been the major adviser for a doctoral student. The results from the dissertation are submitted to a refereed journal, but the professor asks the student to list him as first author. What is the primary ethical dilemma in this situation?
a. Individuals shall continue their professional development throughout their careers
b. Individuals shall use persons in research or as subjects of teaching demonstrations only with their informed consent
c. Individuals shall not participate in professional activities that constitute a conflict of interest
d. Individuals whose professional services are adversely affected by substance abuse or other health-related conditions shall seek professional assistance, and when appropriate, withdraw from the affected areas of practice
e. None of the above

22. An SLP with the CCC works with a licensed physical therapist who is a native of Iran. The SLP mentions to a patient that the physical therapist was recently interviewed by the U.S. Federal Bureau of Investigation (FBI). The patient tells the physical therapist that he is discontinuing services because of a possible connection with terrorists. Specifically, what ethical rule was violated by the SLP in this situation?
a. Individuals shall not discriminate in the delivery of professional services or the conduct of research and scholarly activities on the basis of race or ethnicity, gender, age, religion, national origin, sexual orientation, or disability
b. Individuals shall not discriminate in their relationships with colleagues, students, and members of allied professions on the basis of race or ethnicity, gender, age, religion, national origin, sexual orientation, or disability
c. Individuals whose professional services are adversely affected by substance abuse or other health-related conditions shall seek professional assistance and, when appropriate, withdraw from the affected areas of practice
d. Individuals shall adequately and appropriately secure records of professional services rendered, research, and scholarly activities conducted, and products dispensed and shall allow access to these records only when authorized or when required by law
e. Individuals shall prohibit anyone under their supervision from engaging in any practice that violates the ASHA (2003) Code of Ethics

23. An SLP with a CCC is providing a workshop to a group of professionals about language and literacy development in children. What is most important with regard to documentation?

a. Not to misrepresent credentials of assistants, technicians, or support personnel and to inform those served professionally of the names and professional credentials of persons providing services

b. Not to provide clinical services solely by correspondence

c. To reference the source when using other person's ideas, research, presentations, or productions in written, oral, or any other media presentation summary

d. Not to participate in professional activities that constitute a conflict of interest

e. To provide practice by telecommunication (e.g., telehealth; e-health) when not prohibited by law

24. An SLP with a CCC enters into a cooperative agreement with a pediatrician that children seen by the pediatrician will be referred to the SLP. The SLP realizes it is important to have a physician referral for reimbursement. What is the most important ethical rule for the SLP to follow in this situation?

a. Individuals shall not provide professional services without exercising independent judgment, regardless of referral source or prescription

b. Individuals shall not provide clinical services solely by correspondence

c. Individuals shall delegate the provision of clinical services only to (1) persons who hold the appropriate CCC; (2) persons in the education or certification process who are appropriately supervised by the person who holds the appropriate CCC; or (3) assistants, technicians, or support personnel who are adequately supervised by an individual who holds the appropriate CCC

d. Individuals shall not guarantee the results of any treatment or procedure

e. Individuals shall ensure that all equipment used in the provision of services or to conduct research and scholarly activities is in proper working order and is properly calibrated

25. An SLP with a CCC has become aware that a business partner with the CCC and state license is committing fraud against Medicaid with the billing practices. Of the following principles, which is most important for the SLP witnessing the fraud to remember?

a. Individuals shall not discriminate in their relationships with colleagues, students, and members of allied professions on the basis of race or ethnicity

b. Individuals who have reason to believe that the ASHA (2003) Code of Ethics has been violated shall inform the Board of Ethics for ASHA

c. Individuals shall not engage in dishonesty, fraud, deceit, misrepresentation, sexual harassment, or any other form of conduct that adversely reflects

on the professions or on the individual's fitness to serve persons professionally

d. Individuals shall not misrepresent diagnostic information, research, services rendered, or products dispensed

e. Individuals shall use persons in research or as subjects of teaching demonstrations only with their informed consent

26. Jane, CCC-SLP, has proper documentation to report an ethical violation about another certified SLP regarding clinical services. However, Jane does not want to provide any personal identification to the ASHA Board of Ethics, and she sends a letter without her signature. What ethical violation has Jane committed?

a. Individuals shall not misrepresent diagnostic information, research, services, rendered, or products dispensed; they shall also not engage in any scheme to defraud in connection with obtaining payment or reimbursement for such services and products

b. Individuals shall prohibit anyone under their supervision from engaging in any practice that violates the ASHA (2003) Code of Ethics

c. Individuals shall not discriminate in their relationships with colleagues, students, and members of allied professions on the basis of race, ethnicity, gender, age, religion, national origin, sexual orientation, or disability

d. Individuals shall evaluate the effectiveness of services rendered and of products dispensed and shall provide services or dispense products only when benefit can reasonably be expected

e. Individuals shall comply fully with the policies of the Board of Ethics in its consideration and adjudication of complaints of violations of the ASHA (2003) Code of Ethics

27. Joshua, CCC-SLP, is conducting a research project with young adults, 21 to 26 years old, who have a diagnosis of autism spectrum disorder and language delay. Joshua reviews patient files from the hospital where he is employed and calls the young adults on the phone and asks them if they would like to be in his research study. With this method of research solicitation, what ethical violation is Joshua most likely to be violating at this point?

a. Individuals shall not provide clinical services solely by correspondence

b. Individuals whose professional services are adversely affected by substance abuse or other health-related conditions shall seek professional assistance and, when appropriate, withdraw from the affected areas of practice

c. Individuals shall evaluate the effectiveness of services rendered and of products dispensed and shall provide services or dispense products only when benefit can reasonably be expected

d. Individuals shall use persons in research or as subjects of teaching demonstrations only with their informed consent

e. Individuals shall not provide professional services without exercising independent professional judgment, regardless of referral source or prescription

28. Kim, CCC-SLP, works for a skilled nursing facility and uses a computer to submit progress notes and other reports. Her computer has a password for access. One day while at work, Kim writes down the new password for the computer on a piece of paper and takes it with her to treat a patient. She accidentally leaves the password in the patient's file. Other employees also have access to the file and the patient's family has requested a copy of the most recent progress notes. What ethical violation is Kim most likely to be violating?

a. Individuals may practice telecommunication (e.g., telehealth or e-health), when not prohibited by law

b. Individuals shall provide clinical services solely by correspondence

c. Individuals shall adequately maintain and appropriately secure records of professional services rendered, research and scholarly activities conducted, and products dispensed and shall allow access to these records only when authorized or when required by law

d. Individuals shall ensure that all equipment used in the provision of services or to conduct research and scholarly activities is in proper working order and is properly calibrated

e. Individuals shall not participate in professional activities that constitute a professional conflict of interest

29. Mrs. Noble is obtaining therapy services at a community-based clinic for her 4-year-old daughter, who has a diagnosis of Down syndrome. Mrs. Noble has asked Sarah, CCC-SLP, who treats Mrs. Noble's daughter for a speech and language delay, not to submit an insurance claim for 3 months because, as a result, the deductible will be paid for by other services such as occupational therapy and physical therapy. What is the appropriate course of action for Sarah in this situation?

a. Submit the claims within the appropriate time frame required by the insurance company, but document about half of the sessions as a "no show" and treat the child anyway

b. Collaborate with the occupational therapist to determine which claims may be submitted and reduce the cost of out-of-pocket (i.e., deductible) for Mrs. Noble

c. Submit all claims in the time frame required by the insurance company, but inquire about a patient assistance payment plan from the community-based clinic

d. Ask Mrs. Noble whether she can afford speech-language services at the local university, which has graduate students providing services under faculty with CCC-SLP

e. Convene a committee at work to review policies and procedures

30. Chris, CCC-SLP, is doing a research project with children. Chris administers some language tests and then asks the children to give a description of something they would like to see different at home. What should Chris do if a child reports that people buy drugs at his home and he is afraid of them?

a. Report the information immediately to the local police

b. Ask the child not to say anything about this for 2 weeks and see if it continues

c. Help the child find a foster parent

d. Ask the parent about the response given by the child

e. Ignore the response from the child

31. A certified SLP has been in practice for 25 years and continues to perform all diagnostic testing as it was taught during graduate school. What ethical violation is most likely occurring?

a. Individuals shall continue their professional development throughout their careers

b. Individuals shall not guarantee the results of any treatment or procedure, directly or by implication; however, they may make a reasonable statement of prognosis

c. Individuals whose professional services are adversely affected by substance abuse or other health-related conditions shall seek professional assistance and, when appropriate, withdraw from the affected areas of practice

d. Individuals shall not participate in professional activities that constitute a conflict of interest

e. Individuals' statements to colleagues about professional services, research results, and products shall adhere to prevailing professional standards and shall contain no misrepresentation

32. During a diagnostic interview with Carolyn, CCC-SLP, the mother of a patient reports that there is a family history of bipolar disorder. How should Carolyn respond to this statement?

a. Tell the mother that some research studies have found mental illness and speech-language disorders can co-occur

b. Ask the mother whether she would like to make an appointment with the psychologist working at the same facility

c. Have the mother document any self-injurious behaviors occurring during the past year
d. Have the mother list all medications taken for treatment of the bipolar disorder by any family members
e. Have the mother review the *DSM-IV-TR* (American Psychiatric Association, 2000) manual to indicate specific diagnostic criteria for bipolar disorder

33. Two graduate students working with a certified SLP were assigned to perform only observations by the university. As the semester progressed, the students began helping patients complete case history forms. The students wore name badges identifying their status and introduced themselves as graduate students when they met patients. The patients were told that the certified SLP would review the case history and conduct the testing. What is the appropriate course of action?
    a. The graduate students should complete all case history information and add their written observations when the reports are submitted to the supervisor
    b. The certified SLP should conduct the case history and the students should observe
    c. The university supervisor should be contacted by the students to determine whether they could also be involved while the patients are being tested
    d. The certified SLP should conduct a more thorough orientation for the students and train them how to complete a case history form
    e. The students should be referred to the grievance procedures office at the university

34. Mary, CCC-SLP, uses programming software for an augmentative communication device. The manufacturer reports in the manual that the software can be used successfully by 98% of the patients. Mary should assist all patients in understanding which of the following about the software?
    a. The device is to be used with proper charging of the battery; otherwise, the software will not operate
    b. She would not charge for services to install the software on a communication device
    c. She would hire a technician from the company that wrote the software to conduct the training for patients under her supervision
    d. The effectiveness of services rendered and products dispensed shall be evaluated with no guarantee of results
    e. Show the results of successful applications used by other patients, including phone numbers to follow up

35. Kathy, CCC-SLP, works for a school system as a full-time SLP. Kathy receives a phone call about the mother of a close friend, living in another state, who has had a stroke and is exhibiting poor word recall and "garbled speech." Kathy's close friend asks for advice about treatment strategies. Kathy should point out which of the following to the close friend?
    a. Ensure that her friend's mother has an augmentative means of communicating while in the hospital to convey her wants and needs
    b. Ethically, Kathy can provide general information about how to help her friend's mother but cannot provide any specific treatment recommendations
    c. Provide the friend the listing of a good SLP who lives in the same city
    d. Listen to her friend's mother over the phone and see if she has other speech-language problems related to her stroke
    e. Write a letter to the mother of her friend describing the characteristics of aphasia and dysarthria and how treatment should proceed

36. John is considering opening a private practice in speech-language pathology. He has 4 years of experience working in a skilled nursing facility. He wants to inform the public about his services and credentials through an advertisement in the phone book. Of the following rules, which should he consult when developing the advertisement?
    a. Individuals shall engage in the provision of clinical services when they hold the appropriate CCC or when they are in the certification process and supervised by an individual who holds the appropriate CCC
    b. Individuals' statements to the public—advertising, announcing, and marketing their professional services; reporting research results; and promoting products—shall adhere to prevailing professional standards and shall not contain misrepresentations
    c. Individuals shall prohibit anyone under their supervision from engaging in any practice that can violate a code of ethics
    d. Individuals shall ensure that all equipment in the provision of services or to conduct research and scholarly activities is in proper working order and is properly installed
    e. Individuals shall reference the source when using other person's ideas, research, presentations, or products in written, oral, or any other media presentation or summary

37. Joyce, CCC-SLP, has been employed by a school system for 22 years. A colleague, a classroom teacher, suspects that Joyce has come to work intoxicated a few times within the past 2 months. She reports the situation to Karen, CCC-SLP, the speech-language services coordinator for the school system. What is Karen's priority for this situation?

a. Individuals shall prohibit anyone under their supervision from engaging in any practice that violates the code of ethics

b. Individuals shall not provide professional services without exercising independent professional judgment, regardless of referral source or prescription

c. Individuals shall not discriminate in their relationship with colleagues, students, and members of allied professions on the basis of race, ethnicity, gender, age, religion, national origin, sexual orientation, or disability

d. Individuals shall not engage in dishonesty, fraud, deceit, misrepresentation, sexual harassment, or any other form of conduct that adversely reflects on the professions or on the individual's fitness to serve person professionally

e. Individuals shall continue their professional development throughout their careers

38. Joan, CCC-SLP, is working for a rehabilitation agency that serves several skilled nursing facilities. Patients with Alzheimer disease are referred to Joan, but she has not received any formal training about the disease and related communication disorders. Joan could be reported to the ASHA Board of Ethics and to the state licensure board for what reason?

a. Individuals shall not provide professional services without exercising independent professional judgment, regardless of referral source or prescription

b. Individuals shall evaluate the effectiveness of services rendered and of products dispensed and shall provide services or dispense products only when benefit can reasonably be expected

c. Individuals shall reference the source when using other persons' ideas, research presentations, or products in written, oral, or any other media presentation or summary

d. Individuals shall not provide clinical services solely by correspondence

e. Individuals shall engage only aspects of the professions that are within the scope of their competence, considering their level of education, training, and experience

39. Christopher, CCC-SLP, works at a small hospital in a community where he was born and raised. He is asked by his supervisor to evaluate the young child of an employee of the hospital. After the evaluation, Christopher's supervisor asks about the results of the evaluation and whether he plans to provide treatment. The most important ethical principle for Christopher is:

a. Individuals shall not reveal, without authorization, any professional or personal information about identified person served professionally or identified

participants involved in research and scholarly activities unless required by law to do so or unless doing so is necessary to protect the welfare of the person or of the community or otherwise required by law

b. Individuals shall not provide professional services without exercising independent professional judgment, regardless of referral source or prescription

c. Individuals shall engage in only aspects of the professions that are within the scope of their competence, considering their level of education, training, and experience

d. Individuals shall not charge for services not rendered, and they shall not misrepresent services rendered, products dispensed, or research and scholarly activities conducted

e. Individuals' statements to colleagues about professional services, research results, and products shall adhere to prevailing professional standards and shall contain no misrepresentations

40. A professor at a university with a graduate program in speech-language pathology believes strongly that students should obtain clinical experience with persons who have fluency disorders. The professor, who holds CCC-SLP, has continued to schedule a patient for maintenance services for 3 years so that students can obtain clinical experience with fluency disorders. What should the Clinic Coordinator, who also holds the CCC-SLP, do about the situation?

a. Ask that the patient increase frequency of visits so that more students can be scheduled to obtain clinical experience

b. Discuss with the professor about how students must also obtain clinical experience with children

c. Discuss with the professor how this situation of continuing to schedule the patient for maintenance services solely for the purpose of providing clinical experience with students may be unethical

d. Report the professor to the Program Director as noncompliant with clinical policy and procedures

e. Consult with current coordinator of the special interest division regarding fluency at ASHA

41. Michelle, CCC-SLP, is married to a local physician. Her husband's partner frequently refers patients for swallowing therapy to Michelle, who owns a small private practice. Michelle should be most concerned with which of the following?

a. Individuals shall engage in the provision of clinical services only when they hold the appropriate CCC

b. Individuals shall use persons in research or as subjects of teaching demonstrations only with their informed consent

c. Individuals' statements to colleagues about professional services, research results, and products shall adhere to prevailing professional standards and shall contain no misrepresentation

d. Individuals shall refer those served professionally solely on the basis of the interest of those being referred and not on the basis of any personal financial interest

e. Individuals may practice by telecommunication (e.g., telehealth; e-health), when not prohibited by law

42. An SLP is employed full-time as a clinical supervisor at a university. The SLP also is in a group private practice in the same town. A mother says that she needs to have her child seen for treatment as soon as possible, but the clinic at the university does not have any available slots. The SLP refers the mother to the private practice group but does not have the case assigned to her. What ethical principle and rule is most important for the SLP?

a. Individuals shall refer those served professionally solely on the basis of the interest of those being served and not on the basis of any personal financial interest

b. Individuals shall not provide clinical services solely by correspondence

c. Individuals shall not use persons in research or as subjects of teaching demonstrations only with their informed consent

d. Individuals shall not misrepresent the credentials of assistants, technicians, or support personnel and shall inform those they serve professionally of the name and professional credentials of the person providing services

e. Individuals shall ensure that all equipment used in the provision of services or to conduct research and scholarly activities is in proper working order and is properly calibrated

43. Dr. Williams, CCC-SLP, just received the Doctor of Education in Leadership degree through a distance learning program. In an informational lecture to a group of senior citizens at a hospital seminar on good health, Dr. Williams boasts that as an SLP with a doctoral degree, he can diagnose swallowing disorders without the use of specific equipment or the consultation of an otolaryngologist. How might this be a violation of ethics?

a. The completion of the doctoral degree does not allow Dr. Williams to ignore the use of available equipment and technology

b. Dr. Williams is guaranteeing the results of a treatment or procedure without a reasonable statement of prognosis

c. The situation is not of ethical concern, because Dr. Williams is not actually treating any of the patients in the audience

d. Dr. Williams does not mention to the audience the importance of equipment calibration

e. Dr. Williams is not assigning credit to those who have contributed to the presentation

44. A professor with CCC-SLP wants to enhance the class being taught about treating patients with a laryngectomy. The professor videotapes several patients at the Veterans Affairs hospital. The professor shares the videotapes with graduate students and believes they are improving their knowledge and skills. What ethical violation has occurred in this situation?

a. Individuals may practice by telecommunication (e.g., telehealth; e-health) when not prohibited by law

b. Individuals shall continue their professional development throughout their careers

c. Individuals shall not require or permit their professional staff to provide services or conduct research activities that exceed the staff member's competence, level of education, training, and experience

d. Individuals shall use persons in research or as subjects of teaching demonstrations only with their informed consent

e. Individuals shall not misrepresent their credentials, competence, education, training, experience, or scholarly or research contributions

45. Jeri, clinical fellow–SLP, is working for a rehabilitation company that contracts with a skilled nursing facility. Jeri has received referrals for patients, but very few meet the criteria of receiving benefit from services. One day, Jeri is absent from work, and her clinical fellow supervisor, Mike, comes to the facility, screens several patients, and leaves a note for Jeri that all of these patients screened will need an evaluation and plan of care for treatment. What is the best option for Jeri at this point?

a. Resign the position because Mike is not a good example of a supervisor

b. Review the documentation Mike has left, determine whether she agrees with the results, and then make a decision

c. Report Mike to the Board of Ethics and state licensure board

d. Ask to attend a workshop that will help improve her clinical skills and become more proficient in clinical knowledge and skills

e. Ask for a meeting with the Director of Nursing at the facility regarding how patient services are provided when she is not there

Answers

1. c. According the ASHA (2003) Code of Ethics, Principle I, Rule B, individuals shall use every resource, including referral when appropriate, to ensure that high-quality service is provided. A referral to the appropriate mental health professional is necessary.

2. b. The SLP must first determine whether the child fails or passes a screening regardless of the reason for referral. According to the ASHA (2003) Code of Ethics, Principle I, Rule B, individuals shall use every resource, including referral when appropriate, to ensure that high-quality service is provided. In this case, the child may need a referral to another professional, but first the SLP must determine whether the child passes or fails criteria to warrant a referral. All aspects of communication should be addressed during a screening to ensure that high-quality service is provided.

3. c. The SLP should ask the mother to consult the child's primary care physician to determine the appropriate referral. According the ASHA (2003) Code of Ethics, Principle I, Rule B, individuals shall use every resource, including referral when appropriate, to ensure that high-quality service is provided. Children with ADD may have a speech-language delay or disorder; however, the formal diagnosis for ADD is not within the scope of practice of a certified SLP.

4. c. According to the ASHA (2003) Code of Ethics, Principle I, Rule B, individuals shall use every resource, including referral when appropriate, to ensure that high-quality service is provided. Although John does hold the CCC-SLP from ASHA, the parent should be informed that other SLPs with similar credentials may also provide services to Seth. In consideration of the ASHA Code of Ethics, Principle I, Rule H, John should explain to Seth's mother that additional time for Seth does not guarantee results of any treatment or procedure. John should consult with his employer or state licensure board, or both, regarding the potential for a conflict of interest, inasmuch as he provides services to Seth within the school setting.

5. a. Since the SLP does not possess the knowledge, skills, and judgment abilities to conduct an evaluation of the patient referred for a swallowing disorder, she should refer the patient to an SLP who holds the CCC and does have the proper training. According to the ASHA (2003) Code of Ethics, Principle I,

Rule B, individuals shall use every resource, including referral when appropriate, to ensure that high-quality service is provided. Furthermore, the SLP should abide by the Principle II, Rules B and C, according to which B individuals shall engage in only aspects of the profession that are within the scope of their competence, in view of their level of education, training, and experience, and C individuals shall continue their professional development throughout their careers and seek continuing education activities regarding swallowing disorders.

6. b. The administrator from the State Department of Education should be asked to provide proper documentation regarding her identity. If this can be done, then Kristin should check to see whether the administrator has the proper and legal authority to review confidential records. According to the ASHA (2003) Code of Ethics, Principle I, Rule K, individuals shall adequately maintain and secure records of professional services rendered, research and scholarly activities conducted, and products dispensed and shall allow access to these records only when authorized or when required by law.

7. b. Because the employment of the support personnel is allowed by the state licensing board, it is of primary importance that personnel be adequately trained and supervised by an individual who holds the CCC. According to the ASHA (2003) Code of Ethics, Principle I, Rule E, individuals with CCC may delegate support services to assistants, technicians, support personnel, students, or any other persons only if those services are adequately supervised by an individual who holds the appropriate CCC.

8. d. According to the ASHA (2003) Code of Ethics, Principle IV, Rule C, individuals shall not engage in sexual activities with clients or students over whom they exercise professional authority. The clinician in this question clearly has professional authority for the treatment of the patient. The clinician should also review the code of conduct for the employment setting regarding personal relationships and discuss this with the supervisor.

9. d. According to Principle IV from the ASHA (2003) Code of Ethics, individuals shall honor responsibilities to the professions and their relationships with colleagues, students, and members of allied professions. According to Principle IV, Rule H, individuals shall not discriminate in their

relationships with colleagues, students, and members of allied professions on the basis of race or ethnicity, gender, age, religion, national origin, sexual orientation, or disability.

10. b. Kelley violated Principle I, Rule L, because she told the referring physician in a nonsecured space (the elevator) about her intent to refer John M. to a psychologist because of depression. According to the ASHA (2003) Code of Ethics, Principle I, Rule L, individuals shall not reveal, without authorization, any professional or personal information about identified persons served professionally or identified participants involved in research and scholarly activities unless required by law to do so or unless doing so is necessary to protect the welfare of the person or of the community or is otherwise required by law.

11. d. The SLP should be aware primarily of the ASHA (2003) Code of Ethics, Principle III, Rule B, because there is a potential for a conflict of interest. The SLP has not recommended that the parent purchase the device or specifically use the device by a specific vendor. If the SLP does recommend a device sold by the vendor for which she is a part-time consultant, then the potential for a conflict of interest exists. The SLP should fully inform the mother that she is a part-time consultant and that other vendors have options for her child.

12. a. The SLP could be violating the ASHA (2003) Code of Ethics, Principle III, Rule F, according to which individuals' statements to the public—advertising, announcing, and marketing their professional services; reporting research results; and promoting products—shall adhere to prevailing professional standards and shall not contain misrepresentations. If the SLP did not state anywhere on the Web page that a fee was required for a reply to questions through e-mail, then the SLP could be in violation of Principle III, Rule F. Providing additional links, such as the ASHA Web page and not inquiring about specific information from the person who sent the e-mail would not constitute misrepresentation or conflict with prevailing Health Insurance Portability and Accountability Act (HIPAA) standards.

13. c. Because the patient paid for services and not all of those were rendered, then the SLP could be in violation of the ASHA (2003) Code of Ethics, Principle I, Rule M, according to which individuals shall not charge for services not rendered nor shall they misrepresent services rendered, products dispensed, or research and scholarly activities conducted. The clinic director must establish that patients are charged for services only after they have been rendered and not allow for one "up front" fee for a semester. If this policy change is implemented, the clinic director and other clinical supervisors must prohibit anyone under their supervision from violating the Code of Ethics (option d).

14. b. Because the professional supervising the clinical fellow–SLP employees did not disclose that the CCC had lapsed, this could be a violation of the ASHA (2003) Code of Ethics, Principle III, Rule A, according to which individuals shall not misrepresent their credentials, competence, education, training, experience, or scholarly or research contribution. If the non-CCC SLP collected payment from insurance companies that required the CCC, then this is a violation of misrepresenting credentials. Furthermore, if a state licensure board is applicable to this case, then the board should be contacted regarding future actions by the clinical fellow–SLPs.

15. d. The new employee should first make certain that the patient is referred to a professional with competence, training, and experience with patients who have a tracheotomy. According to the ASHA (2003) Code of Ethics, Principle I, Rule B, individuals shall use every resource, including referral when appropriate, to ensure that high-quality service is provided. The welfare of the patient is paramount, and the new employee must make certain that the patient's needs are met first. The new employee should discuss with the supervisor competence, training, and experience involving a tracheotomy, and then a decision should be made regarding continued employment or misrepresentation by the new employee.

16. a. The SLP conducting the hearing screenings is ultimately responsible for patient care and procedural safeguards. According to the ASHA (2003) Code of Ethics, Principle II, Rule F, individuals shall ensure that all equipment used in the provision of services or to conduct research and scholarly activities is in proper working order and is properly calibrated. The audiometer is to be calibrated annually, and the SLP needs to inform the supervisor that continuing to use the audiometer without calibration is an ethical violation. The supervisor is not bound by the ASHA Code of Ethics, but needs to approve the calibration; otherwise, the hearing screenings will not continue as a service.

17. c. The SLP should list only the credentials that are appropriate for practice within the state. According to the ASHA (2003) Code of Ethics, Principle III, Rule A, individuals shall not misrepresent their credentials, competence, education, training, experience,

or scholarly or research contributions. The CCC-SLP is a national certification, and it is appropriate for the SLP in this case to list that as a credential; however, the hearing aid dispensing license is for another state and is not the equivalent of the CCC for audiology. The SLP should designate that the hearing aid dispensing license is only for a particular state and not list the CCC-A as a credential.

18. b. The SLP has continued professional development by showing the patient the workshops attended and extensive expertise. This information is not misleading or fraudulent because attendance at the trainings is documented. However, the SLP may be violating an ethical rule. According to the ASHA (2003) Code of Ethics, Principle III, Rule F, individuals' statements to the public—advertising, announcing, and marketing their professional services; reporting research results; and promoting products—shall adhere to prevailing professional standards and shall not contain misrepresentations. Providing a listing of all training in aphasia in the past 5 years to the patient does not typically conform to standards within the community. A certificate or proof of completion of a workshop may be on the wall of the office of the SLP; however, most health care providers (including physicians, nurses, physical therapists, and so forth) would not show a list of their training unless requested by the patient or family. The patient and family should be encouraged to visit with SLPs at other clinics in the community and make an independent decision.

19. e. The state licensure board does not have the specialty recognition at the current time; therefore, the SLP must remove it from the advertisement at the next opportunity the phone book is published and must also immediately put a sign disclosing to the public in the lobby or in other forms of correspondence that the state does not have a specialty recognition for a swallowing therapist. According to the ASHA (2003) Code of Ethics, Principle III, Rule F, individuals' statements to the public—advertising, announcing, and marketing their professional credentials; reporting research results; and promoting products—shall adhere to prevailing professional standards and shall not contain misrepresentation. If specialty recognition in dysphagia becomes available from the state licensure board or ASHA, then it would be appropriate for the SLP to list this credential.

20. a. The welfare of the patient is paramount in ethical and clinical decision making and could be compromised if no planning or supervision is provided during the evaluation. The supervisor is ultimately responsible for patient care and ensuring high-quality

services. According to the ASHA (2003) Code of Ethics, Principle I, individuals shall honor their responsibility to hold paramount the welfare of persons they serve professionally or participants in research and scholarly activities. Other choices in this question do not refer to the tenet that the welfare of the patient is paramount.

21. e. According the ASHA (2003) Code of Ethics, Principle IV, Rule D, individuals shall assign credit only to those who have contributed to a publication, presentation, or product. Credit shall be assigned in proportion to the contribution and only with contributor's consent. The doctoral student performed the majority of the work for the dissertation. The major adviser did contribute a significant portion to the dissertation but should not request to be listed as first author. If the student, however, asks that the major adviser be listed as first author, then this is permissible. None of the other choices for this question are referred to in the question.

22. b. The SLP could be discriminating against a professional colleague (i.e., the physical therapist) because of the colleague's national origin. This is specifically prohibited by the ASHA (2003) Code of Ethics, Principle IV, Rule H. Furthermore, the conversation the physical therapist had with the FBI was a confidential matter and should not have been conveyed to anyone else. Moreover, the conversation the SLP had with the patient resulted in discontinuation of the physical therapist's services, which could have adverse effects for the patient, as well as for the therapist.

23. c. The SLP must abide by the ASHA (2003) Code of Ethics, Principle IV, Rule E, according to which individuals shall reference the source when using other person's ideas, research, presentations, or products, in written, oral, or any other media presentation or summary. The SLP should be mindful of the other rules listed for this question, but this case concerns proper referencing of all materials and avoiding plagiarism.

24. a. Although the SLP has a cooperative agreement and a physician referral may be required for reimbursement, the professional should always exercise independent judgment regarding clinical services. According to the ASHA (2003) Code of Ethics, Principle IV, Rule G, individuals shall not provide professional services without exercising independent professional judgment, regardless of referral source or prescription. The SLP should be mindful of the other rules listed for this question, but it is most important to exercise independent judgment in this situation.

25. b. The SLP witnessing the fraud by a business partner must report any possible violation of the ASHA (2003) Code of Ethics to the Board of Ethics, according to the ASHA Code of Ethics, Principle IV, Rule I. Although the fraud by the business partner could have serious financial ramifications for the practice, the SLP must make the referral with proper cause. All other rules are important for the SLP witnessing the fraud; however, informing the Board of Ethics is most important in this scenario.

26. e. Jane must abide by the ASHA (2003) Code of Ethics, Principle IV, Rule J, according to which individuals shall comply fully with the policies of the Board of Ethics in its consideration and adjudication of complaints of violations of the Code of Ethics. Because Jane has documentation and is knowledgeable about the ethical violation of another certified SLP, she must cooperate, including identifying herself as the source for reporting the ethical violation. Also, the licensure board for the state and the state speech-language-hearing association may have ethical rules that require full cooperation. The other choices for this question could be reasons why Jane is reporting the certified SLP, but Jane has the responsibility to uphold Rule J.

27. d. Joshua has contacted the subjects for the research project; however, it is important that he obtain written consent and also give full disclosure about the purpose, expectations, and risks and benefits for the study. Joshua needs to submit his proposal to the appropriate review committee or board at his place of employment to ensure that proper procedures are followed. According to the ASHA (2003) Code of Ethics, Principle I, Rule N, individuals shall use persons in research or as subjects of teaching demonstrations only with their informed consent. Furthermore, because the subjects have a history of autism spectrum disorder and language delay, Joshua may need to have special considerations regarding the methods for documenting informed consent and should consult with the review committee or board.

28. c. Kim, although not intentionally, has not appropriately secured records of professional services and thereby allowed other people to see the new password. Other people may use the password to view patient records. According to the ASHA (2003) Code of Ethics, Principle I, Rule K, individuals shall adequately maintain and appropriately secure records of professional services rendered, research and scholarly activities conducted, and products dispensed and shall allow access to these records only when authorized or when required by law.

29. c. Sarah is required by the ASHA (2003) Code of Ethics, Principle I, Rule M, not to misrepresent diagnostic information, research, services rendered, or products dispensed; Sarah must also not engage in any scheme to defraud in connection with obtaining payment or reimbursement for such services or products. The best option for Sarah is to submit all claims as required but direct Mrs. Noble to the business office at the community clinic, which may offer a discounted fee schedule for services. If Mrs. Noble cannot continue services with Sarah, then the next best option may be for services from the university.

30. d. Chris should follow the ASHA (2003) Code of Ethics, Principle I, Rule L, according to which individuals shall not reveal, without authorization, any professional or personal information about identified persons served professionally or identified participants involved in research and scholarly activities unless required by law to do so or unless doing so is necessary to protect the welfare of the person or of the community or otherwise required by law. In this situation, Chris should tell the parent, who signed the informed consent for the child to be in the study, what was said about the home situation. Chris must also review laws regarding protection of children and use every resource such as a social worker or other professionals (according to Principle I, Rule B) about the laws and take the appropriate action.

31. a. All professionals shall continue professional development throughout their careers, according to the ASHA (2003) Code of Ethics, Principle II, Rule C. The SLP should make every effort to implement current best practices that are available from evidence-based practice.

32. b. Carolyn is mindful of the ASHA Code of Ethics, Principle I, Rule B, according to which individuals shall use every resource, including referral when appropriate, to ensure that high-quality service is provided. A referral to a professional with training and competence within the area of documented mental illness would be the best option at this point.

33. b. The certified SLP should follow the ASHA (2003) Code of Ethics, Principle I, Rule E, according to which individuals who hold the CCC shall not delegate tasks that require the unique skills, knowledge, and judgment that are within the scope of their profession to assistants, technicians, support personnel, students, or any nonprofessionals over whom they have supervisory responsibility. The students were assigned to perform only observations by the

university. The certified SLP needs to meet with families and conduct the case history and have the graduate students observe the process. In addition, the supervisor should allow the students the opportunity to ask follow-up questions at the appropriate time or provide written summaries of their observations and share them with the university supervisor.

34. d. Mary should follow the ASHA (2003) Code of Ethics, Principle I, Rules G and H. According to Rule G, individuals shall evaluate the effectiveness of services rendered and of products dispensed and shall provide services or dispense products only when benefit can be reasonably expected. According to Rule H, individuals shall not guarantee the results of any treatment or procedure. Although the manufacturer of the software states that the success rate is 98%, success cannot be guaranteed.

35. b. Kathy must follow the ASHA (2003) Code of Ethics, Principle I, Rule I, according to which individuals shall not provide clinical services solely by correspondence. Kathy may provide general information (see Principle III, Rule E) about the effects that a stroke may have on speech and language and tell her friend about the ASHA Web site (www.asha.org) as a source for making contact with qualified professionals within the area.

36. b. John needs to review the ASHA (2003) Code of Ethics, Principle III, Rule F, according to which individuals' statements to the public—advertising, announcing, and marketing their professional services; reporting research results; and promoting products—shall adhere to prevailing professional standards and shall not contain misrepresentations.

37. a. First, Karen, who is an ASHA-certified SLP, shall prohibit anyone under her supervision from engaging in any practice that violates the ASHA (2003) Code of Ethics, according to Principle IV, Rule A. Karen must then determine whether Joyce is fit to serve persons professionally. This determination would require additional documentation and investigation.

38. e. Joan's level of education and training are possibly not sufficient for her to provide adequate services to patients with Alzheimer disease. There are specific issues and recommended practices for individuals with Alzheimer's disease and communication disorders. According to the ASHA (2003) Code of Ethics, Principle II, Rule B, individuals shall engage in only those aspects of the professions that are within the scope of their competence, considering

their level of education, training, and experience. Joan also needs to follow this ethical principle to continue her professional development throughout her career.

39. a. Although the request to evaluate the young child came from Christopher's supervisor, he should not reveal, without authorization, any professional or personal information about the child. According to the ASHA (2003) Code of Ethics, Principle I, Rule L, individuals shall not reveal, without authorization, any professional or personal information about identified persons served professionally or identified participants involved in research and scholarly activities unless required by law to do so or unless doing so is necessary to protect the welfare of the person or of the community or otherwise required by law. In this situation, Christopher was not required by law and did not believe that the welfare of the child was at risk. Christopher's supervisor was not authorized to know about the results unless the child's parents signed a form allowing him to disclose his results and treatment plan.

40. c. The professor could be in violation of the ASHA (2003) Code of Ethics, Principle I, Rule G, according to which individuals shall evaluate the effectiveness of services rendered and of products dispensed and shall provide services or dispense products only when benefit can reasonably be expected. The professor must document the rationale for the patient to have treatment with maintenance services for an extended time. The Clinical Coordinator should have a discussion with the professor about a possible ethical violation, ask for documented progress of the patient, and also try to help the professor obtain other patients with fluency issues for services so that students can obtain clinical experiences.

41. d. Michelle should make certain that her husband's partner is providing patients a variety of referral sources and options. According to the ASHA (2003) Code of Ethics, Principle III, Rule B, individuals shall not participate in professional activities that constitute a conflict of interest.

42. a. The SLP should inform the mother about several service providers (schools, hospitals, community clinics, and so forth) that may be available to serve her child. If the SLP lists her private practice group as a referral source, she should fully disclose to the mother her affiliation with the group and that there is no personal financial interest. According to the ASHA (2003) Code of Ethics, Principle III, Rule C, individuals shall refer those served professionally solely

on the basis of the interest of those being referred and not on any personal financial interest.

43. b. Dr. Williams may be qualified to diagnose swallowing disorders without the use of technology or otorhinolaryngological consultation; however, he may be misleading the audience and misrepresenting his credentials. According to the ASHA (2003) Code of Ethics, Principle I, Rule H, individuals shall not guarantee the results of any treatment or procedure directly or by implication; however, they may make a reasonable statement of prognosis. Furthermore, Dr. Williams should specifically document how obtaining a doctoral degree in educational leadership improved his knowledge and skills regarding swallowing disorders.

44. d. Obtaining the videotapes without the informed consent of the patients with a laryngectomy would violate the ASHA (2003) Code of Ethics. According to Principle I, Rule N, individuals shall use persons in research or as subjects of teaching demonstrations only with their informed consent.

45. b. Jeri must first determine whether she agrees with the information left by Mike. Jeri must determine whether there is sufficient documentation to proceed with providing clinical services. According to the ASHA (2003) Code of Ethics, Principle IV, Rule G, individuals (including clinical fellow–SLP) shall not provide professional services without exercising independent professional judgment, regardless of referral source or prescription. Although Mike is Jeri's clinical fellow supervisor and possibly has more clinical knowledge and skills, Jeri must make an independent decision regarding services.

Bibliography

American Psychiatric Association. (2000). *Diagnostic and statistical manual of mental disorders* (4th ed., text revision [DSM-IV-TR]). Washington, DC: Author.

American Speech-Language-Hearing Association. (2003). *Code of ethics.* Available at www.asha.org/policy (accessed July 7, 2009).

Irwin, D. L., Pannbacker, M., Powell, T. W., & Vekovius, G. T. (2007). *Ethics for speech-language pathologists and audiologists: An illustrative casebook.* Clifton Park, NY: Thomson Delmar Learning.

CHAPTER 25

Research Methodology and Psychometrics

Susan Rvachew

1. This question is based on the following hypothetical abstract of a treatment efficacy study.

PURPOSE:

This study was designed to determine whether a classroom-based intervention would improve kindergarten children's emergent literacy skills.

METHOD:

Two kindergarten teachers in a single school volunteered their morning classes to take part. A coin flip was used to randomly assign one class to the intervention ($n = 20$) and the other class to the control condition ($n = 22$). In the control class, the classroom teacher conducted daily story time as usual, reading a different book to the children each day and asking comprehension questions after the reading. In the intervention class, the speech-language pathologist (SLP) conducted the daily story time sessions in the same manner, except that she also incorporated emergent literacy exercises into the story-reading procedure. A study-specific probe of the children's emergent literacy skills (letter knowledge, phonological awareness, and sight word reading) was conducted in September, before the onset of the intervention, and in June, after 36 weeks of the intervention had been completed. Standardized tests of receptive vocabulary skills and nonverbal intelligence were also conducted in September. These assessments were conducted by another SLP, who was unaware of each child's class placement and the purpose of the study.

RESULTS:

The September assessment revealed that the two classrooms were well matched for receptive vocabulary skills, nonverbal intelligence, and emergent literacy skills. The children in the control class were, however, 3 months older, on average, than the children in the intervention class. In June, the children in the intervention condition achieved significantly higher scores on the probe of emergent literacy than did the children in the control condition; the effect size was medium ($d = .61$). Examination of subtest scores revealed that the outcome was explained by improvements in letter knowledge and phonological awareness; sight word reading scores of the two classes were similar.

CONCLUSIONS:

An embedded emergent literacy intervention conducted in the classroom by an SLP can be valuable for kindergarten-aged children.

Of the following, which represents the primary dependent variable used in this study?
  a. Phonological awareness
  b. Nonverbal intelligence
  c. Emergent literacy skills
  d. Receptive vocabulary skills
  e. Sight word reading skills

2. This question is based on the following hypothetical abstract of a treatment efficacy study.

PURPOSE:

This study was designed to determine whether a classroom-based intervention would improve kindergarten children's emergent literacy skills.

METHOD:

Two kindergarten teachers in a single school volunteered their morning classes to take part. A coin flip was used to randomly assign one class to the intervention ($n = 20$) and the other class to the control condition ($n = 22$). In the control class, the classroom teacher conducted daily story time as usual, reading a different book to the children each day and asking comprehension questions after the reading. In the intervention class, the SLP conducted the daily story time sessions in the same manner, except that she also incorporated emergent literacy exercises into the story-reading procedure. A study-specific probe of the children's emergent literacy skills (letter knowledge, phonological awareness, and sight word reading) was conducted in September, before the onset of the intervention, and in June, after 36 weeks of the intervention had been completed. Standardized tests of receptive vocabulary skills and nonverbal intelligence were also conducted in September. These assessments were conducted by another SLP, who was unaware of each child's class placement and the purpose of the study.

RESULTS:

The September assessment revealed that the two classrooms were well matched for receptive vocabulary skills, nonverbal intelligence, and emergent literacy skills. The children in the control class were, however, 3 months older, on average, than the children in the intervention class. In June, the children in the intervention condition achieved significantly higher scores on the probe of emergent literacy than did the children in the control condition; the effect size was medium ($d = .61$). Examination of subtest scores revealed that the outcome was explained by improvements in letter knowledge and phonological awareness; sight word reading scores of the two classes were similar.

CONCLUSIONS:

An embedded emergent literacy intervention conducted in the classroom by an SLP can be valuable for kindergarten-aged children.

Of the following conclusions, which represents the greatest threat to the *internal validity* of this study?
  a. The long interval between prestudy and poststudy testing means that the children's improvement in emergent literacy test scores might be caused largely by the children's greater age in June than in September
  b. The teacher of the intervention class may have been more effective at promoting emergent literacy during the rest of the day than was the teacher of the control class
  c. The children in the intervention class may have been faster learners than the children in the control class
  d. The children are not well described in the abstract, and thus it is impossible to generalize the findings to children outside the study who might be of a different age, ethnicity, language background, and so forth
  e. The outcome measure was assessed with a study-specific probe rather than with a standardized test

3. This question is based on the following hypothetical abstract of a treatment efficacy study.

PURPOSE:

This study was designed to determine whether a classroom-based intervention would improve kindergarten children's emergent literacy skills.

METHOD:

Two kindergarten teachers in a single school volunteered their morning classes to take part. A coin flip was used to randomly assign one class to the intervention ($n = 20$) and the other class to the control condition ($n = 22$). In the control class, the classroom teacher conducted daily story time as usual, reading a different book to the children each day and asking comprehension questions after the reading. In the intervention class, the SLP conducted the daily story time sessions in the same manner, except that she also incorporated emergent literacy exercises into the story-reading procedure. A study-specific probe of the children's emergent literacy skills (letter knowledge, phonological awareness, and sight word reading) was conducted in September, before the onset of the intervention, and in June, after 36 weeks of the intervention had been completed. Standardized tests of receptive vocabulary skills and nonverbal intelligence were also conducted in September. These assessments were conducted by another SLP, who was unaware of each child's class placement and the purpose of the study.

RESULTS:

The September assessment revealed that the two classrooms were well matched for receptive vocabulary skills, nonverbal intelligence, and emergent literacy skills. The children in the control class were, however, 3 months older, on average, than the children in the intervention class. In June, the children in the intervention condition achieved significantly higher scores on the probe of emergent literacy than did the children in the control condition; the effect size was medium ($d = .61$). Examination of subtest scores revealed that the outcome was explained by improvements in letter knowledge and phonological awareness; sight word reading scores of the two classes were similar.

CONCLUSIONS:

An embedded emergent literacy intervention conducted in the classroom by an SLP can be valuable for kindergarten-aged children.

In the body of the report, the investigators use an independent-samples t test to describe the results of the study, stating that "the intervention group achieved a significantly higher mean score ($M = 15.15$, $SD = 2.68$) compared to the control group ($M = 13.32$, $SD = 3.26$) on the probe of emergent literacy [$t(40) = 1.89$, $p = .03$, one-tailed]." In fact, this analysis is not appropriate for this study because of the way in which it was designed. Of the following explanations, which is the correct reason why this analysis is inappropriate for this study?
  a. As a consequence of the random assignment procedure, the unit of analysis is the classroom and not the student, and therefore the total sample size is only 2 (and not 42)
  b. The sample sizes are unequal; therefore, the t test should have been corrected for unequal variances
  c. The control condition might have been as effective as or more effective than the intervention and therefore the t test should have been two-tailed

  d. The more appropriate test would have been an analysis of covariance (ANCOVA) to control for the effects of differences in receptive vocabulary and nonverbal intelligence
  e. A paired-samples t test should have been used because the groups were well matched for receptive vocabulary, nonverbal intelligence, and initial emergent literacy skills

4. This question is based on the following hypothetical abstract of a treatment efficacy study.

PURPOSE:

This study was designed to determine whether a classroom-based intervention would improve kindergarten children's emergent literacy skills.

METHOD:

Two kindergarten teachers in a single school volunteered their morning classes to take part. A coin flip was used to randomly assign one class to the intervention ($n = 20$) and the other class to the control condition ($n = 22$). In the control class, the classroom teacher conducted daily story time as usual, reading a different book to the children each day and asking comprehension questions after the reading. In the intervention class, the SLP conducted the daily story time sessions in the same manner, except that she also incorporated emergent literacy exercises into the story-reading procedure. A study-specific probe of the children's emergent literacy skills (letter knowledge, phonological awareness, and sight word reading) was conducted in September, before the onset of the intervention, and in June, after 36 weeks of the intervention had been completed. Standardized tests of receptive vocabulary skills and nonverbal intelligence were also conducted in September. These assessments were conducted by another SLP, who was unaware of each child's class placement and the purpose of the study.

RESULTS:

The September assessment revealed that the two classrooms were well matched for receptive vocabulary skills, nonverbal intelligence, and emergent literacy skills. The children in the control class were, however, 3 months older, on average, than the children in the intervention class. In June, the children in the intervention condition achieved significantly higher scores on the probe of emergent literacy than did the children in the control condition; the effect size was medium ($d = .61$). Examination of subtest scores revealed that the outcome was explained by improvements in letter knowledge and phonological awareness; sight word reading scores of the two classes were similar.

CONCLUSIONS:

An embedded emergent literacy intervention conducted in the classroom by an SLP can be valuable for kindergarten-aged children.

The investigators developed a study-specific probe of emergent literacy skills in order to assess the outcomes of their study. Of the following procedures, which would be the best recommendation for assessing the reliability of this measure of emergent literacy?

    a. Give the study-specific probe and a standardized test of emergent literacy skills to the same children on the same day and examine the correlation between the two sets of test scores; if the correlation is high, the reliability of the probe is good

    b. Give the study-specific probe and a standardized measure of nonverbal intelligence to the the children in one group on the same day and examine the correlation between the two sets of scores; if the correlation is low, the reliability of the probe is good

    c. Give the study-specific probe to a group of children with normally developing language skills and to a group of children with delayed language skills on the same day; if the children with normally developing language skills score higher than the children with delayed language skills, then the reliability of the probe is good

    d. Give the study-specific probe to the same children two times in the same week and examine the correlation between the two sets of scores. If the correlation is high, the reliability of the probe is good

    e. Give the study-specific probe to a group of children and examine the correlations between the subtests (letter knowledge, phonological awareness, sight word reading). If the correlations are high, the reliability of the probe is good

5. This question is based on the following hypothetical abstract of a treatment efficacy study.

PURPOSE:

This study was designed to determine whether a classroom-based intervention would improve kindergarten children's emergent literacy skills.

METHOD:

Two kindergarten teachers in a single school volunteered their morning classes to take part. A coin flip was used to randomly assign one class to the intervention ($n = 20$) and the other class to the control condition ($n = 22$). In the control class, the classroom teacher conducted daily story time as usual, reading a different book to the children each day and asking comprehension questions after the reading. In the intervention class, the SLP conducted the daily story time sessions in the same manner, except that she also incorporated emergent literacy exercises into the story-reading procedure. A study-specific probe of the children's emergent literacy skills (letter knowledge, phonological awareness, and sight word reading) was conducted in September, before the onset of the intervention, and in June, after 36 weeks of the intervention had been completed. Standardized tests of receptive vocabulary skills and nonverbal intelligence were also conducted in September. These assessments were conducted by another SLP, who was unaware of each child's class placement and the purpose of the study.

RESULTS:

The September assessment revealed that the two classrooms were well matched for receptive vocabulary skills, nonverbal intelligence, and emergent literacy skills. The children in the control class were, however, 3 months older, on average, than the children in the intervention class. In June, the children in the intervention condition achieved significantly higher scores on the probe of emergent literacy than did the children in the control condition; the effect size was medium ($d = .61$). Examination of subtest scores revealed that the outcome was explained by improvements in letter knowledge and phonological awareness; sight word reading scores of the two classes were similar.

CONCLUSIONS:

An embedded emergent literacy intervention conducted in the classroom by an SLP can be valuable for kindergarten-aged children.

Of the following descriptions of the study design, which is the best?

    a. Double-blind, randomized, control group design

    b. Single-blind, randomized, control group design

    c. Double-blind, static group comparison design

    d. Single-blind, time-series design

    e. Single-blind, nonequivalent comparison group design

6. This question is based on the excerpt in Box 25-1 and Figure 25-1 from a hypothetical conference poster describing the results of a study designed to test a treatment for dyslexia. Of the following sentences from the poster, which constitutes the clearest statement of the hypothesis of the study?

    a. "Scotoscopic sensitivity is a form of perceptual dyslexia in which the person has difficulty accommodating different wavelengths of light, which results in text distortions"

    b. "Recent research implicates abnormalities in the magnocellular pathway in the visual cortex as the cause of the scotoscopic sensitivity"

Box 25-1

Introduction: Scotoscopic sensitivity is a form of perceptual dyslexia in which the person has difficulty accommodating different wavelengths of light, which results in text distortions. Recent research implicates abnormalities in the magnocellular pathway in the visual cortex as the cause of the scotoscopic sensitivity. The purpose of this study was to assess the efficacy of a potential cure. It was expected that the wearing of Irlen lenses during reading would improve the sight word reading abilities of three young struggling readers after 3 to 9 weeks of use.

Method: The participants were three fourth grade children attending remedial reading sessions twice per week because they were reading at the 10th percentile on standardized measures of decoding and reading comprehension. Child A was a Spanish-English bilingual boy attending an English Language Learner class; child B was a girl with a speech-sound disorder; and child C was a boy receiving speech therapy for stuttering. Remedial reading activities were continued as usual and the glasses were introduced in a staggered schedule. A 25-item word reading probe was administered at the end of each session.

Results: Dramatic improvements in word reading ability were observed for all three children. Child A learned to read 100% of the words on the word reading probe. Child B and child C learned to read 80% of the words, struggling only with the longest words on the list, although child C's progress was somewhat slower than that of child B.

Conclusions: Irlen lenses helped these children accommodate different wavelengths of light and dramatically improved their reading skills. These specially tinted lenses are a valuable adjunct to reading interventions.

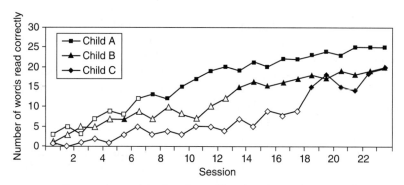

Open markers = baseline phase; Closed markers = treatment phase

Figure 25-1   Sight word probe scores by child and session

c. "The purpose of this study was to assess the efficacy of a potential cure"

d. "It was expected that the wearing of Irlen lenses during reading would improve the sight word reading abilities of three young struggling readers after 3 to 9 weeks of use"

e. "Irlen lenses, special tinted glasses, helped these children accommodate different wavelengths of light and dramatically improved their reading skills"

7. This question is based on the excerpt in Box 25-1 and Figure 25-1 from a hypothetical conference poster describing the results of a study designed to test a treatment for dyslexia. Of the following descriptions, which best matches the research design that was used to test the hypothesis?
   a. Multiple-baseline design
   b. Baseline and intervention (AB) single-case design

c. Reversal design
d. Alternating-treatments design
e. Changing-criterion design

8. This question is based on the excerpt in Box 25-1 and Figure 25-1 from a hypothetical conference poster describing the results of a study designed to test a treatment for dyslexia. Of the following conditions, which represents the greatest threat to the *internal validity* of the study?
   a. Failure to include a reversal phase, in which treatment is withdrawn in order to demonstrate experimental control
   b. Selection of a treatment that has already been judged to be ineffective in previously published systematic reviews of the literature
   c. Selection of research participants whose reading disability was complicated by other factors (speech-sound disorder, stuttering, bilingualism)

d. Failure to include measures of reading comprehension and reading fluency, as well as a measure of sight word reading

e. Observation of an unstable baseline for all three children before the introduction of the treatment

9. This question is based on the excerpt in Box 25-1 and Figure 25-1 from a hypothetical conference poster describing the results of a study designed to test a treatment for dyslexia. Assume that it is true that some studies have described abnormal function of magnocellular pathways in the visual cortex of dyslexic adults in comparison with normal readers. Do the research findings in the current study provide support for the clinical practice of adopting the Irlen lenses as a treatment for dyslexia?

a. Yes, because these findings support the underlying theory that explains why the lenses work

b. No, because the correlation between magnocellular dysfunction and dyslexia does not prove that there is a causal relationship

c. Yes, because evidence-based practice requires that there be a scientific foundation for the use of any clinical intervention

d. Yes, because brain imaging research constitutes the highest level of scientific evidence

e. No, because research with adults reveals nothing about reading acquisition by children

10. This question is based on the excerpt in Box 25-1 and Figure 25-1 from a hypothetical conference poster describing the results of a study designed to test a treatment for dyslexia. Child C shows a great deal of session-to-session variability in the number of correct responses to the sight word reading probe, sometimes improving and other times regressing from one session to the next. Of the following conditions, which is the most likely combination of factors to explain this lack of stability between sessions?

a. Investigator bias, reactive pretest effects, situation factors

b. Investigator bias, statistical regression, situation factors

c. Child characteristics, examiner characteristics, situation factors

d. Child characteristics, examiner characteristics, reactive pretest effects

e. Investigator bias, child characteristics, statistical regression

11. This question is based on Figure 25-2 and the research article (Camarata et al., 1994) from which it was taken. In this study, 21 children with specific language impairment received 24 language therapy sessions, each 50 minutes long and divided equally, in

counterbalanced order, between an imitative treatment procedure and a conversational recasting treatment procedure. The treatments were designed to improve the children's production of grammatical morphemes and complex sentence targets. The investigators coded videotapes of the treatment sessions to count how many times the clinician presented each target before the child's first elicited and first spontaneous production of the target. Of the following descriptions, which best matches the design of this study?

a. Cross-sectional descriptive research

b. Longitudinal descriptive research

c. Between-subjects experimental research

d. Within-subjects experimental research

e. Mixed within-subjects and between-subjects experimental research

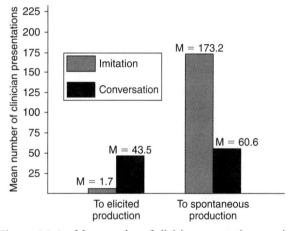

Figure 25-2   Mean number of clinician presentations required for elicited and spontaneous target production under each treatment. (From Camarata, S. M., Nelson, K. E., Camarata, M. N. [1994]. Comparison of conversational recasting and imitative procedures for training grammatical structures in children with specific language impairment. *Journal of Speech and Hearing Research, 37*, 1414–1423.)

12. This question is based on Figure 25-2 and the research article (Camarata et al., 1994) from which it was taken. In this study, 21 children with specific language impairment received 24 language therapy sessions, each 50 minutes long and divided equally, in counterbalanced order, between an imitative treatment procedure and a conversational recasting treatment procedure. The treatments were designed to improve the children's production of grammatical morphemes and complex sentence targets. The investigators coded videotapes of the treatment sessions to count how many times the clinician presented each target before the child's first elicited and first spontaneous production of the target. Figure 25-2 shows the mean number of clinician presentations of the target grammatical structures before the child's first elicited and first spontaneous use of those targets in the imitative and

conversational treatment conditions. Of the following statistical procedures, which is most appropriate to use to evaluate the statistical significance of these results?

a. Factorial analysis of variance
b. Repeated measures *t*-test
c. Standard error of the mean
d. Cohen's *d* measure of effect size
e. Pearson correlation coefficient

13. This question is based on Figure 25-2 and the research article (Camarata et al., 1994) from which it was taken. In this study, 21 children with specific language impairment received 24 language therapy sessions, each 50 minutes long and divided equally, in counterbalanced order, between an imitative treatment procedure and a conversational recasting treatment procedure. The treatments were designed to improve the children's production of grammatical morphemes and complex sentence targets. The investigators coded videotapes of the treatment sessions to count how many times the clinician presented each target before the child's first elicited and first spontaneous production of the target. Figure 25-2 shows the mean number of clinician presentations of the target grammatical structures before the child's first elicited and first spontaneous use of those targets in the imitative and conversational treatment conditions. The outcome measure was coded from videotapes of these treatment sessions. What is the most likely threat to the *internal validity* of this study?

a. History effects
b. Maturation effects
c. Experimenter bias
d. Fatigue effects
e. Practice effects

14. This question is based on Figure 25-2 and the research article (Camarata et al., 1994) from which it was taken. In this study, 21 children with specific language impairment received 24 language therapy sessions, each 50 minutes long and divided equally, in counterbalanced order, between an imitative treatment procedure and a conversational recasting treatment procedure. The treatments were designed to improve the children's production of grammatical morphemes and complex sentence targets. The investigators coded videotapes of the treatment sessions to count how many times the clinician presented each target before the child's first elicited and first spontaneous production of the target. Figure 25-2 shows the mean number of clinician presentations of the target grammatical structures before the child's first elicited and first spontaneous use of those targets in the imitative and conversational treatment conditions. One outcome measure is the number of times the clinician presented the targets before the child's first elicited and spontaneous use of

the targets. The internal validity of the study is dependent partly on the reliability of this outcome measure. Of the following methods, which is the best for determining this reliability?

a. Examine the correlation between the outcome measure and Developmental Sentence Scores for all children in the study
b. Use Cronbach's alpha to estimate the average of all possible split-half correlations for 10% of the coded sessions
c. Have teams of three researchers view each videotape together to derive a consensus coding of each session
d. Require all coders to take a 3-day workshop and pass a test on the coding procedure before they are allowed to begin coding the videotapes
e. Have at least 20% of the sessions coded independently by two coders and then examine the correlation between scores and the range and average of the differences between scores for the two raters

15. This question is based on Figure 25-2 and the research article (Camarata et al., 1994) from which it was taken. In this study, 21 children with specific language impairment received 24 language therapy sessions, each 50 minutes long and divided equally, in counterbalanced order, between an imitative treatment procedure and a conversational recasting treatment procedure. The treatments were designed to improve the children's production of grammatical morphemes and complex sentence targets. The investigators coded videotapes of the treatment sessions to count how many times the clinician presented each target before the child's first elicited and first spontaneous production of the target. Figure 25-2 shows the mean number of clinician presentations of the target grammatical structures before the child's first elicited and first spontaneous use of those targets in the imitative and conversational treatment conditions. One outcome measure is the number of times the clinician presented the targets before the child's first elicited and spontaneous use of the targets. The internal validity of the study is dependent partly on the reliability of this outcome measure. Of the following statements, which is the most accurate conclusion to draw from Figure 25-2?

a. The imitation intervention led to the fewest elicited productions of grammatical targets but the most numerous spontaneous productions of grammatical targets
b. Fewer clinician presentations of the targets were required for spontaneous production (in comparison with elicited production) of the grammatical targets in the conversational-recasting treatment, whereas the reverse effect was observed in the imitative treatment

c. There was a significant main effect of the conversational-recasting treatment that led to greater spontaneous production of the grammatical targets

d. There was a significant main effect of the imitation treatment that led to greater spontaneous use of the grammatical targets

e. There was a significant interaction of grammatical target with type of treatment; therefore, the conversational-recasting treatment is the superior choice for treating children with delayed language skills

16. An important characteristic of any diagnostic test of speech or language is reliability. A test is reliable to the extent to which:

a. The test is measuring the construct that the test is intended to measure

b. The test is sensitive to differences between individuals who have the disorder of interest and individuals who have normal speech and language function

c. The test will yield similar scores when an individual is tested repeatedly in similar circumstances

d. The test will yield a standard score similar to that yielded by another test of the same construct that the original test is intended to measure

e. The error component of the observed scores on the test is systematic rather than randomly distributed

17. When an SLP selects a diagnostic test, it is important to examine the test manual for evidence of test reliability. Of the following patterns of information, which would indicate that a test is reliable?

a. High reliability coefficient and low standard error of measurement

b. Low reliability coefficient and high standard error of measurement

c. High reliability coefficient and high standard error of measurement

d. Low reliability coefficient and low standard error of measurement

e. High reliability coefficient

18. The SLP wishes to assess the phonological memory skills of a 68-year-old patient who recently suffered a mild stroke. The SLP asks the patient to repeat a series of sentences of increasing length, including "George Washington was the first president of the United States." The patient refuses the item, explaining that he knows nothing about the presidents because he did not attend school in North America. This reveals a problem with which of the following forms of validity for this test procedure?

a. Content validity

b. Criterion validity

c. Construct validity

d. Predictive validity

e. Face validity

19. Coplan and Gleason (1988) developed a new screening questionnaire for speech-sound disorders by asking the parents of children aged 1 to 5 years whether their child's speech was 50%, 75%, or 100% intelligible to a stranger. They validated the screening questionnaire by conducting both the screening questionnaire and a formal speech-language assessment with 151 children who were referred for possible developmental delays. The screening questionnaire reportedly had a *sensitivity* of 95%. Of the following statements, which is the best interpretation of this finding?

a. There is a 95% probability that a child with a speech problem will be identified by the screening questionnaire

b. There is a 95% probability that a child with normally developing speech will pass the screening questionnaire

c. If a child fails the screening questionnaire, there is a 95% probability that the child will prove to have a speech problem upon formal testing

d. If a child passes the screening questionnaire, there is a 95% probability that the child will prove to have normal speech development upon formal testing

e. There is a 5% probability that a child who passes the screening questionnaire will prove in formal testing to have normal speech

20. Coplan and Gleason (1988) developed a new screening questionnaire for speech-sound disorders by asking the parents of children aged 1 to 5 years whether their child's speech was 50%, 75%, or 100% intelligible to a stranger. They validated the screening questionnaire by conducting both the screening questionnaire and a formal speech-language assessment with 151 children who were referred for possible developmental delays. The screening questionnaire reportedly had a *positive predictive value* of 95%. Of the following statements, which is the best interpretation of this finding?

a. There is a 95% probability that a child with a speech problem will be identified by the screening questionnaire

b. There is a 95% probability that a child with normally developing speech will pass the screening questionnaire

c. If a child fails the screening questionnaire, there is a 95% probability that the child will prove to have a speech problem upon formal testing

d. If a child passes the screening questionnaire, there is a 95% probability that the child will prove to have normal speech development upon formal testing

e. There is a 5% probability that a child who passes the screening questionnaire will prove in formal testing to have normal speech

21. Coplan and Gleason (1988) developed a new screening questionnaire for speech-sound disorders by asking the parents of children aged 1 to 5 years whether their child's speech was 50%, 75%, or 100% intelligible to a stranger. They validated the screening questionnaire by conducting both the screening questionnaire and a formal speech-language assessment with 151 children who were referred for possible developmental delays. The screening questionnaire reportedly had a *negative predictive value* of 95%. Of the following statements, which is the best interpretation of this finding?
    a. There is a 95% probability that a child with a speech problem will be identified by the screening questionnaire
    b. There is a 95% probability that a child with normally developing speech will pass the screening questionnaire
    c. If a child fails the screening questionnaire, there is a 95% probability that the child will prove to have a speech problem upon formal testing
    d. If a child passes the screening questionnaire, there is a 95% probability that the child will prove to have normal speech development upon formal testing
    e. There is a 5% probability that a child who passes the screening questionnaire will prove in formal testing to have normal speech

22. In deciding whether to use a new treatment technique, it is important to examine the published evidence that supports of the use of the technique. Of the following conditions, which constitutes the *lowest* level of evidence to support clinical decision making about the efficacy of treatment procedures?
    a. Observational study of a cohort without a control group
    b. Nonrandomized, between-groups, controlled trial
    c. Multiple-baseline, single-subject experiment
    d. Retrospective case-control study
    e. Expert opinion

23. What is the role of clinical expertise in evidence-based practice?
    a. Clinical expertise is derived solely from the published research evidence
    b. Clinical expertise is integrated with the best available research evidence
    c. Clinical expertise plays no role in evidence-based practice
    d. Clinical expertise is used when randomized controlled trial (RCT) evidence is not available
    e. Clinical expertise is integrated with the patient's values and preferences

24. An investigator wishes to assess the relative effectiveness of prelinguistic milieu therapy and focused stimulation to increase the expressive vocabulary size of toddlers with global developmental delays. In a large special-needs child care center, Ms. Brown's class has 16 children. These children are randomly assigned to receive one or the other treatment in individual daily 1-hour sessions from an SLP. To assess the children's expressive vocabulary sizes, the children are observed in the classroom, and the words that they produce over a 1-week period are counted. This assessment is conducted by an observer, who was unaware of the conditions, after 4 months of intervention. Is this a properly designed RCT?
    a. No, because the sample was not randomly selected from the center's population
    b. No, because no children were randomly assigned to a "no-treatment" control group
    c. Yes, because the dependent variable was assessed by an observer who was unaware of the conditions
    d. Yes, because the children were randomly assigned to the treatment conditions
    e. No, because the dependent variable is based on a nonstandardized assessment procedure

25. Of the following statements of results, which makes use of inferential statistics?
    a. An analysis of variance revealed no main effect of the lipreading intervention on language comprehension scores, $F(1, 30) = 0.47$, $p = .498$
    b. Computerized script training led to a very large advantage to the treatment group in relation to the control group in self-reported ratings of communicative effectiveness ($d = .85$)
    c. Patients with Alzheimer disease were able to recall more information units in the immediate-recall condition ($M = 7.15$, $SD = 1.67$) than in the delayed-recall condition ($M = 1.25$, $SD = 0.75$)
    d. The results showed that the within-group variances in reaction times for the younger adults ($s^2 = 53$ ms) and the older adults ($s^2 = 152$ ms) were markedly different, and thus all of the statistical analyses were corrected for heterogeneity of variance
    e. Performance of the patients with Parkinson disease on the voice task used in this study was converted to a z score that was based on the mean and standard deviation of scores obtained from an age-matched group of normal control subjects ($M = 4.89$, $SD. = .05$), which resulted in a mean z score of -2.5 for the Parkinson group

26. Inferential statistics are *not* used to:
    a. Provide an estimate of the size of the difference between the experimental group and the control group in an experimental treatment efficacy study
    b. Express the ratio of the between-groups variance to the within-groups variance

c. Describe the amount of variance in the dependent variable that is explained by the independent variable

d. Estimate the value of a population parameter from the sample statistic

e. Describe the characteristics of the experimental sample as precisely as possible

27. Omega-3 fatty acids were found in one RCT to have a positive effect on reading scores in children with developmental coordination disorder. An investigator wishes to assess the use of omega-3 fatty acid supplements for the treatment of dysfluency in preschoolers. Spontaneous speech samples are recorded from all the 3-year-old children in a preschool program, and the three children with the highest rates of dysfluency are provided with a daily omega-3 fatty acid supplement. After 3 months the investigator rerecords spontaneous speech samples from all of the children in the class. The treated children now rank in the middle of the class for amount of dysfluency in relation to their peers. Of the following statements, which does *not* explain why the *internal validity* of the design is threatened?

a. The observed improvement in the children's scores may be caused by statistical regression to the mean

b. The children may be showing spontaneous improvements in fluency as a result of maturation

c. It is unreasonable to think that a treatment that improves reading can be generalized to dysfluency

d. Events occurring in the classroom or at home besides the treatment might be responsible for the change in the children's fluency

e. The observed changes in the children's fluency may be influenced by observer bias

28. In a multiple-baseline, single-subject experiment, what is the purpose of the withdrawal phase of the study?

a. To show that the treatment effect generalizes to untreated behaviors that are similar to the treated behavior

b. To show that changes in the dependent variable are caused by experimental manipulation of the independent variable

c. To demonstrate experimental control by showing that the treatment effect does not generalize to behaviors that are dissimilar to the treated behavior

d. To show that changes in the independent variable are caused by experimental manipulation of the dependent variable

e. To demonstrate experimental control by demonstrating a stable baseline for the dependent variable

29. Consider the following hypothesis from a hypothetical research report: "The purpose of this study was to assess the effect of the Lee Silverman Voice Treatment by using a multiple-baseline design with three patients who had cerebellar dysfunction secondary to thiamine deficiency." What is the most important element that is missing from this statement of the hypothesis?

a. Description of the dependent variable

b. Description of the age and gender of the patients

c. Description of the independent variable

d. Description of the research strategy that will be used

e. Details of the frequency and duration of the treatment

30. The following paragraph was taken from the discussion section of an actual research report:

"This study was experimental in nature and, as such, findings may not generalize directly to clinical situations. For instance, alphabet cues were experimentally imposed on the habitual speech of the persons with dysarthria for this study. In clinical practice, implementation of alphabet supplementation or a combined cueing strategy would require the speaker to point physically to the first letter of each word as he or she speaks it. The physical act of pointing to an alphabet board may have an effect on speech-production skills for some speakers with motor impairment. In addition, learning demands for employing alphabet and topic cues and the actual effectiveness of these strategies in spontaneous speaking situations are unclear. Further research is necessary to generalize findings from the present study to clinical implementation."
(Hustad & Beukelman, 2001, p. 507)

The concerns addressed in this paragraph are about which of the following aspects of the research?

a. Efficacy of the treatment

b. Reliability of the findings

c. External validity of the findings

d. Internal validity of the study

e. Cost-effectiveness of the intervention

31. This question is based on the following abstract from a research article:

"Despite the importance of grammatical morpheme (GM) production for both clinical decision-making and theoretical accounts of child language impairment, evidence concerning developmental expectations for GM use is inadequate. We studied grammatical morpheme production in 15-minute spontaneous language samples from a large (N = 100), sociodemographically diverse group of 4-year-olds. Substantial variability was observed in both the frequency of obligatory contexts (OCs) and in the percentage of correct usage of GMs. For only one morpheme did all 100 samples contain the minimum

number of 3 OCs; for only 7 of the 14 GMs was an adequate number of OCs found in at least half of the 100 samples. Although mean percentages of production from samples with 3 or more OCs were high (> 85%), fewer than 25% of participants contributed to the 'group' means for 6 of the 14 GMs. Results from the present investigation indicate a need for caution in interpreting information on GM production derived from samples of this nature from children at this age; the validity of using such data to identify deficits in inflectional morphology for either clinical or research purposes appears questionable." (Balason & Dollaghan, 2002)

This study is an example of which of the following types of research strategy?
a. Descriptive research
b. Correlational research
c. Survey research
d. Experimental research
e. Comparative research

32. This question is based on the following abstract from a research article:

"Despite the importance of grammatical morpheme (GM) production for both clinical decision-making and theoretical accounts of child language impairment, evidence concerning developmental expectations for GM use is inadequate. We studied grammatical morpheme production in 15-minute spontaneous language samples from a large (N = 100), sociodemographically diverse group of 4-year-olds. Substantial variability was observed in both the frequency of obligatory contexts (OCs) and in the percentage of correct usage of GMs. For only one morpheme did all 100 samples contain the minimum number of 3 OCs; for only 7 of the 14 GMs was an adequate number of OCs found in at least half of the 100 samples. Although mean percentages of production from samples with 3 or more OCs were high (> 85%), fewer than 25% of participants contributed to the 'group' means for 6 of the 14 GMs. Results from the present investigation indicate a need for caution in interpreting information on GM production derived from samples of this nature from children at this age; the validity of using such data to identify deficits in inflectional morphology for either clinical or research purposes appears questionable." (Balason & Dollaghan, 2002)

In their conclusions, the authors express concern about the "validity of using such data to identify deficits in inflectional morphology for either clinical or research purposes." As a clinician, if you were to record a 15-minute spontaneous speech sample from a 4-year-old child with a suspected language impairment and record the child's use of grammatical morphemes (GMs), which

of the following would be your primary concern, in view of the authors' conclusion ?
a. The speech sample might overestimate the child's actual abilities with regard to GM use
b. The frequency of GM use may not be replicable over repeated speech samples
c. The spontaneous speech sampling procedure may not be sensitive to improvements in GM use that occur as a result of language intervention
d. Less than 85% use of the GMs in the child's speech sample might falsely suggest that the child is language impaired in relation to normally developing children
e. Internal consistency of the results would be too poor to yield diagnostically interpretable results

33. This question is based on the following abstract from a research article:

"Despite the importance of grammatical morpheme (GM) production for both clinical decision-making and theoretical accounts of child language impairment, evidence concerning developmental expectations for GM use is inadequate. We studied grammatical morpheme production in 15-minute spontaneous language samples from a large (N = 100), sociodemographically diverse group of 4-year-olds. Substantial variability was observed in both the frequency of obligatory contexts (OCs) and in the percentage of correct usage of GMs. For only one morpheme did all 100 samples contain the minimum number of 3 OCs; for only 7 of the 14 GMs was an adequate number of OCs found in at least half of the 100 samples. Although mean percentages of production from samples with 3 or more OCs were high (> 85%), fewer than 25% of participants contributed to the 'group' means for 6 of the 14 GMs. Results from the present investigation indicate a need for caution in interpreting information on GM production derived from samples of this nature from children at this age; the validity of using such data to identify deficits in inflectional morphology for either clinical or research purposes appears questionable." (Balason & Dollaghan, 2002)

In the method section of this research report, the authors stated that "a second coder independently identified OCs and presence and absence of GMs in 20 randomly selected transcripts. Across all GMs, the percentage of coding decisions agreed upon by both coders was divided by the total number of coding decisions." The purpose of this procedure is to determine:
a. Intrarater reliability
b. Internal consistency
c. Interrater reliability
d. Coefficient of equivalence
e. Criterion validity

34. This question is based on the following abstract from a research article:

Despite the importance of grammatical morpheme (GM) production for both clinical decision-making and theoretical accounts of child language impairment, evidence concerning developmental expectations for GM use is inadequate. We studied grammatical morpheme production in 15-minute spontaneous language samples from a large (N = 100), sociodemographically diverse group of 4-year-olds. Substantial variability was observed in both the frequency of obligatory contexts (OCs) and in the percentage of correct usage of GMs. For only one morpheme did all 100 samples contain the minimum number of 3 OCs; for only 7 of the 14 GMs was an adequate number of OCs found in at least half of the 100 samples. Although mean percentages of production from samples with 3 or more OCs were high (> 85%), fewer than 25% of participants contributed to the 'group' means for 6 of the 14 GMs. Results from the present investigation indicate a need for caution in interpreting information on GM production derived from samples of this nature from children at this age; the validity of using such data to identify deficits in inflectional morphology for either clinical or research purposes appears questionable." (Balason & Dollaghan, 2002)

Of the following statistical procedures, which would be the most appropriate for describing the number of obligatory contexts that occurred for each grammatical morpheme observed across the 100 samples?
a. The *t* test and Cohen's *d*
b. Mean and standard deviation
c. Pearson product-moment correlation coefficient
d. Spearman rho correlation coefficient
e. Analysis of variance

35. This question is based on the following abstract from a research article:

Despite the importance of grammatical morpheme (GM) production for both clinical decision-making and theoretical accounts of child language impairment, evidence concerning developmental expectations for GM use is inadequate. We studied grammatical morpheme production in 15-minute spontaneous language samples from a large (N = 100), sociodemographically diverse group of 4-year-olds. Substantial variability was observed in both the frequency of obligatory contexts (OCs) and in the percentage of correct usage of GMs. For only one morpheme did all 100 samples contain the minimum number of 3 OCs; for only 7 of the 14 GMs was an adequate number of OCs found in at least half of the 100 samples. Although mean percentages of production from samples with 3 or more OCs were high

(> 85%), fewer than 25% of participants contributed to the 'group' means for 6 of the 14 GMs. Results from the present investigation indicate a need for caution in interpreting information on GM production derived from samples of this nature from children at this age; the validity of using such data to identify deficits in inflectional morphology for either clinical or research purposes appears questionable." (Balason & Dollaghan, 2002)

Of the following statements from Balason and Dollaghan's (2002) report, which points to a limitation on the *external validity* of the study?
a. "Interobserver agreement was 91%" (p. 964)
b. "Not a single sample contained 3 or more OCs [obligatory contexts] for the uncontractable auxiliary *be*" (p. 964)
c. "The finding that few and variable numbers of obligatory contexts were present in spontaneous language samples of this length suggests that they are insufficient for measuring GM [grammatical morpheme] production...." (p. 966)
d. "Research assistants [unaware of] the child's OME (otitis media with effusion) status transcribed each sample orthographically using the Systematic Analysis of Language Transcripts conventions, as well as a set of additional conventions to ensure transcription consistency" (p. 963)
e. "In summary, results from the present investigation indicate a need for caution in interpreting information on GM [grammatical morpheme] production derived from 15-min spontaneous language samples from 4-year-old children" (p. 967)

36. A school board with a culturally, linguistically, and sociodemographically diverse student body decides to develop a test of emergent literacy skills that will be administered to all children on entry to first grade. The purpose of the test is to identify children who may need extra services in addition to the regular first grade curriculum in order to achieve success in learning to read during the first grade. The test construction committee is composed of SLPs, educational psychologists, reading specialists, and school principals. The committee decides to develop a *criterion-referenced test*. From a literature review, the committee members learn that emergent literacy abilities at school entry have been shown to be an important predictor of reading skills in later grades. Further research yields information on the domain of skills that compose emergent literacy and typical performance levels achieved by beginning first graders. The committee decides to develop a pool of 45 test items covering phonological awareness, concepts about print, and letter name knowledge, taking care to ensure the cultural and linguistic appropriateness of the items for their student population. Thus far, the

committee's activities have been directed at ensuring which of the following types of validity for the test under development?
a. Predictive validity
b. Criterion-related validity
c. Divergent validity
d. Construct validity
e. Content validity

37. A school board with a culturally, linguistically, and sociodemographically diverse student body decides to develop a test of emergent literacy skills that will be administered to all children on entry to first grade. The purpose of the test is to identify children who may need extra services in addition to the regular first grade curriculum in order to achieve success in learning to read during the first grade. The test construction committee is composed of SLPs, educational psychologists, reading specialists, and school principals. The committee decides to develop a *criterion-referenced test*. In order to validate the items selected for the new test, the committee needs to choose a procedure that serves as a "gold standard" for identifying children who are "emergent readers" versus those children who are "not ready to learn to read" and thus in need of extra services. Of the following procedures, which is most likely to meet this need *and* be appropriate for the diverse student population that will take the test?
a. A standardized norm-referenced test such as the Wide Range Achievement Test
b. A test of nonword repetition ability
c. Informal observation of the child by the teacher in the classroom
d. Dynamic assessment of the child's ability to learn literacy-related skills
e. A commercial screening test of emergent literacy skills

38. A school board with a culturally, linguistically, and sociodemographically diverse student body decides to develop a test of emergent literacy skills that will be administered to all children on entry to first grade. The purpose of the test is to identify children who may need extra services in addition to the regular first grade curriculum in order to achieve success in learning to read during the first grade. The test construction committee is composed of SLPs, educational psychologists, reading specialists, and school principals. The committee decides to develop a *criterion-referenced test*. In October, the entire pool of 45 test items is administered to 300 first graders, selected through stratified random sampling to ensure similarity to the school population with regard to sociodemographic diversity. An item analysis is conducted to select 15 of the items for use in the final version of the criterion-referenced test. Of the following strategies, which would be the most appropriate for the

committee to use when selecting items for inclusion in the final version of the test?
a. Select items passed by all students identified as "emergent readers" and failed by all students identified as "not ready to learn to read"
b. Select items so that the mean difficulty level is .5
c. Select items so that the mean difficulty ranges from .2 to .8 and the mean discrimination index varies from .3 to 1.00
d. Select items for which the proportion of students passing is approximately equal among speakers of Standard American English, speakers of African American English, and English language learners
e. Select items so that the distribution of scores summed across the 15 items is normal for the 300 scores, whereby 68% of obtained scores are within plus or minus one standard deviation of the mean

39. A school board with a culturally, linguistically, and sociodemographically diverse student body decides to develop a test of emergent literacy skills that will be administered to all children on entry to first grade. The purpose of the test is to identify children who may need extra services in addition to the regular first grade curriculum in order to achieve success in learning to read during the first grade. The test construction committee is composed of SLPs, educational psychologists, reading specialists, and school principals. The committee decides to develop a *criterion-referenced test*. In June of the same year, the same 300 first graders receive a sight-word reading test and are judged to pass or fail the test according to state-mandated criteria. Performance on the reading test is compared to their performance on the 15-item emergent literacy test administered in October. The contingency table below shows the proportion of children who passed the two tests.

	Pass Reading Test	Fail Reading Test	Total
Pass Emergent Literacy Test	.59	.09	.68
Fail Emergent Literacy Test	.05	.27	.32
Total	.64	.36	1.00

Of the following statements, which is the best interpretation of the results of this analysis?
a. The emergent literacy test has good concurrent validity
b. The emergent literacy test has poor divergent validity
c. The emergent literacy test has good predictive validity
d. The emergent literacy test has good test-retest reliability
e. The emergent literacy test has good construct validity

40. A school board with a culturally, linguistically, and sociodemographically diverse student body decides to develop a test of emergent literacy skills that will be

administered to all children on entry to first grade. The purpose of the test is to identify children who may need extra services in addition to the regular first grade curriculum in order to achieve success in learning to read during the first grade. The test construction committee is composed of SLPs, educational psychologists, reading specialists, and school principals. The committee decides to develop a *criterion-referenced test*. After developing a criterion-referenced test of emergent literacy that was shown to have good reliability and validity, the committee administered the test to all of the first graders who were enrolled in the school district in the subsequent year. Of the following results, which is the most likely cutoff score used to identify the children who will be referred for extra services?

a. Performance below the 10th percentile
b. Fewer than 12 of 15 correct responses
c. A *z* score less than 0
d. Fewer than 3 of 15 correct responses
e. A standard score less than 85

41. The following question is based on the following abbreviated abstract and the study (Gillam et al., 2008) it describes.

PURPOSE:

An RCT was carried out to compare the language and auditory processing skills of children who received the Fast For-Word Language (FFW-L) intervention with the skills of children assigned to nonspecific or specific language intervention comparison treatments that did not include modified speech.

METHOD:

Two hundred sixteen children between the ages of 6 and 9 years with language impairments were randomly assigned to one of four conditions: (1) FFW-L, (2) academic enrichment, (3) computer-assisted language intervention (CALI), or (4) individualized language intervention (ILI) provided by an SLP. All children received 1 hour and 40 minutes of treatment, 5 days per week, for 6 weeks. Examiners who were unaware of treatment condition administered language and auditory processing measures to the children before treatment, immediately after treatment, 3 months after treatment, and 6 months after treatment.

RESULTS:

The children in all four conditions improved significantly on a global language test and a test of backward masking. Effect sizes, analyses of standard error of measurement, and normalization percentages supported the clinical significance of the improvements on the Comprehensive Assessment of Spoken Language.

CONCLUSION:

FFW-L, the intervention that provided modified speech to address a hypothesized underlying auditory processing deficit, was not more effective at improving general language skills or temporal processing skills than a nonspecific comparison treatment (academic enrichment) or specific language intervention comparison treatments (CALI and ILI) that did not contain modified speech stimuli.

Of the following, which is the independent variable in this study?

a. FFW-L
b. Treatment condition
c. Comprehensive Assessment of Spoken Language
d. Test of backward masking
e. Language and auditory processing measures

42. The following question is based on the following abbreviated abstract and the study (Gillam et al., 2008) it describes.

PURPOSE:

An RCT was conducted to compare the language and auditory processing outcomes of children assigned to receive the FFW-L intervention with the outcomes of children assigned to nonspecific or specific language intervention comparison treatments that did not contain modified speech.

METHOD:

Two hundred sixteen children between the ages of 6 and 9 years with language impairments were randomly assigned to one of four conditions: (1) FFW-L, (2) academic enrichment, (3) CALI, or (4) individualized language intervention (ILI) provided by an SLP. All children received 1 hour and 40 minutes of treatment, 5 days per week, for 6 weeks. Examiners who were unaware of treatment condition administered language and auditory processing measures to the children before treatment, immediately after treatment, 3 months after treatment, and 6 months after treatment.

RESULTS:

The children in all four conditions improved significantly on a global language test and a test of backward masking. Effect sizes, analyses of standard error of measurement, and normalization percentages supported the clinical significance of the improvements on the Comprehensive Assessment of Spoken Language.

CONCLUSION:

FFW-L, the intervention that provided modified speech to address a hypothesized underlying auditory processing deficit, was not more effective at improving general language skills or temporal processing skills than a nonspecific comparison treatment (academic enrichment) or specific language intervention comparison treatments (CALI and ILI) that did not contain modified speech stimuli.

Of the following designs, which is the best description of the one used by Gillam and colleagues (2008)?
   a. Time series design
   b. Solomon randomized four-group design
   c. Within-subjects experimental design
   d. Nonequivalent comparison groups design
   e. Between-subjects experimental design

43. The following question is based on the following abbreviated abstract and the study (Gillam et al., 2008) it describes.

PURPOSE:

An RCT was conducted to compare the language and auditory processing outcomes of children assigned to receive the FFW-L intervention with the outcomes of children assigned to nonspecific or specific language intervention comparison treatments that did not contain modified speech.

METHOD:

Two hundred sixteen children between the ages of 6 and 9 years with language impairments were randomly assigned to one of four conditions: (1) FFW-L, (2) academic enrichment, (3) CALI, or (4) individualized language intervention (ILI) provided by an SLP. All children received 1 hour and 40 minutes of treatment, 5 days per week, for 6 weeks. Examiners who were unaware of treatment condition administered language and auditory processing measures to the children before treatment, immediately after treatment, 3 months after treatment, and 6 months after treatment.

RESULTS:

The children in all four conditions improved significantly on a global language test and a test of backward masking. Effect sizes, analyses of standard error of measurement, and normalization percentages supported the clinical significance of the improvements on the Comprehensive Assessment of Spoken Language.

CONCLUSION:

FFW-L, the intervention that provided modified speech to address a hypothesized underlying auditory processing deficit, was not more effective at improving general language skills or temporal processing skills than a nonspecific comparison treatment (academic enrichment) or specific language intervention comparison treatments (CALI and ILI) that did not contain modified speech stimuli.

The abstract indicates that examiners who were unaware of treatment condition administered the language and auditory processing measures on all four testing occasions. This procedure protects the internal validity of the trial by guarding against which one of the following types of bias?
   a. Selection bias
   b. Attrition bias
   c. Performance bias
   d. Detection bias
   e. Systematic bias

44. The following question is based on the following abbreviated abstract and the study (Gillam et al., 2008) it describes.

PURPOSE:

An RCT was conducted to compare the language and auditory processing outcomes of children assigned to receive the FFW-L intervention with the outcomes of children assigned to nonspecific or specific language intervention comparison treatments that did not contain modified speech.

METHOD:

Two hundred sixteen children between the ages of 6 and 9 years with language impairments were randomly assigned to one of four conditions: (1) FFW-L, (2) academic enrichment, (3) CALI, or (4) individualized language intervention (ILI) provided by an SLP. All children received 1 hour and 40 minutes of treatment, 5 days per week, for 6 weeks. Examiners who were unaware of treatment condition administered language and auditory processing measures to the children before treatment, immediately after treatment, 3 months after treatment, and 6 months after treatment.

RESULTS:

The children in all four conditions improved significantly on a global language test and a test of backward masking. Effect sizes, analyses of standard error of measurement, and normalization percentages supported the clinical significance of the improvements on the Comprehensive Assessment of Spoken Language.

CONCLUSION:

FFW-L, the intervention that provided modified speech to address a hypothesized underlying auditory processing deficit, was not more effective at improving general language skills or temporal processing skills than a nonspecific comparison treatment (academic enrichment) or specific language intervention comparison treatments (CALI and ILI) that did not contain modified speech stimuli.

The results of the study with respect to language outcomes were assessed with a mixed-model ANCOVA, in which the covariate was pretest language scores and the fixed independent variables were treatment condition and postintervention assessment time. The statistical analysis revealed a significant main effect of time but no main effect of treatment condition and no significant interaction of treatment condition and treatment time. Figure 25-3 represents the change that was observed for each group from the pretreatment to the posttreatment assessment on the Comprehensive Assessment of Spoken Language.

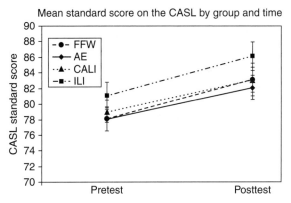

Mean standard score on the CASL by group and time

Figure 25-3 AE, academic enrichment; CALI, computer-assisted language intervention; CASL, Comprehensive Assessment of Spoken Language; FFW, Fast ForWord (intervention); ILI, individualized language intervention. (From Gillam, R. B., Loeb, D. F., Hoffman, L. M., et al. [2008]. The efficacy of Fast ForWord Language Intervention in school-age children with language impairment: A randomized controlled trial. *Journal of Speech, Language, and Hearing Research, 51*, 97–119.)

Of the following statements, which is the most appropriate conclusion to draw from the results of this study?
   a. It is not clear whether the four treatments were equally effective or equally ineffective
   b. The four treatments were equally effective
   c. The four treatments were equally ineffective
   d. The ILI treatment was most effective
   e. The ILI treatment was effective, and the academic enrichment, CALI, and FFW treatments were equally ineffective

45. The following question is based on the following abbreviated abstract and the study (Gillam et al., 2008) it describes.

PURPOSE:

An RCT was conducted to compare the language and auditory processing outcomes of children assigned to receive the FFW-L intervention with the outcomes of children assigned to nonspecific or specific language intervention comparison treatments that did not contain modified speech.

METHOD:

Two hundred sixteen children between the ages of 6 and 9 years with language impairments were randomly assigned to one of four conditions: (1) FFW-L, (2) academic enrichment, (3) CALI, or (4) individualized language intervention (ILI) provided by an SLP. All children received 1 hour and 40 minutes of treatment, 5 days per week, for 6 weeks. Examiners who were unaware of treatment condition administered language and auditory processing measures to the children before treatment, immediately after treatment, 3 months after treatment, and 6 months after treatment.

RESULTS:

The children in all four conditions improved significantly on a global language test and a test of backward masking. Effect sizes, analyses of standard error of measurement, and normalization percentages supported the clinical significance of the improvements on the Comprehensive Assessment of Spoken Language.

CONCLUSION:

FFW-L, the intervention that provided modified speech to address a hypothesized underlying auditory processing deficit, was not more effective at improving general language skills or temporal processing skills than a nonspecific comparison treatment (academic enrichment) or specific language intervention comparison treatments (CALI and ILI) that did not contain modified speech stimuli.

Gillam and colleagues (2008) stated that "the gains in language and auditory processing that were observed across the four conditions of the study may have arisen as a result of practice effects, maturation, regression to the mean, and/or spontaneous recovery (p. 110)." Of the following changes to the design of the study, which might have controlled for these potential threats to the internal validity of the study?
   a. Including a comparison group of normally developing children who received the language tests according to the same assessment schedule as the children enrolled in the trial
   b. Using an intention-to-treat analysis so that even the results for the children who drop out of the trial are included in the final data analysis
   c. Randomly assigning children with language impairment to a no-treatment control condition but assessing their language skills according to the same assessment schedule as the children enrolled in the trial
   d. Including children whose language impairments represent a broader range of severity levels in the study sample
   e. Ensuring that the random allocation list is concealed from the staff who recruit and treat the children so that there is no chance that the most severely impaired children will be assigned to certain treatment conditions

Answers

1. c. Emergent literacy skills is the primary dependent variable. Phonological awareness (option a) is the independent variable; nonverbal intelligence (option b) and receptive vocabulary skills (option d) are covariates. Sight word reading skill (option e) forms part of the measure of the dependent variable but is not the primary dependent variable, as stated in the purpose statement of the abstract.

2. b. A history effect threatens the internal validity of the study because the children in the intervention and control conditions have different experiences all morning at school, in addition to receiving the control and intervention conditions at story time. The maturation threat (option a) applies equally to both classes. The differential subject selection effect (option c) is a plausible threat, although the investigators report that receptive vocabulary and nonverbal intelligence were matched across the two classrooms. The problem of poor subject description (option d) is a threat to the external validity of the study. The use of nonstandardized measures (option e) is not necessarily a threat to internal validity; problems with the instrumentation should apply equally to both classes.

3. a. The independence assumption that underlies the application of the *t* test has been violated in this case (the children are not independent of each other, but the classrooms are, and thus the classroom is the unit of analysis). Unequal sample sizes (option b) do not necessarily lead to unequal variances (although they might). The implied hypothesis is clearly that the intervention will be superior to the control condition, and thus a one-tailed *t* test is most appropriate(option c). ANCOVA (option d) is not necessary in this case, in which there are no between-group differences in these other variables. Paired samples (option e)—with children as the unit of analysis—would have been appropriate only if individual children are matched to each other, not when groups are shown to be matched post hoc.

4. d. Giving the children the probe twice in one week is the procedure for obtaining a measure of test-retest reliability. Measuring scores on the probe and test when given twice in one day (option a) describes convergent validity; testing this way in only one group of children (option b) yields measures of divergent validity. Comparing the scores of children with normal skills with the scores of children with delay skills (option c) also provides evidence of validity rather than reliability. Measuring subtest scores for one

group of children (option e) provides a measure of internal consistency, which is a form of reliability but not well suited to the purpose in this case, especially because consistency across these three aspects of emergent literacy are not necessarily expected (i.e., a child might have good rime awareness but not be able to read any sight words), although consistency within the subtests should be expected.

5. e. In a single-blind nonequivalent comparison group design, there is a control group, but the intervention and control conditions are provided to intact groups and the outcomes are evaluated by an assessor who is unaware of treatment condition. This study was not double-blind (options a and c) because the SLP administering the intervention had to know which treatment she was administering! The children were not randomly assigned individually to conditions (option b). The comparison was between groups, and the measures were conducted only twice (before and after intervention) rather than repeatedly over time (option d).

6. d. The correct answer is the only sentence that states the hypothesis of the study ("It was expected that the wearing of Irlen lenses…would improve the sight word reading abilities") while identifying the independent (Irlen lenses) and dependent (reading sight words) variables.

7. a. The treatment was applied to several children at staggered intervals, so that the baseline phase was lengthened for each successive subject. A multiple-baseline design is a variant of the AB design (option b), but a simple AB design does not have the added control of the multiple baselines. A reversal design (option c) involves the withdrawal of treatment after the treatment phase. The study involved only one treatment; therefore, there could be no alternating between treatments (option d). The treatment was not changed in form or intensity (option e) after the children achieved some criterion level of performance.

8. e. The unstable baselines suggest that the observed improvements in reading performance could have resulted from maturation or history effects rather than from the treatment itself. Although this treatment has been shown to be ineffective in other studies, those prior findings do not preclude the design of an internally valid study to confirm or refute the prior findings (option b). Selection of complex research participants (option c) and simple measures

of reading limit the external validity of the study but do not affect the internal validity of the study. Treatment withdrawal (option a) is not likely to work in this case; the children are not likely to forget how to read the words that they have learned after removing the glasses. Furthermore, a second strategy for demonstrating experimental control (option d) is not strictly necessary when the multiple-baseline strategy has already been implemented; the difficulty in this case is not applying the strategy correctly (i.e., not ensuring a stable baseline before introducing the treatment), which is a requirement for the internal validity of all single-subject designs.

9. b. The implied argument in the poster is that the magnocellular deficit causes scotoscopic sensitivity, which in turn impairs reading and is cured by tinted lenses that fix the text distortions that result from the scotoscopic sensitivity. The argument is not necessarily supported by descriptive research reporting an association between magnocellular dysfunction and dyslexia because this research cannot prove a causal link. For the same reason, the argument that that findings support the underlying theory of why the lenses work (option a) is incorrect. The statements about evidence-based practice (option c) and brain imaging research (option d) are correctly concerned with scientific evidence but identify erroneous levels of evidence to support clinical practice. The statement that research with adults reveals nothing about reading acquisition by children (option e) is not strictly true and not fully relevant to the question.

10. c. Fluctuations in characteristics of the child and examiner and in situation factors might cause session-to-session fluctuations in test scores. Investigator bias (options a, b, and e), reactive pretest (e.g., practice effects; options a and d) and statistical regression (options b and e) are better explanations for the generally upward trend in test scores across the entire study interval than the seemingly random fluctuations in scores from session to session.

11. d. The research is experimental, not descriptive (options a and b), because type of treatment and elicitation condition (the independent variables) were manipulated by the investigators. No between-subjects comparisons (options c and e) were made.

12. a. Factorial analysis of variance enables the researchers to examine the main effects and interaction of the two independent variables on the dependent variable. Although a repeated-measures t test is a within-subjects design, it is not designed to handle two independent variables at once. Standard error of the mean (option c) and Cohen's d measure of effect size

(option d) are descriptive rather than inferential statistics, and the Pearson correlation coefficient (option e) is better suited to descriptive research with continuous predictor variables, rather than experimental research with categorical independent variables.

13. c. Because neither the clinicians who provided the treatment nor the observers who coded the videotapes could be unaware of treatment condition, experimenter bias is the most likely threat to the internal validity of this study. The within-subjects design and the counterbalancing of treatment conditions within sessions control for history (option a), maturation (option b), fatigue effects (option d), and practice effects (option e).

14. e. A procedure for determining interrater reliability is to have at least 20% of the sessions coded independently by two coders and then to examine the correlation between scores and the range and average of the differences between scores for the two raters. Interrater reliability is particularly important in this case because the most likely threat to the internal validity of the study, in view of its otherwise strong design, is observer bias in the measurement of the dependent variable. Examining the correlation between the outcome measure and Developmental Sentence Scores (option a) is related more closely to validity than to reliability. Using Cronbach's alpha to estimate the average of split-half correlations (option b) is a measure of internal consistency, which is not the primary concern and not relevant to a measure that does not involve a standard number of discrete items. A consensus rating (option c) is not the same as reliability. A training workshop and testing of coders (option d) would tend to improve reliability, but it would still be necessary to measure interrater or intrarater reliability, to ensure that it has been achieved.

15. b. The correct answer is option b, the only alternative that correctly identifies the interaction effect and the appropriate dependent variable. The statement about grammatical target (option e) mentions an interaction but identifies an irrelevant variable (grammatical target), and its conclusion implies a main effect of treatment type. It is clear from Figure 25-2 that there are no significant main effects (options c and d). Option a is not correct in stating the findings reported in the graph.

16. c. A reliable test will yield similar scores when an individual is tested repeatedly in similar circumstances. Measuring the correct construct (option a), sensitivity (option b), and yielding scores similar to those on other tests (option d) are all concerned with the

validity of the test. The statement about the error component (option e) is a misstatement of classical test theory.

17. a. A high reliability coefficient indicates that the test yields replicable results, and a low standard error of measurement indicates that the test yields precise or accurate results.

18. e. *Face validity* refers to the extent to which the measure looks valid to the examinee. The examinee in this case believes that he is being unfairly tested on his knowledge of U.S. presidents, even though this is not the SLP's intention. This issue is distinct from the question of whether the measure is actually revealing the patient's phonological memory skills (option c). Criterion validity (option b) and predictive validity (option d) are not relevant to the vignette because no other measures are mentioned. Content validity (option a) is the extent to which a measure or test represents all characteristics of a construct being evaluates as is typically apart of test validation. The case in question is a clinician devised informal measure.

19. a. Sensitivity, or the percentage of true positive results, is the percentage of persons who are at risk for a particular problem or disorder. Specificity, or the percentage of true negative results (option b), is the percentage of persons who are correctly identified as not having a disease or disorder. An appropriate assessment or measure would have satisfactory specificity and sensitivity.

20. c. A 95% probability that a child who fails the screening questionnaire will be identified by formal testing as having a speech problem is an example of positive predictive value.

21. d. A 95% probability that a child who passes the screening questionnaire will be identified by formal testing as having normal speech (option d) is an example of negative predictive value.

22. e. Expert opinion does not constitute scientific evidence by itself. Although the other conditions do not yield the highest levels of evidence provided by meta-analyses and RCTs, they are stronger than expert opinion. On most levels of evidence hierarchies in the medical literature, the highest level of evidence is yielded by a nonrandomized, between-groups, controlled trial (option b); the next highest, by a retrospective case-control study (option d); and the lowest, by an observational study of a cohort without a control group (option a). The use of single-subject experiments (option c) is

controversial in medical circles but allowed by the American Speech-Language-Hearing Association (ASHA) because they yield a relatively high level of evidence if the studies are well designed with good controls for internal validity, such as are afforded by the multiple-baseline design.

23. b. According to Sackett and associates' (1996) seminal definition (from which the ASHA definition is derived), clinical expertise is integrated with the best available research evidence. The statement that it is integrated with the patient's values and preferences (option e) is partially correct but incomplete and missing the critical mention of "evidence." It follows from Sackett and associates' definition that options a, c, and d are incorrect. Clinical expertise is not derived solely from published research evidence (option a), it does play a role in evidence-based practice (option c), and it is not used in place of RCT evidence (option d).

24. d. Random assignment of the unit of analysis (in this case, individual children) to the treatment conditions is the hallmark of an RCT. The use of an observer who is unaware of treatment condition (option c) strengthens the design but does not by itself mean that the study is an RCT. Random selection of participants (option a), standardized outcome measures (option e), and a no-treatment control condition (option b) are not necessary components of an RCT.

25. a. The statement about the analysis of variance (option a) refers to inferential statistics. The statements concerning mean and standard deviation (options c and e) and within-group variance (option d) contain only descriptive statistics, and the effect size measure (option b) is independent of statistical significance.

26. e. Describing the characteristics of the experimental sample as precisely as possible characterizes descriptive statistics.

27. c. It may be true that a treatment that improves reading cannot be generalized to dysfluency, but this statement is more closely related to the external validity of the study (to whom can the findings be generalized?) than the internal validity of the study in question. The reductions in the children's dysfluency beyond the possible effect of the treatment can be explained plausibly by statistical regression to the mean (option a), maturation (option b), events occurring in the classroom or at home (option d), or observer bias (option e); thus, the investigator has failed to control for these threats to the internal validity of the design.

28. b. Questions about generalization (options a and c) cannot be assessed with a multiple-baseline design. The idea that manipulation of the dependent variable could cause changes in the independent variable (option d) represents confusion about the definition of independent and dependent variables. The idea that demonstrating a stable baseline for the dependent variable would demonstrate experimental control (option e) represents confusion of the baseline and withdrawal phases of the study.

29. a. The behavior that the treatment is supposed to affect (the dependent variable) is not mentioned. The independent variable (the Lee Silverman Voice Treatment) is mentioned (option c), as is the research strategy (multiple-baseline design; option d). The gender and age of the patients (option b) and details of the treatment (option e) are omitted, but these omissions are less serious than the complete absence of the dependent variable.

30. c. The concern raised is about the conditions to which the findings can be generalized (external validity). No concerns are expressed about whether the experimental implementation was actually the cause of changes in the patients' speech, and thus efficacy of the treatment (option a) and internal validity of the study (option d) are not addressed in the paragraph. Reliability (option b) is concerned with replicability under similar circumstances rather than generalization to different circumstances. No mention of the cost of the treatment in relation to other treatments (option e) is mentioned.

31. a. The paragraph represents descriptive research. The study does not entail an examination of the relationship between two variables, and so it is not correlational research (option b). The study involves observing a behavior directly rather than asking respondents about the behavior or attitude of interest; therefore, it is not survey research (option c). The independent variable is not directly manipulated, and so it is not experimental research. The study does not involve a comparison of two or more groups of subjects on the variable of interest, so it is not comparative research.

32. d. The primary concern would be a false suggestion of impairment. Overestimation of the child's abilities (option a) also points to the validity of the measure with regard to the child's use of GMs, but the concern expressed in the conclusion is more focused on the validity of the normative data. It is just as likely that the measure will underestimate the child's ability in any case. Questions about replicability (option b), sensitivity (option c), and internal consistency (option e) are directly or indirectly concerned with reliability.

33. c. The calculation of agreements and disagreements for two independent coders is performed to determine interrater reliability. Intrarater reliability (option a) is concerned with a single rater; internal consistency (option b), with responses among items; and coefficient of equivalence (option d), with parallel forms. Criterion validity (option e) pertains to validity, not reliability.

34. b. The mean and standard deviation are descriptive statistics. The t test and Cohen's d (option a) and analysis of variance (option e) are used to compare differences between groups, which does not correspond to the question. The Pearson product-moment correlation coefficient (option c) and the Spearman rho correlation coefficient (option d) are used to describe the relationship between two variables, which also does not correspond to the question.

35. e. The stated need for caution makes it clear that the conclusions relate specifically to 4-year-old children. The statements about interobserver agreement (option a) and what the research assistants used to transcribe data (option d) are concerned with reliability. The statements about what was present in the samples (options b and c) are concerned with the validity of the measurement procedure rather than the external validity of the study itself.

36. e. Content validity is an assessment of the extent to which the test covers the domain of knowledge or skills that the test is intended to measure, on the basis of expert opinion (as opposed to empirical evidence). Predictive (option a), criterion-related (option b), divergent (option c), and construct validity (option d) require that the test be given to a sample of children, along with other assessment procedures, and that the empirical evidence be examined in various ways in order to establish the type of validity in question.

37. d. Dynamic assessment of the child's ability to learn literacy-related skills would fulfill both requirements. A standardized norm-referenced test (option a) and a commercial screening test of emergent literacy skills (option e) are likely to be culturally biased or at least scored on the basis of normative samples or reference samples not similar to the school population that will take the test. Nonword repetition (option b), as a processing-dependent test, is less likely to be culturally biased but has poor content validity and construct validity in this context. Informal observation is likely to have poor reliability and, since the standards that the teacher uses to identify children may not be well known, construct validity may also be poor (e.g., the teacher's

judgment may reflect social maturity rather than emergent literacy skills; Laing & Kamhi, 2003).

38. a. The correct procedure involves selecting items that are passed by 100% of children deemed to be "masters" of the criterion skill and failed by 100% of the children deemed to be "nonmasters" of the criterion skill. Selecting items so that the mean difficulty level is .5 (option b), so that the mean difficulty ranges from .2 to .8 (option b), or so that 68% of obtained scores are within plus or minus one standard deviation of the mean (option c) would be appropriate for norm-referenced tests; in other words, these strategies are designed to produce a varied distribution of test scores that will distinguish among individuals. Selecting items that reflect equal proportions of students who speak standard American English or African American English, or who are English language learners, would guard against cultural bias but might not meet the goal set by the committee, which is to identify children who may not learn to read unless they receive extra services beyond the regular class room curriculum. Some steps have already been taken to ensure a culturally fair test (choosing a criterion- rather than norm-referenced test, selecting a reference group for item analysis from the school board's own culturally diverse student body, and designing test items to be culturally sensitive).

39. c. The emergent literacy test has good predictive validity, which indicates that the test predicts, with a reasonable level of accuracy, which children will be reading at the end of first grade and which children will not be reading at a level deemed satisfactory according to state-mandated standards. Because the two tests were given at different times and do not measure exactly the same construct, concurrent validity (option a) cannot be determined. Because the two tests are concerned with related rather than opposing constructs, divergent validity (option b) cannot be determined. Because two completely different tests were administered, test-retest reliability (option d) cannot be determined. Because the tests were measuring different constructs (emergent literacy versus sight word reading are not the same construct even though there is a predictive relationship between the constructs), construct validity (option e) cannot be measured.

40. b. A score of fewer than 12 of 15 correct responses is a raw score measure that is reasonably but not overly strict and that separates those children who have mastered the skill in question from those who have not. A score of fewer than 3 of 15 correct responses (option d) is also a raw score measure but it is atypically low for a criterion-referenced test and would

not separate those children who have mastered the skill from those who have not. All of the remaining alternatives—a score below the 10th percentile (option a), a z score less than 0 (option c), and a standard score less than 85 (option e)—are norm-referenced scores that describe the test-taker's performance in relation to performance by other children in the reference group.

41. b. The treatment condition was the independent variable because it was manipulated by the experimenter (children were randomly assigned to one of four conditions). FFW-L (option a) was only one of the treatment conditions. The Comprehensive Assessment of Spoken Language (option c), the test of backward masking (option d), and language and auditory processing measures (option e) were dependent variables.

42. e. This study is best described as a between-subjects experimental design because children were randomly assigned to treatment conditions. Each was independently assigned to one of the four treatments; therefore, it is not a within-subjects design (option c). Children were assessed repeatedly over time, but there was more than one group, and so the study was not a time series design (option a). All groups were pretested, and so it was not a Solomon randomized four-group design (option b). Random assignment to conditions means that it was not a nonequivalent comparison groups design (option d).

43. d. In detection bias, assessment of the outcome is biased by knowledge of the participants' group assignment; because the examiners were unaware of treatment condition, detection bias could not occur. Selection bias (option a) is protected against by concealment of the allocation sequence; attrition bias (option b), by an intention-to-treat analysis; and performance bias (option c), by keeping the participant and health care provider unaware of the treatment provided. Internal validity is threatened by any source of systematic error, but there is no form of bias officially called *systematic bias* (option e).

44. a. All groups have made a significant improvement over time, but it is not clear whether the improvement is caused by the treatment (history, maturation, and statistical regression are alternative explanations). In particular, it is not clear that the ILI treatment was most effective (option d) or that the other three treatments were equally ineffective (option e), in view of the overlapping standard error bars in Figure 25-3 and because the results of the statistical analysis indicated no main effect of treatment condition and no interaction of treatment condition with time.

45. c. Randomly assigning children with language impairment to a no-treatment control condition but assessing their language skills at the same times as the other children is a procedure that will control for several potential explanations for the results in this case (practice effects, spontaneous recovery and maturation, and regression toward the mean). This procedure will reveal whether the improvement under treatment is significantly greater than the improvements observed when other children are assessed repeatedly over the same time interval but not treated. Including children with a broader range of impairment (option d) would only eliminate regression toward the mean if average and above-average ability levels were included; however, this does not make sense in this trial, and this practice would not control for maturation and practice effects in any case. A comparison group of normally developing children (option a) does not control for any potential threats to the internal validity of the study. Using an intention-to-treat analysis (option b) is a control for attrition bias. Concealing the random allocation list from recruiting staff (option e) is a control for selection bias.

Bibliography

Balason, D. V., & Dollaghan, C. A. (2002). Grammatical morpheme production in 4-year-old children. *Journal of Speech, Language, and Hearing Research, 45,* 961–969.

Camarata, S. M., Nelson, K. E., & Camarata, M. N. (1994). Comparison of conversational recasting and imitative procedures for training grammatical structures in children with specific language impairment. *Journal of Speech and Hearing Research, 37,* 1414–1423.

Coplan, J., & Gleason, J. R. (1988). Unclear speech: Recognition and significance of unintelligible speech in preschool children. *Pediatrics, 82,* 447–452.

Gillam, R. B., Loeb, D. F., Hoffman, L. M., et al. (2008). The efficacy of Fast ForWord Language intervention in school-age children with language impairment: A randomized controlled trial. *Journal of Speech, Language, and Hearing Research, 51,* 97–119.

Hustad, K. C., & Beukelman, D. R. (2001). Effects of linguistic cues and stimulus cohesion on intelligibility of severely dysarthric speech. *Journal of Speech, Language, and Hearing Research, 44,* 497–510.

Laing, S. P., & Kamhi, A. (2003). Alternative assessment of language and literacy in culturally and linguistically diverse populations. *Language, Speech and Hearing Services in Schools, 34,* 44–55.

Sackett, D. L., Rosenberg, W. M., Gray, J. A., Haynes, R. B., & Richardson, W. S. (1996). Evidence based medicine: What it is and what it isn't. *British Medical Journal, 13: 312*(7023): 71–72.

CHAPTER 26

Standards and Laws

Shelly S. Chabon
Dorian Lee-Wilkerson

1. Lisa is an audiologist working in private practice. She is currently seeing a Medicare beneficiary for auditory rehabilitation following a cochlear implant. She instructed the billing coordinator to bill Medicare for this service. The most likely outcome is:
   a. Medicare will deny this claim because it is for aural rehabilitation
   b. Medicare will pay the complete charge
   c. Medicare will pay some of the charge
   d. Medicare will deny this claim because it only covers services for cases related to prelingual hearing loss
   e. Medicare will deny this claim because Lisa is in private practice

2. Transcutaneous electrical stimulation (TES) has been used by speech-language pathologists (SLPs) in the treatment of individuals with dysphagia. The most appropriate statement regarding the safety and precautions important to the successful use of such a device is:
   a. The American Speech-Language-Hearing Association (ASHA) must approve the device before it can be used with a client
   b. Each state has specific regulations on the use of TES
   c. The use of TES is viewed to be outside of the scope of practice for SLPs
   d. TES devices are subject to U.S. Food and Drug Administration (FDA) regulations
   e. All of the above

3. Reuben and his parents moved to Kansas from Mexico when he was 5½ years old. Reuben and his family had limited exposure to English before he was enrolled in school. Of the following conditions, which best meets the requirements of the No Child Left Behind Act with regard to Reuben and his family?

a. Reuben may be excused from participating in the state assessment

b. Reuben must participate in the state assessment

c. Under the No Child Left Behind Act, Kansas is required to administer the assessment in Spanish

d. Under the No Child Left Behind Act, Kansas is required to delay administration of the test for 6 months

e. Under the No Child Left Behind Act, Kansas is required to delay administration of the test until the child has resided in the state for 1 year

4. Many states and the federal government have enacted student loan forgiveness programs as an incentive for serving high-need schools. Of the following people, who are eligible for state-level funds?

a. Teachers who work in public schools and want to pursue graduate studies in communication service for the deaf (CSD)

b. SLP graduates who agree to work in public schools

c. Both of the above

d. Neither a nor b, because these options are available only when the SLP agrees to work in a high need school

e. Speech-language pathology assistants, regardless of their place of employment

5. Of the following legislative acts, which is credited as beginning the inclusion movement in the public schools?

a. Education of the Handicapped Act (P.L. 91-230) in 1970

b. Individuals with Disabilities Education Act (IDEA) (P.L. 94-142) in 1975

c. The Regular Education Initiative (REI) in 1985

d. The Americans with Disabilities Act (P.L. 101-336) in 1990

e. The Taft-Hartley Act (80 P.L. 101) in 1947

6. Of the following, which established that separation of students on the basis of race or ethnicity was a direct violation of the Fourteenth Amendment of the U.S. Constitution?

a. *Brown v. Board of Education*

b. Individuals with Disabilities Education Act (IDEA)

c. *Mills v. Board of Education*

d. *Guadalupe Argentina v. Tempe Elementary School District #3*

e. *Dred Scott v. Sandford*

7. Maria is a 7-year-old Mexican American child with a diagnosis of attention deficit/hyperactivity disorder (ADHD) who has recently moved into your school district with a 504 plan from the school district in which she was previously enrolled. Of the following recommendations, which is *least* likely to be included in her 504 plan?

a. Ensure that the classroom environment has as few visual and auditory distractions, or both, as possible

b. Encourage Maria's teacher to provide frequent opportunities to select tasks and arrange her own schedule

c. Suggest that Maria's teacher use visual highlighters to make her work more interesting

d. Recommend that Maria be given short and frequent breaks from work

e. Provide a consistent and structured schedule of activities

8. In your school district, English is not the first language for a number of children. You have noticed that a disproportionate number of these children have been referred for speech and language services on the basis of their performance on standardized measures. Of the following statements, which is *not* correct with regard to this situation?

a. According to federal law, only standardized tests may be used to measure language performance

b. All children are entitled to a free and appropriate public education

c. Tests must be administered in the language in which the child is most proficient

d. No single procedure may be used in making a determination about a child's educational program

e. All of the above statements are correct

9. Leo received his Certificate of Clinical Competence (CCC-SLP) in 1999. In 2002, he let his certification lapse to pursue a law degree. In 2008, he decided to return to his first profession and provide clinical services. He was told that he would need to apply for reinstatement. Of the following assertions, which is *not* a requirement of reinstatement?

a. Leo must provide evidence of 30 hours of professional development completed no more than 3 years before the submission of the reinstatement application

b. Leo must meet the certification requirements in effect at the time of his request for reinstatement

c. Leo must repeat all graduate coursework if taken more than 15 years before the submission of the reinstatement application

d. Leo must provide official notification from the Educational Testing Service that he earned a score of 600 or above on the Praxis Examination in speech-language pathology no more than 5 years before submission of the reinstatement application

e. Leo's coursework must have targeted the acquisition of specific knowledge and skills of the profession

10. Nguyen and her parents moved to Missouri from Vietnam. She speaks very limited English even after her first year of school. The No Child Left Behind Act

requires yearly statewide accountability. Of the following accommodations, which may be selected in the assessment of Nguyen's yearly progress?

a. Use an assessment written in Vietnamese that is aligned with the state content and achievement standards

b. Provide audiotaped instructions in Vietnamese

c. Allow Nguyen to provide responses in either Vietnamese or English

d. Allowing Nguyen to utilize certain reading materials in Vietnamese

e. All of the above

11. Of the following statements, which is a principal component of the No Child Left Behind Act of 2001?

a. Importance of accountability for results

b. Importance of expanded parental options

c. Importance of local control and flexibility

d. Importance of demonstrated progress and improvement

e. All of the above are principal components of the No Child Left Behind Act

12. Lisa is beginning graduate school in CSD. A conscientious student, she has already researched requirements for ASHA certification in SLP. Her adviser has assured her that because she is attending a program that holds accreditation by the Council on Academic Accreditation (CAA) in Audiology and Speech-Language Pathology and because she received passing grades in all of her coursework, she does not need to worry. Of the following statements, which best reflects the accuracy of Lisa's adviser's response?

a. It is correct

b. It is incorrect

c. Passing grades are also required in clinical practicum

d. Certification standards no longer specify that the graduate academic program must be accredited

e. Grades of A or B, and not simply passing grades, are required to be eligible for certification

13. Jonathan is preparing to graduate with a master's degree in speech-language pathology. Of the following credentials, which is legally mandatory in most states for the practice of speech-language pathology in different work settings?

a. ASHA certification

b. State licensure

c. State Department of Education certification

d. All of the above

e. National licensure

14. Of the following, which gave legal recognition of social dialects, including, and in particular, African American English?

a. Individuals with Disabilities Education Act (IDEA) (P.L. 99-457)

b. *Lau v. Nichols*

c. *Martin Luther King Jr. Elementary School v. Ann Arbor School District*

d. *Brown v. Board of Education*

e. All of the above

15. A number of accrediting agencies at the national, state and local levels establish and monitor standards for provisions of quality services in settings in which SLPs may be employed. Talya is a certified SLP who works for a private, nonprofit, free-standing agency that serves young children with disabilities. Of the following regulatory agencies, which is *least* likely to play a role in the assessment of Talya's agency?

a. National Association for the Education of Young Children (NAEYC)

b. Commission on Accreditation of Rehabilitation Facilities (CARF)

c. Qualified Rating and Improvement Systems (QRS)

d. Council on Academic Accreditation in Audiology and Speech-Language Pathology of ASHA (CAA)

e. State Department of Education

16. Janice is a certified SLP, licensed to practice in the state of Virginia. One of Janice's clients is moving to West Virginia and asks to continue receiving services from Janice through telepractice. What would be an appropriate response from Janice?

a. "I can provide services to you through telepractice; my Certificate of Clinical Competence from ASHA qualifies me to provide the services you request"

b. "I cannot provide services to you through telepractice; although I am licensed to practice in the state of Virginia, I am not licensed to practice in West Virginia"

c. "I can provide the services as long as I maintain my license in the state where I provide the service and I maintain my ASHA certification"

d. "I cannot provide services to you through telepractice; the requirements for state licensure in West Virginia are different from the requirements for state licensure in Virginia, and there is no reciprocity between the two states"

e. "I cannot provide the services you request because my ASHA certification restricts my clinical practice to the state of my residence"

17. An SLP owns a private practice that specializes in oral motor therapy. She also works part time as a clinical instructor in a university clinic. Can this SLP refer the university clinic's patients to her private practice?

a. No, because such a referral would violate federal law

b. Yes, because the university clinic cannot accept any more clients for treatment

c. Yes, if the SLP allows students to obtained clinical hours at her private practice

d. No, because the referral would create an atmosphere of distrust between full-time and part-time clinical instructors

e. No, because directors of university clinics are always looking to recruit new clients so that students may earn their clinical clock hours

18. Julie is hired as a clinical fellow by the local school system. At the first meeting with her clinical supervisor, Julie is given her caseload assignment and the curriculum guides for kindergarten through second grade. Why would Julie need the curriculum guides?

a. The Americans with Disabilities Act requires that children be given access to the curriculum

b. IDEA requires school-based SLPs to be knowledgeable of how disability affects a child's access to the general curriculum

c. The No Child Left Behind Act is designed to ensure that children with special needs make functional gains in academic and nonacademic settings

d. ASHA requires SLPs to write treatment objectives that are aligned with the state's educational curriculum

e. Julie does not need the curriculum guides; the clinical supervisor is being overzealous because Julie is a clinical fellow

19. Six-year-old Lydia was referred for a speech-language evaluation by the Individualized Education Plan (IEP) team during the month of October. Lydia was evaluated and enrolled in speech therapy, beginning in January. When Lydia's parents received her report card in February, they were astonished to see that Lydia was receiving speech therapy in addition to her special class placement for a learning disability. The parents complained to the Superintendent's Office that rules of due process were violated. Due process provides for:

a. The right to be notified of the need for evaluation and treatment

b. The opportunity to participate and provide input during eligibility meetings

c. The right to appeal educational placement decisions

d. The right to nondiscriminatory testing

e. a, b, and c

20. Frank, an SLP, needs evidence to support his use of oral-motor training to facilitate /r/ production by school-aged children. To gather this evidence, Frank includes oral-motor training as part of the therapy plan for two clients and does not include oral-motor training as part of the therapy for two other clients. Of the following legal standards, which must apply?

a. Right to refuse participation

b. Right to informed consent

c. Right to confidentiality

d. All of the above

e. b and c only

21. Ms. Jones noticed that the SLP washed his hands before and after every treatment session with her son. She wondered if he took special precautions to wash his hands because she and her son were seropositive for the human immunodeficiency virus (HIV). What is the most likely reason for the therapist's consistent hand washing?

a. The therapist is following the Centers for Disease Control and Prevention (CDC) guidelines for the control and prevention of disease

b. The therapist is being overly cautious because of personal biases

c. The therapist is being cautious to protect himself, his family, and his other clients

d. The therapist is following regulations specified in the Americans with Disabilities Act

e. The therapist is following the facility's policy of identifying all clients with infectious diseases and ensuring that infection control procedures are used when these clients are being provided services

22. Ms. Taylor is a certified SLP with expertise in augmentative and alternative communication. She has recently been hired by her home state to develop and implement a comprehensive, statewide assistive technology program for school-aged children. Of the following legislative acts, which is most likely to provide funding for such a program?

a. IDEA

b. Technology Assistance for Individuals with Disabilities Act

c. The Bilingual Education Act

d. All of the above

e. a and b

23. Which law provides all individuals with the right of access to all educational programs, including those *not* receiving federal funding?

a. IDEA

b. The Rehabilitation Act

c. No Child Left Behind Act

d. Americans with Disabilities Act (ADA)

e. Family Education Rights and Privacy Act (FERPA)

24. Collaborative consultation as a service delivery model requires school-based SLPs to provide therapeutic services in the classroom whenever possible. Of the following legislative provisions, which is probably responsible for an increase in the use of the collaborative consultation model?

a. Least restrictive environment

b. Free and appropriate public education

c. Cultural competency

d. Evidence-based practice

e. Extended school year

25. HIPAA ensures that:
    a. Treatment decisions made by insurance companies are grounded in evidence-based clinical practice
    b. All individuals have access to affordable health insurance that covers medical and rehabilitation costs
    c. Individuals have specific rights regarding the use and disclosure of their health information
    d. Health insurance companies are held liable for all costs associated with a patient's medical and rehabilitative care
    e. All of the above

26. Julie's private practice is growing at a steady pace. She sees a variety of patients, and much of her revenue comes from third-party payers. Unfortunately, the storage space at Julie's facility is limited. She decides to discard the records of all patients that have been discharged. Of the following regulations, which might Julie be violating?
    a. Medicare regulations
    b. HIPAA regulations
    c. State Department of Health regulations
    d. All of the above
    e. None of the above; each agency is free to develop and implement its own policies regarding medical record retention

27. Dr. Bell routinely uses case information from clients enrolled in the University Speech and Hearing Clinic to teach assessment and treatment principles in her introductory course on clinical practice. Before sharing the case information with the class, Dr. Bell meticulously removes all identifying information, including names, addresses, phone numbers, birth dates, dates of service, and case file numbers. Is this teaching practice permissible in light of stringent regulations regarding client privacy and confidentiality?
    a. No; the sharing of case file information is a violation of HIPAA regulations
    b. Yes; once the identifying information has been removed, the information is no longer protected information
    c. Yes; teachers must use actual cases to help students acquire clinical problem-solving skills
    d. Yes; if Dr. Bell has administrative permission to share the case information
    e. No; health information remains protected regardless of the practice to exclude personal identifiers before use as teaching material

28. Isabel's early intervention center accepts Medicaid patients in its practice but wishes to waive the copayment, which is 20% of the fee, to ease the financial burden that many of the families face. Is this policy acceptable under Medicaid regulations?
    a. The policy is acceptable as long as there is documentation that this policy is applied equally to all patients
    b. The policy is acceptable if the center bills Medicaid for 80% of the discounted fee, rather than 80% of the full fee
    c. The policy is acceptable if the center informs Medicaid of the copayment waiver
    d. The policy is discouraged; if the policy is used, Medicaid will reimburse only the waived copayment, not the full fee
    e. The policy is unacceptable

29. Conner received his master's degree in speech-language pathology from an accredited program. He took the national examination 1 month later, earning a score of 750. Then, Conner decided to take a few years off, to pursue his passion for travel. That pursuit lasted 5½ years. When he returned to begin his career as an SLP, he was hired to work in a private practice as a clinical fellow. After Conner completed the 36 weeks of his clinical fellowship, he applied for initial certification. Of the following requirements for initial certification, which has Conner failed to meet?
    a. Degree requirement
    b. Coursework requirement
    c. National examination requirement
    d. Clinical fellow requirement
    e. Clinical clock hours requirement

30. All ASHA-certified SLPs must demonstrate a commitment to continuing professional development by obtaining 3.0 ASHA continuing education units, 30 certification maintenance hours, or 2 semester hours of academic credit to maintain their ASHA certification. Cheryl earned her initial ASHA certification in May 2007. Her first interval for demonstrating maintenance of continuing education would be:
    a. January 2007 to December 2010
    b. January 2008 to December 2010
    c. January 2012 to January 2017
    d. January 2008 to December 2013
    e. January 2009 to December 2012

1. a. Medicare covers only diagnostic audiology services, regardless of whether the deafness is prelingual or postlingual or where the service is provided.

2. d. The FDA regulates food, medicine, electronics that emit radiation, biological agents, cosmetics, veterinary products, and medical devices. Electrical stimulation devices are therefore subject to FDA regulations. ASHA does not participate in this regulation or act as a clearinghouse for medical devices for patient use.

3. b. States must include all English language learners in their state assessments. No exceptions are allowed on the basis of English proficiency. If it is determined that administration of a native language assessment would be more reliable than administration of the test in English, the state should make every effort to develop and administer such a test; however, states are not required to do so. A student who is learning English must be assessed in English after 3 consecutive years of attending school in the United States.

4. c. Various types of loan forgiveness programs specifically designate SLPs and audiologists as eligible participants. However, each program has different eligibility criteria, such as the length of commitment required and different levels of loan forgiveness, ranging from a mandatory cap to complete repayment. Many loan forgiveness programs are not restricted to high-need schools.

5. c. The REI emerged as a result of research supporting the benefits of mainstreaming for children with special needs and mandated the integration of these children in regular schools and classrooms. P.L. 91-230 (option a) was the first law to establish minimum education requirements for children with disabilities. P.L. 94-142 (option b) amended P.L. 91-230 and called for free appropriate public education for all children with disabilities aged 5 to 21 in the least restrictive environment. P.L. 101-336 (option d) provided definitions of those practices considered discriminating and illegal and sought to ensure reasonable accommodations for individuals with disabilities. The Labor Management Relations Act, informally known as the Taft-Hartley Act (option e), restricted the activities of labor unions.

6. a. *Brown v. Board of Education* was a landmark case in which the Supreme Court ruled that separation of students on the basis of race or ethnicity was in direct violation of the Fourteenth Amendment of the U.S. Constitution. The Fourteenth Amendment specified that no state shall "deny any person within its jurisdiction the equal protection of the laws." Segregated or separate education for students of color was judged to be unequal education. IDEA (option b) focused on early intervention services for children with disabilities. *Mills v. Board of Education* (option c) established that students with disabilities must receive special education services regardless of the school district or financial capability. The Guadalupe consent decree (option d) mandated the assessment of students in their primary language or through the use of nonverbal measures. In the Dred Scott case (option e), the Supreme Court ruled that slaves were not protected under the U.S. Constitution and could not be citizens.

7. b. Section 504 of the Rehabilitation Act of 1993 guarantees certain rights to individuals with disabilities, including ADHD. Parents may request a 504 plan to help meet their child's needs in the classroom. According to Section 504, no persons "shall, solely by reason of his or her disability, be excluded from the participation in, be denied the benefit of, or be subjected to discrimination under any program or activity receiving Federal Financial Assistance." Thus, the 504 plan is implemented by the classroom teacher to help a student succeed in the general education classroom, which does not mean allowing the child to select tasks and arrange her own schedule. Students with ADHD tend to benefit from a more structured classroom environment with a predictable schedule.

8. a. Federal law requirements regarding the assessment of communication in children in the public schools does not exclude subjective, qualitative, or alternative assessment techniques. Although historically many SLPs have used standardized tests, the choice of assessment procedures is left to the educator as long as the measures used for assessment are non-biased (or least biased) materials and procedures.

9. c. Requirements for reinstatement do not specify that previously taken courses expire after a certain period of time. It is true, however, that all coursework must be of sufficient depth and breadth to achieve the knowledge and skills outcomes outlined in the 2005 certification requirements. Under the 2005 certification standards, the focus is on the acquisition of knowledge and skills, not on completion of specific courses.

10. e. Each state may determine the accommodations appropriate. Accommodations should have been scientifically researched and should not change the validity of the assessment.

11. e. The landmark legislation known as the No Child Left Behind Act of 2001 requires states to implement statewide accountability systems covering all public schools and students. Accountability for results, expanded parental options, local control and flexibility, and demonstrated progress and improvement are all important components of the Act. The Act also emphasizes the need for schools to use scientific research to support assessment decisions.

12. b. A passing grade in a course may or may not be considered as evidence of a particular knowledge or skill. A grade by itself does not demonstrate which knowledge or skill has been mastered. Each academic program will have determined the specific learning outcomes and the methods used to assess the acquisition of knowledge and skills. Furthermore, no specific courses in SLP are required for certification. There has been no change in the requirement that all graduate level coursework and graduate level clinical practicum for ASHA certification be initiated and completed in a program accredited by the CAA in Audiology and speech-language pathology.

13. b. A state license is a state-regulated credential issued by the government and is thus the mandatory legal credential that permits practice in a particular state. Licensure provides the state with the legal authority to intervene in cases of misconduct and can prohibit an individual from practicing. ASHA certification is a voluntary professional credential that provides national recognition of the SLP's professional affiliation and expertise. Only individuals who choose to be certified are bound by the ASHA Code of Ethics. The revocation of an ASHA certification has no bearing on the status of the license or the ability to practice professionally. State Departments of Education issue credentials that are mandatory for SLPs who work in the public schools.

14. c. In the "Ann Arbor Decision," concerned parents of African American preschool and elementary school children living in Ann Arbor, Michigan, petitioned the court to require the school board to adopt a policy to ensure that teachers be more sensitive to the influence of a native dialect on learning Standard English. The court ruled that the school board had violated Section 1703 of Title 20 of the U.S. Code, which stipulated that educational agencies are requested to remove all language barriers that impede equal participation in educational programs. The court's decision provided recognition of African

American English as a true dialect. In *Lau v. Nichols* (option b), the Supreme Court decided that educational programs must be designed to meet the specific language needs of non–English-speaking (in this case, Chinese) children, who should have equal protection under the law. This case paved the way for the passage of the Bilingual Education Act and Ann Arbor Decision. P.L. 99-457 (option a) extended services required in P.L. 94-142; instead of covering 3 to 21 years, services covered birth to 21 years of age. Thus, its primary focus was on early intervention with infants and toddlers. *Brown v. Board of Education* (option d) produced the ruling that separate but equal schools denied African Americans equal opportunity for education.

15. d. Accreditation is an important sign of accountability and quality for human service organizations. The CAA is the single nationally recognized accreditation volunteer group for the professions of audiology and speech-language pathology within the discipline of CSD. The CAA accredits master's and clinical programs in speech-language pathology and audiology. It does not offer oversight of professional service delivery programs. The NAEYC (option a) establishes national professional standards for early childhood education programs. Similarly, the QRS (option c) use state regulation and licensing in their focus on continuous quality improvement in early childhood education. CARF (option b) standards address outcomes and the satisfaction of persons served across several categories including child and youth services. All three of these accrediting bodies provide accreditation services for agencies such as the one described in this scenario. Since the agency is a private entity, state department of education requirements would not apply (option e).

16. b. Telepractice across state lines requires that the SLP be licensed in the state where the client is receiving the service. Therefore, the SLP would also be required to hold a West Virginia license.

17. a. The Ethics in Patient Referral Acts of 1989, a federal law, prohibits health care professionals from referring patients to entities in which they have a financial interest.

18. b. IDEA requires that all children with a disability, including those with a communication, hearing, or swallowing impairment, be evaluated and treated in terms of how the disability affects their ability to access the general curriculum and meet the academic standards of their state. Julie needs the curriculum guides to understand the academic learning requirements for children on her caseload.

19. e. Due process is a civil right that is upheld in IDEA. Due process ensures that parents have the right to participate in all school decisions regarding the identification, evaluation, and educational placements for their children. Due process also affords parents the right to appeal decisions made by schools.

20. d. Common law standards apply. Individuals have the right to refuse participation in research activities (option a), and they have the right to informed consent (option b). Regulations for protection of human participants in research also apply. The National Research Act of 1974 and the FDA regulations uphold the rights of individuals to refuse participation in research, delineate the requirements for obtaining informed consent from individuals or their guardians, and define requirements for protection of participant confidentiality (option c). In addition, the Health Insurance Portability and Accountability Act (HIPAA) ensures protection of individuals' medical privacy and confidentiality. Informed consent or some other legal authority must be obtained before client information may be used for research.

21. a. According to CDC recommendations concerning standard precautions, "Assume that every person is potentially infected or colonized with an organism that could be transmitted in the healthcare setting and apply…infection control practices during the delivery of health care." These practices include, but are not limited to, hand hygiene; use of gloves; use of mouth, nose, and eye protection; respiratory hygiene; cough etiquette; and care of patient equipment and instruments.

22. b. The Technology Assistance for Individuals with Disabilities Act defines assistive technology devices and services and provides funding for all 50 states to develop permanent, comprehensive statewide technology-assistance programs for children and adults. IDEA (option a) outlines the school's responsibility to provide assistive technology. The Bilingual Education Act of 1968 provided funding to local school districts for the establishment of educational programs for children with limited English language skills.

23. d. The Americans with Disabilities Act (ADA) extends civil rights legislation by prohibiting discrimination in the public and private sector. All students, regardless of ability or disability, have the right of access to all educational programs, including those *not* receiving federal funding.

24. a. The provision of least restrictive environment specifies that children with disabilities are to be educated, to the greatest extent possible, in classrooms with children who do not have disabilities. This provision also ensures that all children have equal access to the general curriculum.

25. c. HIPAA contains guidelines designed to protect the private information of patients. Some guidelines specify what is protected health information, and some guidelines specify how protected health information may be used or disclosed to others.

26. d. Most state departments of health (option c) have regulations regarding retention of medical records. These regulations vary from state to state, so it is important to contact the state department of health to learn about regulations governing patient records. Medicare regulations (option a) require that in the absence of state regulations, medical records be kept for a minimum of 5 years after the date of discharge. HIPAA regulations (option b) specify that medical records be retained for 6 years after discharge or 2 years after a patient's death. ASHA (2004) recommended that professionals develop and implement medical record retention policies that meet the standards of the "most stringent" regulations in their clinical practice setting.

27. b. The teaching practice is acceptable. HIPAA's Privacy Rule does prohibit the use or disclosure of patient health information without patient authorization or other legal authority. Patient health information has been defined by HIPAA as including individual identifiers, health demographics, treatment provided, and payment history. Individual identifiers include names, addresses, dates related to the individual, contact information, account numbers, medical record and case file numbers, health insurance information, and photographs. Once individual identifiers have been removed, however, this material is no longer viewed as protected health information. HIPAA regulations do not apply in Dr. Bell's case.

28. b. When a health care provider waives the copayment, federal regulations require the provider to bill Medicaid at the discounted rate. For example, if the service is typically billed at $100.00, then the patient is expected to pay 20% ($20) and Medicaid pays 80% ($80.00). If the provider waives the 20% copayment, then the actual charge is $80.00, and the provider can bill Medicaid only 80% that charge ($64.00). However, Medicaid regulations discourage the waiver of copayments and deductibles. These regulations are designed to involve patients in the cost of their care and to discourage overuse of health care services.

29. c. Even though Conner earned a passing score ($\geq$600) on the national examination in speech-language

pathology, his score was obtained 52½ years before his application for initial certification. The test must be taken no more than 5 years prior to receipt of an applicant's certification application.

30. b. ASHA stipulates that all CCC holders earn 30 hours of continuing education within a 3-year cycle to maintain their certification. Because Cheryl earned her initial certification in 2007, her certification maintenance interval would begin in January 2008 and end in December 2010. Maintenance of certification is an ongoing process that lasts until retirement or until a professional no longer wishes to remain certified. Once a certification maintenance interval is completed, another is assigned. The next maintenance interval is determined by (1) timely completion of professional development hours, (2) timely completion of certification maintenance form, (3) keeping current on dues every year, and (4) the possibility that the professional may request a one-time change of their maintenance interval (causing the next interval to begin sooner than previously scheduled). Failure to complete requirements by the deadline may result in a lapse of certification. If the professional chooses to reinstate his or her certification, a new interval would be determined.

Bibliography

American Speech-Language-Hearing Association. (2008a). *2005 Standards and implementation procedures for the certificate of clinical competence in speech-language pathology.* Available at http://www.asha.org/certification/slp_standards.htm (accessed August 4, 2009).

American Speech-Language-Hearing Association. (2008b). *Medical record retention.* Available at http://www.asha.org/does/html/RP1994.00206.html

Guilford, A. M., Graham, S. V., & Scheuerle, J. (2007). *The speech-language pathologist: From novice to expert.* Columbus, OH: Allyn & Bacon.

Horner, J., & Wheeler, M. (2005). HIPAA: Impact on clinical practice. *The ASHA Leader,* 10–11, 22–23. Available at http://www.asha.org/publications/leader/archives/2005/050906/f050906b.htm (accessed August 4, 2009).

Lubinski, R., Golper, L., & Frattali, C. (2007). *Professional issues in speech-language pathology* (3rd ed.). Clifton Park, NJ: Thomson Delmar Learning.

McCarthy, J. (2006). Billing policies: What's legal, what's not. *The ASHA Leader,* 11(10), 1, 20. Available at http://www.asha.org/publications/leader/archives/2006/060905/060905a.htm (accessed August 4, 2009).

Siegel, J., Rhinehart, E., Jackson, M., et al. Healthcare Infection Control Practices Advisory Committee. *Guideline for isolation precautions: 2007. Preventing transmission of infectious agents in healthcare settings 2007. Education and training.* Atlanta: Centers for Disease Control and Prevention. Available at http://www.guideline.gov/summary/summary.aspx?doc_id=10984&nbr=005764&string=2007+AND+guidelines+AND+isolation+AND+precautions (accessed August 4, 2009).

Torrens, J. (2007). Technology as a professional issue. In R. Lubinski, L. Golper, & C. Frattali (Eds.), *Professional Issues in Speech-Language Pathology* (3rd ed pp. 510–541). Clifton Park, NJ: Thomson Delmar Learning.

Index

Note: Page numbers followed by *f* refer to figures; page numbers followed by *b* refer to boxes.